Let's Code It!

2019–2020 CODE EDITION

Procedure

Shelley C. Safian, PhD, RHIA

MAOM/HSM/HI, CCS-P, COC, CPC-I, HCISPP,

AHIMA-Approved ICD-10-CM/PCS Trainer

Mary A. Johnson, MBA-HM-HI, CPC

Central Carolina Technical College

Mc
Graw
Hill

LET'S CODE IT! 2019–2020 CODE EDITION PROCEDURE

Published by McGraw-Hill Education, 2 Penn Plaza, New York, NY 10121. Copyright © 2021 by McGraw-Hill Education. All rights reserved. Printed in the United States of America. Previous edition © 2019. No part of this publication may be reproduced or distributed in any form or by any means, or stored in a database or retrieval system, without the prior written consent of McGraw-Hill Education, including, but not limited to, in any network or other electronic storage or transmission, or broadcast for distance learning.

Some ancillaries, including electronic and print components, may not be available to customers outside the United States.

This book is printed on acid-free paper.

1 2 3 4 5 6 7 8 9 LMN 24 23 22 21 20

ISBN 978-1-260-48117-4 (bound edition)
MHID 1-260-48117-4 (bound edition)
ISBN 978-1-260-48125-9 (loose-leaf edition)
MHID 1-260-48125-5 (loose-leaf edition)

Executive Portfolio Manager: *William Lawrensen*
Senior Product Developer: *Michelle Flomenhoft*
Executive Marketing Manager: *Roxan Kinsey*
Content Project Managers: *Sandy Wille/Brent dela Cruz/Karen Jozefowicz*
Senior Buyer: *Laura Fuller*
Senior Designer: *Egzon Shaqiri*
Content Licensing Specialist: *Sarah Flynn*
Cover Image: *©antishock/Shutterstock*
Compositor: *SPi Global*

All credits appearing on page or at the end of the book are considered to be an extension of the copyright page.

Library of Congress Cataloging-in-Publication Data

Names: Safian, Shelley C., author. | Johnson, Mary A. (Medical record
    coding program manager), author.
Title: Let's code it! : 2019-2020 code edition : procedure / Shelley C.
    Safian, PhD, RHIA, MAOM/HSM, CCS-P, CPC-H, CPC-I, AHIMA-Approved
    ICD-10-CM/PCS Trainer, Mary A. Johnson, CPC, Central Carolina Technical College.
Description: 2nd edition. | Dubuque : 2020.
Identifiers: LCCN 2019027483 | ISBN 9781260481174
Subjects: LCSH: Medicine–Terminology–Code numbers. | Nosology–Code numbers.
Classification: LCC R123 .S185 2020 | DDC 610.1/4–dc23
LC record available at https://lccn.loc.gov/2019027483

The Internet addresses listed in the text were accurate at the time of publication. The inclusion of a website does not indicate an endorsement by the authors or McGraw-Hill Education, and McGraw-Hill Education does not guarantee the accuracy of the information presented at these sites.

mheducation.com/highered

Shelley C. Safian

Shelley Safian has been teaching medical coding and health information management for more than 15 years, at both on-ground and online campuses. In addition to her regular teaching responsibilities at University of Maryland Global Campus and Colorado State University-Global, she volunteers with the AHIMA Foundation Research Network (AFRN) and the Central Florida Health Information Management Association (CFHIMA). She regularly presents webinars/seminars and writes about coding for the *Just Coding* newsletter. Safian is the course author for multiple distance education courses on various coding topics, including ICD-10-CM, ICD-10-PCS, CPT, and HCPCS Level II coding.

Safian is a Registered Health Information Administrator (RHIA) and a Certified Coding Specialist–Physician-based (CCS-P) from the American Health Information Management Association and a Certified Outpatient Coder (COC) and a Certified Professional Coding Instructor (CPC-I) from the American Academy of Professional Coders. She is also a Health Care Information Security and Privacy Practitioner (HCISPP) and a Certified HIPAA Administrator (CHA) and has earned the designation of AHIMA-Approved ICD-10-CM/PCS Trainer.

Safian completed her Graduate Certificate in Health Care Management at Keller Graduate School of Management. The University of Phoenix awarded her the Master of Arts/Organizational Management degree and a Graduate Certificate in Health Informatics. She earned her Ph.D. in Health Care Administration with a focus in Health Information Management.

Courtesy of Shelley C. Safian

Mary A. Johnson

Mary Johnson is the Medical Record Coding Program Director at Central Carolina Technical College in Sumter, South Carolina. She is also an adjunct faculty member for Southern New Hampshire University. Her background includes corporate training using both on-campus and online platforms. Johnson also designs and implements customized coding curricula. Johnson received her Bachelor of Arts dual degree in Business Administration and Marketing from Columbia College, and earned a Masters of Business Administration with a dual focus in Healthcare Management and Health Informatics from New England College. Johnson is a Certified Professional Coder (CPC) credentialed through the American Academy of Professional Coders (AAPC).

Dedications

—This book is dedicated to all of those who have come into my life sharing encouragement and opportunity to pursue work that I love; for the benefit of all of my students: past, present, and future.—*Shelley*

Courtesy of Mary A. Johnson

—This book is dedicated in loving memory of my parents, *Dr. and Mrs. Clarence J. Johnson Sr.,* for their love and support. Also, to those students with whom I have had the privilege to work and to those students who are beginning their journey into the world of medical coding.—*Mary*

BRIEF CONTENTS

Let's Code It! 2019–2020 Code Edition: Procedure is part of the comprehensive Let's Code It! series. This product was specifically chosen for your course, and you will notice that Part II is not included, along with the corresponding chapters and pages. This is intentional and please know that you are not missing any content

CONTENTS

GUIDED TOUR

Let's Code It! was developed with student success in mind: success in college, success taking the certification exam, and success in their future health care career.

Chapter Openers

Each chapter begins by clearly identifying the **Learning Outcomes** students need to master along with the **Key Terms** that they need to learn.

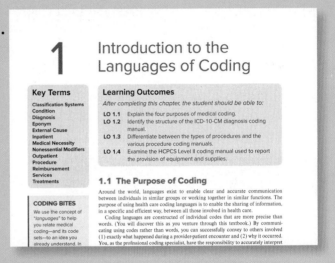

Coding Bites

These appear throughout the text to highlight key concepts and tips to further support understanding and learning.

CODING BITES

This is just an overview to help you orient yourself to the structure of the code book. You will learn, in depth, how to use the ICD-10-CM code set to report any and all of the reasons *why* a patient needs the care of a health care professional in *Part II: Reporting Diagnoses*.

Examples, Let's Code It! Scenarios, and You Code It! Case Studies

Examples are included throughout each chapter to help students make the connection between theoretical and practical coding. **Let's Code It! Scenarios** walk students through abstracting and the coding process, step-by-step, to determine the correct code. And **You Code It! Case Studies** provide students with hands-on practice coding scenarios and case studies throughout each chapter. In addition, **You Interpret It!** questions present opportunities for students to use critical-thinking skills to identify details needed for accurate coding.

EXAMPLES

C82.07	Follicular lymphoma grade I, spleen
C82.16	Follicular lymphoma grade II, intrapelvic lymph nodes

These two codes are examples of those with code descriptions that require you to check the physician's documentation and pathology reports to identify the grade

LET'S CODE IT! SCENARIO

Abby Shantner, a 41-year-old female, comes to see Dr. Branson to get the results of her bi____ that Abby has an alpha cell adenoma of the pancreas. Dr. Branson spends 30 minutes dis____

Let's Code It!

Dr. Branson has diagnosed Abby with an *alpha cell adenoma of the pancreas*. You h____ Dr. Branson as his coder for a while, so you know that an adenoma is a neoplasm, but w____ it—benign or malignant? To help you determine this, instead of going to *neoplasm*, let's ____ the Alphabetic Index under *adenoma*. When you find *adenoma*, the book refers you to ____

Adenoma (*see also* Neoplasm, benign, by site)

This tells you an adenoma is a benign tumor. Or you can continue down this list to the i____

Adenoma
  alpha-cell
    pancreas D13.7

Turn to the Tabular List and read the complete description of code category D13:

☑ **D13**   Benign neoplasm of other and ill-defined parts of digestive system

YOU INTERPRET IT!

What is the mode of transmission for each condition?
1. Hepatitis B _____   4. Insect bites
2. Measles _____   5. Influenza
3. Cholera _____

Guidance Connections

Each of these boxes connects the concepts students are learning in the chapter to the related, specific Official Guidelines in order to further students' knowledge and understanding of coding resources.

 GUIDANCE CONNECTION

Read the ICD-10-CM Official Guidelines for Coding and Reporting, section **I. Conventions, General Coding Guidelines and Chapter-**

End-of-Chapter Reviews

Most chapters end with the following assessment types to reinforce the chapter learning outcomes: Let's Check It! Terminology; Let's Check It! Concepts; Let's Check It! Guidelines; Let's Check It! Rules and Regulations; and You Code It! Basics.

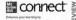
Real Abstracting Practice with You Code It! Practice, You Code It! Application, and Capstone Case Studies Chapters

Gain real-world experience by using actual patient records (with names and other identifying information changed) to practice ICD-10-CM, ICD-10-PCS, CPT, and HCPCS Level II coding for both inpatients and outpatients. *You Code It! Practice* exercises give students the chance to practice coding with short coding scenarios. *You Code It! Application* exercises give students the chance to review and abstract physicians' notes documenting real patient encounters in order to code those scenarios. Both of these types of exercises can be found at the end of most chapters. *Capstone Chapters* come at the end of Parts II–V and include 15 additional real-life outpatient and inpatient case studies to help students synthesize and apply what they have learned through hands-on coding practice with each code set.

In addition, all of the exercises in the Chapter Review can be assigned through Connect. Of particular note are the *You Code It! Practice* exercises, which offer our unique **CodePath** option. In Connect, students are presented with a series of questions to guide them through the critical thinking process to determine the correct code.

 YOU CODE IT! Application

The following exercises provide practice in abstracting physician documentation from our health care facility, Prader, Bracker, & Associates. These case studies are modeled on real patient encounters. Using the techniques described in this chapter, carefully read through the case studies and determine the most accurate ICD-10-CM code(s) for each case study. Remember to include external cause codes, if appropriate.

PRADER, BRACKER, & ASSOCIATES

A Complete Health Care Facility

159 Healthcare Way • SOMEWHERE, FL 32811 • 407-555-6789

PATIENT: Kassandra, Kelly

ACCOUNT/EHR #: KASSKE001

DATE: 09/16/19

Attending Physician: Oscar R. Prader, MD

S: Pt is a 19-year-old female who has had a sore throat and cough for the past week. She states that she had a temperature of 101.5 F last night. She also admits that it is painful to swallow. No OTC medication has provided any significant relief.

O: Ht 5'5" Wt. 148 lb. R 20. T 101 F. BP 125/82. Pharynx is inspected, tonsils enlarged. There is pus noted in the posterior pharynx. Neck: supple, no nodes. Chest: clear. Heart: regular rate and rhythm without murmur.

A: Acute pharyngitis

P: 1. Send pt for Strep test

   2. Recommend patient gargle with warm salt water and use OTC lozenges to keep throat moist

   3. Rx if needed once results of Strep test come back

   4. Return in 2 weeks for follow-up

ORP/pw D: 9/16/19 09:50:16 T: 9/18/19 12:55:01

Determine the most accurate ICD-10-CM code(s).

WESTON HOSPITAL

629 Healthcare Way • SOMEWHERE, FL 32811 • 407-555-6541

PATIENT: DAVIS, HELEN

ACCOUNT/EHR #: DAVIHE001

DATE: 10/21/19

Attending Physician: Renee O. Bracker, MD

Patient, an 82-year-old that presents today to see Dr. Newson. Dr. Newson saw this patient 10 days ago in office, where she was diagnosed with a UTI and prescribed nitrofurantoin po. Today she presents with the complaints of dysuria, low back pain, abdominal pain, nausea, and diarrhea. After a positive UA she was admitted to Weston Hospital.

Welcome to *Let's Code It!* This product is part of a multipart series that instructs students on how to become proficient in medical coding—a health care field that continues to be in high demand. The Bureau of Labor Statistics notes the demand for health information management professionals (which includes coders) will continue to increase incredibly through 2024 and beyond.

Let's Code It! provides a 360-degree learning experience for anyone interested in the field of medical coding, with strong guidance down the path to coding certification. Theory is presented in easy-to-understand language and accompanied by lots of examples. Hands-on practice is included with real-life physician documentation, from both outpatient and inpatient facilities, to promote critical thinking analysis and evaluation. This is in addition to determination of accurate codes to report diagnoses, procedures, and ancillary services. All of this is assembled to support the reader's development of a solid foundation upon which to build a successful career after graduation.

The Safian/Johnson Medical Coding series includes the following products:

> *Let's Code It!*
> *Let's Code It! ICD-10-CM*
> *Let's Code It! ICD-10-CM/PCS*
> *Let's Code It! Procedure*
> *You Code It! Abstracting Case Studies Practicum, 3e*

The different solutions are designed to fit the most common course content selections. *Let's Code It!* is the comprehensive offering with coverage of ICD-10-CM, ICD-10-PCS, CPT, and HCPCS Level II.

These products are further designed to give your students the medical coding experience they need in order to pass their first medical coding certification exams, such as the CCS/CCS-P or CPC/COC. The products offer students a variety of practice opportunities by reinforcing the learning outcomes set forth in every chapter. The chapter materials are organized in short bursts of text followed by practice—keeping students active and coding!

What's new for the 2019-2020 Code Edition: All codes within the text, as well as the Instructor Manual answer keys, have been updated to be compliant with the 2019 code sets: ICD-10-CM, CPT, HCPCS Level II, and ICD-10-PCS. Updates based on the 2020 code sets have been made as feasible. Updates will continue to be made to the answer keys and Connect exercises on an annual basis. The product content has been refined and polished based on customer feedback.

Here's What You Can Expect from *Let's Code It!*

- Each of the six parts of this product includes an Introduction to provide students with an overview of the information within that part and how they can use this knowledge.
  - Part I: Medical Coding Fundamentals
  - Part II: Reporting Diagnoses
  - Part III: Reporting Physicians Services and Outpatient Procedures
  - Part IV: DMEPOS & Transportation
  - Part V: Inpatient (Hospital) Reporting
  - Part VI: Legal, Ethical, and Reimbursement Issues

- **Part I: Medical Coding Fundamentals** helps students build a strong theoretical foundation regarding the various code sets. The chapters teach students how and when each code set is used and how to abstract documentation. These chapters also teach them how to use a solid coding process, including the importance of queries, how to write a legal query, exposure to the Official Guidelines, and confirmation of medical necessity.

- **Part II: Reporting Diagnoses** provides students with an incremental walkthrough of the ICD-10-CM code set.

- **Part III: Reporting Physicians Services and Outpatient Procedures** provides students with a progressive learning experience for using CPT® procedure codes.

- **Part IV: DMEPOS & Transportation** gives students insight into, and hands-on practice using, the HCPCS Level II code set to report the provision of durable medical equipment, prosthetics, orthotics, and other medical supplies.

- **Part V: Inpatient (Hospital) Reporting** shows students how to build an accurate ICD-10-PCS code to report inpatient procedures, services, and treatments.

- The coding chapters in Parts II–V all include real-life scenarios, as well as physician documentation mainly in the form of procedure notes and operative reports (both inpatient and outpatient) for students to practice abstracting and coding.
    - *Let's Code It! Scenarios* provide step-by-step instruction so students can learn to use their critical-thinking skills throughout the coding process to determine the correct code.
    - *You Code It! Case Studies* provide students with hands-on practice coding scenarios and case studies throughout each chapter.
    - *You Interpret It!* questions present additional opportunities for students to use critical-thinking skills to identify details required for accurate coding.
    - *Chapter Reviews* include assessments of chapter concepts:
        - Let's Check It! Terminology
        - Let's Check It! Concepts
        - Let's Check It! Guidelines
        - Let's Check It! Rules and Regulations
        - You Code It! Basics
        - You Code It! Practice Case Studies
        - You Code It! Application Case Studies

- *Examples* are included throughout each chapter to help students make the connection between theoretical and practical coding.

- *Coding Bites* highlight key concepts and tips to further support understanding and learning.

- *Guidance Connection* features point to the specific Official Guideline applicable for the concept being discussed.

- *Capstone Chapters* come at the end of Parts II–V with 15 additional real-life outpatient and inpatient case studies to help students synthesize and apply what they have learned through hands-on coding practice with each code set.

- **Part VI: Legal, Ethical, and Reimbursement Issues** provides a concise overview connecting these broad topics to a professional coding specialist's job requirements.

- *Examples* again take students through real-life scenarios to help them understand how they will use this information.

- *Coding Bites* provide tips and highlight key concepts.

- This part also includes material to teach students how to access credible resources on the Internet.

- *Codes of Ethics* from both AHIMA and AAPC are discussed as well as information on compliance plans.

- *You Interpret It!* questions present students with opportunities to use critical-thinking skills to identify details required for accurate job performance.
- *Chapter Reviews* include assessments of chapter concepts:
  - Let's Check It! Terminology
  - Let's Check It! Concepts
  - Let's Check It! Which Type of Insurance?
  - Let's Check It! Rules and Regulations
  - You Code It! Application Case Studies

SUPPORT AT every step

Effective, efficient studying.

Connect helps you be more productive with your study time and get better grades using tools like SmartBook 2.0, which highlights key concepts and creates a personalized study plan. Connect sets you up for success, so you walk into class with confidence and walk out with better grades.

Study anytime, anywhere.

Download the free ReadAnywhere app and access your online eBook or SmartBook 2.0 assignments when it's convenient, even if you're offline. And since the app automatically syncs with your eBook and SmartBook 2.0 assignments in Connect, all of your work is available every time you open it. Find out more at **www.mheducation.com/readanywhere**

"I really liked this app—it made it easy to study when you don't have your text-book in front of you."

- Jordan Cunningham, Eastern Washington University

Calendar: owattaphotos/Getty Images

No surprises.

The Connect Calendar and Reports tools keep you on track with the work you need to get done and your assignment scores. Life gets busy; Connect tools help you keep learning through it all.

Learning for everyone.

McGraw-Hill works directly with Accessibility Services Departments and faculty to meet the learning needs of all students. Please contact your Accessibility Services office and ask them to email accessibility@mheducation.com, or visit **www.mheducation.com/about/accessibility** for more information.

Top: Jenner Images/Getty Images, Left: Hero Images/Getty Images, Right: Hero Images/Getty Images

CONNECT FOR LET'S CODE IT!

McGraw-Hill Connect for *Let's Code It!* includes:

- All end-of-chapter questions.
- CodePath versions of You Code It! practice questions, in which students are presented with a series of questions to guide them through the critical thinking process to determine the correct code.
- Interactive Exercises, such as Matching, Sequencing, and Labeling activities.
- Testbank questions.
- Lecture-style videos, which provide additional guidance on challenging coding questions. With the 2019–2020 Code Edition, the videos are now assignable through the Question Bank with new assessment questions for students to complete after each video. The videos are also available in the Connect Media Bank.

INSTRUCTORS' RESOURCES

You can rely on the following materials to help you and your students work through the material in the book; all are available in the Instructor Resources under the Library tab in *Connect* (available only to instructors who are logged in to *Connect*).

Supplement	Features
Instructor's Manual (organized by Learning Outcomes)	• Lesson plans • Answer keys for all exercises
PowerPoint Presentations (organized by Learning Outcomes)	• Key terms • Key concepts • Accessible
Electronic Testbank	• Computerized and Connect • Word version • Questions are tagged with learning outcomes; level of difficulty; level of Bloom's taxonomy; feedback; and ABHES, CAAHEP, and CAHIIM competencies.
Tools to Plan Course	• Correlations by learning outcomes to accrediting bodies such as ABHES, CAAHEP, and CAHIIM • Sample syllabi • Asset map—recap of the key instructor resources as well as information on the content available through *Connect*

Want to learn more about this product? Attend one of our online webinars. To learn more about them, please contact your McGraw-Hill learning technology representative. To find your McGraw-Hill representative, go to www.mheducation.com and click "Get Support," select "Higher Ed" and then click the "Get Started" button under the "Find Your Sales Rep" section.

Need help? Contact the McGraw-Hill Education Customer Experience Group (CXG). Visit the CXG website at www.mhhe.com/support. Browse our frequently asked questions (FAQs) and product documentation and/or contact a CXG representative.

ACKNOWLEDGMENTS

Digital Products

Several instructors helped review the digital content for Connect.

Julie Alles-Grice, DHA, RHIA, Grand Valley State University

Erika Bailey, MBA, RHIA, Grand Valley State University

Laura A. Diggle, MS, CMA (AAMA), Ivy Tech Community College

Terri Fleming, EdD, Ivy Tech Community College

Savanna Garrity, MPA, CPC, Madisonville Community College

Susan H. Holler, MSEd, CPC,CCS-P, CMRS, Bryant & Stratton College

Janis A. Klawitter, AS, CPC, CPB, CPC-I, Provider Audits/Analytics, Bakersfield Family Medical Center

Beverly Marquez, MS, RHIA, State Fair Community College

Tracey A. McKethan, MBA, RHIA, CCA, Springfield Technical Community College

Janna Pacey, DHA, RHIA, Grand Valley State University

Kristi Perillo-Okeke, DC, CMRS, Bryant & Stratton College

Sharon Turner, MS, CMC, CMIS, CHI, CBCS, CMAA, CEHRS, Brookhaven College

Digital Tool Development

Special thanks to the instructors who helped with the development of Connect and SmartBook.

Tammy L. Burnette, PhD, CPC, CPB, Tyler Junior College

Judith Hurtt, MEd, East Central Community College

Shauna Phillips, RMA, AHI, CCMA, CMAA, CPT, PIMA Medical Institute

Patricia A. Saccone, MA, RHIA, CCS-P, Waubonsee Community College

Board of Advisors

A select group of instructors participated in our Coding Board of Advisors to help develop the first editions of the series. They provided timely and focused guidance to the author team on all aspects of content development. We are extremely grateful for their input on this project.

Christine Cusano, CMA (AAMA), CPhT, Lincoln Technical Institute

Gerry Gordon, BA, CPC, CPB, Daytona College

Shalena Jarvis, RHIT, CCS

Janis A. Klawitter, AS, CPC, CPB, CPC-I, San Joaquin Valley College

Tatyana Pashnyak, CHTS-TR, Bainbridge State College

Patricia Saccone, MA, RHIA, CCS-P, Waubonsee Community College

Stephanie Scott, MSHI, RHIA, CDIP, CCS, CCS-P, Moraine Park Technical College

First Edition Reviewers

Many instructors reviewed the manuscript while it was in development and provided valuable feedback that directly affected the product's development. Their contributions are greatly appreciated.

Julie Alles-Grice, MSCTE, RHIA

Alicia Alva, AS, San Joaquin Valley College

Kelly Berge, MSHA, CPC, CCS-P, Berkeley College

Valerie Brock, EdS, MBA, RHIA, CDIP, CPC, Tennessee State University

William Butler, MHA, UNC Healthcare

Heather Copen, RHIA, CCS-P, Ivy Tech Community College

Gerard Cronin, MS, DC, Salem Community College

Christine Cusano, CMA (AAMA), CPhT, Lincoln Technical Institute

Patti Fayash, CCS, ICD-10-CM/PCS AHIMA Approved Trainer, Luzerne County Community College

Rashmi Gaonkar, BS, MS, MHA/Informatics, ASA College

Savanna Garrity, MPA, CPC, Madisonville Community College

Deborah Gilbert, RHIA, MBA, CMA, Dalton State College

Terri Gilbert, MS, ECPI University

Gerry Gordon, BA, CPC, CPB, Daytona College

Michelle A. Harris, CPC, CPB, CPC-I, Bossier Parish Community College

Susan Hernandez, B.S.B.A., San Joaquin Valley College

Judith Hurtt, MEd, East Central Community College

Beverlee Jackson, BA, RHIT, CCS, AHIMA Ambassador, Central Oregon Community College

Shalena Jarvis, RHIT, CCS

Mary Z. Johnston, RN, BSN, RHIA, CPC, CPC-H, CPC-I, Ultimate Medical Academy

Janis A. Klawitter, AS, CPC, CPB, CPC-I, San Joaquin Valley College

Jennifer Lamé, MPH, RHIT, Southwest Wisconsin Technical College

Jorell Lawrence, MSA, CPC, Stratford University

Tracey Lee, MSA, CPC, Vista College

Angela Leuvoy, AAS, CMA, CPT, CBCS, Fortis College

Glenda Lloyd, MBA, BS, RHIA, Rasmussen College, Vista College

Lynnae Lockett, RN, RMA, CMRS, MSN, Bryant & Stratton College

Marta Lopez, MD, BXMO, RMA, Miami Dade College

JanMarie Malik, MBA, RHIA, CCS-P, National University

Barbara Marchelletta, BS, CMA (AAMA), CPT, CPC, AHI, Beal College

David Martinez, MHSA, RHIT, RMA, University of Phoenix

Jillian McDonald, BS, RMA (AMT), EMT, CPT(NPA)

Cheryl Miller, MBA/HCM, Westmoreland County Community College

Robin Moore, CPC, CCMA, Davis College

Lisa Nimmo, CPC, CFPC, Central Carolina Technical College

Melissa Oelfke, RHIA, HIT Program Coordinator, Rasmussen College

Barbara Parker, CPC, CCS-P, CMA (AAMA), Olympic College

Brenda Parks-Brown, MHS, HCA, CCS, CMA, Miller-Motte Technical College

Tatyana Pashnyak, CHTS-TR, Bainbridge State College

Staci Porter, AA, San Joaquin Valley College

Terri Randolph, MBA/HCM, CAHI, CBCS, CEHRS, Eagle Gate College

Lisa Riggs, CPC, CPC-I, Ultimate Medical Academy

Rolando Russell, MBA, RHIA, CPC, CPAR, Ultimate Medical Academy

Patricia A. Saccone, MA, RHIA, CCS-P, Waubonsee Community College

Georgina Sampson, RHIA, Anoka Technical College

Stephanie Scott, MSHI, RHIA, CDIP, CCS, CCS-P, Moraine Park Technical College

Mary Jo Slater, MS, MIE, Community College of Beaver County

Karen K. Smith, MEd, RHIA, CDIP, CPC, University of Arkansas for Medical Sciences

Kameron Stutzman, MEd, CMBS, IBMC College

Stephanie Vergne, MAEd, RHIA, CPC, Hazard Community & Technical College

PART I

MEDICAL CODING FUNDAMENTALS

INTRODUCTION

Coding is not like anything you have ever studied before. No courses that you experienced in elementary, middle, or high school have prepared you for learning this skill. Biology and your science classes began your education that your anatomy and physiology class continued. Other courses you are taking as part of this program also typically connect to something, in some way, you have previously learned.

As you begin this educational journey, you will use your critical thinking skills as well as some experiences you may have had as a patient yourself (or as the loved one of a patient). For the most part, though, this will be different, so prepare yourself for a new learning experience.

In Part I, the chapters Introduction to the Languages of Coding, Abstracting Clinical Documentation, and The Coding Process share an overview of the concepts and skills you will apply in the chapters that follow. You will be introduced to the tools you have and will need to use as a professional coding specialist. Together, these three chapters create the foundation, the first layer, of a multilayered approach to learning coding. Then, the remaining parts will share with you, one by one, the best practices for how to use each of these tools correctly. You will then be given many opportunities for hands-on practice so that you can build your skills and reinforce the knowledge you have obtained.

1 Introduction to the Languages of Coding

Learning Outcomes

After completing this chapter, the student should be able to:

LO 1.1 Explain the four purposes of medical coding.
LO 1.2 Identify the structure of the ICD-10-CM diagnosis coding manual.
LO 1.3 Differentiate between the types of procedures and the various procedure coding manuals.
LO 1.4 Examine the HCPCS Level II coding manual used to report the provision of equipment and supplies.

CODING BITES

We use the concept of *"languages"* to help you relate medical coding—and its code sets—to an idea you already understand. In the health care industry, however, the various code sets, such as ICD-10-CM or HCPCS Level II, are referred to as **Classification Systems**.

Classification Systems
The term used in health care to identify ICD-10-CM, CPT, ICD-10-PCS, and HCPCS Level II code sets.

CODING BITES

A **diagnosis** explains WHY the patient requires the attention of a health care provider and a **procedure** explains WHAT the physician or health care provider did for the patient.

1.1 The Purpose of Coding

Around the world, languages exist to enable clear and accurate communication between individuals in similar groups or working together in similar functions. The purpose of using health care coding languages is to enable the sharing of information, in a specific and efficient way, between all those involved in health care.

Coding languages are constructed of individual codes that are more precise than words. (You will discover this as you venture through this textbook.) By communicating using codes rather than words, you can successfully convey to others involved (1) exactly what happened during a provider-patient encounter and (2) why it occurred. You, as the professional coding specialist, have the responsibility to accurately interpret health care terms and definitions (medical terminology) into numbers or number-letter combinations (alphanumeric codes) that specifically convey **diagnoses** and **procedures**.

Why is it so critical to code diagnoses and procedures accurately? The coding languages, known as **classification systems**, communicate information that is key to various aspects of the health care system, including

- Medical necessity
- Statistical analyses
- Reimbursement
- Resource allocation

Medical Necessity

The diagnosis codes that you report explain the justification for the procedure, service, or treatment provided to a patient during his or her encounter. Every time a health care professional provides care to a patient, there must be a valid medical reason. Patients certainly want to know that health care professionals performed procedures or provided care for a specific, justified purpose, and so do third-party payers! This is referred to as **medical necessity**. Requiring medical necessity ensures that health care providers are not performing tests or giving injections without a good medical reason. Diagnosis codes explain *why* the individual came to see the physician and support the physician's decision about *what* procedures to provide.

Medical necessity is one of the reasons why it is so very important to code the diagnosis accurately and with all the detail possible. If you are one number off in your code selection, you could accidentally cause a claim to be denied because the diagnosis, identified by your incorrect code, does not justify the procedure.

Let's analyze an example:

> **EXAMPLE**
>
> Dr. Justini performs a colonoscopy on Shoshanna because a lab test identified that she had blood in her feces (melena).

A colonoscopy involves the insertion of a camera, with surgical tools, into the patient's anus, rectum, and up through the large intestine. If you are Shoshanna, or if you are the one paying for this procedure, you want to make certain that this colonoscopy was done to support Shoshanna's good health and not any other reason. This is clearly communicated when you report the code K92.1 Melena (the presence of blood in feces). Now, whether for resource allocation or reimbursement, it is understood that Dr. Justini was caring properly for Shoshanna and her good health.

Statistical Analyses

Research organizations and government agencies statistically analyze the data provided by codes to develop programs, identify research areas, allocate funds, and write public health policies that will best address areas of concern for the health of our nation. For example, we can only know that a disease such as Alzheimer's needs diagnostic tests, treatments, and possibly a vaccine or a cure by studying statistics to see what individual signs and symptoms are being identified and treated around the country and around the world.

Reimbursement

In most cases, there are three parties involved in virtually every encounter: the health care provider, the patient, and the person or organization paying for the care provided (frequently, a health care insurance company). However, the insurance company is not always an actual insurance company, so the broader term "third-party payer" is used. Third-party payers use our coding data to determine how much they should pay health care professionals for the attention and services they provide patients. This is the role that coding plays in the **reimbursement** process. The codes make it easier for the organizations involved to evaluate and manage all their data.

Resource Allocations

Whether a health care facility is a one-physician office or a large hospital, there are not unlimited resources available. Administrators and managers must ensure that all resources are employed in the most efficient and effective manner. Computer programs can easily and quickly organize data (the codes) to identify the largest patient population's diagnoses and the most frequently provided treatments and services. With these details, staff members, equipment, and money can be directed to those patients and locations that need them the most.

1.2 Diagnosis Coding

When a person goes to see a health care provider, he or she must have a reason—a health-related reason. After all, as much as you might like your physician, you probably wouldn't make an appointment, sit in the waiting room, and go through all the paperwork just to say, "hello." Whether the reason is a checkup, a flu shot, or something more serious, there is always a reason *why*. The physician will create notes, either written or dictated, recounting the events of the visit. The diagnosis,

Diagnosis
A physician's determination of a patient's condition, illness, or injury.

Procedure
Action taken, in accordance with the standards of care, by the physician to accomplish a predetermined objective (result); a surgical operation.

Medical Necessity
The assessment that the provider was acting according to standard practices in providing a procedure or service for an individual with a specific diagnosis.

> **CODING BITES**
>
> The WHY justifies the WHAT.

Reimbursement
The process of paying for health care services after they have been provided.

> **CODING BITES**
>
> In most cases, there are three parties involved in reimbursement:
>
> - The health care provider = First party
> - The patient = Second party
> - The insurance company or other organization financially responsible = Third-party payer

or diagnostic statement, in these notes will explain the reason *why* the patient was seen and treated.

The physician's notes explain, in writing, the reasons *why* the encounter occurred. The notes may document a specific condition or illness, the signs or symptoms of a yet-unnamed problem, or another reason for the encounter, such as a preventive service. As a coding specialist, it is your job to translate this explanation into a diagnosis code (or codes) so that everyone involved will clearly understand the issues of a particular patient at a particular time.

The International Classification of Diseases – 10th Revision – Clinical Modification (ICD-10-CM) code book contains all of the codes from which you will choose to report the reason *why* the health care professional cared for the patient during a specific encounter.

Overview of the International Classification of Diseases – 10th Revision – Clinical Modification (ICD-10-CM) Code Book Sections

The ICD-10-CM code book (whether paper or electronic) is made up of several sections. Here is an overview of its parts and how you will utilize the information in these sections to determine the most accurate code or codes to report the reasons *why* an encounter occurred.

Index to Diseases and Injuries [aka Alphabetic Index]

The Alphabetic Index [Index to Diseases and Injuries] lists, in alphabetic order, the terms used by the physician to describe the reasons why the patient required attention from a health care professional.

The Alphabetic Index lists all diagnoses and other reasons to provide health care by their basic description alphabetically from A to Z (see Figure 1-1). Diagnostic descriptions are listed by

- **Condition** (e.g., infection, fracture, and wound)
- **Eponym** (e.g., Epstein-Barr syndrome and Cushing's disease)
- Other descriptors (e.g., personal history, family history)

So, whichever type of words you read in the documentation, you should be able to find them in the Alphabetic Index in one form or another.

The Alphabetic Index can only suggest a possible code to report the patient's diagnosis, and you will use this suggestion to guide you to the correct page or subsection in the

Condition
The state of abnormality or dysfunction.

Eponym
A disease or condition named for a person.

Abnormal, abnormality, abnormalities (*see also* Anomaly)

- acid-base balance (mixed) E87.4
- albumin R77.0
- alphafetoprotein R77.2
- alveolar ridge K08.9
- anatomical relationship Q89.9
- apertures, congenital, diaphragm Q79.1
- auditory perception H93.29
- diplacusis — *see* Diplacusis
- hyperacusis — *see* Hyperacusis
- recruitment — *see* Recruitment, auditory
- threshold shift — *see* Shift, auditory threshold
- autosomes Q99.9

FIGURE 1-1 ICD-10-CM Alphabetic Index, partial listing under main term Abnormal

B67 Echinococcosis

INCLUDES *hydatidosis*

B67.0 Echinococcus granulosus infection of liver

B67.1 Echinococcus granulosus infection of lung

B67.2 Echinococcus granulosus infection of bone

B67.3 Echinococcus granulosus infection, other and multiple sites

B67.31 Echinococcus granulosus infection, thyroid gland

B67.32 Echinococcus granulosus infection, multiple sites

B67.39 Echinococcus granulosus infection, other sites

B67.4 Echinococcus granulosus infection, unspecified

Dog tapeworm (infection)

FIGURE 1-2 ICD-10-CM Tabular List, partial list of codes included in code category B67 Echinococcosis

Tabular List (see the next subsection of this text, *Tabular List of Diseases and Injuries*). The Official Guidelines require you to always find a suggested code in the Tabular List to confirm it is accurate, or to find another code that might be better.

Tabular List of Diseases and Injuries

The Tabular List provides you with each and every available code in the ICD-10-CM code book, in order of the code characters—alphanumeric order. You need to carefully read the descriptions, beginning at the top of the three-character code category. When you begin reading at this point, you can make certain that you find the best code, to the highest level of specificity, according to the physician's documentation.

You will find that the Tabular List section shows all ICD-10-CM codes, first in alphabetic order and then in numeric order: A00 through Z99.89 (see Figure 1-2), along with additional details (notations and symbols) that guide you to the accurate code.

Ancillary Sections of ICD-10-CM

Neoplasm Table

The Neoplasm Table (Figure 1-3) itemizes all of the anatomical sites in the human body that may develop a tumor (neoplasm). Columns in this table further describe the type of neoplasm and suggest a code that may be accurate. As with other codes suggested by the Alphabetic Index, you will need to go to the Tabular List to look up any code found on the Neoplasm Table to confirm accuracy, additional characters required, and other details before you can determine the accurate code to report.

You will learn how to use the Neoplasm Table to report diagnoses of benign, malignant, and other types of neoplasms in the *Coding Neoplasms* chapter.

Table of Drugs and Chemicals

The Table of Drugs and Chemicals (Figure 1-4) lists pharmaceuticals and chemicals that may cause poisoning or adverse effects in the human body. The multiple columns in this table categorize the intent of how or why the patient became ill from the drug or chemical to suggest a possible code. As with all of these, this suggested code must be reviewed in the Tabular List to ensure completeness and accuracy before you can report it.

You will learn how to use the Table of Drugs and Chemicals in the chapter *Coding Injury, Poisoning, and External Causes.*

CODING BITES

Notations in the Tabular List help make your coding process more accurate and a bit easier. For example, as you can see in Figure 1-2, the condition represented by code category B67 is Echinococcosis. Now, read the INCLUDES note directly below B67; it reads . . . INCLUDES hydatidosis. This notation lets you know that, if the physician wrote "echinococcosis" or "hydatidosis" in the documentation, this is the correct code category.

In ICD-10-CM, the INCLUDES note provides you with alternative words or phrases that the physician might use that mean the same condition. In English, they are known as synonyms. In ICD-10-CM, they are known as **nonessential modifiers**.

You will learn more about notations in the *Introduction to ICD-10-CM* chapter.

Nonessential Modifiers
Descriptors whose inclusion in the physician's notes are not absolutely necessary and that are provided simply to further clarify a code description; optional terms.

Neoplasm, neoplastic	Malignant Primary	Malignant Secondary	Ca in situ	Benign	Uncertain Behavior	Unspecified Behavior
Neoplasm, neoplastic	C80.1	C79.9	D09.9	D36.9	D48.9	D49.9
-abdomen, abdominal	C76.2	C79.8-	D09.8	D36.7	D48.7	D49.89
--cavity	C76.2	C79.8-	D09.8	D36.7	D48.7	D49.89
--organ	C76.2	C79.8-	D09.8	D36.7	D48.7	D49.89
--viscera	C76.2	C79.8-	D09.8	D36.7	D48.7	D49.89
--wall (see also Neoplasm, abdomen, wall, skin)	C44.509	C79.2-	D04.5	D23.5	D48.5	D49.2
---connective tissue	C49.4	C79.8-	-	D21.4	D48.1	D49.2
---skin	C44.509	-	-	-	-	-
----basal cell carcinoma	C44.519	-	-	-	-	-
----specified type NEC	C44.599	-	-	-	-	-
----squamous cell carcinoma	C44.529	-	-	-	-	-

FIGURE 1-3 The Neoplasm Table from ICD-10-CM, listings for abdominal neoplasms

Substance	Poisoning, Accidental (Unintentional)	Poisoning, Intentional Self-harm	Poisoning, Assault	Poisoning, Undetermined	Adverse Effect	Underdosing
Acefylline piperazine	T48.6X1	T48.6X2	T48.6X3	T48.6X4	T48.6X5	T48.6X6
Acemorphan	T40.2X1	T40.2X2	T40.2X3	T40.2X4	T40.2X5	T40.2X6
Acenocoumarin	T45.511	T45.512	T45.513	T45.514	T45.515	T45.516
Acenocoumarol	T45.511	T45.512	T45.513	T45.514	T45.515	T45.516
Acepifylline	T48.6X1	T48.6X2	T48.6X3	T48.6X4	T48.6X5	T48.6X6
Acepromazine	T43.3X1	T43.3X2	T43.3X3	T43.3X4	T43.3X5	T43.3X6
Acesulfamethoxypyridazine	T37.0X1	T37.0X2	T37.0X3	T37.0X4	T37.0X5	T37.0X6
Acetal	T52.8X1	T52.8X2	T52.8X3	T52.8X4	—	—
Acetaldehyde (vapor)	T52.8X1	T52.8X2	T52.8X3	T52.8X4	—	—
- liquid	T65.891	T65.892	T65.893	T65.894	—	—
P-Acetamidophenol	T39.1X1	T39.1X2	T39.1X3	T39.1X4	T39.1X5	T39.1X6
Acetaminophen	T39.1X1	T39.1X2	T39.1X3	T39.1X4	T39.1X5	T39.1X6

FIGURE 1-4 The Table of Drugs and Chemicals from ICD-10-CM, listings from Acefylline piperazine to Acetaminophen
Source: *ICD-10-CM Official Guidelines for Coding and Reporting,* The Centers for Medicare and Medicaid Services (CMS) and the National Center for Health Statistics (NCHS)

Index to External Causes

External Cause
An event, outside the body, that causes injury, poisoning, or an adverse reaction.

The Index to **External Causes** (Figure 1-5) lists the causes of injury and poisoning. These codes are used to explain *how* a patient got injured and *where* (place of occurrence) he or she was when the injury happened.

As with the other content in the Alphabetic Index, the code or codes shown here are only suggestions and must be confirmed in the Tabular List before you are permitted to report them. You will learn about the importance of reporting these codes as you progress through your learning experience, particularly in the chapter *Coding Injury, Poisoning, and External Causes.*

FIGURE 1-5 The Index to External Causes, first listings including main terms Abandonment, Abuse, and Accident

The Format of ICD-10-CM Codes

A complete, valid ICD-10-CM code will always begin with a three (3)-character code category: a letter of the alphabet followed by a minimum of two (2) characters (either letters or numbers).

E54	**Ascorbic acid deficiency (scurvy)**
L26	**Exfoliative dermatitis**

A majority of the codes will require additional characters to communicate more specific information about the patient's condition. When an additional character is needed to complete the code, a symbol to the left of the code in the Tabular List will identify that additional characters are necessary. The symbol may be a bullet ● or it may be a box with a check mark ☑4, depending upon the publisher of your code book. You will find a legend to explain the meaning of each symbol at the bottom of the page in your code book. As you evaluate the options available for the additional character, make certain to place a dot (period) between the third and fourth characters.

Let's take a look at an example together:

☑4 **M17 Osteoarthritis of knee**
    M17.0 Bilateral primary osteoarthritis of knee

The symbol to the left of code M17 alerts you that this code requires a fourth (4th) character. In looking at the second line of this example (M17.0), you can see that this fourth character shares additional, important information about the patient's condition. It is not enough to communicate that the patient has been diagnosed with osteoarthritis of the knee. You must explain the specific location (from our example, bilateral = both knees) and specific type of condition (from our example, primary osteoarthritis).

ICD-10-CM codes can be as short as three (3) characters and can add additional characters containing more specificity about the patient's condition . . . up to a total of seven (7) characters. These additional characters ensure that as much detail as possible about the patient's condition is communicated accurately and completely.

CODING BITES

When additional characters are required, those codes with fewer characters are invalid. The need for additional characters is mandatory, not a suggestion.

CODING BITES

You will learn many more details about reporting diagnoses in *Part II: Reporting Diagnoses,* with more in-depth introduction to ICD-10-CM as well as details by body system.

 ## LET'S CODE IT! SCENARIO

MCGRAW GENERAL HOSPITAL

DATE OF ADMISSION: 05/27/19

DATE OF DISCHARGE: 05/28/19

PATIENT: YOUNG, MATTHEW JAMES

HISTORY: Neonate is male, delivered 05/27/2019 at 1915 hours by C-section due to previous C-section. Mother is:

- gravida 2, para 2, AB 1
- blood type B positive
- GBS negative
- hepatitis B surface antigen negative
- rubella immune
- VDRL nonreactive

VITAL SIGNS:
Weight: 6 pounds 9 ounces
Height: 19-1/2 inches
Head circumference: 14 inches

GENERAL:
APGAR = 10 @1 min., 10 @ 5 min
SKIN: Portwine nevus on right ankle
NEUROLOGIC: Alert, vigorous cry, good tone, nonfocal

DISPOSITION:
The neonate was discharged to his mother. I instructed the mother to phone me PRN. I told her that I want to see both in my office in 10 days for a follow-up.

Let's Code It!

Dr. Michaels delivered Matthew James Young and examined him. Being born is the confirmed reason why the baby needed Dr. Michael's time and expertise. You need to translate the reason *why* into an ICD-10-CM diagnosis code. So, begin in the Alphabetic Index of your ICD-10-CM manual. What should you look up? Matthew needed to be examined right after being born, so let's look up:

Birth . . . nothing here that matches.
Next, try: Newborn. We have a match!
Newborn (infant) (liveborn) (singleton) Z38.2

Turn in the Tabular List to this code and begin by reading at the three-character code category:

☑4 Z38 Liveborn infants according to place of birth and type of delivery

> NOTE: This category is for use as the principal code on the initial record of a newborn baby. It is to be used for the initial birth record only. It is not to be used on the mother's record.

You know that Matthew was just born, so this note confirms you are in the right place in the code book. Notes, notations, symbols, and other marks in the code book are there to help point you in the right direction and to support your determination of the correct code.

Our next step is to look at the mark to the left of the code . . . it may be a box with a check mark ☑4, it may be a dot ●, or the following lines may just be indented. However your copy of the code book alerts you, it is clear . . . this code needs an additional character. And this is not a suggestion; it is mandatory.

There are three options for a fourth character:

☑5 Z38.0   Single liveborn infant, born in hospital
Z38.1   Single liveborn infant, born outside hospital
Z38.2   Single liveborn infant, unspecified as to place of birth

You can see in the record above that Matthew was born in McGraw General Hospital and, therefore, Z38.0 is the most accurate.

But we aren't done yet. There is a symbol to the left of code Z38.0. It is telling you that an additional character is required. Let's look at the two options:

Z38.00   Single liveborn infant, delivered vaginally
Z38.01   Single liveborn infant, delivered by cesarean

Go back to the documentation and read the information provided by the doctor. He noted that Matthew was born via a C-section (the C stands for cesarean).

There are no more symbols or notations here in the Tabular List. Next, double-check the **Official Guidelines, Section 1C. Chapter 21, subsection 12) Newborns and Infants** as well as **Chapter 16, subsection 6) Code all clinically significant conditions.** It appears that there are no further details or codes needed . . . so this is the code.

Good job! You were able to determine that code Z38.01 most accurately reports Matthew's birth. You did it!

1.3 Procedure Coding

Once the physician has determined the patient's condition or problem, he or she can then establish a treatment plan. Generally, there are three terms used to describe actions that the physician can take to support a patient's good health or to improve a current condition:

Procedures are actions, or a series of actions, taken to accomplish an objective (result). For example, surgically removing a mole or resectioning the small intestine.

Services are actions that will most often involve counseling, educating, and advising the patient, such as discussing test results or sharing recommendations for risk reduction.

Treatments are typically an application of a health care service, such as radiation treatments for tumor reduction or acupuncture.

Services
Spending time with a patient and/or family about health care situations.

Treatment
The provision of medical care for a disorder or disease.

These actions provided by the physician, or other health care professional, are done for one of three reasons:

Diagnostic tests or procedures are performed to provide the physician with additional information required to determine a confirmed diagnosis.

Preventive procedures and services are provided to keep a healthy patient healthy. In other words . . . to avoid illness or injury. These also include early detection testing, known as screenings.

Therapeutic procedures, treatments, and services are performed with the intention of removing, correcting, or repairing an abnormality or condition.

There are three different code sets available for you to use to translate health care procedures, services, and treatments into codes. These three code sets are

Current Procedural Terminology (CPT)

International Classification of Diseases - 10th Revision - Procedure Coding System (ICD-10-PCS)

Healthcare Common Procedure Coding System (HCPCS) Level II

Current Procedural Terminology (CPT)

CPT codes are used to describe procedures performed by a physician in any location. These services range from speaking with a patient about test results to performing surgery or determining a treatment plan. In addition, CPT codes are used to report the contribution made by **outpatient** facilities (a physician's office, a clinic, an ambulatory surgical center, or the emergency department of a hospital) such as a sterile procedure room, trained nursing and support staff, etc.

The Organization of the CPT Code Book

The CPT book has two parts, which in turn have many sections.

The CPT book (see Figure 1-6) has six sections, which are generally presented in numeric order by code number:

- Evaluation and Management: 99201–99499
- Anesthesia: 00100–01999 and 99100–99140

Outpatient

An **outpatient** is a patient who receives services for a short amount of time (less than 24 hours) in a physician's office or clinic, without being kept overnight. An **outpatient facility** includes a hospital emergency room, ambulatory care center, same-day surgery center, or walk-in clinic.

pancreas, 49180 for abdominal or retroperitoneal mass, 50200 for kidney, 54500 for testis, 54800 for epididymis, 60100 for thyroid, 62267 for nucleus pulposus, intervertebral disc, or paravertebral tissue, 62269 for spinal cord)

(For evaluation of fine needle aspirate, see 88172, 88173)

Integumentary System

Skin, Subcutaneous, and Accessory Structures

Introduction and Removal

⊙ 10030   Image-guided fluid collection drainge by catheter (eg. abscess, hematoma, seroma, lymphocele, cyst), soft tissue (eg. extremity, abdominal wall, neck), percutaneous

CPT Changes: An Insider's View 2014
CPT Assistant Fall 13:6, May 14:3, 9
Clinical Examples in Radiology Summer 14:9

(Report 10030 for each individual collection drained with a separate catheter)

(Do not report 10030 in conjunction with 75989, 76942, 77002, 77003, 77012, 77021)

Incision and Drainage

(For excision, see 11400, et seq)

10040   Acne surgery (eg, marsupialization, opening or removal of multiple milia, comedones, cysts, pustules)
CPT Assistant Fall 92:10, Feb 08:8

10060   Incision and drainage of abscess (eg, carbuncle, suppurative hidradenitis, cutaneous or subcutaneous abscess, cyst, furuncle, or peronychia); simple or single
CPT Assistant Sep 12:10

10061   complicated or multiple
CPT Assistant Sep 12:10

10080   Incision and drainage of pilonidal cyst; simple
CPT Assistant Fall 92:13, Dec 06:15, May 07:5

10081   complicated
CPT Assistant Fall 92:13, Dec 06:15. May 07:5

(For excision of pilonidal cyst, see 11770-11772)

10120   Incision and removal of foreign body, subcutaneous tissues; simple
CPT Assistant Sep 12:10, Apr 13:10, Dec 13:16

10121   complicated
CPT Assistant Spring 91:7, Dec 06:15. Sep 12:10, Dec 13:16

(To report wound exploration due to penetrating trauma without laparotomy or thoracotomy, one 20100-20103, as appropriate)

FIGURE 1-6 CPT main section, showing codes 10030–10121   Source: American Medical Association, *CPT Professional Manual*

- Surgery: 10021–69990
- Radiology: 70010–79999
- Pathology and Laboratory: 80047–89398, 0001U–0061U
- Medicine: 90281–99199, 99500–99607

The second part of the CPT book also contains several sections, including

- *Category II codes:* used for supplemental tracking of performance measurements. These codes are not reimbursable but support research on specific physician actions taken on behalf of a patient's health.
- *Category III codes:* temporary codes used to report emerging technological procedures. Technology and health care are innovating and improving every day. These codes enable tracking physician adoption and the frequency of use to identify what should stay and what will be deleted.
- *Appendixes A–P:* modifiers and other relevant additional information.
- *Alphabetic Index:* all the CPT codes in alphabetical order by code description, presented in four types of entries (see Figure 1-7):
  a. Procedures or services, such as bypass, decompression, insertion.
  b. Anatomical site or organ, such as brain stem, spinal cord, lymph nodes.
  c. Condition, such as pregnancy, fracture, abscess.
  d. Eponyms, synonyms, or abbreviations, such as Potts-Smith Procedure or EEG.

CODING BITES

CPT codes and sections run, generally, in numeric order; however, there are exceptions throughout. Bottom line . . . *read carefully and completely.*

CODING BITES

More information about Category II and Category III codes will be covered in the chapter *Introduction to CPT.*

The Formats of CPT Codes

Each code listed in the various CPT sections has a different structure:

CPT codes (Category I codes) are five-digit codes. They have all numbers (no letters, no punctuation). Example: 51100 Aspiration of bladder; by needle.

Category II codes are five-character codes, with four numbers followed by the letter "F." Example: 2001F Weight recorded (PAG).

Activity, Glomerular Procoagulant   **Alanine Transaminase**

Activity, Glomerular Procoagulant	**Labial**
See Thromboplastin	Lysis................................56441
Acupuncture	**Liver**
with Electrical Stimulation.........97813, 97814	Lysis................................58660
without Electrical Stimulation.......97810, 97811	**Lungs**
Acute Poliomyelitis	Pneumonolysis.............32174, 32940
See Polio	**Nose**
	Lysis................................30560
Acylcarnitines........82016, 82017	**Pelvic**
Adamantinoma, Pituitary	Lysis...................58660, 58740
See Craniopharyngioma	**Penile**
Addam Operation	Lysis
See Dupuytren's Contracture	Post-circumcision.................54162
Adductor Tenotomy of Hip	**Preputial**
See Tenotomy. Hip, Adductor	Lysis................................54450
	Urethral
Adenoidectomy	Lysis................................53500
See Adenoids. Excision	**Adipectomy**
Adenoids	*See* Lipectomy
Excision........................42830, 42836	**ADL**
with Tonsils.................42820, 42821	*See* Activities of Daily Living
Unlisted Services and Procedures.........42999	**Administration**
Adenoma	Immunization
Pancreas	Each Additional Vaccine/Toxoid 90472, 90474
Excision...........................48120	with Counseling...................90461
Parathyroid	One vaccine/Toxoid............90471, 90473
Localization	with Counseling...................90460
Injection Procedure.................78808	Occlusive Substance...................31634
Thyroid Gland Excision.................60200	Pharmacologic Agent..................93463
	ADP
	See Adenosine Diphosphate

Adult T Cell Leukemia Lymphoma Virus I
See HTLV-I
Advanced Life Support
Physician/Health Care Professional Direction 99288
Advancement
Genioglossus...........................21199
Tendon
Tibia..............................28238
Advancement Flap
See Skin, Adjacent Tissue Transfer
Aerosol Inhalation
See Pulmonology, Therapeutic
Pentamidine.......................94642
AFB
See Acid-Fast Bacilli (AFB)
Afferent Nerve
See Sensory Nerve
AFP
See Alpha-Fetoprotein (AFP)
After Hours Medical Services..99050
Agents, Anticoagulant
See Clotting Inhibitors
Agglutinin
Cold............................86156, 86157
Febrile..............................86000

FIGURE 1-7 CPT Alphabetic Index, partial listings from Activity, Glomerular Procoagulant to Agglutinin Source: American Medical Association, *CPT Professional Manual*

LET'S CODE IT! SCENARIO

Corey Carter, a 55-year-old male, came to the McGraw Ambulatory Surgery Center, an outpatient facility, so Dr. Lucano could perform a percutaneous core needle biopsy on his thyroid. Corey's primary care physician referred him to Dr. Lucano after noting a lump on his thyroid during an annual physical.

Let's Code It!

Open your CPT book to the Alphabetic Index. Which term should you look up? Let's dissect the scenario:

    Biopsy = the procedure
    Percutaneous core needle = the type of biopsy
    Thyroid = the anatomical site

Let's begin by finding Biopsy in the Alphabetic Index:

    Biopsy
    See Brush Biopsy; Needle Biopsy
    Abdomen 49000, 49321

Notice that Abdomen is the beginning of a long list of anatomical sites on which a biopsy can be done. Read down the list to find:

    Thyroid 60100

Now, turn into the Main Section of CPT to find code 60100. You can see:

    60100 Biopsy thyroid, percutaneous core needle

This matches Dr. Lucano's documentation perfectly—you can report this procedure code with confidence!

CODING BITES

You will learn many more details about reporting procedures in *Part III: Reporting Physician Services and Outpatient Procedures.*

Category III codes are five-character codes. These codes also have four numbers; however, Category III codes are followed by the letter "T." Example: 0208T Pure tone audiometry (threshold), automated; air only.

Modifiers (listed in Appendix A of your CPT code book) are two characters: two numbers, two letters, or one letter and one number. Modifiers are appended to CPT codes under special circumstances, such as the use of unusual anesthesia, two surgeons working on the same patient at the same time, or a multipart procedure performed over time. When required, a modifier is added after the main CPT code with a hyphen. Example: 47600-54 Cholecystectomy, surgical care only.

International Classification of Diseases – 10th Revision – Procedure Coding System (ICD-10-PCS)

The International Classification of Diseases – 10th Revision – Procedure Coding System (ICD-10-PCS) codes are used to describe the contribution made by the hospital to a procedure provided to an **inpatient** (a patient admitted into an acute care facility). These are known as "facility charges" because they report what the hospital provided during a specific procedure, service, or treatment, such as the skilled nursing staff, the operating room, the equipment, and whatever else is required.

ICD-10-PCS contains an Alphabetic Index and a Tables section (Figure 1-8). The Alphabetic Index is used in the same way you use this part of the other code books—to get an idea of where in the Tables section to find codes. However, the Tables section of this code set is very different. Rather than a listing of the codes in numeric or alphanumeric order, you will find Tables listing various characters and their meanings. Then, you will actually build the code, according to the physician's documentation.

The Format of ICD-10-PCS Codes

ICD-10-PCS codes have seven (7) characters and are alphanumeric (both letters and numbers). Each of the seven positions in the code represents a specific piece

---

Inpatient
An individual admitted for an overnight or longer stay in a hospital.

Section	0	Medical and Surgical
Body System	2	Heart and Greater Vessels
Operation	5	Destruction: Physical eradication of all or a portion of a body part by the direct use of energy, force, or a destructive agent

Body Part	Approach	Device	Qualifier
Character 4	**Character 5**	**Character 6**	**Character 7**
4 Coronary Vein **5** Atrial Septum **6** Atrium, Right **8** Conduction Mechanism **9** Chordae Tendineae **D** Papillary Muscle **F** Aortic Valve **G** Mitral Valve **H** Pulmonary Valve **J** Tricuspid Valve **K** Ventricle, Right **L** Ventricle, Left **M** Ventricular Septum **N** Pericardium **P** Pulmonary Trunk **Q** Pulmonary Artery, Right **R** Pulmonary Artery, Left **S** Pulmonary Vein, Right **T** Pulmonary Vein, Left **V** Superior Vena Cava **W** Thoracic Aorta, Descending **X** Thoracic Aorta, Ascending/Arch	**0** Open **3** Percutaneous **4** Percutaneous Endoscopic	**Z** No Device	**Z** No Qualifier
7 Atrium, Left	**0** Open **3** Percutaneous **4** Percutaneous Endoscopic	**Z** No Device	**K** Left Atrial Appendage **Z** No Qualifier

FIGURE 1-8 Table 025, one of the tables from the ICD-10-PCS Tables section

of information relating to a procedure, service, or treatment provided. These meanings change for each section of the codebook. But don't worry. No memorization is required . . . the code book provides you with what you need to know. All you have to do is read carefully.

For example, in the Medical and Surgical Section, each character reports the:

1. *Section* of the ICD-10-PCS code set.

2. *Body system* upon which the procedure or service was performed.

3. *Root operation,* which explains the category or type of procedure.

4. *Body part,* which identifies the specific anatomical site involved in the procedure.

5. *Approach,* which reports which method was used to perform the service or treatment.

6. *Device,* which reports, when applicable, what type of device was involved in the service or procedure.

7. *Qualifier,* which adds any additional detail.

Whereas in the Imaging Section, each character reports the:

1. *Section* of the ICD-10-PCS code set.
2. *Body system* upon which the procedure or service was performed.
3. *Root type,* which explains the type of imaging, such as MRI or CT scan.
4. *Body part,* which identifies the specific anatomical site imaged and recorded.
5. *Contrast,* which reports if contrast materials were used in the imaging process.
6. *Qualifier,* which adds any additional detail.
7. *Qualifier,* which adds any additional detail.

 ## LET'S CODE IT! SCENARIO

Marlena Takamoto, a 37-year-old female, contracted hepatitis seven years ago. The disease severely damaged her liver. She was admitted to Carolina Brookdale Hospital today so Dr. Lewis and his team can perform a liver transplantation, open approach. The liver donor was killed in a car accident early this morning.

Let's Code It!

The physicians will transplant a liver, using an open approach, from the donor to Marlena. The coder who works for Dr. Lewis will use CPT codes to report his services provided to Marlena. You work as the coder for Carolina Brookdale Hospital, so you need to use ICD-10-PCS to report the hospital's contribution in this surgery (the operating room, the support staff [surgical nurses, technicians, etc.], and other equipment).

The procedure is a transplant, so let's start by looking in the Alphabetic Index in ICD-10-PCS for transplant. In the index, we find

Transplantation
Liver 0FY00Z-

In this particular case, the Alphabetic Index provides you with the first six of the required seven characters. In other cases, you may find the Alphabetic Index will only provide you with three or four characters. Regardless, you must find this Table in the Tables section to complete the seven (7) characters. Using the first three characters provided by the Alphabetic Index, turn in the Tables section to the Table that begins with **OFY** (see below):

Section	0	Medical and Surgical
Body System	F	Hepatobiliary System and Pancreas
Operation	Y	Transplantation: Putting in or on all or a portion of a living body part taken from another individual or animal to physically take the place and/or function of all or a portion of a similar body part

Body Part	Approach	Device	Qualifier
0 Liver **G** Pancreas	**0** Open	**Z** No Device	**0** Allogeneic **1** Syngeneic **2** Zooplastic

Now, with all of this information, let's build the correct code:

1. *Section* of the ICD-10-PCS code set = *Medical and Surgical 0*
2. *Body system* upon which the procedure was performed = *Hepatobiliary F*

   Remember, the liver is an organ that is part of the Hepatobiliary System.

3. *Root operation:* the type of procedure = *Transplantation Y*
4. *Body part:* the specific anatomical site involved in the procedure = *Liver 0*
5. *Approach:* method used to perform the transplant = *Open 0*
6. *Device,* when applicable = *No Device Z*
7. *Qualifier:* any additional detail = *Allogeneic 0*

Before reporting this code . . . check the **Official Guidelines,** specifically **B3.16 Transplantation vs. Administration.** This confirms that you used the correct root operation term of Transplantation.

Good job! Now you have built the ICD-10-PCS code for this procedure: **0FY00Z0.**

It would not be unusual for one patient encounter, for a patient admitted into the hospital, to ultimately require interpretation into all three coding languages: ICD-10-CM, CPT, and ICD-10-PCS.

EXAMPLE

Injured in an accident, Terence McCarthy was admitted into McGraw General Hospital with a major contusion of the spleen. Terence was brought into the operating room, he was placed in the supine position, and general anesthesia was administered by Dr. London. Dr. Berring performed a total splenectomy.

Together, let's review all of the codes that will be reported for this surgical procedure:

- The professional coding specialist for Dr. Berring, the surgeon, will report:

S36.021A	**Major contusion of spleen, initial encounter**
38100	**Splenectomy; total**

- The professional coding specialist for Dr. London, the anesthesiologist, will report:

S36.021A	**Major contusion of spleen, initial encounter**
00790-P1	**Anesthesia for intraperitoneal procedures in upper abdomen including laparoscopy; not otherwise specified**

- The professional coding specialist for McGraw General Hospital, the facility, will report:

S36.021A	**Major contusion of spleen, initial encounter**
07TP0ZZ	**Splenectomy, open approach**

HCPCS Level II Procedure Codes

In some cases, you might determine that the CPT code set does not contain a code that accurately and completely reports a procedure or service. It is possible that a HCPCS Level II code may do the job.

CODING BITES

Use a medical dictionary whenever you do not know the meaning of a term:

Allogeneic means coming from a different individual of the same species.

Syngeneic means coming from a genetic identical, such as from an identical twin.

Zooplastic means the tissue or organ is coming from a donor of another species into a human.

CODING BITES

You will learn many more details about reporting inpatient procedures in *Part V: Inpatient (Hospital) Reporting.*

HCPCS (pronounced "hick-picks") is the abbreviation for Healthcare Common Procedure Coding System.

- HCPCS Level I codes are actually called CPT codes. While CPT codes are maintained by the American Medical Association (AMA), this code set was adopted by our industry as the first level of HCPCS.
- HCPCS Level II codes are referred to as HCPCS Level II codes.

For the most part, health care services are listed in the HCPCS Level II section titled Procedures/Professional Services (Temporary) G0008–G0151 [but not exclusively, so be certain to check the Alphabetic Index first]. As always, reading carefully and completely is required. However, as you scan the codes and their descriptions in this section of HCPCS Level II, you may find some are very close to CPT code descriptions. But . . . not exactly. Let's look at the simple repair of a 2.1 cm superficial laceration on the patient's left hand being repaired with tissue adhesive.

In CPT, under REPAIR (CLOSURE), the in-section guidelines state: "*Use the codes in this section to designate wound closure utilizing sutures, staples, or tissue adhesives, either singly or in combination with each other or in combination with adhesive strips.*"

The definition in CPT of a simple repair includes "*. . . requires simple one layer closure.*" With this scenario, this would lead to code

12001   **Simple repair of superficial wounds of scalp, neck, axillae, external genitalia, trunk and/or extremities (including hands and feet); 2.5 cm or less**

Compare this with the most appropriate HCPCS Level II code:

G0168   **Wound closure utilizing tissue adhesive(s) only**

Which code reports the repair more accurately? You must go back to the documentation and read carefully, looking for the additional details included in the definition of Simple Repair in CPT. Was a one-layer closure performed? Was local anesthesia used? Was anything else done by the physician in addition to the application of the tissue adhesive?

If the answer to any of these questions is Yes, then you need to report the CPT code 12001. If the answers to all of these questions are No, then report G0168.

Let's look at an example that is perhaps a bit less complex. Compare and contrast these two codes, both of which are used for reporting speech therapy services:

92507   **Treatment of speech, language, voice, communication, and/or auditory processing disorder; individual**
S9128   **Speech therapy, in the home, per diem**

CODING BITES

Learn about the other types of HCPCS Level II codes in the section *Equipment and Supplies* in this chapter.

And learn more about the HCPCS Level II code set in the chapter *HCPCS Level II*.

These two codes report similar services: speech therapy provided to an individual. However, they differ with regard to location, length of the session, and possibly the professional providing the therapy. Be certain to read the CPT in-section guidelines related to the reporting of 92507 (and other codes in this subsection) before you decide. And, of course, you need to carefully abstract the details within the documentation from which you are coding and compare the specifics to each of the code descriptions, and perhaps to any others available. Then, and only then, can you determine which code to report.

Don't worry . . . one item, one detail, one concept at a time. It will take time, but we are confident you will be able to understand, learn, and master coding for health care services.

1.4 Equipment and Supplies

A large number of components of health care extend beyond what are usually referred to as procedures, services, and treatments you learned about earlier in Section 1.3

of this chapter. This includes equipment that is provided for a patient's use at home, supplies that are not already included in other codes, and transportation services not described in the CPT book at all. HCPCS Level II also contains codes you can use to report them.

HCPCS Level II codes cover specific aspects of health care services, including

- Durable medical equipment (e.g., a wheelchair or a humidifier).
- Pharmaceuticals administered by a health care provider (e.g., a saline solution or a chemotherapy drug).
- Medical supplies provided for the patient's home use (e.g., an eye patch or gradient compression stockings).
- Dental services (e.g., all services provided by a dental professional).
- Transportation services (e.g., ambulance services).
- Vision and hearing services (e.g., trifocal spectacles or a hearing aid).
- Orthotic and prosthetic procedures (e.g., scoliosis brace or prosthetic arm).

HCPCS Level II codes are listed in sections, grouped by the type of service, the type of supply item, or the type of equipment they represent. However, you should not assume that a particular item or service is located in a specific section. Use the Alphabetic Index (Figure 1-9) to direct you to the correct section or subsection in the Alphanumeric Listing of the code book. One type of service or procedure might be located under several different categories depending upon the details.

Medicare and Medicaid want you to use HCPCS Level II codes; however, not all insurance carriers accept these codes. It is your responsibility, as a coding specialist, to find out whether each third-party payer with which your facility works will permit the reporting of HCPCS Level II codes on a claim form. If not, you should ask for the payer's policies on reporting the services and supplies covered by HCPCS Level II so you don't have a claim delayed or denied.

The Format of HCPCS Level II Codes

The codes listed in the HCPCS Level II code book are all structured the same way: one letter followed by four numbers. No dots, no dashes (Figure 1-10).

A0225	**Ambulance service, neonatal transport, base rate, emergency transport, one way**
E0130	**Walker, rigid (pickup), adjustable or fixed height**
J3480	**Injection, potassium chloride, per 2 mEq**
L0130	**Cervical, flexible, thermoplastic collar, molded to patient**
V5050	**Hearing aid, monaural, in the ear**

Cyclosporine, J7502, J7515, J7516
Cytarabine, J9100
Cytarabine liposome, J9098
Cytomegalovirus immune globulin (human), J0850

D

Dacarbazine, J9130
Daclizumab, J7513
Dactinomycin, J9120

FIGURE 1-9 HCPCS Level II Alphabetic Index, partial listing from Cyclosporine to Dactinomycin

J7512 Prednisone, immediate release or delayed release, oral, 1 mg

J7513 Daclizumab, parenteral, 25 mg
Use this code for Zenapax.
CMS: 100-2,15,50.5; 100-4, 17, 80.3
AHA: 2Q, '05, 11

J7515 Cyclosporine, oral, 25 mg
Use this code for Neoral, Sandimmune, Gengraf, Sangcya.
CMS: 100-4, 17, 80.3

J7516 Cyclosporine, parenteral, 250 mg
Use this code for Neoral, Sandimmune, Gengral, Sangcya.
CMS: 100-4, 17, 80.3

J7517 Mycophenolate mofetil, oral, 250 mg
Use this code for CeliCept.
CMS: 100-4, 17, 80.3

J7518 Mycophenolic acid, oral, 180 mg
Use this code for Mytoxtic Delayed Release.
CMS: 100-4, 17, 80, 3.1
AHA: 2Q, '05, 11

J7520 Sirolimus, oral, 1 mg
Use this code for Rapamune.
CMS: 100-2, 15, 50.5; 100-4, 17, 80.3

J7525 Tacrolimus, parenteral, 5 mg
Use this code for Prograt.
CMS: 100-2, 15, 50.5; 100-4, 17, 80.3

J7527 Everolimus, oral, 0.25 mg
Use this code for Zortress, Afinitor.

J7599 Immunosuppressive drug, not otherwise classified
Determine if an alternative HCPCS Level II or a CPT code Better describes the service being reported. This code should be used only if a more specific code is unavailable.
CMS: 100-2, 15, 50.5; 100-4, 17, 80.3
AHA: 2Q, '13, 3

Inhalation Drugs

J7604 Acetylcysteine, Inhalation solution, compounded product, administered through DME, unit dose form, per g

J7605 Arformoterol, inhalation solution, FDA approved final product, noncompounded, administered through DME, unit dose form, 15 mcg

J7611 Albuterol, inhalation solution, FDA-approved final product, noncompounded, administered through DME, unit dose, 1 mg
Use this code for Acouneb, Proventil, Respirol, Ventelin.
AHA: 2Q, '08, 10; 2Q, '07, 10

J7612 Lavalbuterol, inhalation solution, FDA-approved final product, noncompounded, administered through DME, unit dose, 0.5 mg
Use this code for Xopenex.
CMS: 100-3, 200.2
AHA: 2Q, '08, 10; 2Q, '07, 10

J7615 Levalbuterol, inhalation solution, compounded product, administered through DME, unit dose, 0.5 mg
CMS: 100-3, 200.2

J7620 Albuterol, up to 2.5 mg and ipratropium bromide, up to 0.5 mg, FDA-approved final product, noncompounded, administered through DME

J7622 Betclomethasone, inhalation solution, compounded product, administered through DME, unit dose form, per mg
Use this code for Beclovent, Beconase.
AHA: IQ, '02, 5

J7624 Betamethasone, inhalation solution, compounded product, administered through DME, unit dose form, per mg
AHA: IQ, '02, 5

J7626 Budesonide, inhalation solution. FDA-approved final product, noncompounded, administered through DME, unit dose form, up to 0.5 mg
Use this code for Pulmicort, Pulmicort Flexhaler, Pulmicort Respules, Vanceril.
AHA: IQ, '02, 5

J7627 Budesonide, Inhalation solution, compounded product, administered through DME, unit dose form, up to 0.5 mg

J7628 Bitolterol mesylate, inhalation solution, compounded product, administered through DME, concentrated form, per mg

Drugs Administered Other Than Oral method

J7512 — J7628

CODING BITES

You will learn many more details about using the HCPCS Level II code set in *Part IV: DMEPOS & Transportation.*

FIGURE 1-10 One page from the HCPCS Level II Alphanumeric Listing, showing codes J7512–J7628 Source: Center for Medicare and Medicaid Services (CMS)

LET'S CODE IT! SCENARIO

Rita Widden, a 92-year-old female, was being transferred from Hampton Medical Center to the Sunflower Nursing Home across town. Cosentti Ambulance Service provided nonemergency transportation prepared with basic life support (BLS) services.

Let's Code It!

Cosentti Ambulance Service provided nonemergency BLS (basic life support) transportation for Rita. After looking carefully in your CPT and ICD-10-PCS code books, you find that this type of service is not represented. Therefore, you need to look in the HCPCS Level II code set.

Begin in the Alphabetic Index, and find:

Transportation
    Ambulance, A0021–A0999

This code set often will require some patience as you read through all of the code options, which were suggested by the Alphabetic Index, until you find the one that matches the services for which you are reporting:

A0428   **Ambulance service, basic life-support, nonemergency transport, (BLS)**

Good work! You got it!

Chapter Summary

Essentially, the process of coding begins with the physician's documentation stating why the patient needed care and what was done for this patient during this visit. As a professional coding specialist, you will interpret the documentation in the patient's record from medical terminology into codes: diagnosis codes to explain *why,* along with *how* and *where* if the patient is injured; and procedure codes to report *what* the physician or facility did for the patient during this encounter. You will need to confirm that the diagnosis code or codes support medical necessity for the procedures, services, and treatments provided. As you proceed through this textbook, read carefully and completely. Coding is like nothing you have experienced before, and you want to learn how to be proficient.

CODING BITES

ICD-10-CM . . . Diagnosis Codes

- Used by all health care providers and facilities
- Report WHY the patient needed care [medical necessity]
- ICD-10-CM diagnosis codes = A12.3K5A (up to seven (7) alphanumeric)

CPT . . . Procedure Codes

- Used by physicians to report services provided at any/all facilities
- Also used by outpatient care facilities [i.e., ambulatory surgery centers, hospital emergency rooms, hospital outpatient surgery centers, etc.]
- Report WHAT was done for the patient
- CPT procedure codes = 12345 (five numbers always)

ICD-10-PCS . . . Procedure Codes

- Used only by hospitals for reporting facility services to inpatients
- ICD-10-PCS procedure codes = 012B4LZ (seven characters always)

HCPCS Level II . . . Services and Supplies Codes

- Used to report services and supplies not already represented by a code in CPT [i.e., transportation, drugs administered by a health care professional, durable medical equipment, etc.]
- Used by any facility or provider
- Not all third-party payers accept the use of HCPCS Level II codes
- HCPCS Level II codes = A1234 (one letter, four numbers always)

CHAPTER 1 REVIEW
Introduction to the Languages of Coding

Enhance your learning by completing these exercises and more at mcgrawhillconnect.com!

Let's Check It! Terminology

Match each key term to the appropriate definition.

1. **LO 1.3** The provision of medical care for a disorder or disease.

2. **LO 1.2** The state of abnormality or dysfunction.

3. **LO 1.1** The determination that the health care professional was acting according to standard practices in providing a particular procedure for an individual with a particular diagnosis.

4. **LO 1.1** The process of paying for health care services after they have been provided.

A. Classification System

B. Condition

C. Diagnosis

D. Eponym

E. External Causes

F. Inpatient

5. LO 1.2 The explanation of how a patient became injured or poisoned, as well as other necessary details about the event; a health concern caused by something outside of the body.

6. LO 1.1 A physician's determination of a patient's condition, illness, or injury.

7. LO 1.1 Action taken, in accordance with the standards of care, by the physician to accomplish a predetermined objective (result); a surgical operation.

8. LO 1.1 The category term used in health care to identify ICD-10-CM, CPT, ICD-10-PCS, and HCPCS Level II code sets.

9. LO 1.3 A patient admitted into a hospital for an overnight stay or longer.

10. LO 1.3 Spending time with a patient and/or family about health care situations.

11. LO 1.3 Health care services provided to individuals without an overnight stay in the facility.

12. LO 1.2 A disease or condition named for a person.

G. Medical Necessity
H. Outpatient
I. Procedure
J. Reimbursement
K. Services
L. Treatment

Let's Check It! Concepts

Choose the most appropriate answer for each of the following questions.

1. LO 1.1 Coding languages communicate information that is key to which of the following aspect(s) of the health care system?

   a. medical necessity   b. reimbursement   c. resources allocation   d. all of these

2. LO 1.1 Coding is accurately interpreting health care terms and definitions into _____ that specifically convey diagnoses and procedures.

   a. letter combinations
   b. number combinations
   c. number-letter combinations
   d. numbers or number-letter combinations

3. LO 1.1 A diagnosis explains

   a. what the provider did for the patient.
   b. who the policyholder is.
   c. why the patient requires attention of the provider.
   d. where the patient was seen by the provider.

4. LO 1.1 A procedure explains

   a. where the patient was seen by the provider.
   b. what the provider did for the patient.
   c. why the patient requires attention of the provider.
   d. who the policyholder is.

5. LO 1.2 Which code book contains all of the codes to report the reason why the health care provider cared for the patient during a specific encounter?

   a. ICD-10-CM code book
   b. ICD-10-PCS code book
   c. CPT code book
   d. HCPCS Level II code book

6. LO 1.2 What part of the ICD-10-CM code book do you use to confirm that a diagnostic code is accurate?

   a. the Alphabetic Index
   b. the Index to External Causes
   c. the Tabular List
   d. the Neoplasm Table

7. LO 1.2 Diagnostic descriptions are listed by

   a. conditions such as fractures.
   b. eponyms such as Epstein-Barr syndrome.
   c. other descriptors such as family history.
   d. all of these.

8. LO 1.2 Which of the following would be an example of an eponym?

   a. infections
   b. wounds
   c. Arnold-Chiari disease
   d. family history

9. LO 1.2 The Index to External Causes lists the causes of

   a. injuries and poisoning
   b. diseases and syndromes
   c. injuries
   d. poisoning

10. **LO 1.2** An example of an ICD-10-CM code is
    a. H2031   **b.** 85460   **c.** H61.022   **d.** 08NTXZZ

11. **LO 1.1** When ICD-10-CM codes support medical necessity, this means that
    a. there was a valid medical reason to provide care.
    b. a preexisting condition was treated.
    c. the patient was seen in a hospital.
    d. a licensed health care professional was involved.

12. **LO 1.1** The why justifies the
    a. who   **b.** where   **c.** what   **d.** when

13. **LO 1.3** Surgical removal of a skin tag is an example of a
    a. treatment   **b.** procedure   **c.** service   **d.** diagnosis

14. **LO 1.3** _____ tests or procedures are performed to provide the physician with additional information to support the determination of a confirmed diagnosis.
    a. Diagnostic   **b.** Preventive   **c.** Therapeutic   **d.** Conditional

15. **LO 1.3** The code set(s) available for the coding specialist to use to translate health care procedures, services, and treatments into codes is/are
    a. CPT code book.   **b.** ICD-10-PCS code book.
    c. HCPCS Level II code book.   **d.** all of these.

16. **LO 1.3** The main body of the CPT book has _____ sections.
    a. 5   **b.** 6   **c.** 7   **d.** 8

17. **LO 1.3** An example of a Category II code is
    a. 89398   **b.** 1134F   **c.** V95.9   **d.** 0241T

18. **LO 1.3** The code set used for hospital facility reporting of procedures, services, and treatments provided to a patient who has been admitted as an inpatient is
    a. ICD-10-CM code book.   **b.** CPT code book.
    c. ICD-10-PCS code book.   **d.** HCPCS Level II code book.

19. **LO 1.4** HCPCS Level II codes are presented as
    a. five numbers.   **b.** one letter followed by four numbers.
    c. four numbers followed by two letters.   **d.** one letter, a dash, and four numbers.

20. **LO 1.4** An example of a HCPCS Level II code is
    a. J3285   **b.** D7056ZZ   **c.** 58940   **d.** T84.010D

Let's Check It! Rules and Regulations

Please answer the following questions from the knowledge you have gained after reading this chapter.

1. **LO 1.1** Explain what is meant by a third-party payer.
2. **LO 1.2** Describe the Tabular List of Diseases and Injuries, including its format and why it is important.
3. **LO 1.3** Explain the difference between diagnostic testing, preventive procedures, and therapeutic procedures.
4. **LO 1.1** Discuss medical necessity and its importance.
5. **LO 1.4** Do all insurance carriers accept HCPCS Level II codes, and what is the responsibility of the coding specialist in regards to billing third-party payers?

Design elements: ©McGraw-Hill

2 Abstracting Clinical Documentation

Key Terms

Abstracting
Assume
Co-morbidity
Demographic
Interpret
Manifestation
Query
Sequela
Signs
Symptoms

Learning Outcomes

After completing this chapter, the student should be able to:

LO 2.1 Identify which health care professional for whom you are coding.

LO 2.2 Describe the process of abstracting physician documentation and operative notes.

LO 2.3 Recognize the terms used to describe diagnoses in documentation.

LO 2.4 Distinguish between co-morbidities, manifestations, and sequelae.

LO 2.5 Determine those conditions that require external cause codes to be reported.

LO 2.6 Recognize the terms used to describe procedures, services, and treatments provided.

LO 2.7 Create a legal query to obtain documentation about a missing, ambiguous, or contradictory component in the existing documentation.

2.1 For Whom You Are Reporting

Most people do not realize how many coders are involved in reporting one patient's surgical procedure or other type of encounter. Let's look at a scenario and dissect it:

Carly Camden, a 27-year-old female, was admitted into the hospital to have surgery on her broken leg.

- The surgeon will have a coder to report what he does for Carly.
- The anesthesiologist will have a coder to report administration of anesthesia.
- The facility will have a coder to report what the hospital did for Carly (providing the nursing and other support staff, equipment, and room, etc.). In this case, the facility is an acute care hospital. In other cases, the facility may be a same day surgery center, a skilled nursing facility, an imaging center, or another health care organization.
- The radiologist will have a coder to report for any imaging (e.g., x-rays, MRI, CT scan, etc.).
- The pathologist will have a coder to report for any blood work or lab tests provided.

Therefore, the first question you, as the professional coder, will need to ask is . . . for whom are you reporting? Only then will you know which key terms to look for as you abstract the operative notes, the physician's notes, and the reports.

CODING BITES

Patient = *Who* is provided with care

Physician = *Who* is the health care provider you are representing

Diagnosis = *Why* the provider is caring for this individual during this encounter

External Cause = *How* and *Where* the patient became injured

Procedure = *What* the provider did for the individual

Facility = *Where* the services were provided

There may also be many professionals providing different types of care for one patient for different reasons. For example . . .

Allen Davidson, a 59-year-old male, was admitted to the hospital due to a myocardial infarction (heart attack). Allen has type 2 diabetes mellitus.

- A cardiologist (heart specialist) will diagnose and treat Allen's heart problem.
- An endocrinologist will diagnose and treat Allen's diabetes mellitus.
- The facility, such as a hospital, will provide care for Allen and all of his health concerns.

For all professionals involved in the care of a patient, the reason or reasons *why* (diagnosis code or codes) care was required are critical to establishing medical necessity for the *what* (specific procedures, services, and treatments) provided. Yet, in a location, such as an acute care facility (hospital), there may be many issues for you to evaluate and connect.

2.2 The Process of Abstracting

You are learning that documentation about the encounter between physician and patient will be your primary source for details that you will use to determine the most accurate codes to report. Physicians, though, do not write their documentation solely for coding; therefore, there will be pieces of information included that you will not use in your coding process. Reading the entire patient record and pulling out the details necessary for determining the correct codes is known as **abstracting**.

Assume or Interpret

Always keep in mind the professional coding specialists' motto: "*If it isn't documented, it didn't happen. If it didn't happen, you can't code it!*"

If it <u>is</u> documented appropriately, there is no reason for you to **assume** any details; you only need to **interpret** what is documented.

One of the most challenging aspects of coding is the very fine line between assuming and interpreting. Yes, professional coding specialists must interpret the physician's documentation. This does not include assuming in any way. Assuming is making up details, filling in the blanks with your own specifics, guessing, or substituting your own knowledge for missing facts. Interpreting is an exact science; it involves changing information from one language to another. Just like *casa* = house (Spanish-to-English), fine needle aspiration = 10021 (medical terminology-to-CPT). This is why coding can be so challenging. We are responsible for not only translating from one language (medical terminology) to another (medical codes) but also for accurately figuring out into *which* language (CPT or ICD-10-CM or ICD-10-PCS or HCPCS Level II) medical terminology must be translated. Another major factor is that no one is a natural-born speaker of medical terminology, so you are required to learn a new language to understand the languages of medical coding. Imagine if you were born speaking English, but you had to learn to speak French before achieving your ultimate goal of interpreting French words into Spanish.

Source Documents

The patient's health care record is at the center of health information management in general as well as the primary focus for you, as the professional coding specialist. Within this record, whether it is written on paper or typed into an electronic health record (EHR), are several important components that you will use to gather details necessary to determine the correct code or codes.

Abstracting
The process of identifying the relevant words or phrases in health care documentation in order to determine the best, most appropriate code(s).

Assume
Suppose to be the case, without proof; guess the intended details.

Interpret
Explain the meaning of; convert a meaning from one language to another.

CODING BITES

Keep a medical dictionary by your side so that the minute you come upon a word you don't understand for an absolute fact, you can look it up right away. If you don't understand what you are reading, you will not be able to interpret it accurately.

EXCELLENT RESOURCE:
MedlinePlus, an online medical dictionary and encyclopedia, is an excellent and reliable source created and maintained by the US National Library of Medicine.

Virtually every patient record should include all, or most, of these pages or sections:

- *Patient's Registration Form:* This document or section includes the patient's **demographic** information, as well as health insurance policy numbers and the name of the individual who will be financially responsible for the patient's care.

- *Referral Authorization Form:* If another physician or health care provider referred this patient for a consultation, you will need to know this to determine the correct evaluation and management code.

- *Physician's Notes/Operative Reports:* Written documentation of what occurred during the encounter between physician and patient is also known as clinical documentation. The physician's notes or operative reports are your most important source for details required to determine the most accurate code or codes. Your job is to interpret the words—medical terminology—into codes. Your ability to interpret accurately is dependent upon your knowledge of anatomy and physiology, as well as medical terminology.

- *Pathology and Laboratory Reports:* Results of testing performed on blood, tissue, and other specimens hold important keys to the patient's condition. The results can provide you with important details necessary for you to determine a specific, accurate code.

- *Imaging Reports:* Similar to pathology reports, these are reports written by a radiologist containing his or her interpretations of images taken of the patient [e.g., x-ray, CT scan, MRI, etc.].

- *Medication Logs:* If the facility is residential, such as an acute care hospital, skilled nursing facility, long-term care facility, etc., the nursing staff must record every time they administer a medication to a patient, including the drug name, dosage, time administered, and route used for administration. All data must be reported.

- *Allergy List:* This list is included for the patient's safety so health care professionals can avoid giving the patient any substance to which he or she may be allergic.

- *History and Physical (H&P):* Essentially, this document, written by the admitting physician, explains the background and current issues used to make the decision to admit the patient into the hospital.

- *Consultation Reports:* When a specialist is asked by an attending physician to evaluate a patient's condition, a report is written and sent over to be included in the patient's medical record in the requesting physician's files, as well as those belonging to the consulting physician.

- *Discharge Summary:* At the time a patient is released from a facility, such as a hospital, the Discharge Summary provides the conclusions and results of the patient's stay in the facility in addition to follow-up advice.

CODING BITES

Principles of Documentation for Medical Records

Adapted from the Centers for Medicare and Medicaid Services

1. The documentation of each patient encounter should include:
   - the date;
   - the reason for the encounter;
   - appropriate history and physical exam in relationship to the patient's chief complaint;
   - review of lab, x-ray data, and other ancillary services, where appropriate;
   - assessment; and
   - a plan for care (including discharge plan, if appropriate).
2. Past and present diagnoses should be accessible.

3. The reasons for—and results of—x-rays, lab tests, and other ancillary services should be documented or included in the medical record.

4. Relevant health risk factors should be identified.

5. The patient's progress, including response to treatment, change in treatment, change in diagnosis, and patient noncompliance, should be documented.

6. The written plan for care should include, when appropriate:
   - treatments and medications, specifying frequency and dosage;
   - any referrals and consultations;
   - patient/family education; and
   - specific instructions for follow-up.

7. The documentation should support the intensity of the patient evaluation and/or the treatment, including thought processes and the complexity of medical decision making as it relates to the patient's chief complaint for the encounter.

8. All entries to the medical record should be dated and authenticated.

9. The CPT/ICD-10-CM/ICD-10-PCS/HCPCS Level II codes reported on the claim form should be supported by the documentation in the medical record.

Abstracting the Documentation

Abstracting is the first step in the coding process. You must read all clinical documentation related to the specific encounter all the way through, slowly and carefully. Whether the encounter was a short visit in a physician's office, an hours-long surgical procedure documented in operative reports, or a five-day stay in a hospital, you cannot expect that one sentence will give you a clear and complete picture of *what* occurred (the procedures or services) and *why* they were provided (the diagnosis or diagnoses). You learned about understanding the *why* and *what* in the *Introduction to the Languages of Coding* chapter. You are required to code all conditions documented to be relevant during this encounter or hospital stay, not just those in the official diagnostic statement. The same stands for the procedures.

Reasons That Are Not Illness; Procedures That Are Not Actions

There are times when an individual comes to see a health care provider without having a particular illness or injury. In such cases, you might assign a diagnosis code that explains *why* the patient was seen that is not a current health condition or injury. A healthy person might go to see a physician for preventive care, for routine and administrative exams, or for monitoring care and screenings for someone with a personal history or family history of a condition. As you read through the documentation, you may discover that the reason *why* the encounter was necessary may be wellness, rather than illness or injury.

In the same fashion, the description of *what* the physician provided may not be a procedure, service, or treatment. It may be advice or a second opinion. The physician and patient may meet to discuss previously done test results, a recommendation for a specific treatment plan, suggestions for risk-factor reduction (e.g., stop smoking), or a referral to another physician or facility.

2.3 Deconstructing Diagnostic Statements

Diagnosis codes, for either reimbursement or statistical purposes, will report only those conditions addressed by the provider during a specific encounter and not the patient's entire health history. When there is no confirmed diagnosis to provide

CODING BITES

One suggestion is to use scrap paper so you can jot down details as you read them, which may point toward *why* the patient required the attention of the physician (e.g., signs, symptoms, confirmed diagnoses), as well as *what* was provided (e.g., specific procedures, services, and treatments).

CODING BITES

Every health care professional/patient encounter must have at least one reportable [codeable] reason *why* and at least one reportable [codeable] explanation of *what*.

Signs
Measurable indicators of a patient's health status.

Symptoms
A subjective sensation or departure from the norm as related by the patient.

medical necessity for a procedure, service, or treatment performed, determining the diagnosis code to report will vary slightly, depending on whether you are coding for an inpatient or outpatient encounter.

- In an outpatient encounter, if there is no confirmed diagnostic statement, you will code the patient's **signs** and/or **symptoms** that led to the physician's decision for the next step in care.
- When an inpatient (admitted into the hospital) is being discharged without a confirmed diagnosis, you will code the suspected conditions listed on the discharge summary as if they were confirmed. You will not code the signs and symptoms.

Dissect the Diagnostic Statement

Now that you have identified all of the statements in the documentation that explain *why* the patient was cared for, take each statement apart to determine which word identifies the disease, illness, condition, or primary reason for the visit (also known as the "main term"). Separate this term from any words that may simply describe the type of condition or the location of the condition (anatomical site/body site). Keep a medical dictionary close by so you can look up any terms you don't clearly understand. Remember, if you do not completely understand the terms, how can you possibly interpret them?

Why is the physician caring for the patient? Many diagnostic statements are made up of multiple words, with each providing additional information. As you analyze the examples below, dissect the condition for which the physician is seeing the patient and separate out those terms used to provide more detail about that condition.

- *Herpes zoster* . . . The disease is "herpes" and "zoster" is the type of herpes.
- *Acute bronchospasm* . . . The condition is a "spasm" (muscle contraction) of the bronchus (a part of the lungs) and the term "acute" (which means severe) describes what type of bronchospasm the patient has.
- *Personal history of lung cancer* . . . The issue of concern is "history"—why the patient is being seen. The type of history is "personal" and the secondary descriptor is "malignant neoplasm of the lung (lung cancer)" to explain "a history of what?"
- *Myocardial infarction* . . . The condition is "infarction" (area of dead tissue) and "myocardial" (heart muscle) is the anatomical site of the infarction.
- *Congenital pneumothorax* . . . The condition is "pneumothorax" (air in the chest cavity) and the term "congenital" (present at birth) describes the cause of the condition.
- *Family history of renal failure* . . . The issue of concern is "history"—why the patient is being seen. The type of history is "family" and the secondary descriptor is "renal failure" (loss of function of the kidneys) to explain "a history of what?"

CODING BITES

A diagnostic term might have a suffix like:

Dermatitis	*derma* = skin + *-itis* = inflammation (a condition)
Acrophobia	*acro* = heights + *-phobia* = fear (a condition)

A procedural term might have a suffix like:

Pancreatectomy	*pancreat* = pancreas + *-ectomy* = to surgically remove (an action)
Conjunctivoplasty	*conjunctivo* = conjunctiva (part of the eye) + *-plasty* = to repair (an action)

LET'S CODE IT! SCENARIO

Dr. Olivera diagnosed Kathleen Belsara with ulcerative blepharitis of the right upper eyelid. He treated her with an injection of gentamicin 80 mg, IM, and gave her a prescription for gentamicin ointment 0.3% q.i.d. for 7 to 10 days.

Let's Code It!

Why did Dr. Olivera care for Kathleen? *ulcerative blepharitis of the right upper eyelid.*

The condition is: *blepharitis*

The type of blepharitis: *ulcerative*

Anatomical site affected: *right upper eyelid*

NOTE: These first three steps will get you started when it comes to determining the correct diagnosis code in ICD-10-CM. You will learn more about this beginning in the chapter *Introduction to ICD-10-CM.*

Also . . .

What did Dr. Olivera do for Kathleen? *an injection of gentamicin 80 mg, IM*

The drug: *gentamicin*

The dosage: *80 mg*

The route of administration: *IM (intramuscular) injection*

NOTE: These first three steps will get you started when it comes to determining the correct drug code in HCPCS Level II. You will learn more about this beginning in the chapter *HCPCS Level II.*

Recognize Inclusive Signs and Symptoms

As you abstract the documentation, you will need to identify any signs and symptoms that are already part of the description of a confirmed diagnosis. Physicians are trained in medical school to add all of the data (history, signs, symptoms, test results, etc.) together, almost like a math equation, to arrive at a diagnosis. This sign + that symptom = this diagnosis. These equations are based on the standards of care accepted by the health care industry around the world.

Think about it: *John comes to see Dr. Finch. John complains of chest congestion, runny nose, sneezing, headaches, being achy all over. Dr. Finch examines John, does a quick lab test, and tells John he has the flu.*

It is a fact that "chest congestion, runny nose, sneezing, headaches, being achy all over" are signs and symptoms of the flu. Therefore, when you report the code for the flu, there is no reason to also code the signs and symptoms of the flu . . . it is redundant.

GUIDANCE CONNECTION

Read the ICD-10-CM Official Guidelines for Coding and Reporting, section **I. Conventions, General Coding Guidelines and Chapter-Specific Guidelines;** subsections

- **B.4 *Signs and Symptoms***
- **B.5 *Conditions that are an integral part of a disease process***
- **B.6 *Conditions that are not an integral part of a disease process***

LET'S CODE IT! SCENARIO

Ralph Carbonna, a 61-year-old male, came into the Emergency Department of McGraw General Hospital. Earlier in the day, Ralph felt lightheaded and a little dizzy. In addition, he complained that his heart was beating so wildly that he thought he may have had a heart attack. When interviewed by the nurse, Ralph revealed his previous diagnosis of type 1 diabetes mellitus, prompting Dr. Geller to order a blood glucose test. Dr. Geller also ordered an EKG (ECG) to check Ralph's heart. After getting the results of the tests, Dr. Geller determined that Ralph's lightheadedness and dizziness were a result of his abnormal glucose level. He spoke with Ralph about how to bring his diabetes mellitus under control and informed Ralph that the EKG was negative [normal], meaning there were no signs of a heart attack.

Let's Code It!

Dr. Geller confirmed that Ralph's *type 1 diabetes mellitus,* specifically his abnormal glucose level, caused his feelings of dizziness. Diabetes seems to be the only confirmed diagnosis in Dr. Geller's notes. You can report this with confidence, and this condition justifies performing the blood glucose test.

Dr. Geller also ordered an EKG (ECG). A diagnosis for diabetes does not provide any medical rationale for doing an EKG. In addition, the test was negative and, therefore, provided no diagnosis.

You still need a diagnosis code to report that there was a medical necessity to run the EKG. Why did Dr. Geller order the EKG? Because Ralph complained of a *rapid heartbeat.* A rapid heartbeat provides the medical necessity for performing the EKG.

Before you confirm any codes, be certain to read all notations and symbols and check the Official Guidelines. Now, you can continue with confidence.

For the encounter, you have one confirmed diagnosis (the diabetes) and one symptom unrelated to the confirmed diagnosis (rapid heartbeat).

 GUIDANCE CONNECTION

Read the ICD-10-CM Official Guidelines for Coding and Reporting, section **I. Conventions, General Coding Guidelines and Chapter-Specific Guidelines;** subsection **B.18. Use of Sign/Symptom/Unspecified Codes.** *"If a definitive diagnosis has not been established by the end of the encounter, it is appropriate to report codes for sign(s) and/or symptoms in lieu of a definitive diagnosis."*

Section **II. Selection of Principal Diagnosis,** subsection **H. Uncertain Diagnosis.** *"If the diagnosis documented at the time of discharge is qualified as 'probable', 'suspected', 'likely', 'questionable', 'possible', or 'still to be ruled out', or other similar terms indicating uncertainty, code the condition as if it existed or was established."* NOTE: This guideline is applicable only to inpatient admissions to short-term, acute, long-term care, and psychiatric hospitals.

2.4 Identifying Manifestations, Co-morbidities, and Sequelae

Manifestations

Manifestation
A condition that develops as the result of another, underlying condition.

There are some diseases (also known as *underlying conditions*) that actually cause patients to develop other conditions. This second condition, directly the result of the first condition, is known as a **manifestation**. In these cases, scientific evidence proves that the patient would not have the manifested disease or problem if the first condition had not already been present. The cause-and-effect relationship between the two conditions must be documented by the physician and supported by medical research to be coded as a manifestation.

A manifestation is a second condition CAUSED by a first condition. Let's use diabetes mellitus as an example. Diabetes is known to cause problems with patients' eyes. The physician determined that the patient has diabetic retinopathy with macular edema. This documentation confirms that diabetes CAUSED the retinopathy to develop. You often will find combination codes in ICD-10-CM. These codes report both the underlying condition and the manifestation. In our example, the combination code is

E11.3513   Type 2 diabetes mellitus with proliferative diabetic retinopathy with macular edema, bilateral

This one code, E11.3513, tells the whole story about this patient's condition. However, not all conditions and their manifestations have combination codes from which to choose. When an appropriate combination code is not available, you will need to select two codes (or more) to clearly communicate the complete story of a patient's diagnosis. One example is a patient who is admitted to the hospital with pulmonary histoplasmosis, a documented manifestation of the patient's HIV-positive status. In this case, there is no combination code, so two codes are needed to tell the whole story of this patient's condition.

B20   Human immunodeficiency virus [HIV] disease

B39.0   Acute pulmonary histoplasmosis capsulati

Co-morbidities

A **co-morbidity** is a condition that is present in the same body at the same time as another problem or disease, but the two conditions are unrelated—there is no documented cause-and-effect relationship. These "other diagnoses" may be referred to in the physician's documentation. However, only those conditions that the physician has specifically evaluated, treated, or ordered additional testing for or those requiring additional monitoring, nursing care, or more time in the hospital should be reported with a code.

Co-morbidity
A separate diagnosis existing in the same patient at the same time as an unrelated diagnosis.

EXAMPLE

Lindsey, 28-weeks pregnant, fell and broke her leg. So, the pregnancy and the fracture are co-morbidities—they are two conditions present in the same patient at the same time. You know that being pregnant does not cause a fracture and a fracture does not cause pregnancy.

Which code will you report first? The code that is the reason for the encounter with the physician. You are coding for Dr. Kessler, an orthopedist, and Lindsey comes in because her leg hurts. Dr. Kessler confirms her leg is fractured, so the fracture will be reported first because this is Dr. Kessler's primary concern—caring for the fracture. However, Dr. Kessler MUST take the pregnancy into consideration because pregnancy is a systemic condition and will impact the treatment plan for the fracture. The pregnancy code also will be reported (after the fracture code).

EXAMPLE

Mary-Ellen's history includes asthma. She is here to see the dermatologist to have a benign mole removed from her arm. Dr. Callen does not ask about Mary-Ellen's asthma. The asthma does not have any relationship at all to the benign mole or the care/treatment of the mole. You will only determine the correct diagnosis code for the benign mole. The asthma will NOT be reported at all.

EXAMPLE

Paul's history includes asthma. He is here to see Dr. Hannah, his family physician, for his annual checkup. Dr. Hannah asks Paul about his asthma and writes a prescription for a refill for his inhaler. In addition to the annual exam code, you also will need to report the code for the asthma because the physician paid attention to it during this encounter.

Sequelae

Sequela

A cause-and-effect relationship between an original condition that has been resolved with a current condition; also known as a late effect.

A **sequela** is the residual impact of a previous condition or injury that may need the attention of a physician. When the patient has come to see the health care professional for the treatment of a sequela (also known as a late effect), you must code the particular problem as a sequela only in the following situations:

- Scarring.
- Nonunion of a fracture.
- Malunion of a fracture.
- When the connection is specifically documented by the physician or health care professional confirming the new condition as a sequela (a late effect) of a previous condition.

Coding a sequela requires at least two codes, in the following order:

1. The sequela condition, which is the condition that resulted and is being treated, such as a scar or paralysis.
2. The sequela (late effect) or original-condition code with the seventh character "S."

CODING BITES

You will learn a lot more about reporting co-morbidities, manifestations, and sequelae in *Part II: Reporting Diagnoses.*

EXAMPLE

Jenna Malaletto, an 18-year-old female, was using a hydrofluoric acid mixture to etch glass for an art class last spring and got some on her left forearm, causing a corrosion burn of the third degree. She came in today to see Dr. Rosen to discuss treatment options for the adherent scarring.

Dr. Rosen is discussing treatment options of the scars that were left behind after the third-degree corrosion burn had healed. This is known as a sequela, and it is the reason for this encounter. However, as you learned, you also will need to report what caused the scar—the corrosion burn.

L90.5 Scar conditions and fibrosis of skin (adherent scar)
T22.712S Corrosion of third degree of left forearm, sequela

2.5 Reporting External Causes

You learned in the *Introduction to the Languages of Coding* chapter that in addition to the *why* and the *what,* if a patient is injured, you will need to abstract details about *how* and *where* the patient became injured. As you learn more about determining external cause codes, you will discover that a simple statement such as "the patient was hurt in a car accident" does not contain enough information to determine the accurate external cause code. The details of the accident are very important. For example:

- Was the patient the driver, a passenger, or outside of the vehicle?
- Was the vehicle a car, a pick-up truck, a van, or a heavy transport vehicle?
- Did the vehicle collide with another vehicle, a nonmotor vehicle, or a stationary object?
- Was this a traffic accident or a nontraffic accident?

LET'S CODE IT! SCENARIO

Victor Lamza, a 13-year-old male, was brought into the Emergency Department complaining of pain after he banged his head. Dr. Farxia diagnosed him with a contusion of the scalp. When asked by Dr. Farxia what he was doing immediately before he got hurt, he reluctantly admitted that he had made a bet with his friends at Space Camp. They wanted to see who could stay the longest in the weightlessness simulator; Victor was in there for 6 hours.

Let's Code It!

Dr. Farxia documented that Victor's staying too long in the weightlessness simulator caused the contusion of his scalp. You will need to code why Dr. Farxia cared for Victor (his injury), how he became injured, and where he was when the injury occurred.

S00.03XA	**Contusion of scalp, initial encounter**
X52.XXXA	**Prolonged stay in weightless environment, initial encounter**
Y92.838	**Other recreation area as the place of occurrence of the external cause**
Y93.89	**Activity, other specified**
Y99.8	**Other external cause status (recreation or sport not for income or while a student)**

There are thousands of different ways a patient can become injured, and there is a different code for almost every incident: the typical, the silly, the unusual, and the surprising.

ICD-10-CM provides a separate *Index to External Causes,* usually found between the Index to Diseases and Injuries (Alphabetic Index) and the beginning of the Tabular List. This index will point you to the correct subsection in the Tabular List, within the code range of V00–Y99.

You will learn more details about how to code external causes later in this textbook in the chapter *Coding Injury, Poisoning, and External Causes.*

2.6 Deconstructing Procedural Statements

In addition to abstracting the terms from the documentation related to the diagnosis code or codes, you also will need to identify those terms that relate to what was done for the patient.

Due to the structure of medical terminology, you might find that the word or term mentioned in the documentation describing what was done for the patient is a combination term identifying both the action taken and the anatomical site on which the action was performed.

EXAMPLES

i. Neuroplasty: *neuro* = nerves + *-plasty* = repair

ii. Thrombolysis: *thrombo* = blood clot + *-lysis* = dissolving

iii. Gastrectomy: *gastr* = stomach + *-ectomy* = surgical removal

Other times, the procedure will be identified by its name. This name may be

- a description of the action, such as ablation, debridement, or injection.

- an eponym (named after the individual who invented it), such as Abbe-Estlander procedure, Swan-Ganz catheter, or Dupuy-Dutemps operation.

- an abbreviation or acronym, such as ECG = electrocardiography; GTT = glucose tolerance test; PET = positron emission tomography; TAVR = transcatheter aortic valve replacement.

CODING BITES

Only the procedures, services, and treatments actually provided during a specific encounter, by a specific physician, health care professional, or facility, will be coded.

Review and practice your medical terminology and keep a medical dictionary close at hand. As you gain more experience, the process of deconstructing the statements in the various types of documentation will become easier (not really easy, but easier). You learned about the part of this career that involves interpreting and you cannot interpret the words if you don't know what they mean.

Interpreting for Each Code Set

You will find that you not only need to understand medical terminology overall to interpret the physician's documentation into codes; each code set may require you to interpret them differently.

 LET'S CODE IT! SCENARIO

McGRAW GENERAL HOSPITAL

DATE OF PROCEDURE: 08/18/2019

PATIENT: Christine Gordon

PREOPERATIVE DIAGNOSIS: Acute right lower abdominal pain.

POSTOPERATIVE DIAGNOSIS: Acute appendicitis.

OPERATION PERFORMED: Laparoscopic appendectomy.

SURGEON: Charles E. Manchester, MD

SEDATION: General endotracheal anesthetic.

PROCEDURE:

This 47-year-old female presented with signs and symptoms consistent with acute appendicitis. Preoperative CT scan indicates an inflamed appendix, rupture not probable. Patient signed written consent for a laparoscopic appendectomy.

Let's Code It!

The documentation created by Dr. Manchester clearly provides us with the details of what occurred during this encounter with this patient, Christine Gordon. She was having lower right side abdominal pain, which was determined to be appendicitis (*why* reported with ICD-10-CM code K35.80 Acute Appendicitis Not Otherwise Specified) and the doctor performed a surgical laparoscopic appendectomy (*what*). Seems very straightforward, doesn't it?

A good place to begin is the CPT Alphabetic Index; look up:

Appendectomy

Appendix Excision. 44950, 44955, 44960

Laparoscopic 44970

Turn to the Main Section of CPT to find code 44970 because Dr. Manchester specifically documented that the appendectomy was done laparoscopically. So, now you have found the correct code to report for Dr. Manchester's work:

44970   Laparoscopy, surgical, appendectomy

--*

Now, if you were the coder for the hospital at which the surgery occurred, you would need to report this same procedure using the ICD-10-PCS code set.

Dr. Manchester performed this surgical procedure on Christine Gordon in the hospital. The hospital provided the support staff (nurses, technicians, etc.), as well as the equipment, the room, etc. You learned earlier that the hospital's coder would use ICD-10-PCS codes to report their participation and care for this patient. Let's look at the documentation again . . .

"the doctor performed a surgical laparoscopic appendectomy"

In the ICD-10-PCS code book's Alphabetic Index, you will see:

Appendectomy

see Excision, Appendix 0DBJ

see Resection, Appendix 0DTJ

Which is correct? The ICD-10-PCS code book includes the definitions right in the front of the code book:

Excision: Cutting out or off, without replacement, a portion of a body part

Resection: Cutting out or off, without replacement, all of a body part

You learned in medical terminology class that appendectomy = surgical removal of the appendix. Therefore, you have documentation that the entire appendix was surgically removed, and this is called "*Resection*" by ICD-10-PCS. Terrific! Now we will turn to the 0DT Table in ICD-10-PCS.

First character: Section: **Medical and Surgical 0**

This is correct because this was a surgical procedure.

Second character: System: **Gastrointestinal System D**

You know this is correct because you learned in anatomy class that the appendix is part of the gastrointestinal system.

Third character: Root Operation: **Resection T**

You confirmed this by reading the root operation term definition for "resection" and comparing it with the physician's documentation.

Fourth character: Body Part: **Appendix J**

The documentation clearly states the appendix is the body part that was removed.

Fifth character: Approach: **Percutaneous Endoscopic 4**

The documentation states that this procedure was performed laparoscopically. A laparoscope is an endoscope passed through the skin of the abdomen using small slits (percutaneously). Therefore, you know that this procedure was done using a percutaneous endoscopic approach.

Sixth character: Device: **None Z**

Seventh character: Qualifier: **None Z**

Great! So, if you were the coder for the hospital where Dr. Manchester performed surgery, you would report ICD-10-PCS code

0DTJ4ZZ Resection of the appendix, via percutaneous endoscope

Good work!

You can see how the two procedure code sets, CPT and ICD-10-PCS, use different terms to describe and report the same procedure. Use your resources, like a medical dictionary, and you will be able to interpret all of the terms correctly.

2.7 How to Query

Query
To ask.

Once you have completed abstracting the documentation, you may find that details needed to determine a specific code are not included. Should this happen, you should **query** the physician who wrote the documentation to ask him or her to provide clarification or additional specifics. Every day, coders and health information management specialists find documentation with information that is

- Missing or incomplete
  - for example, *What specific type of fracture?*
- Ambiguous or inconsistent
  - for example, *Procedure notes state a single lead pacemaker was inserted; however, the equipment list states the pacemaker was dual lead.*
- Contradictory
  - for example, *In first paragraph, notes state, "Patient denies any cough or chest congestion."; however, last paragraph states patient was prescribed Tessalon (a cough suppressant).*

In Section 2.2, *The Process of Abstracting,* you learned the difference between assuming and interpreting. Therefore, you will need to ask the physician to add the details you need to the patient's record so you can move forward and determine the correct code. This process is known as creating a query, and it must be done in a very specific manner so as not to break the law.

Writing the Query

Remember that one important use of codes is to determine reimbursement. Different codes are paid at different amounts. [You will learn more about this in the *Reimbursement* chapter.] When writing a query, the law does not permit you to prompt or promote a specific response so you don't inadvertently influence the physician to opt for the higher-paying detail rather than the truth. This means you must ask for the details in a nonleading manner. Asking open-ended questions and providing multiple options for the answer are the best approaches.

EXAMPLES

Dr. Osage saw Jose Ramirez and documented him to have a displaced fracture of the metatarsal bone of the right foot.

After rereading the operative notes again, and reviewing the entire patient record, you discover that the detail of which specific bone was fractured is missing. Therefore, you need to query Dr. Osage.

Open-ended query:

Which metatarsal bone was fractured?

Multiple-choice query:

Which metatarsal bone was fractured?

A. First
B. Second
C. Third
D. Fourth
E. Fifth

*_*_*

Dr. Stabler performed a total hysterectomy on Melinda Blaudon.

After rereading the operative notes again, and reviewing the entire patient record, you discover that the detail of which approach was used to perform the hysterectomy is missing. Therefore, you need to query Dr. Stabler.

Open-ended query:

What approach was used in the surgery?

Multiple-choice query:

What approach was used in the surgery?

A. Open
B. Percutaneous endoscopic [Laparoscopic]
C. Via natural orifice

The query you write to request the specific details needed should be accompanied by the pertinent clinical information from the patient's chart. You want to make it clear to the physician what you need clarified or supported with more details. There are many query templates available and often larger organizations have their own versions, already approved by attorneys.

Query Pathways

The specific details will need to be added to the chart in a time-efficient manner; therefore, the way you deliver the query to the physician is important. Most facilities have an existing process for delivering a query to the attending physician. Certainly, in a physician's office or small clinic, it may be easier than in a hospital to connect with the physician to ask a question or questions and obtain a response or responses.

Some electronic health record software programs include a query feature. Alternatively, using a secure, encrypted e-mail system can provide a swift route for asking for the details required as well as a written response. Remember our creed: "*If it's not documented, it didn't happen. If it didn't happen, you cannot code it!*" This reinforces the importance of obtaining those additional specifics in writing from the physician.

For those facilities still using paper patient records, query notes should be attached to the front of charts, so all relevant information about that patient, for that encounter, is at hand and easy for the physician to reference and annotate.

Chapter Summary

In preparation for you to learn the process of determining the specific code or codes, you must be able to gather the required information from the clinical documentation. You must read through the clinical documentation in the patient's record and understand everything you read so you can collect the specifics you need. If details are missing, ambiguous, or conflicting, you will need to query the physician to have the documentation amended. This is your responsibility and a critical part of the coding process.

CHAPTER 2 REVIEW
Abstracting Clinical Documentation

Enhance your learning by completing these exercises and more at mcgrawhillconnect.com!

Let's Check It! Terminology

Match each key term to the appropriate definition.

1. LO 2.2 Suppose to be the case, without proof; guess the intended details.
2. LO 2.3 A patient's subjective description of feeling.
3. LO 2.7 To ask; an official request to the attending physician for more specific information related to a patient's condition or treatment.
4. LO 2.3 Measurable indicators of a patient's health status.
5. LO 2.2 The patient's name, address, date of birth, and other personal details, not specifically related to health.
6. LO 2.2 Explain the meaning of; convert a meaning from one language to another.
7. LO 2.4 A cause-and-effect relationship between an original condition that has been resolved with a current condition; also known as a late effect.
8. LO 2.4 A condition that develops as the result of another, underlying condition.
9. LO 2.2 Identifying the key words or terms needed to determine the accurate code.
10. LO 2.4 A separate condition or illness present in the same patient at the same time as another, unrelated condition or illness.

A. Abstracting
B. Assume
C. Co-morbidity
D. Demographic
E. Interpret
F. Manifestation
G. Query
H. Sequela
I. Signs
J. Symptoms

Let's Check It! Concepts

Choose the most appropriate answer for each of the following questions.

1. LO 2.1 The first question you, as the professional coder, will need to ask is
   a. does the patient have health insurance?
   b. is there a preexisting condition?
   c. for whom are you reporting?
   d. is this encounter to treat a sequela?

2. LO 2.1 The _____ will have a coder to report for any imaging procedures.
   a. anesthesiologist
   b. radiologist
   c. cardiologist
   d. pathologist

3. LO 2.1 Which of the following is an acute care facility?
   a. The physician's office
   b. A nursing facility
   c. A hospital
   d. An assisted-living facility

4. LO 2.2 Converting a meaning from one language to another is called
   a. assuming.
   b. interpreting.
   c. querying.
   d. supposing.

5. LO 2.2 The most important source for details required for the coding specialist to determine the most accurate code or codes is found in which part of the patient's record?
   a. Patient's Registration Form
   b. Referral Authorization Form
   c. Physician's Notes/Operative Reports
   d. Imaging Reports

6. LO 2.2 What is the best way to begin abstracting clinical documentation?
   a. Listen to the nurse explain the encounter.
   b. Read all the way through the clinical documentation for the specific encounter.

c. Talk to the technician.

d. Read the patient's registration form.

7. **LO 2.2** Every patient encounter must have at least _____ reportable [codeable] reason(s) *why* and at least _____ reportable [codeable] explanation(s) of *what*.

    a. 1, 1   **b.** 2, 1   **c.** 1, 2   **d.** 3, 1

8. **LO 2.3** All of the following would be considered a diagnostic "main term" except

    a. herpes.   **b.** acute.   **c.** spasm.   **d.** infarction.

9. **LO 2.3** The patient has been diagnosed with hypersecretion of thyroid stimulating hormone. Identify the condition.

    a. hormone   **b.** thyroid   **c.** stimulating   **d.** hypersecretion

10. **LO 2.3** Which official guideline is concerned with conditions that are an integral part of a disease process?

    a. Section I.B.4   **b.** Section I.B.5   **c.** Section I.B.6   **d.** Section I.B.7

11. **LO 2.4** A manifestation is a _____ condition caused by the _____ condition.

    a. first, second   **b.** third, fourth   **c.** second, first   **d.** second, third

12. **LO 2.4** Coding a sequela requires at least _____ code(s).

    a. 1   **b.** 2   **c.** 3   **d.** 4

13. **LO 2.5** External causes explain _____ and _____ the patient became injured.

    a. why, what   **b.** what, where   **c.** how, where   **d.** why, how

14. **LO 2.5** Which of the following would be an example of an external causes code?

    a. H26.053   **b.** M62.831   **c.** S00.03A   **d.** Y92.838

15. **LO 2.6** The suffix *-plasty* means

    a. to dissolve.   **b.** to repair.   **c.** to crush.   **d.** to remove.

16. **LO 2.6** The abbreviation *ECG* stands for

    a. electrocardiography.   **b.** electroencephalography.

    c. electroconvulsive therapy.   **d.** electrocautery.

17. **LO 2.7** When you find missing or incomplete information in the physician's notes, you should

    a. place the file at the bottom of the pile.

    b. figure out the information yourself; you should know what the doctor is thinking.

    c. ask a coworker.

    d. query the physician.

18. **LO 2.7** Before using an unspecified or NOS (not otherwise specified) code(s), you should

    a. code the case as unspecified and move to the next file.

    b. assume what the missing information is.

    c. query the physician to gain the details needed to use a more specific code.

    d. leave it for your coworker to do.

19. **LO 2.3** Tom is diagnosed with herpes zoster, conjunctivitis. Which ICD-10-CM diagnosis code would you assign?

    a. B02.9   **b.** B02.31   **c.** B02.0   **d.** B02.1

20. **LO 2.6** Judith presents for a unilateral mammography. Which procedural (CPT) code would you assign?

    a. 77053   **b.** 77054   **c.** 77065   **d.** 77066

Let's Check It! A Diagnosis or Procedure

First, identify the following statements as a diagnosis or a procedure, and then identify the main term.

Example: Factitial dermatosis:

    a. diagnosis or procedure: <u>diagnosis</u> *b.* main term: <u>dermatosis</u>

1. LO 2.3 Sprained wrist, left, initial encounter:

    a. diagnosis or procedure: _____ **b.** main term: _____

2. LO 2.6 Tympanic neurectomy:

    a. diagnosis or procedure: _____ **b.** main term: _____

3. LO 2.3 Acute bronchitis:

    a. diagnosis or procedure: _____ **b.** main term: _____

4. LO 2.6 Cerebral thrombolysis:

    a. diagnosis or procedure: _____ **b.** main term: _____

5. LO 2.3 Newborn circulatory failure:

    a. diagnosis or procedure: _____ **b.** main term: _____

6. LO 2.6 Laryngeal web laryngoplasty:

    a. diagnosis or procedure: _____ **b.** main term: _____

7. LO 2.3 Cutaneous abscess of chest wall, initial encounter:

    a. diagnosis or procedure: _____ **b.** main term: _____

8. LO 2.6 Planned tracheostomy:

    a. diagnosis or procedure: _____ **b.** main term: _____

9. LO 2.3 Stenosis of the esophagus:

    a. diagnosis or procedure: _____ **b.** main term: _____

10. LO 2.6 Ulna osteomyelitis:

    a. diagnosis or procedure: _____ **b.** main term: _____

Let's Check It! Rules and Regulations

Please answer the following questions from the knowledge you have gained after reading this chapter.

1. LO 2.2 What is the professional coding specialists' motto?

2. LO 2.2 Explain the difference between assuming and interpreting.

3. LO 2.3 Explain the ICD-10-CM Official Guidelines concerning Signs and Symptoms—Section I.B.4; include where the guideline directs you.

4. LO 2.4 Discuss the ICD-10-CM Official Guidelines concerning Sequela—Section I.B.10; include where the guideline directs you.

5. LO 2.4 Discuss co-morbidity and the correct coding sequence for the encounter.

Design elements: ©McGraw-Hill

The Coding Process

Key Terms

Alphabetic Index
Alphanumeric
Alphanumeric Section
Coding Process
Linking
Main Section
Notations
Official Guidelines
Symbols
Tables
Tabular List

3.1 The Coding Process Overview

There are six specific actions that you should take as part of the **coding process**. As you gain experience, it will take you less time to go through these tasks. However, remember that time is not the number one consideration when coding—no matter what anyone says, accuracy is the most important factor. Following all of these actions every time you code will support your development of habits that will maintain accuracy throughout your career.

Action 1. Abstract the documentation

- Read completely through the documentation for the encounter, from beginning to end.
- Then, reread the documentation and identify the main words regarding the diagnoses (*why*) and procedures (*what*) of the encounter.
- Remember, if the patient was injured, you will need to identify the external causes (*how* and *where*) as well.

Action 2. Query, if necessary

- Make a list of any questions you have regarding unclear or missing information necessary to code the encounter. Query the health care provider who cared for the patient. Never assume or guess. You are only allowed to code what you know from actual documentation. *If it is not documented, it did not happen. If it didn't happen, you cannot code it!*
- Create a query using nonleading questions, with open-ended or multiple-option formatting, to have the physician amend the documentation, so you can use those added details to determine the accurate code or codes. *NOTE:* In school, your queries should go to your instructor.

Action 3. Code the diagnosis or diagnoses

- Code each diagnosis and/or appropriate signs or symptoms describing *why* the health care provider treated this patient during this encounter, as documented in the notes, to tell the whole story. Use the best, most accurate code or codes available based on that documentation.

Coding Process
The sequence of actions required to interpret physician documentation into the codes that accurately report what occurred during a specific encounter between health care professional and patient.

- Read the symbols and notations around the code in the Tabular List.
- Go to the Official Guidelines to review any coding rules with which you must comply.

NOTE: Part II: Reporting Diagnoses of this textbook *will share with you everything you need to know to determine the accurate diagnosis code or codes.*

Action 4. Code the procedure or procedures

- Determine for whom you are reporting: physician, outpatient facility, or inpatient facility. This way, you will know which code set to use: CPT or ICD-10-PCS.
- Code each procedure, service, or treatment, as stated in the notes, describing what the provider did for the patient during this encounter. You should not code any procedures that are simply recommended, suggested, or ordered; you can only code those that have already been provided to the patient during the encounter for which you are reporting. Use the best, most accurate codes available based on the documentation.
- Read the symbols and notations around the code in the Main Section. Check for guidelines (in front of this section as well as in the subsection) to review any coding rules with which you must comply.
- In some cases, you will also need to report a code or codes using the HCPCS Level II code set. You will learn more about this code set in *Part IV: DMEPOS & Transportation.*

NOTE: Part III: Reporting Physician Services and Outpatient Procedures of this textbook *will share with you everything you need to know to determine the accurate procedure code or codes. This chapter is just an introduction.*

Action 5. Confirm medical necessity

- Ensure that each and every procedure code is supported by at least one diagnosis code to verify medical necessity.

Action 6. Double-check your codes

You, as the professional coding specialist, have a responsibility to ensure that you are submitting only accurate, truthful information, supported by the physician's documentation. Yet, we are all human and anyone can make a mistake. *Now* is the time to build the habit of double-checking your work before you hit that submit button.

- Go back into the code books you have used and reread the full descriptions, all notations, and symbols for the codes you have assigned. Compare these details, once more, with the original documentation—just to be certain you did not misread anything.
- Read carefully, one letter at a time, one number at a time, so you can catch and correct any typos before your work becomes official.

Taking action to code precisely will result in a greater number of your claims getting paid quickly, and your reports will represent accurate data. You owe this to your facility, your patients, and yourself.

3.2 The Alphabetic Indexes

Alphabetic Index
The section of a code book showing all codes, from A to Z, by the short code descriptions.

Once you have abstracted the main terms that describe the diagnosis (*why*) and the procedure (*what*) from within the physician documentation or operative reports, the next action is to determine the codes that accurately report these details. You will begin by matching those main terms to an entry in the appropriate code book's **Alphabetic Index**.

In the *Introduction to the Languages of Coding* chapter, you learned to connect the details you abstracted from the medical documentation to the correct code set:

Diagnoses (*why*) = ICD-10-CM code set

Physician services (*what*) = CPT code set

Outpatient facility services (*what*) = CPT code set

Inpatient (hospital) facility services (*what*) = ICD-10-PCS code set

Transportation, equipment, drugs (*what*) = HCPCS Level II code set

Each of these code set books includes a section, or part, that is called the Alphabetic Index. Each Alphabetic Index lists all of the main terms that are represented by codes within its set, in alphabetic order (A to Z). So . . .

In ICD-10-CM's Alphabetic Index, you will see terms such as:

Abscess

Carcinoma

Hyperemia

Pneumonia

Shock

Ulcer

In CPT's Alphabetic Index, you will see terms such as:

Angioplasty

Bypass

Discography

Insertion

Psychotherapy

Reconstruction

In ICD-10-PCS's Alphabetic Index, you will see terms such as:

Cannulation

Detachment

Extraction

Laryngoplasty

Repair

Supplement

In HCPCS Level II's Alphabetic Index, you will see terms such as:

Commode

IPPB machine

Nebulizer

Wheelchair

Once you find the main term that matches the word or words that you abstracted from the medical documentation, you may find an indented list containing adjectives providing more detail about that specific main term. It may be an additional description, such as chronic or laparoscopic, or it may be the anatomical site that was involved.

EXAMPLES
ICD-10-CM: ABDOMINAL ABSCESS
   Abscess
      Abdominal

(continued)

Often, you will find that further details will be necessary, and options will be provided in another list, indented from the previous indented list.

EXAMPLES

ICD-10-CM: ABSCESS IN THE WALL OF THE ABDOMINAL CAVITY
Abscess
   Abdominal
      Cavity
      Wall

CPT: PERCUTANEOUS INSERTION OF GASTROSTOMY TUBE
Insertion
   Gastrostomy Tube
      Laparoscopic
      Percutaneous

ICD-10-PCS: REPAIR OF THE RIGHT MANDIBLE
Repair
   Mandible
      Left
      Right

HCPCS LEVEL II: NON-DISPOSABLE NEBULIZER FILTER
Nebulizer
   Filter
      Disposable
      Non-disposable

You are required to keep making choices, matching the documentation, all the way to the most specific detail. Once at the most specific level, you will see that the Alphabetic Index will suggest a code or codes.

EXAMPLES

ICD-10-CM: ABSCESS IN THE WALL OF THE ABDOMINAL CAVITY
Abscess
   Abdominal
      Cavity K65.1
      Wall L02.211

CPT: PERCUTANEOUS INSERTION OF GASTROSTOMY TUBE
Insertion
   Gastrostomy Tube

(continued)

```
        Laparoscopic 43653
        Percutaneous 43246

ICD-10-PCS: REPAIR OF THE RIGHT MANDIBLE
    Repair
        Mandible
            Left 0NQV
            Right 0NQT

HCPCS LEVEL II: NON-DISPOSABLE NEBULIZER FILTER
    Nebulizer
        Filter
            Disposable A7013
            Non-disposable A7014
```

You are not done with the coding process yet. These codes will guide you to find the suggested code in the Main Section, Tabular List, or Tables of that code book. You are not permitted, by law, to report a code from the Alphabetic Index without first confirming that it is the best possible option in the Tabular List, Main Section, or Tables.

3.3 The Tabular List, Main Section, Tables, and Alphanumeric Section

Think of the Alphabetic Index as a very cheap GPS mapping app. You cannot count on it to give you accurate information because it is not designed to get you to your precise destination. Sometimes, yes, it will get you to the correct front door. Sometimes, however, it will mistakenly take you to the house down the block, and you will have to look at all of the houses and all of the addresses in the area to see which one is correct. You begin with a suggested code from the Alphabetic Index to get you to the correct neighborhood. However, you cannot report this code until you have confirmed it is correct and complete, using the ICD-10-CM's **Tabular List**, CPT's **Main Section**, ICD-10-PCS's **Tables** section, or HCPCS Level II's **Alphanumeric Section** of the appropriate code book.

These sections list all of the codes available in that code set, only this time, they are listed in numeric or **alphanumeric** order by the code first, followed by the words describing exactly what that code represents. Here, you will find several things to help you get to absolute accuracy.

Full Code Descriptions

In these sections, you will be able to read the full code description, not the shortened version used in the Alphabetic Index. Let's continue with our examples from the previous section, Section 3.2, *The Alphabetic Indexes:*

EXAMPLES
ICD-10-CM
The Alphabetic Index gave you:

    Abscess, Abdominal, Cavity K65.1
    Abscess, Abdominal, Wall L02.211

The Tabular List gives you:

        K65.1 Peritoneal abscess (mesenteric abscess)
        L02.211 Cutaneous abscess of abdominal wall

(continued)

Symbols
Marks, similar to emojis, that provide additional direction to use codes correctly and accurately.

Notations
Alerts and warnings that support more accurate use of codes in a specific code set.

Tabular List
The section of the ICD-10-CM code book listing all of the codes in alphanumeric order.

Main Section
The section of the CPT code book listing all of the codes in numeric order.

Tables
The section of the ICD-10-PCS code book listing all of the codes in alphanumeric order, based on the first three characters of the code.

Alphanumeric Section
The section of the HCPCS Level II code book listing all of the codes in alphanumeric order.

Alphanumeric
Containing both letters and numbers.

CPT

The Alphabetic Index gave you:

Insertion, Gastrostomy Tube, Laparoscopic 43653
Insertion, Gastrostomy Tube, Percutaneous 43246

In the Main Section, you will read:

43653 Laparoscopy, surgical; gastrostomy, without construction of gastric tube (e.g., Stamm procedure)
43246 Esophagogastroduodenoscopy, flexible, transoral; with directed placement of percutaneous gastrostomy tube

ICD-10-PCS

The Alphabetic Index gave you:

Repair, Mandible, Left 0NQV
Repair, Mandible, Right 0NQT

In the Tables Section, you must build the code out to seven (7) characters based on the additional details in the operative notes:

0NQV0ZZ Repair of mandible, left side, open approach
0NQTXZZ Repair of mandible, right, external approach

HCPCS LEVEL II

The Alphabetic Index gave you:

Nebulizer, Filter, Disposable A7013
Nebulizer, Filter, Non-disposable A7014

In the Alphanumeric List, you will read:

A7013 Filter, disposable, used with aerosol compressor or ultrasonic generator
A7014 Filter, non-disposable, used with aerosol compressor or ultrasonic generator

Look at all the additional details provided in the complete code descriptions. As you can see with just our few examples, there are specifics that may require you to go back to the documentation to confirm these additional details are still accurate. While you are here, you also need to read the complete code descriptions for all of the other codes in this code category. It is not uncommon that you may find another code that is a better match for the documentation.

Conventions (Notations and Symbols)

In addition to full code descriptions, you also will find conventions (notations and symbols) in the Tabular List (ICD-10-CM) and Main Section (CPT) that include tips and hints pointing you toward the correct code. This section is a preview of more in-depth discussions about symbols that will come in future chapters. So, for now, just a little glance.

ICD-10-CM

In the Tabular List above K65.1 is a notation that states:

Use additional code **to identify infectious agent**
K65.1 Peritoneal abscess (mesenteric abscess)

A "*Use additional code*" notation reminds you that you will need to include a second code reporting the detail identified in the notation. This notation helps you ensure you are reporting complete information about a patient's diagnosis that will support medical necessity for the appropriate treatment.

CPT

In the Main Section to the left of code 97803 is a star symbol:

★ 97803   Medical nutrition therapy; re-assessment and intervention, individual, face-to-face with the patient, each 15 minutes

Both at the bottom of the page in CPT and in the "Introduction" in the front of the CPT code book, you can see that this symbol ★ informs you, the coder, that if this service was provided using audio/video synchronous equipment (i.e., Skype, FaceTime), you will need to append modifier 95 to this code. This small symbol helps you avoid committing fraud.

ICD-10-PCS

The majority of the codes suggested in the Alphabetic Index of ICD-10-PCS are not complete codes. This fact will not let you forget that you have to go into the Tables section to build the code out to seven (7) characters (based on the additional details in the operative notes). To report a complete, valid code, you must go into the Tables section.

0NQV0ZZ Repair of mandible, left side, open approach
0NQRXZZ Repair of maxilla, external approach

NOTE: Even in those occasions when the Alphabetic Index provides you with all seven characters for the code, you still should go to the appropriate Table to confirm. It will only take a few seconds, and you can be certain you are reporting the complete and accurate code.

HCPCS LEVEL II

In the Alphanumeric Section, to the left of code J8705 is a symbol:

☑   J8705 Topotecan, oral, 0.25mg

The symbol ☑, in some versions of the HCPCS Level II book, alerts you that this code description includes a specific quantity. When seeing this, you should confirm the quantity documented with the quantity in the code description. The code may need to be reported multiple times.

3.4 The Official Guidelines

With all these code sets and all these codes, you can see that the process to get from documentation to code is more complicated than simply finding a word here and a code there. Coding is important work, so you want to get it accurate every time. To accomplish this, it is essential to have help and support exactly when you need it. And you have that help right at your fingertips within each code set's book. Always there, just the turn of a few pages, is the guidance from those who created these code sets and who oversee their legal and correct use. These are the published **Official Guidelines** with which you must comply. You don't need to memorize them; you just need to remember they are there and refer to them every time you are working to determine a code.

ICD-10-CM

Usually in the front of this code book, you will find the section titled "*ICD-10-CM Official Guidelines for Coding and Reporting.*"

CPT

In the front of each individual main section, you will find the guidelines applicable to that part of the CPT codes. So, in front of the *Evaluation and Management (E/M)*

CODING BITES

You will learn more about ICD-10-CM conventions, notations, and symbols in the chapter titled *Introduction to ICD-10-CM.*

CODING BITES

You will learn more about CPT conventions, notations, and symbols in the chapter titled *Introduction to CPT.*

CODING BITES

You will learn more about ICD-10-PCS conventions in the chapter titled *Introduction to ICD-10-PCS.*

CODING BITES

You will learn more about HCPCS Level II conventions, notations, and symbols in the chapter titled *HCPCS Level II.*

Official Guidelines
A listing of rules and regulations instructing how to use a specific code set accurately.

Services codes are the pages containing the ***Evaluation and Management (E/M) Services Guidelines;*** in front of the *Anesthesia* code section are the ***Anesthesia Guidelines;*** etc.

In addition, it is important to note that the CPT book also includes official guidelines within the sections, at some subsections, with advice and direction for accurate coding of just those procedures, services, and treatments. This means you must get in the habit of reading from the beginning of each section *and* the beginning of the subsection before determining a code. It only takes a few seconds, and it can make the difference between accuracy and fraudulent reporting.

ICD-10-PCS

Usually in the front of this code book, you will find the section titled "***ICD-10-PCS Official Guidelines for Coding and Reporting.***"

Guidance Connection

Throughout this book, you will see special boxes titled **GUIDANCE CONNECTION** that will point you to a specific guideline in that particular code set directly related to whatever concept or aspect is being discussed. Take a minute and turn to that guideline in your personal code book and read it, think about it, and identify how you would apply this guideline to your work as a professional coding specialist. There is no need to memorize these details because they will always be there for you, right inside your code book, at your fingertips.

 LET'S CODE IT! SCENARIO

DATE OF PROCEDURE: 08/18/2019

PATIENT: ARTHUR FERGUSON

PREOPERATIVE DIAGNOSIS: Acute upper abdominal pain

POSTOPERATIVE DIAGNOSIS: Liver tumor

OPERATION PERFORMED: Diagnostic laparoscopy; Laparoscopic ablation, using radiofrequency

SURGEON: Harrison Brusk, MD

SEDATION: General endotracheal anesthetic

ESTIMATED BLOOD LOSS: Minimal.

COMPLICATIONS: None.

INDICATIONS FOR PROCEDURE:
This 57-year-old male presented with signs and symptoms consistent with liver malfunction. Laparoscopic investigation to confirm suspected liver tumor, and if so, ablation. The informed consent form was signed.

DESCRIPTION OF OPERATION:
The patient was brought to the operating room and placed in a supine position on the operating table. After administration of general anesthetic, I prepped and draped the upper abdomen in the usual sterile fashion.

A small incision was made into the umbilicus through which a bladeless 11 mm trocar was inserted without difficulty. After the pneumo-peritoneum was established, the patient was moved into the Trendelenburg position. Two additional 5 mm trocar insertions were made. The liver was visualized and two tumors were identified, one on the distal portion of the liver and one on the proximal surface. The diagnostic laparoscopy was then converted to a surgical procedure so we could remove the tumors. Using radiofrequency techniques, both tumors were successfully ablated.

(continued)

The documentation created by Dr. Brusk clearly provides us with the details of what occurred during this encounter with this patient, Arthur Ferguson. He was having upper abdominal pain that was determined to be two liver tumors (*why* reported with ICD-10-CM code *D13.4 Benign neoplasm of liver*) and the doctor performed a diagnostic laparoscopy, followed by a surgical laparoscopic ablation of liver tumors (*what*). Seems very straightforward, doesn't it?

A good place to begin: in the CPT Alphabetic Index, look up:

Ablation

Liver (Tumor)

Cryosurgical 47381, 47383

Laparoscopic 47370, 47371

Radiofrequency 47380-47382

Turn to the Main Section of CPT to find code 47370 because Dr. Brusk specifically documented that the ablation was done laparoscopically. Directly above code 47370 are some official guidelines that provide important direction:

"Surgical laparoscopy always includes diagnostic laparoscopy. To report a diagnostic laparoscopy (peritoneoscopy) (separate procedure), use 49320."

Without this direction, you might have gone to the trouble to report both 49320 and 47370. So, now you saved yourself some time and found the correct code to report for Dr. Brusk's work:

47370   Laparoscopy, surgical, ablation of 1 or more liver tumor(s); radiofrequency

If you had reported both codes, this could constitute overcoding—which would be fraud.

See . . . the guidelines help you code accurately, and legally.

Good work!

3.5 Confirming Medical Necessity

No one believes physicians or other health care professionals should be permitted to do whatever they want to a patient without a valid reason. In our industry, this valid reason is known as medical necessity, and you learned about it in the *Introduction to the Languages of Coding* chapter. The code or codes that you report to identify the reasons *why* the patient required the attention of a health care professional justify *what* the physician or health care professional did to the patient or for the patient . . . but only when they are in accordance with the standards of care.

Outpatient Settings

In an outpatient setting, once you have determined the accurate diagnosis codes and procedure codes, you must confirm that you are reporting at least one diagnosis code to identify medical necessity by **linking** it to at least one procedure code. Multiple procedure codes can link to one diagnosis code, and multiple diagnosis codes can link to one procedure code. But there must be at least one of each to support the encounter.

You must take this action to ensure that the diagnosis codes you are reporting accurately represent the documented reasons *why* the physician made the decisions he or she made and provided care to this patient, based on those reasons. You must make certain you did not miss anything in the documentation. You must make certain you did not jot down, or enter, the code incorrectly [a typo?].

Linking
Confirming medical necessity by pairing at least one diagnosis code to at least one procedure code.

LET'S CODE IT! SCENARIO

Ahmed Obodeh, a 23-year-old male, came in to see Dr. Starkey because he hit his head on a cabinet and has had a headache for 2 days nonstop. Dr. Starkey examined Ahmed and ordered an MRI of his brain to be taken. Just before the nurse took him down to imaging, Ahmed told Dr. Starkey that he also banged his left knee and was having pain when walking. So Dr. Starkey told the nurse to have radiology take an x-ray of his left knee while he was there. Afterwards, Dr. Starkey gave Ahmed instructions for care of a mild concussion, and suggested an ace bandage for his knee and over-the-counter pain relievers for 1 week.

Let's Code It!

Dr. Starkey diagnosed Ahmed with a mild concussion and provided an MRI of the brain and an x-ray of the left knee. Let's analyze this. The concussion is a traumatic impact of the brain and skull. This matches with the MRI of the brain. Perfect.

But there is no diagnosis to justify the x-ray of the knee. Did Dr. Starkey order an unnecessary test? Was he trying to cheat the insurance company and take advantage of Ahmed? No. He is a good doctor, and he was doing a good job by ordering the x-ray of Ahmed's knee. How will you communicate that he was properly caring for his patient?

Go back to the documentation. What was written about Ahmed's knee? *"was having pain when walking"* The report of pain by a patient is a symptom and a valid reason for the provision of an x-ray. Therefore, you will determine the diagnosis code to explain that pain in the knee was the medical necessity.

Diagnosis		Procedure
Brain concussion [S06.0X0A]	–Links to–	MRI brain [70551]
Pain in left knee [M25.562]	–Links to–	X-ray of knee, left [73560-LT]

You are really learning!

Inpatient Setting

In an inpatient setting, the diagnosis code or codes reported must support the medical necessity for the patient to require acute care in a hospital setting—24-hour care from trained health care professionals.

For example, *uncomplicated mild intermittent asthma* [J45.20], occasional narrowing of the bronchi causing diminished breathing, relieved with a prescription inhaler, is not a reason to admit a patient into the hospital to receive round-the-clock care; however, *mild intermittent asthma with status asthmaticus* [J45.22], a life-threatening asthma attack that is not responding to normal treatments such as an inhaler or nebulizer, certainly might be.

LET'S CODE IT! SCENARIO

DATE OF ADMISSION: 09/18/2019

ADMITTING DIAGNOSIS: Suspected bowel obstruction

CHIEF COMPLAINT: Severe abdominal pain, vomiting, bloating

HISTORY OF PRESENT ILLNESS: Patient is a 29-year-old male with a history of Crohn's disease of the large intestine. The patient came to the ER for an episode of vomiting, continuous, 36 hours. Patient states crampy abdominal pain and

(continued)

bloating. Abdominal ultrasound shows thickening of the bowel wall resulting in acute stricture of the descending colon. Patient is admitted with suspected Crohn's disease with bowel obstruction. Consult with gastroenterology is requested.

Let's Code It!

The admitting diagnosis appears to be clear:

K50.112   **Crohn's disease of large intestine with intestinal obstruction**

You could see the problem getting reimbursed for this hospital stay if, by mistake, this code was reported:

K50.10   **Crohn's disease of large intestine without complications**

The little details are important!

CHAPTER SUMMARY

In this chapter, you learned how to take the data culled from the physician's documentation and interpret the data into another language, a medical code (ICD-10-CM, CPT, HCPCS Level II, or ICD-10-PCS). Following each and every one of the six actions required will help you ensure that you are accurately interpreting what occurred between physician and patient during a specific encounter or during a patient's stay in a hospital. In the next part of this book, you will delve more deeply into diagnosis coding using the language of ICD-10-CM.

CODING BITES

Action 1. Abstract the documentation
Action 2. Query, if necessary
Action 3. Code the diagnosis or diagnoses
Action 4. Code the procedure or procedures
Action 5. Confirm medical necessity
Action 6. Double-check your codes

CHAPTER 3 REVIEW
The Coding Process

Let's Check It! Terminology

Match each key term to the appropriate definition.

1. LO 3.2 The section of a code book showing codes, from A to Z, by the short code descriptions.

2. LO 3.3 The section of the ICD-10-PCS code book listing all of the codes in alphanumeric order, based on the first three characters of the code.

3. LO 3.1 The sequence of actions required to interpret physician documentation into the codes that accurately report what occurred during a specific encounter between health care professional and patient.

4. LO 3.3 A code consisting of both numbers and letters.

5. LO 3.5 Confirming medical necessity by pairing at least one diagnosis code to at least one procedure code.

6. LO 3.3 The section of the CPT code book listing all of the codes in numeric order.

7. LO 3.4 A listing of rules and regulations instructing how to use a specific code set accurately.

8. LO 3.2 Alerts and warnings that support more accurate use of codes in a specific code set.

9. LO 3.2 Marks, similar to emojis, that provide additional direction to use codes correctly and accurately.

10. LO 3.3 The section of the ICD-10-CM code book listing all of the codes in alpha-numeric order.

A. Alphabetic Index
B. Alphanumeric
C. Coding Process
D. Official Guidelines
E. Linking
F. Main Section
G. Notations
H. Symbols
I. Tables
J. Tabular List

Let's Check It! Concepts

Choose the most appropriate answer for each of the following questions.

1. LO 3.1 There are _____ specific actions that you should take to construct your proper coding process.
   a. 3   b. 4   c. 5   d. 6

2. LO 3.1 The most important factor in coding is
   a. speed of the coding process.   b. accuracy of codes.
   c. level of codes   d. quantity of codes.

3. LO 3.1 *Abstract the documentation* is Action _____ in the coding process.
   a. 1   b. 2   c. 3   d. 4

4. LO 3.1 Action 5 in the coding process is to
   a. code the diagnosis or diagnoses.   b. code the procedure or procedures.
   c. confirm medical necessity.   d. double-check your codes.

5. LO 3.1 Every encounter between patient and health care professional must have at least _____ diagnosis code(s) and at least _____ procedure code(s).
   a. 2, 2   b. 1, 2   c. 1, 1   d. 2, 1

6. LO 3.2 After abstracting the main terms, a coder will go next to the
   a. external cause codes.   b. Tabular listings.
   c. Alphabetic Index.   d. Appendix C.

7. **LO 3.2** Pneumonia would be an example of a term found in which Alphabetic Index?

    a. ICD-10-CM

    b. CPT

    c. ICD-10-PCS

    d. HCPCS Level II

8. **LO 3.2** IPPB machine would be an example of a term found in which Alphabetic Index?

    a. ICD-10-CM

    b. CPT

    c. ICD-10-PCS

    d. HCPCS Level II

9. **LO 3.2** The Main Section and Tabular List of the code books all contain additional _____ and _____ to help you determine the most accurate code.

    a. notations, modifiers

    b. symbols, notations

    c. figures, icons

    d. transformers, symbols

10. **LO 3.3** Which of the following code books lists the codes in numeric order?

    a. ICD-10-CM   **b.** HCPCS Level II   **c.** CPT   **d.** ICD-10-PCS

11. **LO 3.3** Which of the following is a full code description?

    a. Carbuncle of trunk L02.23

    b. Furuncle of trunk L02.22

    c. Cutaneous abscess of chest wall L02.213

    d. Impetigo L01.0

12. **LO 3.3** In the ICD-10-CM Tabular List above code K70.31 there is a notation. What is the notation?

    a. Use additional code to identify alcohol abuse and dependence

    b. Code first underlying diseases

    c. Code also, if applicable, viral hepatitis

    d. Code first poisoning due to drug or toxin, if applicable

13. **LO 3.3** If you see this symbol + in the CPT code book's main section beside a code, it tells you that

    a. the code is a revised code.

    b. moderate sedation is included in this code.

    c. the code is an add-on code.

    d. the code is a new code.

14. **LO 3.3** Which code set requires you, the coder, to build the code out to seven characters?

    a. ICD-10-CM

    b. HCPCS Level II

    c. CPT

    d. ICD-10-PCS

15. **LO 3.3** What is the correct ICD-10-PCS code for the repair of maxilla, left side, open approach?

    a. 0NQT0ZZ

    b. 0NQRXZZ

    c. 0NQR0ZZ

    d. 0NQV0ZZ

16. **LO 3.3** What is the correct CPT code for a Laparoscopy, surgical; gastrostomy, without construction of gastric tube?

    a. 43246

    b. 43653

    c. 48001

    d. 43830

17. **LO 3.4** Official _____ is(are) a listing of rules and regulations instructing you how to use a specific code set accurately.

    a. Guidelines

    b. linking

    c. tables

    d. appendix

18. **LO 3.4** The Official Guidelines for ICD-10-CM can usually be found in the

    a. back of the code book.

    b. Alphabetic Index.

    c. Tabular List.

    d. front of the code book.

19. **LO 3.5** The why justifies the _____

    a. where.

    b. who.

    c. what.

    d. when.

20. LO 3.5 _____ confirm(s) medical necessity by pairing at least one diagnosis code to at least one procedure code.

a. Tables

b. Linking

c. Guidelines

d. Appendix

Let's Check It! Guidelines

Part I

Refer to the ICD-10-CM Official Guidelines and match each section number to the corresponding guideline.

1. Diagnostic Coding and Reporting Guidelines for Outpatient Services.

2. Selection of Principal Diagnosis.

3. Conventions, general coding guidelines and chapter-specific guidelines.

4. Reporting Additional Diagnoses.

A. Section I

B. Section II

C. Section III

D. Section IV

Part II

Refer to the ICD-10-CM Official Guidelines and match each section number to the corresponding guideline.

1. LO 3.4 Sequela (Late Effects)

2. LO 3.4 Format and Structure

3. LO 3.4 Abbreviations – Tabular List abbreviations

4. LO 3.4 Etiology/manifestation convention ("code first", "use additional code" and "in diseases classified elsewhere" notes)

5. LO 3.4 "Code Also" note

6. LO 3.4 Conditions that are an integral part of a disease process

7. LO 3.4 Placeholder character

8. LO 3.4 Conditions that are not an integral part of a disease process

9. LO 3.4 Signs and symptoms

10. LO 3.4 Laterality

A. Section I.A.2

B. Section I.A.4

C. Section I.A.6.b

D. Section I.A.13

E. Section I.A.17

F. Section I.B.4

G. Section I.B.5

H. Section I.B.6

I. Section I.B.10

J. Section I.B.13

Let's Check It! Rules and Regulations

Please answer the following questions from the knowledge you have gained after reading this chapter.

1. LO 3.1 List the six actions of the coding process and explain each action in your own words.

2. LO 3.2 Discuss the Alphabetic Index and the role it plays in the coding process.

3. LO 3.3 Explain the ICD-10-CM Tabular List, how the codes are listed, and why it is important.

4. LO 3.4 Describe what the Official Guidelines are, why they are important, where they are located, and if you are required to comply with these guidelines.

5. LO 3.5 Discuss the importance of linking a diagnosis code to a procedure code.

Design elements: ©McGraw-Hill

PART III

REPORTING PHYSICIAN SERVICES AND OUTPATIENT PROCEDURES

INTRODUCTION

Now that you have learned to better understand the reasons why *a patient may need the attention and care from a physician or other health care provider, the next phase—layer 2—of your learning will be about reporting* what *is done for this patient.*

Procedures, services, and treatments are essentially all-inclusive to cover anything and everything a health care provider can do to, or for, someone. These actions may be preventive in nature, such as a vaccination; diagnostic such as an x-ray; or therapeutic—something done to fix or repair an existing problem.

While you think of all the actions a physician may perform in care of the patient, keep in mind that this includes advice and recommendations. Most of us rely on our health care providers for guidance related to improving our health. As the professional coder, a "service" might be conversation with the patient. This counts, too!

Introduction to CPT

Learning Outcomes

After completing this chapter, the student should be able to:

LO 21.1 Recognize the main terms for procedure codes.
LO 21.2 Distinguish the various sections of CPT and how to use them.
LO 21.3 Analyze complete code descriptions.
LO 21.4 Recall the meanings of notations and symbols within CPT.
LO 21.5 Interpret accurately the Official Guidelines, shown before sections and in-section.
LO 21.6 Utilize Category II and Category III codes, as required.

 STOP! Remember, you need to follow along in your CPT code book for an optimal learning experience.

21.1 Abstracting for Procedure Coding

Procedures, **services**, and **treatments** are the terms used for anything and everything that occurs between a health care professional and a patient. Remember, you learned about distinguishing *what* the provider did for the patient and reporting them in the chapter *Introduction to the Languages of Coding*. CPT is one of the languages—the terminologies—we use to communicate these details.

CPT stands for **C**urrent **P**rocedural **T**erminology and lists services, procedures, and treatments provided by all types of health care professionals. Services such as counseling, treatments such as the application of a cast, and procedures such as the surgical removal of a mole are each assigned a special code to simplify reporting for purposes of reimbursement and statistical analysis. In addition, ancillary services, such as imaging (x-rays, CT scans, magnetic resonance imaging), pathology, and laboratory (biopsy analysis, blood tests, cultures), also are reported using CPT codes. These services may range from intense surgical procedures, such as a heart transplant, to everyday treatments or services, such as removing a splinter or providing professional advice regarding a treatment plan or preventive service.

When you are coding for a physician or other health care professional, or on behalf of an **outpatient** facility, you will use CPT codes to report the actions taken for the health and well-being of a patient.

An **outpatient facility** may be in the same building as a hospital, for example, an emergency room, ambulatory care center, or same-day surgery center, or it may be a free-standing facility, such as a physician's office, a walk-in clinic, or an independent same-day surgery center.

Procedure
Action taken, in accordance with the standards of care, by the physician to accomplish a predetermined objective (result); a surgical operation.

Services
Spending time with a patient and/or family about health care situations.

Treatment
The provision of medical care for a disorder or disease.

Outpatient
An **outpatient** is a patient who receives services for a short amount of time (less than 24 hours) in a physician's office or clinic, without being kept overnight.

Outpatient facility
An **outpatient facility** includes a hospital emergency room, ambulatory care center, same-day surgery center, or walk-in clinic.

EXAMPLES

Outpatient Facilities
- Physicians' offices
- Urgent care and walk-in clinics

(continued)

- Ambulatory care centers
- Same-day surgery centers
- Emergency departments

When you are abstracting the physician's documentation to collect the details, you need to determine the codes that report what actions the physician accomplished for the patient during this encounter. This is a different perspective from when you are abstracting for diagnosis coding. As you read through the case, look for action verbs: inserted; excised; administered; discussed; dilated; and many, many more. Then, you will be able to identify which terms to interpret into CPT codes.

YOU INTERPRET IT!

Identify the term in the sentence that describes WHY the physician treated the patient and the term that describes WHAT the physician did for the patient.

1. Liam O'Connor fractured his thumb when building a bookshelf in his house. Dr. Brazinski placed a cast on Liam's hand.
2. Emma Burgeron has been using tobacco for 20 years, and she wants to quit, once and for all. Dr. Spencer discussed with her several ways to help her.
3. Jacob Treviani was found to have cholelithiasis (gallstones), so Dr. Myverson performed a cholecystectomy.

21.2 CPT Code Book

The Organization of the CPT Book

The CPT book has two parts, each of which has many sections.

1. The main body of the CPT book has six sections, presented in numeric order (generally speaking) by code number:

   - Evaluation and Management: 99201–99499
   - Anesthesia: 00100–01999 and 99100–99140
   - Surgery: 10021–69990
   - Radiology: 70010–79999
   - Pathology and Laboratory: 80047–89398, 0001U–0138U
   - Medicine: 90281–99199, 99500–99607

   You may notice that, while each section within itself is in numeric order (for the most part), the sections are also in numeric order, for the most part. Bottom line . . . _read carefully._

2. The second part of the CPT book contains several sections, including:

   - _Category II codes:_ for supplemental tracking of performance measurement.
   - _Category III codes:_ temporary codes for emerging technological procedures.
   - _Appendixes A–P:_ modifiers and other relevant additional information.
   - _Alphabetic Index:_ all the CPT codes in alphabetical order by code description, presented in four classes of entries:
     a. Procedures or services, such as removal, implantation, or debridement.
     b. Anatomical site or organ, such as heart, mouth, or pharynx.

c. Condition, such as miscarriage, cystitis, or abscess.

d. Eponyms, synonyms, or abbreviations, such as Baker's cyst or EKG.

As you prepare to learn and improve your knowledge about medical procedures, and build your skills for interpreting the documentation into CPT codes, you will find that your education in medical terminology will be very useful.

YOU INTERPRET IT!

Identify the term that explains WHAT the physician did for the patient and from which SECTION that would be reported.

4. Dr. Harper excised a mole from Katrina's arm.

5. Dr. Aubrey administered general anesthesia prior to the beginning of the surgery.

6. Dr. Davine took and evaluated the MRI images of Lawrence's head after the car accident.

CPT Resequencing Initiative

The American Medical Association (AMA) was faced with the challenge of fitting new codes for evolving health care innovation and technology into a preexisting set of numbers. So, the AMA determined that resequencing codes would be easier, and less confusing, than renumbering the entire code set. (That certainly would have caused havoc!)

Therefore, when new codes needed to be added to CPT and there were no more available numbers in the correct sequence, the next available code number was assigned. Different publishers of CPT books present this new information in various ways.

In the AMA-published CPT book, the new code is listed in two places:

1. In its correct numeric sequence. The code is shown in the correct numeric sequence with a notation that informs you where to find the code in its topic-related location.

EXAMPLE

Directly after code 46200 is code

46220   Code is out of numerical sequence. See 46200–46255

You can actually find code 46220 with its description between codes 46946 and 46230.

2. In its correct topic-related location. The code is placed with the other codes that report the same procedure or service based on the specific code description. This is highlighted by a symbol to the left of the code number—# (the hashtag sign)—to bring your attention to the fact that this code is not in numeric order.

EXAMPLES

The codes in the subsection for Anus, Excision are listed:

46221	Hemorrhoidectomy, internal, by rubber band ligation(s)	
# 46945	Hemorrhoidectomy, internal, by ligation other than rubber band; single hemorrhoid column/group	
# 46946	2 or more hemorrhoid columns/groups	

As you can see, it makes much more sense for all of the hemorrhoidectomy codes to be in the same place so that you can read through all of the code descriptions and choose the one that most accurately matches the physician's notes. If the new codes were just placed in numeric order, you would need to keep flipping back and forth.

21.3 Understanding Code Descriptions

As you look through the CPT book, both the numeric listings and the Alphabetic Index show their data in columns. Notice that some information is indented under other descriptions or terms. An indented description or term attaches to the description or term that appears at the margin of the column above, or before, the indented words.

In the Alphabetic Index

The Alphabetic Index uses a *list with an indented list* as a space-saving format. Take a look at this example:

> **EXAMPLE**
>
> Find "excision" in the Alphabetic Index:
>
> **Excision**
> Abdomen
>   Tumor 49203-49205

Look at the words at the margin and those indented.

The term *Excision,* a type of procedure, is the heading of this part of the index. This heading is at the margin of the column, in bold. Beneath this, also at the margin of the column, is the word *Abdomen,* to indicate the anatomical site where the excision was performed. Underneath this, indented, is the word *Tumor,* to report what specifically was being excised, followed by a short range of suggested codes. Read backward and you have *Tumor, Abdomen, Excision.* The physician's notes are more likely to read:

<u>Excision</u> of a <u>tumor</u> in the <u>abdomen</u>

Just as with the descriptions in the numeric listing, you must be careful as you read and connect the indented words and phrases. Using a ruler or other straight edge may make it easier to see which words are indented and which are at the margins.

Notice that the CPT Alphabetic Index will not necessarily direct you toward one code. Very often, there will be multiple or a range of codes suggested. Take a look at the example for the *Excision* of an abdominal tumor; the Index suggests the range of codes 49203–49205. This means that you are required to investigate ALL of these codes before making a decision as to which code will accurately report *what* the physician did.

As you compare these three code descriptions in the *Main Section* of CPT, you can identify which additional specific detail or details you will need to abstract from the documentation. Continue to the *Main Section* as you learn the steps to determine an accurate CPT code.

In the Main Section (Numeric Listing)

Turn to the *Main Section* of CPT and find the first code suggested by the Alphabetic Index:

49203	**Excision or destruction, open, intra-abdominal tumors, cysts, or endometriomas, 1 or more peritoneal, mesenteric, or retroperitoneal primary or secondary tumors; largest tumor 5 cm diameter or less**

Look carefully. Do you see that this description is set at the inner margin of the column? The positioning indicates that it is the complete description of this code. Now, let's look right below this code, at the next two codes listed, which were included in the Alphabetic Index's suggested range.

49203	Excision or destruction, open, intra-abdominal tumors, cysts, or endometriomas, 1 or more peritoneal, mesenteric, or retroperitoneal primary or secondary tumors; largest tumor 5 cm diameter or less
49204	largest tumor 5.1–10.0 cm diameter
49205	largest tumor greater than 10.0 cm diameter

You can see that the descriptions next to codes 49204 and 49205 are both indented, not in line at the inner margin of the column. This means you must not only read 49204 or 49205's description but also attach it to the description above. How do you know what parts or how much? Look at the punctuation of the first code:

| 49203 | Excision or destruction, open, intra-abdominal tumors, cysts, or endometriomas, 1 or more peritoneal, mesenteric, or retroperitoneal primary or secondary tumors; largest tumor 5 cm diameter or less |

Notice the *semicolon (the dot over the comma)* after the word *tumors.* The semicolon is very important. When you read the description for a code that has an indented term or phrase, attach it to the description of the code above, but only the part of the description *up to the semicolon.* Read it as shown by the colored text:

| 49203 | Excision or destruction, open, intra-abdominal tumors, cysts, or endometriomas, 1 or more peritoneal, mesenteric, or retroperitoneal primary or secondary tumors; largest tumor 5 cm diameter or less |
| 49204 | largest tumor 5.1–10.0 cm diameter |

Putting both lines together means that the actual complete description of code 49204 is

| 49204 | Excision or destruction, open, intra-abdominal tumors, cysts, or endometriomas, 1 or more peritoneal, mesenteric, or retroperitoneal primary or secondary tumors; largest tumor 5.1–10.0 cm diameter |

Now that you know the trick to reading these code descriptions, you can understand the precise details reported by each of these three codes, and how they differ:

49203	Excision or destruction, open, intra-abdominal tumors, cysts, or endometriomas, 1 or more peritoneal, mesenteric, or retroperitoneal primary or secondary tumors; largest tumor 5 cm diameter
49204	Excision or destruction, open, intra-abdominal tumors, cysts, or endometriomas, 1 or more peritoneal, mesenteric, or retroperitoneal primary or secondary tumors; largest tumor 5.1–10.0 cm diameter
49205	Excision or destruction, open, intra-abdominal tumors, cysts, or endometriomas, 1 or more peritoneal, mesenteric, or retroperitoneal primary or secondary tumors; largest tumor greater than 10.0 cm diameter

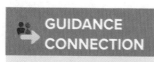

GUIDANCE CONNECTION

Read the CPT **Introduction,** subsection **Instructions for Use of the CPT Codebook—Format of the Terminology.**

 LET'S CODE IT! SCENARIO

Dr. Cragen performed a subtotal pericardiectomy using cardiopulmonary bypass on Lucy Brockton.

Let's Code It!

The procedure performed by Dr. Cragen was a pericardiectomy. Let's begin in the CPT Alphabetic Index, and read

   Pericardiectomy, Subtotal 33030, 33031

(continued)

Turn in the *Main Section* of CPT, and find these codes:

33030   Pericardiectomy, subtotal or complete; without cardiopulmonary bypass
33031   with cardiopulmonary bypass

To determine the complete description for 33031, put it together, as you learned earlier. Remember, use the part of the first code description ***up to the semicolon*** + the indented information:

33030   Pericardiectomy, subtotal or complete; without cardiopulmonary bypass
33031   Pericardiectomy, subtotal or complete; with cardiopulmonary bypass

Dr. Cragen documented that this pericardiectomy was performed with a cardiopulmonary bypass. Now, you know exactly which code to report!

33031   Pericardiectomy, subtotal or complete; with cardiopulmonary bypass

Good job!

Unlisted Procedure or Service

On rare occasions, the physician for whom you are coding may perform a service or procedure that does not yet have a designated CPT Category I or CPT Category III code. When this is the case, you may find it necessary to report an **unlisted code**. There is one of these codes at the end of almost every section or subsection.

Unlisted Codes
Codes shown at the end of each subsection of the CPT used as a catch-all for any procedure not represented by an existing code.

EXAMPLES

You will typically find an unlisted procedure code at the end of each section or subsection.

01999   Unlisted anesthesia procedure(s)
19499   Unlisted procedure, breast
78699   Unlisted nervous system procedure, diagnostic nuclear medicine

In these situations, report the unlisted code and attach a special report to the claim that includes the specific details of the procedure or service. Make certain you, as the professional coder, have done everything possible, including querying the physician, to confirm there are no other codes that will sufficiently or accurately report what was done.

21.4 Notations and Symbols

Throughout the CPT book, you will see notations and symbols. Let's review them together.

See

A "*see*" reference is found under a heading in the Alphabetic Index. Let's review an example to better understand this reference.

EXAMPLE

Leukocyte
See White Blood Cell

In this example, under the heading "Leukocyte," the notation "*See* White Blood Cell" provides an alternate term that the physician may have used in his or her notes. The CPT book is suggesting that, if you cannot find a match to the documentation under "Leukocyte," you might find it under the heading "White Blood Cell."

GUIDANCE CONNECTION

Read the CPT **Introduction,** subsection **Instructions for Use of the CPT Codebook— Add-on Codes.**

+ Plus Sign

The plus symbol (+) identifies an *add-on code.* An add-on procedure is most often performed with a main procedure. These services or treatments are in addition to, and associated with, the main procedure and are never performed or reported alone (without the main procedure). Due to this relationship with the main procedure, add-on codes *never* use the modifier 51 Multiple Procedures. (You will learn all about modifiers later in this book.) All the add-on codes are grouped and listed in the CPT code book's Appendix D for additional reference.

EXAMPLE

Add-On Code Listing—the Plus Symbol

+22328   each additional fractured vertebra or dislocated segment (List separately in addition to code for primary procedure)

(List Separately in Addition to Code for Primary Procedure)

This notation can be seen at the end of the description of an add-on code and reminds you that the code represents a procedure that is done as a part of another procedure, reported separately. Again, this should also remind you that this code cannot be used by itself.

EXAMPLE

Add-On Code Listing—the Parenthetical Notations

22630   Arthrodesis, posterior interbody technique, including laminectomy and/or discectomy to prepare interspace (other than for decompression), single interspace; lumbar

+22632   each additional interspace (List separately in addition to code for primary procedure)

(Use 22632 in conjunction with 22612, 22630, or 22633 when performed at a different level.)

(Use . . . in Conjunction with . . .)

The notation "*Use . . . in conjunction with . . .*" is found below the description of an add-on code. Here, the CPT book is going one step further. In addition to the + symbol and the notation "List separately," the book states the primary procedure code or codes with which the add-on code may be reported.

● Bullet Symbol

The bullet symbol (●) identifies a new code, one that is in the CPT book for the first time. During the annual update of the CPT book, various codes and guidelines are added, deleted, or revised. The new, updated, printed version of CPT is effective every January 1.

▲ Triangle Symbol

The triangle symbol (▲) distinguishes a code whose description has been changed, or revised, since the last edition of CPT.

▶◀ Double Sideways Triangles

The double sideways triangles (▶◀) mark the beginning and end of text that has been revised or is being shown for the first time in this year's CPT book. This symbol may highlight code descriptions, guidelines, and/or instructional paragraphs throughout the CPT book.

★ Star Symbol

The star symbol (★), new beginning with the 2017 edition of CPT, is placed to the left of those procedure codes that are permitted to be reported when the service has been provided using synchronous telemedicine services, and appended with modifier 95. These synchronous (real-time) telemedicine services engage physician and patient by use of equipment with functioning audio and video. These codes are listed in the CPT code book's Appendix P.

⊘ Open Circle with Slash

The symbol of a circle with a slash through it (⊘), also called the Forbidden Symbol, identifies codes that are _not_ permitted to be appended with modifier 51 Multiple

---

CODING BITES

If a claim form is received listing codes that have been deleted or changed, the claim will be rejected for the use of invalid codes.

GUIDANCE CONNECTION

Read the CPT **Introduction,** subsection **Instructions for Use of the CPT Codebook—Code Symbols.** Also, be certain to check across the bottom of each page throughout the book. A legend will help remind you about the meaning for the symbols.

Procedures. These codes are procedures that are sometimes done at the same time as another procedure (like an add-on code) but also can be performed alone (unlike an add-on code). Consequently, when such a procedure is performed along with other procedures, you are not allowed to attach the multiple procedure modifier. All codes that are modifier 51 exempt are grouped and listed in the CPT code book's Appendix E. There will be a lot more about modifiers as you go through this text.

> **EXAMPLE**
>
> ⊘ 44500   Introduction of long gastrointestinal tube (e.g., Miller-Abbott) (separate procedure)

Hashtag

When you see this symbol, a hashtag (#), to the left of a CPT code, this identifies a code that has been added and placed into the code set out of numeric order. For more on this, see the section on the *CPT Resequencing Initiative* in the section *CPT Code Book* of this chapter.

○ Open Circle

An open circle (○) identifies a recycled or reinstated code, which is a code that was previously deleted and now is found to be necessary, so it has been reactivated.

↺ Arrow in a Circle

Some versions of the CPT book may also include a circle with an arrow symbol (↺). This symbol (↺) points you toward an AMA-published reference that may be of additional guidance. The notation may direct you toward a particular edition of either the *CPT Assistant* newsletter or the book *CPT Changes: An Insider's View*. The American Medical Association (AMA) describes this subscription-only publication, *CPT Assistant,* as *"instrumental to many in their appeal of insurance denials, validating coding to auditors, training their staff and simply making answering day-to-day coding questions second nature."*

CODING BITES

There is a legend across the bottom of the pages throughout the CPT code book to remind you what each symbol represents, so you don't have to worry about memorizing all of these notations and symbols.

LET'S CODE IT! SCENARIO

Kevin Kewly was in a fight with a member of his rival company's softball team. The other player took out a knife and stabbed him. When he arrived at the Emergency Department, Dr. Jarrenson repaired his 12 cm laceration, including debridement and retention sutures, on his lower right arm.

Let's Code It!

Dr. Jarrenson stitched a 12 cm laceration on Kevin's arm. You learned in medical terminology class that this is known in health care services as a wound repair. Turn to the Alphabetic Index in your CPT code book and find

Wound

Read down the list to find Repair, and indented beneath this, Arms.

Wound
Repair
   Arms

      Complex. 13120–13122
      Intermediate. . . 12031, 12032, 12034–12037
      Simple. 12001, 12002, 12004–12007

(continued)

Do you know whether Kevin's wound required a simple repair, intermediate repair, or complex repair? Not yet (you will learn), so for now, let's turn to the first code—12001—and see what we can find out.

Look at the in-section guidelines that are here, in the Repair (Closure) subsection, above code 12001. As you read the descriptions of the three types of repairs, notice that debridement and retention sutures are mentioned in both the case scenario and the description of Complex Repair.

Turn to the subsection Repair—Complex and find

13120	**Repair, complex, scalp, arms and/or legs; 1.1 cm to 2.5 cm**
13121	**2.6 cm to 7.5 cm**
+ 13122	**each additional 5 cm or less (List separately in addition to code for primary procedure)**

Look back at the case scenario. It states the wound was 12 cm. You learned earlier in this chapter that the plus sign (+) means you will need two codes because code 13122 cannot be reported alone. So, you will have to do some addition.

Code 13121 reports the first 7.5 cm, and you also will need to report 13122 for the additional 4.5 cm to total 12 cm.

That completes the story. Now, you can report Dr. Jarrenson's procedure performed on Kevin with confidence . . .

13121	**Repair, complex, scalp, arms and/or legs; 2.6 cm to 7.5 cm**
13122	**each additional 5 cm or less (List separately in addition to code for primary procedure)**

Good job!

21.5 Official Guidelines

Section Guidelines

The Official Guidelines you will use to ensure that you are coding procedures correctly are presented right in your CPT code book. Notice the pages in front of each of the six sections of the main part of the book.

- Evaluation and Management Guidelines
- Evaluation and Management Numerical Listings
- Anesthesia Guidelines
- Anesthesia Numerical Listings
- Surgery Guidelines
- Surgery Numerical Listings
- Radiology Guidelines
- Radiology Numerical Listings
- Pathology and Laboratory Guidelines
- Pathology and Laboratory Numerical Listings
- Medicine Guidelines
- Medicine Numerical Listings

The guidelines identify important rules and directives that coders must follow when assigning codes from each section—for example:

- Evaluation and management services guidelines include the definitions of commonly used terms.

FIGURE 21-1 A portion of the Surgery Guidelines in the CPT code book, including the CPT Surgical Package Definition Source: *CPT Professional Manual,* American Medical Association

- Surgery guidelines include a listing of services that are bundled into the surgical package definition (see Figure 21-1).

- Medicine guidelines include instructions on how to code multiple procedures and the proper use of add-on codes.

In-Section Guidelines

There are additional guidelines and instructions throughout each section, shown in paragraphs under various subheadings. These instructional notations, ranging from a short sentence to several paragraphs, provide specific information regarding the proper coding appropriate to that anatomical site or type of procedure. (See Figure 21-2.)

EXAMPLES

Instructional Notations in a Subsection

Biopsy

Directly above code 11102 is more than a page of guidance containing important details for coders preparing to report a code from this subsection.

(continued)

Stereotactic Radiation Therapy

Thoracic stereotactic body radiation therapy (SRS/SBRT) is a distinct procedure which may involve collaboration between a surgeon and radiation oncologist. The surgeon identifies and delineates the target for therapy. The radiation oncologist reports the appropriate code(s) for clinical treatment planning, physics and dosimetry, treatment delivery and management from the Radiation Oncology section (see 77295, 77331, 77370, 77373, 77435). The same physician should not report target delineation services with radiation treatment management codes (77427-77499).

Target delineation involves specific determination of tumor borders to identify tumor volume and relationship with adjacent structures (eg, chest wall, intraparenchymal vasculature and atelectatic lung) and previously placed fiducial markers, when present. Target delineation also includes availability to identify and validate the thoracic target prior to treatment delivery when a fiducial-less tracking system is utilized.

Do not report target delineation more than once per entire course of treatment when the treatment requires greater than one session.

32701 Thoracic target(s) delineation for stereotactic body radiation therapy (SRS/SBRT), (photon or particle beam), entire course of treatment

➔ CPT Changes: An Insider's View 2013

(Do not report 32701 in conjunction with 77261-77799)

(For placement of fiducial markers, see 31626, 32553)

FIGURE 21-2 In-section guidelines from the Surgery section of the CPT code book related to reporting Stereotactic Radiation Therapy Source: *CPT Professional Manual, American Medical Association*

Remember, the CPT code book will actually support your efforts to code accurately. The Official Guidelines are right there at your fingertips, and it is your obligation to read them before you confirm a code is ready to be reported. This is to your benefit . . . as you will improve your accuracy!

YOU INTERPRET IT!

Identify the pre-section or in-section guideline that you need to report the procedure accurately.

7. Dr. Singer documented that he debrided Jesse's abdominal wall. What specific details do you need to know to determine this code?

8. Dr. Trenton documented performing a sleep study with simultaneous recording of vital signs for Kent Burlington. The CPT code description is

95807 Sleep study, simultaneous recording of ventilation, respiratory effort, ECG or heart rate, and oxygen saturation, attended by a technologist

What does "attended by" mean?

9. Dr. Obatunda completed his documentation on his evaluation of Adam. To determine the correct Evaluation and Management code, you must determine the level of history documented in the notes. What exactly is included in a problem-focused history?

21.6 Category II and Category III Coding

Category I Codes
The codes listed in the main text of the CPT book, also known as CPT codes.

Category II Codes
Codes for performance measurement and tracking.

Category III Codes
Codes for emerging technology.

In the chapter *Introduction to the Languages of Coding*, you learned about the three categories of codes located in the CPT code book: **Category I codes** in the main text of the CPT book, **Category II codes**, and **Category III codes**. Let's briefly review how Category II and Category III codes are used.

Category II Codes

Category II codes are used for statistical purposes—to track and measure performance and the quality of care provided in a health care facility.

While the number of Category II codes is small, these codes identify specific services that have been proven to be connected to quality patient care. Category II codes have five characters: four numbers followed by the letter *F*.

EXAMPLES

0015F   Melanoma follow-up completed (includes assessment of all of the following components): history obtained regarding new or changing moles, complete physical skin exam performed, and patient counseled to perform a monthly self-skin examination.

1220F   Patient screened for depression

As you can see from these examples, Category II codes provide detailed information about the encounter between physician and patient . . . details that are important to research.

Each code's description explains clinical fundamentals (such as vital signs), lab test results, patient education, or other facets that might be provided within a typical office visit. However, individually, these component services do not have any billable value and, therefore, are not assigned a code from Category I CPT codes. Assigning Category II codes simply is a way for the health care researchers to specifically calculate how often these services are being provided.

Merit-Based Incentive Payment System (MIPS)

Beginning in 2017, the Merit-Based Incentive Payment System (MIPS) was launched by the Centers for Medicare and Medicaid Services (CMS) to provide a way to reward participating providers with a performance-based payment adjustment to their earned Medicare reimbursements. This program replaces the Physician Quality Reporting System (PQRS) program. Coders are instructed to report when designated sets of quality measures are provided by an eligible professional (EP), using CPT Category II codes on a standard claim form, with a charged amount of $0.00 (zero) or $0.01 (zero dollars and one cent).

 LET'S CODE IT! SCENARIO

Michael Catapano, a 71-year-old male, comes to see Dr. Sheridan, his primary care physician for the last 5 years, for his annual checkup. Michael has a family history of cardiac disease, so Dr. Sheridan takes extra care to examine Michael and speak with him about angina (severe acute chest pain caused by inadequate supply of oxygen to part of the heart). Dr. Sheridan documents that angina is absent.

Let's Code It!

As the coder for Dr. Sheridan, you will report a preventive medicine evaluation and management (E/M) code for the annual physical, along with codes for any specific tests or exams that she ordered to make certain Dr. Sheridan is properly reimbursed for her work. Dr. Sheridan was a good health care professional taking the time to discuss angina with Michael, and to carefully confirm that angina is not present. How can you, as the coder, report this service to Medicare?

Turn to the Category II code section in your CPT book.

Under the heading *Patient History,* find the code that identifies this patient does not have angina. You will see this code:

1012F   Angina absent

So your report for this encounter will include two codes to tell the whole story about this encounter:

99397   **Periodic comprehensive preventive medicine reevaluation and management of an individual including an age and gender appropriate history, examination, counseling/participatory guidance/risk factor reduction interventions, and the ordering of laboratory/diagnostic procedures; 65 years and older**
1012F   **Angina absent**

*NOTE: You will learn more about annual physical exam coding in the chapter *CPT Evaluation and Management Coding,* section on *Preventive Medicine Services.*

Category III Codes

Category III codes offer the opportunity to collect detailed information on the use of new technological advancements, services, and procedures at their entry point into the practice of health care throughout the United States. Each code identifies an innovative procedure that is at the forefront of the health care industry but not yet widely used or accepted as a standard of care. It is why the codes in this section of the CPT book are considered temporary.

GUIDANCE CONNECTION

Read the additional explanation in the guidelines directly under the section heading **Category III Codes** in your CPT book.

Category III codes may eventually become Category I codes (the codes in the main text of the CPT book). New procedures and services are assigned a Category III code so that actual usage can be accurately measured. They are placed in this section of the CPT book and assigned a code that has five characters: four numbers followed by the letter *T* (for *temporary*) in the fifth position.

EXAMPLES

0184T Excision of rectal tumor, transanal endoscopic microsurgical approach (ie. TEMS), including muscularis propria (i.e., full thickness)

0509T Electroretinography (ERG) with interpretation and report, pattern (PERG)

The use of Category III codes is mandatory, as appropriate, according to the physician's notes. If there aren't any accurate Category I codes in the CPT book to report the physician's services, you must check the Category III section for an appropriate code *before* you are permitted to use a Category I **unlisted code**. The good news is that the CPT book will continue to help you. Category III codes *are* included in the Alphabetic Index. In addition, there are notations throughout the main sections that will direct you to a Category III code, if applicable.

It is important that you are aware of the fact that Category III codes represent up-and-coming technology. Because of this, the third-party payers from whom you seek reimbursement may consider some services **experimental**. When you work in a health care facility that uses any procedures or services reported with a Category III code, it is critical that you determine the carrier's rules and coverage with regard to the treatment or test. Should the carrier exclude it and refuse to pay, both the patient and your facility are better off knowing this as soon as possible.

Keep good communication open with the physicians for whom you code. There are multiple benefits for this, including you finding out about a new technique or procedure before it is provided to any patient. Then, you can determine if this procedure will require a Category III code. Knowing this before a patient is involved will give you time. You may be able to petition the payer to convince it of the medical necessity and the cost efficiency of the new technology, and you may receive an approval after all. Waiting for a denial notice is not an efficient way to handle the situation. That is also not respectful to the patient.

A particular Category III code, once assigned, is reserved for 5 years, whether the code is upgraded to a Category I code or deleted altogether. It allows for the fact that certain technologies or procedures may take time to find acceptance.

Unlisted Codes
Codes shown at the end of each subsection of the CPT used as a catch-all for any procedure not represented by an existing code.

Experimental
A procedure or treatment that has not yet been accepted by the health care industry as the standard of care.

 YOU CODE IT! CASE STUDY

Grace Emerson, a 55-year-old female, had a heart transplant 2 months ago. She has not been feeling well, so Dr. Rasmussen performs a breath test for heart transplant rejection. This test is experimental, but it is noninvasive.

You Code It!

Go through the steps of coding, and determine the code(s) that should be reported for this test provided by Dr. Rasmussen to Grace Emerson.

Step #1: Read the case carefully and completely.

Step #2: Abstract the scenario. Which key words or terms describe what service the physician provided to the patient during this encounter?

(continued)

Step #3: Are there any details missing or incomplete for which you would need to query the physician? [If so, ask your instructor.]

Step #4: Determine the correct CPT procedure code or codes to explain the details about what was provided to the patient during this encounter.

Step #5: Check for any relevant guidance, including reading all of the symbols and notations.

Step #6: Do you need to append any modifiers to ensure complete and accurate information is provided?

Step #7: Double-check your work.

Answer:

Did you determine this to be the code?

0085T   **Breath test for heart transplant rejection**

Good job!

Chapter Summary

In this chapter, you learned about the important role that coding plays in our health care system, with specific focus on procedure codes used to report physician services and outpatient facility services. As an up-and-coming professional coding specialist, you must strive to accurately report the procedure, services, and treatments provided to every patient using CPT codes. Health care professionals are responsible for ensuring that the supporting documentation is complete so that you have the information necessary to find the most accurate code or codes.

CODING BITES

Steps to Coding Procedures

Step #1: Read the case carefully and completely.

Step #2: Abstract the scenario. Which key words or terms describe what service the physician provided to the patient during this encounter?

Step #3: Are there any details missing or incomplete for which you would need to query the physician? [If so, ask your instructor.]

Step #4: Determine the correct CPT procedure code or codes to explain the details about what was provided to the patient during this encounter.

Step #5: Check for any relevant guidance, including reading all of the symbols and notations.

Step #6: Do you need to append any modifiers to ensure complete and accurate information is provided?

Step #7: Double-check your work.

You Interpret It! Answers

1. Fracture = diagnosis code reported to explain why; Cast = CPT code reported to explain what Dr. Brazinski did for Liam. **2.** Tobacco use = diagnosis code reported to explain why; Discuss = CPT code reported to explain what Dr. Spencer did for Emma. **3.** Cholelithiasis = diagnosis code reported to explain why; Cholecystectomy = CPT code reported to explain what Dr. Myverson did for Jacob. **4.** Excision = surgical removal . . . report a code from the Surgery section. **5.** Anesthesia . . . report a code from the Anesthesia section. **6.** MRI (Magnetic Resonance Imaging) = imaging . . . report a code from the Radiology section. **7.** Inside the Surgery section of CPT, above the many codes available to report debridement, are in-section guidelines that include *Debridement.* Wound debridements (11042–11047) are reported by depth of tissue that is removed and by surface area of the wound. **8.** 95807 Sleep study, simultaneous recording of ventilation, respiratory effort, ECG or heart rate, and oxygen saturation, attended by a technologist. What does "attended by" mean? The CPT book includes this definition right there, along with in-section guidelines for Sleep Medicine Testing: "*Attended: a technologist or qualified health care professional is physically present.*" **9.** Turn to the Evaluation and Management (E/M) Services Guidelines directly in front of the Evaluation and Management code section in the CPT book and find this subsection: "**Determine the Extent of History Obtained** . . . *Problem focused:* Chief complaint; brief history of present illness or problem."

CHAPTER 21 REVIEW
Introduction to CPT

Let's Check It! Terminology

Match each term to the appropriate definition.

1. LO 21.1 The provision of care for a patient using advice, recommendations, or discussion.

2. LO 21.1 A treatment or service provided by a health care professional.

3. LO 21.1 A patient who receives services for a short term (less than 1 day) in a physician's office or clinic, without being kept overnight.

4. LO 21.1 The provision of medical care for a disorder or disease.

5. LO 21.6 Codes for performance measurement and tracking.

6. LO 21.6 The codes listed in the main text of the CPT book, also known as CPT codes.

7. LO 21.6 Codes for emerging technology.

8. LO 21.6 A procedure or treatment that has not yet been accepted by the health care industry as the standard of care.

9. LO 21.3 Codes shown at the end of each subsection of the CPT used as a catch-all for any procedure not represented by an existing code.

A. Category I

B. Category II

C. Category III

D. Experimental

E. Outpatient

F. Procedure

G. Service

H. Treatments

I. Unlisted Code

Let's Check It! Concepts

Choose the most appropriate answer for each of the following questions.

1. LO 21.1 CPT stands for

   a. Current Procedural Trailers.

   b. Classification of Procedural Techniques.

   c. Current Procedural Terminology.

   d. Classification of Procedural Terms.

2. LO 21.2 The main body of the CPT book has _____ sections, presented in numeric order (for the most part) by code number.

   a. 2   **b.** 4   **c.** 6   **d.** 8

3. **LO 21.3** When reading a code description, the rule is to read the part of the code _____ and then attach the indented description to it.

    a. up to the comma   **b.** up to the semicolon

    c. up to the period   **d.** up to the hyphen

4. **LO 21.5** CPT guidelines

    a. must be memorized by professional coders.

    b. can be found in the front of every CPT section.

    c. can be found in a separate guidelines book.

    d. change every 2 months.

5. **LO 21.4** The ✚ plus symbol identifies

    a. a new code.   **b.** a revised code.

    c. an add-on code.   **d.** a code that includes conscious sedation.

6. **LO 21.4** The ★ star symbol identifies

    a. a new code.   **b.** an add-on code.

    c. a revised code.   **d.** a telemedicine encounter.

7. **LO 21.4** The ● bullet symbol identifies

    a. a new code.   **b.** an add-on code.

    c. a revised code.   **d.** a code that includes conscious sedation.

8. **LO 21.4** The # hashtag symbol identifies

    a. a reinstated or recycled code.   **b.** a product pending FDA approval.

    c. an out-of-numeric-sequence code.   **d.** an exemption from modifier 51.

9. **LO 21.3** An unlisted code should only be used when

    a. an accurate Category I code is not available.

    b. an accurate Category I code is not available *and* an accurate Category III code is not available.

    c. an accurate Category III code is not available.

    d. an accurate Category I code is not available *or* an accurate Category III code is not available.

10. **LO 21.6** The _____ program provides for a bonus payment to those eligible professionals who meet the criteria for successful reporting, and a negative payment adjustment is applied when reporting is not submitted as required.

    a. MIPS   **b.** AMA   **c.** RVU   **d.** PQRS

Let's Check It! Symbols and Sections

Part I

Match each symbol to the appropriate definition.

    1. **LO 21.4** Add-on code   **A.** ▲

    2. **LO 21.4** New or revised text   **B.** ○

    3. **LO 21.4** Telemedicine   **C.** ●

    4. **LO 21.4** Out-of-numeric-sequence code   **D.** ★

    5. **LO 21.4** New code   **E.** ⊘

    6. **LO 21.4** Revised code   **F.** ✚

    7. **LO 21.4** Exempt from modifier 51   **G.** ►◄

    8. **LO 21.4** Reinstated or recycled code   **H.** #

Part II

The main body of the CPT book has six sections. Match the code range to the correct section name.

1. LO 21.2 Surgery
2. LO 21.2 Pathology and Laboratory
3. LO 21.2 Evaluation and Management
4. LO 21.2 Medicine
5. LO 21.2 Anesthesia
6. LO 21.2 Radiology

A. 99201–99499
B. 00100–01999 and 99100–99140
C. 10021–69990
D. 70010–79999
E. 80047–89398, 0001U–0138U
F. 90281–99199, 99500–99607

Let's Check It! Rules and Regulations

Please answer the following questions from the knowledge you have gained after reading this chapter.

1. LO 21.1 Explain what is meant by *outpatient*. Include three examples of an outpatient facility.
2. LO 21.2 Explain the CPT Resequencing Initiative.
3. LO 21.3 Discuss unlisted procedure or service codes, when it is appropriate to use them, and any attachment that should be included.
4. LO 21.4 What does the arrow in a circle symbol identify?
5. LO 21.6 Differentiate between a CPT Category I code, Category II code, and Category III code, including any special characteristics of how they are identified.

YOU CODE IT! Basics

First, identify the procedural main term in the following statements; then code the procedure or service.

Example: Drainage of eyelid abscess

a. main term: *Drainage*   b. procedure: *67700*

1. Ligation salivary ducts, intraoral:
   a. main term: _____   b. procedure: _____
2. Carpal scaphoid fracture manipulation:
   a. main term: _____   b. procedure: _____
3. Thoracotomy with cardiac massage:
   a. main term: _____   b. procedure: _____
4. Ureter meatotomy:
   a. main term: _____   b. procedure: _____
5. Intraocular pressure monitoring for 36 hours:
   a. main term: _____   b. procedure: _____
6. Tendon sheath incision, finger:
   a. main term: _____   b. procedure: _____
7. Immunoassay antigen detection influenza B:
   a. main term: _____   b. procedure: _____

8. Anesthesia for ear biopsy:
   a. main term: _____   b. procedure: _____
9. Data analysis of implantable defibrillation, wearable device:
   a. main term: _____   b. procedure: _____
10. Keratoplasty, anterior lamellar:
    a. main term: _____   b. procedure: _____
11. Lower arm x-ray:
    a. main term: _____   b. procedure: _____
12. Kidney cyst injection:
    a. main term: _____   b. procedure: _____
13. Lithotripsy with cystourethroscopy:
    a. main term: _____   b. procedure: _____
14. Percutaneous spinal cord biopsy:
    a. main term: _____   b. procedure: _____
15. Pediatric gastroenteritis education, individual:
    a. main term: _____   b. procedure: _____

YOU CODE IT! Practice

Using the techniques described in this chapter, carefully read through the case studies and determine the most accurate CPT code(s) for each case study.

1. Kelley Gaylord, a 7-year-old female, saw Dr. Roberts for a screening audiologic function test, pure tone, air only, to check her hearing.

2. Marlene Carrington, a healthy 42-year-old female, was taken to the operating room (OR) for an anterior cervical discectomy with decompression of a single interspace of the spinal cord and nerve roots and including osteophytectomy.

3. Rosa Phillips, a 34-year-old female, presents today for a percutaneous breast biopsy, needle core.

4. Sandra Lewis, a 55-year-old female, has been experiencing pain in her lower left back that wraps around to her inner thigh. Dr. Janson does a renal ultrasound, limited, real time with image documentation.

5. Hoyt Markum, a 78-year-old male, was taken to the OR for a single lung transplant with a cardiopulmonary bypass. Dr. Cannelloni was concerned because Hoyt was not expected to survive without the transplant.

6. Sunshine Thomas, an otherwise healthy 24-year-old female, was taken to the OR for a total thyroidectomy to remove a left thyroid mass.

7. Elaine Coker, an otherwise healthy 41-year-old female, was admitted to the same-day surgery center after having an abnormal shoulder x-ray in the clinic the week before. Dr. Logan decided to do a diagnostic arthroscopy.

8. Dr. Unentl inserted a nontunneled centrally inserted central venous catheter into Kevin Lorenzi, a 4-year-old male.

9. Anna Mourning, a 24-year-old female who is an amateur gymnast, was brought to the OR for the insertion of a plate with screws to assist the healing of the malunion of a humeral shaft fracture, open treatment.

10. Viviana Shank, a 5-month-old female, was taken to the OR for an excision, radical resection, of a 1.3-cm malignant neoplasm on the soft tissue of her left cheek right below her eye. It is expected that the carcinoma was caught before any spread. The patient is in otherwise healthy condition.

11. Nancy Hansen, an 18-year-old female, was brought to the OR for a c-section. Anesthesia was administered. She has type 1 diabetes that is currently under control. Dr. Klackson came to perform the cesarean delivery only. Code Dr. Klackson's procedure.

12. Ted Garrison, a 37-year-old male, was rushed to the hospital by ambulance and taken directly to the OR for an appendectomy for a ruptured appendix and generalized peritonitis. The patient is otherwise healthy.

13. Dr. Simmons performed a spigelian hernia repair in the lower abdomen on Drew Avalino, a 7-month-old male.

14. Barbara Cannin, an 18-year-old female, came to see her physician, Dr. Cordoba. She had something in her eye, and it was irritating her. Nothing she did could get it out. Dr. Cordoba took a problem-focused history and examined the area. He then applied a topical anesthetic and removed the foreign body from the superficial conjunctiva of her eye. Code the removal of the foreign body only.

15. Michael Munsey, an 84-year-old male, was seen by his physician at an ambulatory surgical center for the insertion of a temporary transvenous single-chamber cardiac electrode. The patient tolerated the procedure well.

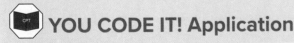 **YOU CODE IT! Application**

The following exercises provide practice in the application of abstracting the physicians' notes and learning to work with SOAP notes from our textbook's health care facility, Prader, Bracker, & Associates. These case studies (SOAP notes) are modeled on real patient encounters. Using the techniques described in this chapter, carefully read through the case studies and find the most accurate CPT code(s) for each case study.

(continued)

SOAP notes are a standardized documentation method used by health care providers to build a patient's chart. The SOAP note has four parts and each part will vary in length depending on the patient's encounter for that day.

So, what does the acronym SOAP stand for?

S = subjective
O = objective
A = assessment
P = plan

What does the **subjective** portion of the SOAP note include?

The chief complaint, a short statement in the patient's own words as to the reason for the encounter.

What does the **objective** portion of the SOAP note include?

The results of the physical examination and any measurable result; a few examples are vital signs, height, weight, and lab and diagnostic results.

What does the **assessment** portion of the SOAP note include?

A brief summation of the physician's diagnosis.

What does the **plan** portion of the SOAP note include?

The physician's plan of care (treatment) for the patient's encounter.

PRADER, BRACKER, & ASSOCIATES

A Complete Health Care Facility

159 Healthcare Way • SOMEWHERE, FL 32811 • 407-555-6789

PATIENT: MURRAY, CARMEL

ACCOUNT/EHR #: MURRCA001

DATE: 07/23/19

Attending Physician: Oscar R. Prader, MD

S: This new patient is a 32-year-old female who comes in with a complaint of severe neck pain and difficulty turning her head. She states she was in a car accident 2 days ago; her car was struck from behind when she was driving home from work.

O: PE reveals tightness upon palpitation of ligaments in neck and shoulders, most pronounced C3 to C5. X-rays are taken of the cervical vertebrae, three views (AP, Lat, and PA). Radiologic review denies any fracture.

A: Anterior longitudinal cervical sprain

P: 1. Prescribed cervical collar to be worn during all waking

   2. Rx Vicodin (hydrocodone) 500 mg po prn

   3. 1,000 mg aspirin

   4. Pt to return in 2 weeks for follow-up

ORP/mg   D: 07/23/19 09:50:16   T: 07/24/19 12:55:01

Determine the most accurate CPT code(s) for the x-ray(s).

PRADER, BRACKER, & ASSOCIATES

A Complete Health Care Facility

159 Healthcare Way • SOMEWHERE, FL 32811 • 407-555-6789

PATIENT: AUSTIN, BRUCE

ACCOUNT/EHR #: AUSTBR001

DATE: 08/09/19

Attending Physician: Renee O. Bracker, MD

Preoperative Dx: Orbital mass, OD

Postoperative Dx: Herniated orbital fat pad, OD

Procedure: Excision of lesion and repair, right superior conjunctiva

Surgeon: Marc Zammarrelli, MD

Anesthesia: Local

PROCEDURE: After proparacaine was instilled in the eye, it was prepped and draped in the usual sterile manner and 2 percent lidocaine with 1:200,000 epinephrine was injected into the superior aspect of the right orbit. A corneal protective shield was placed in the eye. The eye was placed in down-gaze.

The upper lid was everted and the fornix examined. The herniating mass was viewed and measured at 0.75 cm in diameter. Westcott scissors were used to incise the fornix conjunctivae. The herniating mass was then clamped, excised, and cauterized. It appeared to contain mostly fat tissue, which was sent to pathology.

The superior fornix was repaired using running suture of 6-0 plain gut. Bacitracin ointment was applied to the eye followed by an eye pad. The patient tolerated the procedure well and left the OR in good condition.

ROB/mg   D: 08/09/19 09:50:16   T: 08/10/19 12:55:01

Determine the most accurate CPT code(s) for the excision of the lesion.

WESTON HOSPITAL

629 Healthcare Way • SOMEWHERE, FL 32811 • 407-555-6541

PATIENT: WOODARD, HOPE

ACCOUNT/EHR #: WOODHO001

DATE: 3/19/19

Attending Physician: Oscar R. Prader, MD

The patient is a 54-year-old female with a very long history of schizoaffective disorder with numerous hospitalizations who was brought in by ambulance due to increasing paranoia; increasing arguments with other people; and, in general, an exacerbation of her psychotic symptoms, 14-day duration.

I am here to provide psychoanalysis.

Initially, the patient was very agitated and uncooperative. She refused medications. A 2PC* was done and the patient had a court hearing that results in retention. Eventually, the patient agreed to a trial of

*2PC stands for "two physicians certify"—a medical certification testifying that an individual requires involuntary treatment at a psychiatric facility.

(continued)

Risperdal; she fairly rapidly improved once she was started on Risperdal 2 mg twice daily. At the time of discharge compared with admission, the patient is much improved. She is usually pleasant and cooperative, with occasional difficult moments and some continuing mild paranoia. She has no hallucinations. She has no thoughts of harming herself or anyone else. She has been compliant with her medication until she recently refused hydrochlorothiazide. She is irritable at times, but overall she is redirectable and is considered to be at or close to her best baseline. She is considered no imminent danger to herself or to others at this time.

FINAL DX: Schizoaffective disorder; hypothyroidism; hypercholesterolemia; borderline hypertension.

Prescriptions for 30-day supplies were given:

Ativan 2 mg po tid; Celexa 40 mg po daily; Risperdal 2 mg po bid; Synthroid 0.088 mg po qam; Zocor 40 mg po qhs

ORP/mg   D: 03/19/19 09:50:16   T: 03/20/19 12:55:01

Determine the most accurate CPT code(s) for the psychoanalysis.

PRADER, BRACKER, & ASSOCIATES

A Complete Health Care Facility

159 Healthcare Way • SOMEWHERE, FL 32811 • 407-555-6789

PATIENT: JOHNS, CHARLENE

ACCOUNT/EHR #: JOHNCH001

DATE: 08/09/19

Attending Physician: Renee O. Bracker, MD

S: This patient is a 34-year-old female who I have not seen in 6 months. She has a history of recurrent sinus infections. She has been well until 6 days ago. She presents with fever, severe frontal headache, facial pain, and runny nose. Patient states she has been having difficulty concentrating.

O: PE reveals: T 101.5°. HEENT: Tenderness over frontal and left maxillary sinuses. Nasal congestion visible. CT scan of the maxillofacial area, without contrast, reveals opacification of both frontal, left maxillary, and sphenoid sinuses and a possible large nonenhanced lesion in the brain.

A: Epidural abscess with frontal lobe lesions caused by significant compression on frontal lobe.

P: Recommendation for surgery to evacuate the abscess. Patient will think about it and call in a day or two.

Rx: Amoxil 875 mg q12h

   Sudafed 120 mg q12h

ROB/MG   D: 08/09/19 09:50:16   T: 08/10/19 12:55:01

Determine the most accurate CPT code(s) for the CT scan.

PRADER, BRACKER, & ASSOCIATES

A Complete Health Care Facility

159 Healthcare Way • SOMEWHERE, FL 32811 • 407-555-6789

PATIENT: PYKE, JOEL

ACCOUNT/EHR #: PYKEJO001

DATE: 05/26/19

Diagnosis: Primary cardiomyopathy with chest pain

Procedure: Arterial catheterization

Physician: Oscar R. Prader, MD

Anesthesia: Local

Procedure: The patient was placed on the table in supine position. Local anesthesia was administered. Once we were assured that the patient had achieved no nervous stimuli, the incision was made and the catheter was introduced percutaneously. The incision was sutured with a simple repair. The patient tolerated the procedure well and was transferred to the recovery room.

ORP/mg   D: 5/26/19 09:50:16   T: 05/27/19 12:55:010

Determine the most accurate CPT code(s) for the catheterization.

22

CPT and HCPCS Level II Modifiers

Key Terms

Alphanumeric
Ambulatory Surgery
　Center (ASC)
AMCC
Category II Modifiers
Class A Finding
Class B Finding
Class C Finding
Clinical Laboratory
　Improvement
　Amendment (CLIA)
CPT Code Modifier
Early and Periodic
　Screening,
　Diagnostic, and
　Treatment (EPSDT)
End-Stage Renal
　Disease (ESRD)
HCPCS Level II
　Modifier
Liters per Minute
　(LPM)
Locum Tenens
　Physician
Modifier
Nonphysician
Parenteral Enteral
　Nutrition (PEN)
Personnel Modifier
Physical Status
　Modifier
Service-Related
　Modifier
Supplemental Report
Urea Reduction Ratio
　(URR)

Modifier
A two-character code that
affects the meaning of
another code; a code addendum that provides more
meaning to the original code.

Learning Outcomes

After completing this chapter, the student should be able to:

LO 22.1 Recognize the purpose of procedure code modifiers.
LO 22.2 Apply personnel modifiers per the guidelines.
LO 22.3 Correctly use anesthesia Physical Status Modifiers.
LO 22.4 Implement ambulatory surgery center modifiers.
LO 22.5 Append anatomical site modifiers, as required.
LO 22.6 Identify circumstances that require a service-related modifier.
LO 22.7 Analyze the guidelines to correctly sequence multiple modifiers.
LO 22.8 Determine when a supplemental report is necessary.

 STOP! Remember, you need to follow along in your CPT and HCPCS Level II code books for an optimal learning experience.

22.1 Modifiers Overview

In addition to the code for the specific procedure or service provided to the patient, there may be times when you will have to append a **modifier**. Modifiers are two-character codes that add clarification and additional details to the procedure code's original description, as written in the main portion of the *Current Procedural Terminology* (CPT) book.

Sometimes, the modifier provides necessary explanation to the third-party payer that directly relates to the reimbursement that the facility or physician should receive. It might explain that

- A service or procedure had both a professional component and a technical component.
- A service or procedure was performed by more than one physician.
- A service or procedure was performed in more than one location.
- A service or procedure was not performed in total (only part of it was done).
- The provider has special qualifications or training.
- An optional extra service was performed.
- A bilateral procedure was performed.
- A service or procedure was performed more than once.
- Unusual events arose.

One of the most important reasons to properly report a procedure code with a modifier is to provide more information about that procedure—additional details that need to be added to the code description to make certain you are completely and accurately reporting what was *actually* provided to the patient during the encounter. Some modifiers will result in the physician or facility getting paid more money because the circumstances resulted in their having to do more work than usual. For example, modifier 22 Increased Procedural Service reports that the procedure was more complex than usual.

Some modifiers will result in the physician or facility getting paid less money for the typical procedure but truthfully and accurately report that less work than usual was provided. For example, modifier 52 Reduced Services reports fewer services were provided.

Other modifiers will prevent a claim for reimbursement from being denied because it brings attention to the fact that unusual circumstances required unusual work. For example, modifier 23 Unusual Anesthesia alerts that a procedure that typically only uses a local anesthetic, for example, required general anesthesia. In these cases, you also will need to provide a supplemental report to explain what those circumstances were so that they will understand because you are telling the *whole* story.

As you go through the lists, you will find there are modifiers that have no effect at all on reimbursement but provide specific details about the procedure that will be important for continuity of care, as well as for research and statistics. An example is modifier RC Right Coronary Artery to identify the specific anatomical site upon which the procedure was completed.

You will find many modifiers listed in their own section of the CPT code book's *Appendix A*. Listed in numeric order, each modifier is shown by category, accompanied by an explanation of when and how you should use that modifier. The rest can be found in the separate HCPCS Level II code book.

Types of Modifiers

There are five categories of modifiers:

- **CPT code modifiers** are two characters that can be attached to regular codes from the main portion of the CPT book and to HCPCS Level II codes.

> ### EXAMPLE
> **CPT Modifiers**
>
> | 23 | Unusual Anesthesia |
> |----|-------------------|
> | 66 | Surgical Team |

- Anesthesia **Physical Status Modifiers** consist of two characters and are **alphanumeric.** They are used only with CPT codes reporting anesthesia services.

> ### EXAMPLE
> **Physical Status Modifiers**
>
> | P1 | A normal healthy patient |
> |----|-------------------------|
> | P3 | A patient with severe systemic disease |

- **Ambulatory surgery center (ASC)** hospital outpatient modifiers are two digits and are used only when reporting services provided at this type of outpatient facility.

> ### EXAMPLE
> **ASC Modifiers**
>
> | 27 | Multiple outpatient hospital E/M encounters on the same date |
> |----|--|
> | 73 | Discontinued outpatient procedure prior to anesthesia |

GUIDANCE CONNECTION

Read the CPT **Introduction,** subsection **Instructions for Use of the CPT Codebook— Modifiers** on how to properly use modifiers.

CODING BITES

Bookmark *Appendix A* in your CPT code book. This is the section containing the CPT modifiers and their full descriptions. It is important that you reference these prior to using any modifier. Your HCPCS Level II book has its own section that lists those modifiers with their complete descriptions.

CPT Code Modifier
A two-character code that may be appended to a code from the main portion of the CPT book to provide additional information.

Physical Status Modifier
A two-character alphanumeric code used to describe the condition of the patient at the time anesthesia services are administered.

Alphanumeric
Containing both letters and numbers.

Ambulatory Surgery Center (ASC)
A facility specially designed to provide surgical treatments without an overnight stay; also known as a *same-day surgery center.*

- **HCPCS Level II modifiers** are two characters and alphabetic or alphanumeric. They are used to provide additional information about services when appended to CPT and HCPCS Level II codes.

EXAMPLE

HCPCS Level II Modifiers

E1	Upper left eyelid
RT	Right side (of body)

- **Category II modifiers** are two characters: a number followed by the letter P. Only appended to Category II codes, these modifiers provide explanations as to why a particular service should not be included in the qualifications for a specific performance measure.

EXAMPLES

1P	Performance Measure Exclusion Modifier due to Medical Reasons
2P	Performance Measure Exclusion Modifier due to Patient Reasons

Using Modifiers

Using modifiers is, most often, a judgment that you, the coding specialist, will have to make as you review the details of each case. As you analyze the descriptions of the procedures performed, as documented by the physician, and compare them with the descriptions of the codes in the CPT book, you may find that there is more to the story than the code description provides. This is important because it is a coding professional's job to relate the *whole story* of the encounter.

EXAMPLE

Dr. Kennedy determined that Patricia's tear ducts were blocked. He dilated and irrigated both the right and left eyes.

[Remember from medical terminology class, the medical term for the tear duct = lacrimal punctum (plural = puncta). If you don't remember, it is important to use your medical dictionary to ensure you can determine the accurate code or codes.]

CPT Modifier Notation

68801 Dilation of lacrimal punctum, with or without irrigation
(To report a bilateral procedure, use 68801 with modifier 50)

Modifier 50 is used to identify that a service or procedure was performed bilaterally (both sides). If the physician's documentation states that this procedure was done on both sides, you can see that the code description does not include this detail. Therefore, you must add a modifier . . . to tell the whole story.

EXAMPLE

Jason has been deaf in his left ear since he was 16. Today, Dr. Sangar is performing a Bekesy audiometry screening test on his right ear.

92560 Bekesy audiometry; screening

(continued)

Does this code report the test on one ear or two ears? It doesn't state this important detail. How do you know how to report this accurately? The CPT in-section guidelines give you the answer.

CPT Instructional Paragraph

Paragraph above code 92550:

Audiologic Function Tests

". . . All services include testing of both ears. Use modifier 52 if a test is applied to one ear instead of two ears. . . ."

Modifier 52 indicates that the service or procedure, as described, was not completed in full. If both ears are included in the code, but only one ear was tested, then a reduced service was provided. This is why it is so very important to read all of these in-section guidelines, in addition to the those in the front of the section, to help you code accurately. Therefore, if the physician's documentation states that only one ear was examined during this encounter, you must append modifier 52 to tell the whole story.

GUIDANCE CONNECTION

Read the **in-section** Official Guidelines, in the subsection **Repair (Closure),** including paragraph **2. When multiple wounds are repaired.**

LET'S CODE IT! SCENARIO

Dinah Chen, a 21-year-old female, came into the emergency clinic with two lacerations: one on her right hand and the second on her right arm. Dr. Padmore debrided and provided a complicated repair of the 3.1-cm laceration on her upper right arm and a layered closure of a 2.5-cm laceration on her right hand, proximal to the second digit.

Let's Code It!

What exactly did Dr. Padmore do for Dinah Chen? *A complicated repair of a laceration on her upper arm + a layered repair on her hand.* Begin in the CPT Alphabetic Index, and look up

Repair . . . Arm, Upper would make sense, but wait a minute. Dr. Padmore did not actually repair Dinah's arm, with regard to its muscles or tendons, etc. He repaired the laceration. Check this out . . .

Repair . . . Laceration does not work either. None of the anatomical sites listed beneath match arm or hand. Pull out your medical dictionary and check the meaning of laceration: a wound or cut in the tissue. Let's try . . .

Repair . . . Wound—this has possibilities. The three terms showing—Complex, Intermediate, Simple—make sense, and Dr. Padmore did provide a "complicated repair," which could translate to Complex. The Alphabetic Index suggests codes in the range 12001–13160. Turn in the CPT *Main Section* to find code **12001 Simple repair.** How do you know what actually constitutes a complex, intermediate, or simple repair?

Directly above this first code [12001] are Official Guidelines under the subheading **Repair (Closure).** These in-section guidelines explain the definitions of **Simple Repair, Intermediate Repair,** and **Complex Repair**, along with other important details that you need to report these repairs accurately.

The chapter *CPT Surgery Section* will provide you with more in-depth instruction about this.

For this chapter, on Modifiers, you want to focus on paragraph 2 of these *in-section guidelines.* It tells you that, when multiple wounds are repaired, reported with different levels of repair, you will need to append modifier **59 Distinct Procedural Service** to the second code and all thereafter. This will help you understand that, to report Dr. Padmore's services to Dinah Chen, you will submit these codes:

13121	Repair, complex, scalp, arms, and/or legs; 2.6 cm to 7.5 cm
12041-59	Repair, intermediate, wounds of neck, hands, feet and/or external genitalia; 2.5 cm or less, distinct procedural service

22.2 Personnel Modifiers

Personnel Modifier
A modifier adding information about the professional(s) attending to the provision of this procedure or treatment to the patient during this encounter.

As you read through the descriptions of the modifiers, most of them will seem very straightforward. **Personnel modifiers** explain special circumstances relating to the health care professionals involved in the treatment of the patient. These modifiers specifically identify the qualifications of the health care professional who provided the service reported by the code to which this modifier is being attached, while other modifiers identify the provider's special training. You will note that some of the modifier descriptions also include a location as a part of their meaning.

EXAMPLES
Personnel Modifier

62 Two Surgeons

66 Surgical Team

80 Assistant Surgeon

GF **Nonphysician** services in a critical access hospital

AQ Physician providing a service in an unlisted health professional shortage area (HPSA)

Nonphysician
A nonphysician can be a nurse practitioner, certified registered nurse anesthetist, certified registered nurse, clinical nurse specialist, or physician assistant.

Modifier 62 Two Surgeons clearly is used when the operative notes indicate that two surgeons worked side by side, both as primary surgeons, during a procedure. If the modifier is not there to explain that there *were* two primary surgeons involved, how else could the insurance carrier know that receiving two separate claim forms for the same patient on the same day is legitimate? The insurance carrier would certainly think that one of the physicians is fraudulently billing for work done by another. The second claim filed, and possibly even the first one, might be denied or set aside for further determination to find out why the second claim was submitted, and/or the carrier may even initiate a fraud investigation. This little two-digit modifier tells the insurance carrier that no one is cheating and both surgeons actually did provide for the patient.

The same scenario works for other CPT personnel modifiers:

- 66 Surgical Team
- 80 Assistant Surgeon
- 81 Minimum Assistant Surgeon
- 82 Assistant Surgeon (when qualified resident surgeon not available)

Locum Tenens Physician
A physician who fills in, temporarily, for another physician.

Using any of these modifiers, or any of the HCPCS Level II modifiers (see Table 22-1), provides an explanation, very directly and simply, why more than one health care professional is claiming reimbursement for providing service to the same patient on the same date, or the specific qualifications of that professional.

TABLE 22-1 HCPCS Level II Personnel Modifiers

AE	Registered dietitian
AF	Specialty physician
AG	Primary physician
AH	Clinical psychologist
AI	Principal physician of record
AJ	Clinical social worker

AK	Nonparticipating physician
AM	Physician, team member service
AQ	Physician providing service in unlisted HPSA
AR	Physician provider services in a physician scarcity area
AS	Physician assistant, nurse practitioner, or clinical nurse specialist services for assistant at surgery
DA	Oral health assessment by professional other than a dentist
GC	Service performed in part by a resident under the direction of a teaching physician
GE	Service performed by a resident without the presence of a teaching physician under the primary care exception
GF	**Nonphysician** services in a critical access hospital
GJ	"Opt out" physician or practitioner emergency or urgent service
GV	Attending physician not employed or paid under arrangement by the patient's hospice provider
HL	Intern
HM	Less than bachelor degree level
HN	Bachelor's degree level
HO	Master's degree level
HP	Doctoral level
HT	Multidisciplinary team
Q4	Service for ordering/referring physician that qualifies as a service exemption
Q5	Service furnished by a substitute physician under a reciprocal billing arrangement
Q6	Service furnished by a **locum tenens physician**
SA	Nurse practitioner rendering service in collaboration with a physician
SB	Nurse midwife
SD	Services provided by registered nurse with specialized, highly technical home infusion training
SW	Services provided by a certified diabetic educator
TD	Registered nurse (RN)
TE	Licensed practical nurse (LPN) or LVN

 LET'S CODE IT! SCENARIO

Valerie Ferguson, a 43-year-old female, has been diagnosed with endometriosis and is admitted to Midtown Hospital to have Dr. Lissard perform a vaginal, radical hysterectomy. While Valerie is in the operating room (OR) and under anesthesia, Dr. Rasmussen is going to perform an open sling operation for stress incontinence on her bladder, and Dr. Barlow is an assistant surgeon who is there to assist Dr. Lissard. She tolerates both procedures well and is taken back to her room.

Let's Code It!

The codes for these procedures are 58285 and 57288. You will learn more about how to determine these codes in the following chapters. For now, let's focus on the modifiers.

The CPT procedure codes explain what was done for Valerie during this procedure. Afterwards, Dr. Lissard's coder will submit a claim and send it to Valerie's health insurance company, including the services provided for both Dr. Lissard and Dr. Barlow. The coder forgets to append any modifiers.

(continued)

Dr. Rasmussen's coder sent the claim for her work performed for Valerie 2 days later. This claim also fails to include any modifiers.

Now, Bernice Cannaloni, claims adjuster for Valerie's health insurance company, looks at Dr. Rasmussen's claim. Wait a minute. We just paid a claim for two other physicians who stated a totally different surgical procedure was provided to the same patient on the same date! Perhaps someone is trying to defraud this company! An investigation begins, delaying payment by several months until it is all straightened out.

If there were modifiers that could explain what role each of these surgeons played, working side-by-side to care for this patient, the entire fraud investigation and delay in payment could be prevented.

Open your CPT code book to **Appendix A** and read through the list of modifiers to see if any might enable Dr. Lissard's coder and Dr. Rasmussen's coder to more clearly explain the whole story. Take a look at

> **62**   **Two Surgeons:** When 2 surgeons work together as primary surgeons performing distinct part(s) of a procedure, each surgeon should report his/her distinct operative work by adding modifier 62 to the procedure code. . .

This looks perfect to explain this unusual situation, doesn't it?

Now what about Dr. Barlow? How do we explain his role during this procedure? Review the modifiers in **Appendix A** to determine if there are any that will help explain. Take a look at

> **80**   **Assistant Surgeon:** Surgical assistant services may be identified by adding modifier 80 to the usual procedure number(s).

So, Dr. Lissard's coder would report this code:

> **58285-62**   **Vaginal hysterectomy, radical (Schauta type operation); two surgeons**

And Dr. Rasmussen's coder would report this code:

> **57288-62**   **Sling operation for stress incontinence; two surgeons**

And Dr. Barlow's coder would report this:

> **58285-80**   **Vaginal hysterectomy, radical (Schauta type operation); assistant surgeon**

Good job!

Anesthesia Personnel Modifiers

The following modifiers (see Table 22-2), used only with anesthesia codes, are actually HCPCS Level II modifiers. You can see that they provide specific details about the personnel administering the anesthetic to the patient. These details are important for reimbursement as well as responsibility.

TABLE 22-2 Anesthesia Personnel Modifiers

AA	Anesthesia services that are performed personally by anesthesiologist
AD	Medical supervision by a physician: more than four concurrent anesthesia procedures
G8	Monitored anesthesia care (MAC) for deep complex, complicated, or markedly invasive surgical procedure
G9	Monitored anesthesia care for patient who has history of severe cardiopulmonary condition
QK	Medical direction of two, three, or four concurrent anesthesia procedures involving qualified individuals
QS	Monitored anesthesia care (MAC) service
QX	Qualified nonphysician anesthetist with medical direction by a physician
QY	Medical direction of one qualified nonphysician anesthetist by an anesthesiologist
QZ	CRNA service without medical direction by a physician

YOU CODE IT! CASE STUDY

Dr. Charleston, an anesthesiologist, was asked to provide anesthesia care while Dr. Ablione performed a needle biopsy of the pleura of Rosalind Bowman's left lung. Gerald Mathinson, a CRNA, will administer the anesthesia for this procedure, with Dr. Charleston's supervision.

You Code It!

Gerald Mathinson is administering this anesthesia, but he is not an anesthesiologist. Dr. Charleston is not administering the anesthesia for this procedure; however, his presence and expertise are still needed. The procedure code for this anesthesia service is this:

> **00522**   **Anesthesia for closed chest procedures; needle biopsy of pleura**

Good. Now, you must find a way to explain that this was not an anesthesiologist who provided the service, but a CRNA (Certified Registered Nurse Anesthetist), with direction by Dr. Charleston. The code description is correct. You just need to clearly communicate what health care professionals were actually involved in this procedure. A modifier can provide this additional explanation.

Answer:

Did you determine this to be the correct modifier?

> **00522-QX**   **Anesthesia for closed chest procedures; needle biopsy of pleura, CRNA service: with medical direction by a physician**

Good job!!

22.3 Anesthesia Physical Status Modifiers

Anesthesia Physical Status Modifiers are two-character alphanumeric codes: the letter *P* followed by a number. These modifiers identify the condition of the patient at the time anesthesia services were provided and highlight health circumstances that might dramatically affect the anesthesiologist's ability to successfully care for the patient. An explanation of the patient's health level at the time the anesthesiologist administers the service helps the third-party payer get a better understanding of how hard this physician (anesthesiologist) had to work.

For example, if a patient has uncontrolled hypertension at the time anesthesia is administered, the anesthesiologist must monitor the patient more carefully, must perhaps use a different type of anesthetic, and must watch for possible complications that would not be an issue with an otherwise healthy patient. This status modifier, for the most part, does not relate to the reason the patient is having the anesthesia administered but is indicative of the patient's overall health. You can see that, without understanding the difference between treatment issue and overall health, it might be hard for you to identify a patient as "P1 A normal healthy patient" when the person is in your facility to have a diseased gallbladder removed. However, if the patient is *otherwise healthy,* P1 is the correct status modifier.

The Physical Status Modifiers, P1–P6, may be appended *only* to codes from the Anesthesia section of the CPT book, codes 00100–01999.

EXAMPLE

Use of a Physical Status Modifier

Anesthesia for a diagnostic arthroscopy of the knee on a 67-year-old male with diabetes mellitus, controlled well with medication.

     01382-P2

 GUIDANCE CONNECTION

Read the anesthesia Physical Status Modifiers and their descriptions in the **Official Guidelines** located immediately prior to the **Anesthesia** code section in the main part of CPT and/or in **Appendix A.**

All anesthesia codes and *only* anesthesia codes are appended with a Physical Status Modifier, immediately following the anesthesia code.

There may be a case when a CPT modifier must also be used with an anesthesia code. When this is done, the Physical Status Modifier is to be placed closest to the anesthesia code.

> ### EXAMPLE
>
> **Using a Physical Status Modifier with a CPT Modifier**
>
> Anesthesia for a third-degree burn excision, 5% of total body surface area, for a patient with uncontrolled diabetes. The procedure was discontinued due to sudden onset of arrhythmia.
>
> **01952-P3-53**
>
> Modifier **P3** reports that this patient has a severe systemic disease [the uncontrolled diabetes mellitus].
>
> Modifier **53** reports a Discontinued Procedure.

You will read more about the anesthesia Physical Status Modifiers in the chapter *CPT Anesthesia Section*.

 ## LET'S CODE IT! SCENARIO

Carson Crosby, a healthy and fit 18-year-old male, fell from a girder on a construction site, fracturing three ribs and two vertebrae, and sustaining a hairline fracture of his pelvis. Dr. Pollack, an anesthesiologist, was brought in to administer general anesthesia so the body cast could be applied by Dr. Abrams, an orthopedist.

Let's Code It!

You are the professional coding specialist for Dr. Pollack, the anesthesiologist. Our focus in this case is the application of anesthesia modifiers; however, you will need a code to which to append that Physical Status Modifier. So, let's begin with the Alphabetic Index:

Anesthesia

The long list beneath includes mostly anatomical sites. Hmmm. You have two terms: body + cast, so try these. There is listing for *Body;* however, there are two listings for *Cast:*

Cast
 Knee 01420
Cast Application
 Forearm, Wrist, and Hand . . .01860
 Leg 01490
 Pelvis .01130
 Shoulder 01680

Cast Application matches the documentation; however, none of these anatomical areas match. The scenario did mention Carson's pelvis being fractured, so let's start with that code.

01130   **Anesthesia for body cast application or revision**

This is perfect! Now, you learned that all codes from the Anesthesia section require a Physical Status Modifier. So, turn to **Appendix A** and find the heading **Anesthesia Physical Status Modifiers** [it is after modifier **99 Multiple Modifiers**]. Go back to the documentation and look for a description of Carson's current health. This is in regard to his overall health, not in relation to this specific issue. Did you read that the scenario states, "*Carson Crosby, a healthy and fit 18-year-old male*"? Healthy and fit! Review all of the Physical Status Modifier descriptions and determine which is most accurate about Carson's condition during this encounter.

P1   **A normal healthy patient**

(continued)

Good job! Now put them together and you can report this, with confidence, to communicate what Dr. Pollack did for Carson during this session:

01130-P1   **Anesthesia for body cast application or revision; a normal healthy patient**

22.4 Ambulatory Surgery Center Hospital Outpatient Use Modifiers

When you are reporting the code or codes for procedures provided to a patient in a same-day surgery center or outpatient surgery center, you might determine that a modifier may be necessary. In these cases, you will append modifiers from those provided specifically for these locations. The Ambulatory Surgery Center (ASC) Hospital Outpatient Use Modifiers are shown in *Appendix A* of your CPT book, in their own subsection. Some of the modifiers in this subheading are the same as the CPT modifiers. However, there are three additional modifiers specifically for ASC coders. Open your CPT book to *Appendix A* and read along as we review some of these modifiers.

Modifier 27

> **27 Multiple Outpatient Hospital E/M Encounters on the Same Date:** For hospital outpatient reporting purposes, utilization of hospital resources related to separate and distinct E/M encounters performed in multiple outpatient hospital settings on the same date may be reported by adding modifier 27 to each appropriate level outpatient and/or emergency department E/M code(s). This modifier provides a means of reporting circumstances involving evaluation and management services provided by physician(s) in more than one (multiple) outpatient hospital setting(s) (e.g., hospital emergency department, clinic).

Using modifier 27 will not be a common occurrence, but still, it can be complex. So, let's use an example scenario to work through together:

CODING BITES

Many hospitals have outpatient departments providing same-day or outpatient surgical procedures. If the patient is "admitted" and "discharged" the same day, this is coded as an outpatient procedure, using CPT and, when necessary, this group of modifiers.

EXAMPLE

Alexandra Benson, a 41-year-old female, cut her hand and went to the Mulford General Hospital clinic. After Dr. Williams evaluated her hand, he sent her to the emergency department (ED) because the cut was so deep it needed more intense care. Dr. Kinsey evaluated the injury and repaired Alexandra's laceration in the ED.

As the coding specialist for the hospital, you would be responsible for coding the services provided in all your facilities, including the clinic as well as the ED. Alexandra Benson was seen in two different facilities on the same day for the same injury. First, you would code the services that Dr. Williams did—the E/M of Alexandra's injury and his decision to send her to the ED for a higher level of care. Second, you would report the services that Alexandra received in the ED, which certainly included additional evaluation and then the repair of her wound.

    For Dr. Williams, report: 99201-27
    For Dr. Kinsey, report: 99281-27

Without the use of modifier 27, you would have difficulty in getting the claim paid because the third-party payer may think that this is a case of duplicate billing, an error, or fraud.

Modifiers 73 and 74

Occasionally, a planned surgical event is not performed due to circumstances that might put the patient in jeopardy. In such cases, all the preparation was done, the team was ready, and your facility needs to be reimbursed, even though you have not performed the service or treatment. Modifiers 73 and 74 will identify these unusual circumstances.

73 **Discontinued Outpatient Hospital/Ambulatory Surgery Center (ASC) Procedure Prior to the Administration of Anesthesia:** Due to extenuating circumstances or those that threaten the well-being of the patient, the physician may cancel a surgical or diagnostic procedure subsequent to the patient's surgical preparation (including sedation when provided, and being taken to the room where the procedure is to be performed), but prior to the administration of anesthesia (local, regional block(s) or general). Under these circumstances, the intended service that is prepared for but canceled can be reported by its usual procedure number and the addition of modifier 73.

74 **Discontinued Outpatient Hospital/Ambulatory Surgery Center (ASC) Procedure After Administration of Anesthesia:** Due to extenuating circumstances or those that threaten the well-being of the patient, the physician may terminate a surgical or diagnostic procedure after the administration of anesthesia (local, regional block(s) or general), or after the procedure was started (incision made, intubation started, scope inserted, etc.). Under these circumstances, the procedure started, but terminated can be reported by its usual procedure number and the addition of modifier 74.

The extenuating circumstances mentioned are generally accepted situations that would be reasonable to stop a procedure at this late point in time. Prior to the administration of anesthesia, it might be that the nurse, while taking the patient's vital signs, documents that the patient has a fever. It is the standard of care to avoid surgical procedures on a patient with a fever, so the proper thing to do would be to postpone. Once the patient is in the procedure room, and anesthesia has been administered, there may be a need to stop the procedure, such as the patient experiencing a seizure or dramatic drop in blood pressure. Make certain that you not only append one of these modifiers, when appropriate, but also include a special report to explain exactly what happened to make cancelling the procedure the right action to take.

 LET'S CODE IT! SCENARIO

Cole Dennali, a 59-year-old male, was brought into Room 5 to be prepared for a bunionectomy. He changed into a gown, he got into bed, and the nurse took his vital signs. Cole's breathing was labored—it appeared he was having an asthma attack. Dr. Fraumann ordered respiratory therapy to come in and provide a nebulizer treatment. Because general anesthesia could not be administered, the bunionectomy was canceled.

Let's Code It!

Dr. Fraumann and her team were prepared and ready to perform a bunionectomy. However, it is not wise to administer general anesthesia to a patient having difficulty breathing, so the procedure had to be canceled in the best interest of the patient. The facility still deserves to be reimbursed for its time, materials and supplies, and efforts. Therefore, the facility will submit a claim form to Cole's insurance carrier with the code for the bunionectomy and the modifier 73 to indicate that the procedure was canceled *prior to the administration of anesthesia:*

28292-73 **Correction, hallux valgus (bunionectomy), with sesamoidectomy, when performed; with resection of proximal phalanx base, when performed, any method, Discontinued Out-Patient Hospital/Ambulatory Surgery Center (ASC) Procedure Prior to the Administration of Anesthesia**

22.5 Anatomical Site Modifiers

Anatomical site modifiers (see Table 22-3) provide additional specific detail about the target of the service or procedure not provided by the code. These pieces of information are important to include for those providing continuity of care as well as for reimbursement purposes.

- E1–E4 identify right/left/upper/lower eyelids
- F1–FA identify each of the 10 fingers
- T1–TA identify each of the 10 toes
- LC–LD identify portions of the left coronary artery
- RC identifies the right coronary artery
- LT = left
- RT = right

EXAMPLE

28008   Fasciotomy, foot and/or toe

Adding a modifier such as T7 would include very important information for the claim, especially if the patient had a preexisting condition involving a different toe.

T7   Right foot, third digit

Therefore, you would report: **28008-T7 Fasciotomy, right foot, third digit.**

TABLE 22-3 Anatomical Site Modifiers

E1	Upper left eyelid
E2	Lower left eyelid
E3	Upper right eyelid
E4	Lower right eyelid
FA	Left hand, thumb
F1	Left hand, second digit
F2	Left hand, third digit
F3	Left hand, fourth digit
F4	Left hand, fifth digit
F5	Right hand, thumb
F6	Right hand, second digit
F7	Right hand, third digit
F8	Right hand, fourth digit
F9	Right hand, fifth digit
LC	Left circumflex coronary artery
LD	Left anterior descending coronary artery
LT	Left side (i.e., left side of the body)

(continued)

TABLE 22-3 Anatomical Site Modifiers *(continued)*

RC	Right coronary artery
RT	Right side (i.e., right side of the body)
TA	Left foot, great toe
T1	Left foot, second digit
T2	Left foot, third digit
T3	Left foot, fourth digit
T4	Left foot, fifth digit
T5	Right foot, great toe
T6	Right foot, second digit
T7	Right foot, third digit
T8	Right foot, fourth digit
T9	Right foot, fifth digit

 YOU CODE IT! CASE STUDY

Beatrice Burmuda, a 37-year-old female, came to the Upton Ambulatory Surgery Center so that Dr. Thomas could excise a benign tumor from her left foot's big toe (known medically as the great toe). She tolerated the procedure well and was discharged.

You Code It!

Go through the steps to determine the procedure code(s) that should be reported for this encounter between Dr. Thomas and Beatrice Burmuda.

Step #1: Read the case carefully and completely.

Step #2: Abstract the scenario. Which key words or terms describe what service the physician provided to the patient during this encounter?

Step #3: Are there any details missing or incomplete for which you would need to query the physician? [If so, ask your instructor.]

Step #4: Determine the correct CPT procedure code or codes to explain the details about what was provided to the patient during this encounter.

Step #5: Check for any relevant guidance, including reading all of the symbols and notations.

Step #6: Do you need to append any modifiers to ensure complete and accurate information is provided?

Step #7: Double-check your work.

Answer:

The procedure code is 28108. Did you determine the correct modifier?

28108-TA   **Excision or curettage of bone cyst or benign tumor, phalanges of foot, left foot, great toe**

Terrific!

22.6 Service-Related Modifiers

As you learn and expand your abilities to accurately report procedures, services, and treatments provided to the patients of your facility, you will discover that to tell the complete story about what was done, you may need to add a detail or two to the existing code description. Modifiers are created to enable this.

Telemedicine Synchronous Services

We live in a world integrated with technology, enabling us to improve patient care. Now, Skype and other synchronous, interactive, audiovisual software programs permit an encounter between physician and patient who are not in the same room—sometimes not even in the same city.

In the CPT code book's *Appendix P*, you will find a list of 79 CPT codes permitted to be appended with modifier **95** when the service is performed using synchronous electronic communications equipment. These codes are primarily located in the E/M and Medicine sections of CPT, marked with a star (★) symbol to the left of the code.

The documentation for these encounters must confirm that the content of the physician/patient meeting is sufficient to meet the requirements for the code to be reported whether the service was provided face-to-face or with the use of synchronous telemedicine services (as indicated by the appending of modifier 95).

95 **Synchronous Telemedicine Service Rendered Via a Real-Time Interactive Audio and Video Telecommunications System:** Synchronous telemedicine service is defined as a real-time interaction between a physician or other qualified health care professional and a patient who is located at a distant site from the physician or other qualified health care professional. The totality of the communication of information exchanged between the physician or other qualified health care professional and the patient during the course of the synchronous telemedicine service must be of an amount and nature that would be sufficient to meet the key components and/or other requirements of the same service when rendered via a face-to-face interaction. Modifier 95 may only be appended to the services listed in Appendix P. Appendix P is the list of CPT codes for services that are typically performed face-to-face, but may be rendered via a real-time (synchronous) interactive audio and video telecommunications system.

EXAMPLES

Dr. Lappin has been working with Louisa providing psychotherapy to help her deal with panic attacks. Today, they had a good, 30-minute session in the office.

90832 **Psychotherapy, 30 minutes with patient**

Dr. Lappin has been working with Louisa providing psychotherapy to help her deal with panic attacks. Today, Louisa is on a plane, traveling to visit her parents in another state. As she feels a panic attack coming on, she uses the airplane's WiFi system to Skype with Dr. Lappin. They spend 30 minutes talking things through and helping Louisa get through.

90832-95 **Psychotherapy, 30 minutes with patient, synchronous telemedicine service rendered via a real-time interactive audio and video telecommunications system**

By appending modifier 95, you are clearly communicating the difference in Dr. Lappin's service to her patient.

TABLE 22-4 Modifiers for Multiple Wounds

A1	Dressing for one wound
A2	Dressing for two wounds
A3	Dressing for three wounds
A4	Dressing for four wounds
A5	Dressing for five wounds
A6	Dressing for six wounds
A7	Dressing for seven wounds
A8	Dressing for eight wounds
A9	Dressing for nine or more wounds

Wound Care

Typically, a dressing change is required for a wound many times throughout the healing process. In addition, it is not unusual that a patient might have more than one wound that needs care at the same time. Therefore, to make the coding process easier and more efficient, one modifier can explain the extent of such care so that listing the same code multiple times is not necessary. The list in Table 22-4 contains the modifiers for multiple wounds.

  LET'S CODE IT! SCENARIO

Ted Kercher, a 33-year-old male, is a firefighter who sustained partial-thickness burns the entire length of his right arm when something exploded. He comes in to see Dr. Taggert to have the dressings changed on four wounds.

Let's Code It!

Ted comes in to have his *dressings changed* on *four* burn wounds. First, you must find the CPT code for the procedure; second, you can address the modifier. Let's go to the Alphabetic Index and look up *dressings*. You find

Dressings
Burns 16020–16030
Change
    Anesthesia 15852

You know that Dr. Taggert is changing Ted's dressings; however, there is nothing in the notes that states anesthesia was involved. In addition, Ted's wounds are burns, so let's turn to the numeric listing and carefully read the descriptions for the codes shown next to *burns*. Do you agree that this is the best code?

16025   **Dressings and/or debridement of partial-thickness burns, initial or subsequent; medium (e.g., whole face or whole extremity, or 5% to 10% total body surface area)**

The notes indicate that Dr. Taggert changed the dressings for *four wounds*. So rather than just list this code four times, we can use a modifier to communicate this fact: 16025-A4 tells the whole story clearly.

16025-A4   **Dressings and/or debridement of partial-thickness burns, initial or subsequent; medium (e.g., whole face or whole extremity, or 5% to 10% total body surface area); four wounds dressed**

Good work!

TABLE 22-5 ESRD/Dialysis Modifiers

CB	Service ordered by a renal dialysis facility (RDF) physician as part of the beneficiary's benefit is not part of the composite rate and is separately reimbursable
CD	**AMCC** test has been ordered by an ESRD facility or MCP physician that is part of the composite rate and is not separately billable
CE	AMCC test has been ordered by an ESRD facility or MCP physician that is a composite rate test but is beyond the normal frequency covered under the rate and is separately reimbursable based on medical necessity
CF	AMCC test has been ordered by an ESRD facility or MCP physician that is not part of the composite rate and is separately billable
EM	Emergency reserve supply (for ESRD benefit only)
G1	Most recent **urea reduction ratio (URR)** reading of less than 60
G2	Most recent URR reading of 60 to 64.9
G3	Most recent URR reading of 65 to 69.9
G4	Most recent URR reading of 70 to 74.9
G5	Most recent URR reading of 75 or greater
G6	ESRD patient for whom less than six dialysis sessions have been provided in a month

Ophthalmology/Optometry

Sometimes, when ophthalmic or optometric services are provided, more detail is necessary to ensure proper reimbursement. Following are the HCPCS Level II modifiers used with these services:

AP Determination of refractive state was not performed in the course of diagnostic ophthalmologic examination
LS FDA-monitored intraocular lens implant
PL Progressive addition lenses
VP Aphakic patient

ESRD/Dialysis

Dialysis and other services for a patient with renal conditions, including those with **end-stage renal disease (ESRD)**, may involve extenuating circumstances requiring further explanation. The dialysis modifiers in Table 22-5 provide that information.

AMCC
Automated Multi-Channel Chemistry—Automated organ disease panel tests performed on the same patient, by the same provider, on the same day.

Urea Reduction Ratio (URR)
A formula to determine the effectiveness of hemodialysis treatment.

End-Stage Renal Disease (ESRD)
Chronic, irreversible kidney disease requiring regular treatments.

  LET'S CODE IT! SCENARIO

Amie Gander, a 39-year-old female, was diagnosed with ESRD. Dr. Linnger prescribed her treatments to begin on May 29 at the Southside Dialysis Center (SDC). Code for the services provided at SDC for the month of May.

Let's Code It!

End-stage renal disease (ESRD) services are billed on a monthly basis. However, Amie only received 3 days of services during the month of May (May 29, May 30, and May 31) from Southside Dialysis Center. In the Alphabetic Index, you will find:

End-Stage Renal Disease Services
Dialysis 90951-90970
   Inpatient 90935, 90937, 90945, 90947
   Home 90963-90966
   Outpatient 90951-90962
Less Than a Full Month 90967-90970

(continued)

After reading the complete code descriptions in the suggested range, you find the best procedure code to be this:

90970 **End-stage renal disease (ESRD) related services (less than full month), per day; for patients twenty years of age and over**

This means you will have to list the code three times because the code description says per day. Are there any modifiers than can help you communicate this situation?

G6 **ESRD patient for whom less than six dialysis sessions have been provided in a month**

The modifier that will complete this report is G6 because she has had fewer than six sessions in 1 month: **90970-G6; 90970-G6; 90970-G6** *or* **90970-G6 × 3**.

Good job!

Habilitative and Rehabilitative Services

In the 2018 CPT code set, two modifiers were added:

96 **Habilitative Services**
97 **Rehabilitative Services**

These modifiers would most often be appended to codes from the *Physical Medicine and Rehabiliation* subsection of the Medicine section. More about this in the chapter *CPT Medicine Section.*

Pharmaceuticals

Pharmaceuticals, the industry term for medications, are items that must be monitored very carefully: the purchase, the storage, and the dispensing. The modifiers in Table 22-6 provide important information that must be tracked.

Modifier RD Drug provided to beneficiary, but not administered "incident to" indicates that a particular pharmaceutical was provided to the patient but not administered. For example, the nurse brings the patient's pills into his room to administer them when she notices he has a rash. She notifies the physician on call and he orders the medication stopped to investigate if the patient is allergic. Once the pills have been taken out of the pharmacy, they cannot be returned. If the patient does not take them, they must be discarded but still accounted for in the system and billing.

Liters per Minute (LPM)
The measurement of how many liters of a drug or chemical are provided to the patient in 60 seconds.

TABLE 22-6 Pharmaceutical Modifiers

JW	Drug amount discarded/not administered to any patient
KD	Drug or biological infused through DME
KO	Single drug unit dose formulation
KP	First drug of a multiple drug unit dose formulation
KQ	Second or subsequent drug of a multiple drug unit dose formulation
QE	Prescribed amount of oxygen is less than 1 **liter per minute (LPM)**
QF	Prescribed amount of oxygen exceeds 4 LPM and portable oxygen is prescribed
QG	Prescribed amount of oxygen is greater than 4 LPM
QH	Oxygen-conserving device is being used with an oxygen delivery system
RD	Drug provided to beneficiary, but not administered "incident to"
SL	State-supplied vaccine
SV	Pharmaceuticals delivered to patient's home but not utilized

TABLE 22-7 Items/Services Modifiers

AU	Item furnished in conjunction with a urologic, ostomy, or tracheostomy supply
AV	Item furnished in conjunction with a prosthetic device, prosthetic or orthotic
BA	Item furnished in conjunction with **parenteral enteral nutrition (PEN)** services
BL	Special acquisition of blood and blood products
BO	Orally administered nutrition, not by feeding tube
EY	No physician or other licensed health care provider order for this item or service
FX	X-ray taken using film
GK	Reasonable and necessary item/item associated with GA or GZ modifier
GL	Medically unnecessary upgrade provided instead of standard item, no charge, no advance beneficiary notice (ABN)
GY	Item or service statutorily excluded or does not meet the definition of any Medicare benefit, not a contract benefit
GZ	Item or service expected to be denied as not reasonable and necessary
KS	Glucose monitor supply for diabetic beneficiary not treated with insulin
KZ	New coverage not implemented by managed care
Q1	Routine clinical service provided in a clinical research study that is in an approved clinical research study
QW	**Clinical Laboratory Improvement Amendment (CLIA)** waived test
SC	Medically necessary service or supply
SF	Second opinion ordered by a professional review organization (PRO)
SM	Second surgical opinion
SN	Third surgical opinion
SQ	Item ordered by home health

Modifier SV Pharmaceuticals delivered to patient's home but not utilized might be used by a mail-order pharmaceutical service to show that the medications were shipped and delivered to the patient's house but have nothing to do with how, when, or if the patient uses those drugs.

Parenteral Enteral Nutrition (PEN)
Nourishment delivered using a combination of means other than the gastrointestinal tract (such as IV) in addition to via the gastrointestinal tract.

EXAMPLES

RD   Drug provided to beneficiary, but not administered "incident to"
SV   Pharmaceuticals delivered to patient's home but not utilized

Clinical Laboratory Improvement Amendment (CLIA)
Federal legislation created for the monitoring and regulation of clinical laboratory procedures.

Items/Services

The modifiers in Table 22-7 cover a variety of circumstances relating to the provision of an item or a service.

  LET'S CODE IT! SCENARIO

Oscar Barkley, a 57-year-old male, was diagnosed with type 2 diabetes mellitus. Dr. Habersham wants to try a new medication to control Oscar's blood glucose levels and delay, or avoid, putting him on insulin. Dr. Habersham gives Oscar the prescription for the medication and a second prescription for a home blood glucose monitor.

(continued)

The code you will report for the provision of the home glucose monitor is this:

E0607   **Home blood glucose monitor**

Now, you need a way to explain that this monitor is for a patient who is a non-insulin-dependent diabetic. Sounds like the perfect job for a modifier!

Did you determine this to be the correct modifier?

E0607-KS   **Home blood glucose monitor; Glucose monitor supply for diabetic beneficiary not treated with insulin**

Purchase/Rental Items

Often, when durable medical equipment (DME) is supplied, the patient has a choice to rent the equipment or purchase it outright. This will depend upon the patient's personal situation. A modifier (see Table 22-8) provides important details, especially to the payor.

 YOU CODE IT! CASE STUDY

Darryl Rosen, an 81-year-old male, fell and broke his hip last winter. Even though it healed, Darryl is still experiencing difficulty walking long distances. Dr. Sorrel prescribed a power wheelchair for him. Darryl decided to purchase a lightweight, portable, motorized/power wheelchair from Hammermill Medical Supply Systems.

You Code It!

Go through the steps of coding, and determine the code or codes that should be reported for the supply of Darryl Rosen's new equipment. [*NOTE:* The wheelchair is reported with an HCPCS Level II code.]

Step #1: Read the case carefully and completely.

Step #2: Abstract the scenario. Which key words or terms describe what service the physician provided to the patient during this encounter?

Step #3: Are there any details missing or incomplete for which you would need to query the physician? [If so, ask your instructor.]

Step #4: Determine the correct CPT procedure code or codes to explain the details about what was provided to the patient during this encounter.

Step #5: Check for any relevant guidance, including reading all of the symbols and notations.

Step #6: Do you need to append any modifiers to ensure complete and accurate information is provided?

Step #7: Double-check your work.

Answer:

The code for the provision of the wheelchair is K0012. Did you determine this to be the correct modifier?

K0012-KH   **Lightweight portable motorized/power wheelchair; DMEPOS item, initial claim, purchase or first month rental**

Good work!

TABLE 22-8 Purchase/Rental Items Modifiers

BP	The beneficiary has been informed of the purchase and rental options and has elected to purchase the item
BR	The beneficiary has been informed of the purchase and rental options and has elected to rent the item
BU	The beneficiary has been informed of the purchase and rental options and after 30 days has not informed the supplier of his/her decision
KH	DMEPOS item, initial claim, purchase or first month rental
KI	DMEPOS item, second or third month rental
KJ	DMEPOS item, parenteral enteral nutrition (PEN) pump or capped rental, months four to fifteen
KR	Rental item, billing for partial month
LL	Lease/rental (use when DME rental payments are to be applied against the purchase price)
MS	Six-month maintenance and servicing fee for reasonable and necessary parts and labor not covered under any manufacturer or supplier warranty
NR	New when rented
RR	Rental DME

Deceased Patient

Should a patient expire (die) while services are in the process of being rendered, certainly the situation changes and there must be some indication of the death. The following modifiers are used in such circumstances:

CA   Procedure payable only in the inpatient setting when performed emergently on an outpatient who expires prior to admission

QL   Patient pronounced dead after ambulance called

Claims and Documentation

The modifiers shown in Table 22-9 directly provide additional information relating to the claims and documentation involved in certain health care encounters.

  YOU CODE IT! CASE STUDY

Jonny Craig, a 45-year-old male, had a mass on his left upper eyelid. Dr. Neilsen performed a biopsy on the eyelid. The pathology report determined it was a benign neoplasm. Gwen Sanders, the professional coding specialist, mistakenly put code 68710-E1 on the claim form instead of 67810-E1. She didn't realize this until the claim came back denied.

You Code It!

What additional modifier should Gwen append to code 67810-E1 on the second claim form, which she needs to submit as a corrected claim?

Answer:

Did you determine this to be the correct code?

> **67810-E1-CC**   **Incisional biopsy of eyelid skin including lid margin; upper left, eyelid, Procedure code change because an incorrect code was filed**

Good job!!

TABLE 22-9 Claims and Documentation Modifiers

CC	Procedure code change (used to indicate that a procedure code previously submitted was changed either for an administrative reason or because an incorrect code was filed)
GA	Waiver of liability statement issued, individual case
GB	Claim being resubmitted for payment because it is no longer covered under a global payment
KB	Beneficiary requested upgrade for ABN, more than four modifiers identified on claim
KX	Requirements specified in the medical policy have been met
QP	Documentation is on file showing that the laboratory test(s) was ordered individually or ordered as a CPT-recognized panel other than automated profile codes 80002–80019, G0058, G0059, and G0060

TABLE 22-10 Family Services Modifiers

EP	Service provided as part of Medicaid early periodic screening diagnosis and treatment (EPSDT) program
FP	Service provided as part of family planning program
G7	Pregnancy resulted from rape or incest or pregnancy certified by physician as life threatening
TL	Early intervention/individualized family service plan (IFSP)
TM	Individualized education plan (IEP)
TR	School-based individualized education program (IEP) services provided outside the public school district responsible for the student

TABLE 22-11 Treatments/Screenings Modifiers

GG	Performance and payment of a screening mammogram and diagnostic mammogram on the same patient, same day
GH	Diagnostic mammogram converted from screening mammogram on same day
SH	Second concurrently administered infusion therapy
SJ	Third, or more, concurrently administered infusion therapy

Family Services

Early and Periodic Screening, Diagnostic, and Treatment (EPSDT)
A Medicaid preventive health program for children under 21.

Services provided under Medicaid's **Early and Periodic Screening, Diagnostic, and Treatment (EPSDT)** program must be identified with the EP modifier, shown in Table 22-10. In addition, other family services may benefit from further explanation by the use of one of the modifiers found in that list.

Treatments/Screenings

The modifiers shown in Table 22-11 are directly related to the provision of mammography and infusion therapeutic services.

 LET'S CODE IT! SCENARIO

Cheryl Baxett, a 41-year-old female, came into the hospital for her annual screening mammogram. Dr. Ogden ordered the screening to be completed with computer-aided detection, due to a prior history of breast cancer. Later that day, after the images were analyzed, Dr. Ogden diagnosed her with a considerable mass in her left breast.

Let' Code It!

Cheryl came in for a screening mammogram with computer-aided detection on her left breast. Let's go to the Alphabetic Index of the CPT book and find the best, most appropriate procedure code:

(continued)

77067 Screening mammography, bilateral (two view film study of each breast), including computer-aided detection (CAD) when performed

Once the results of the mammogram became the basis for a decision to have surgery, the screening mammogram became a diagnostic mammogram. Cheryl's insurance carrier accepts HCPCS Level II codes and modifiers, so you must adapt the definition of the mammogram from screening to diagnostic by appending a modifier: 77065-GH. The **GH** modifier means that a **diagnostic mammogram was converted from a screening mammogram on the same day.**

77065-GH-LT Diagnostic mammography, including computer-aided detection (CAD) when performed; unilateral, diagnostic mammogram converted from screening mammogram on same day, left side

77067-52-RT Screening mammography, bilateral (two view film study of each breast), including computer-aided detection (CAD) when performed, reduced services, right side

Great job!

Transportation

Table 22-12 has the modifiers that provide additional details with relation to transportation services provided to patients.

Funded Programs

When a service or treatment is provided under the terms or conditions of a formalized program or plan, the services must be identified so that statistical tracking can be accomplished accurately and reimbursement is not received from two sources. The modifiers shown in Table 22-13 enable such tracking.

TABLE 22-12 Transportation Modifiers

GM	Multiple patients on one ambulance trip
LR	Laboratory round trip
QM	Ambulance service provided under arrangement by a provider of services
QN	Ambulance service furnished directly by a provider of services
TK	Extra patient or passenger, non-ambulance
TP	Medical transport, unloaded vehicle
TQ	Basic life support transport by a volunteer ambulance provider

TABLE 22-13 Funding Modifiers

GN	Services delivered under an outpatient speech language pathology plan of care
GO	Services delivered under an outpatient occupational therapy plan of care
GP	Services delivered under an outpatient physical therapy plan of care
H9	Court-ordered

(continued)

TABLE 22-13 Funding Modifiers   *(continued)*

HA	Child/adolescent program
HB	Adult program, nongeriatric
HC	Adult program, geriatric
HE	Mental health program
HF	Substance abuse program
HG	Opioid addiction treatment program
HH	Integrated mental health/substance abuse program
HI	Integrated mental health and mental retardation/developmental disabilities program
HJ	Employee assistance program
HK	Specialized mental health programs for high-risk populations
HU	Funded by child welfare agency
HV	Funded by state addictions agency
HW	Funded by state mental health agency
HX	Funded by county/local agency
HY	Funded by juvenile justice agency
HZ	Funded by criminal justice agency
SE	State and/or federally funded programs/services

Individual/Group

Most often, modifiers for individuals or groups are going to be used in conjunction with psychiatric and psychotherapeutic codes to clarify how many patients were involved in the session. The modifiers shown in Table 22-14 relate to the number, and sometimes the type, of patient(s) being helped at one time.

Prosthetics

When services are provided relating to the supply or adjustment of a prosthetic device, you might have to include additional information by using one of the modifiers shown in Table 22-15.

TABLE 22-14 Individual/Group Modifiers

HQ	Group setting
HR	Family/couple with client present
HS	Family/couple without client present
TJ	Program group, child and/or adolescent
TT	Individualized service provided to more than one patient in same setting
UN	Two patients served
UP	Three patients served
UQ	Four patients served
UR	Five patients served
US	Six or more patients served

TABLE 22-15 Prosthetics Modifiers

K0	Lower extremity prosthesis functional level 0—does not have the ability or potential to ambulate or transfer safely with or without assistance and prosthesis does not enhance his or her quality of life or mobility
K1	Lower extremity prosthesis functional level 1—has the ability or potential to use a prosthesis for transfers or ambulation on level surfaces at fixed cadence, typical of the limited and unlimited household ambulatory
K2	Lower extremity prosthesis functional level 2—has the ability or potential for ambulation with the ability to traverse low-level environmental barriers such as curbs, stairs, uneven surfaces, typical of limited community ambulatory
K3	Lower extremity prosthesis functional level 3—has the ability or potential for ambulation with variable cadence. Typical of the community ambulatory who has the ability to traverse most environmental barriers and may have vocational, therapeutic, or exercise activity that demands prosthetic utilization beyond simple locomotion
K4	Lower extremity prosthesis functional level 4—has the ability or potential for prosthetic ambulation that exceeds the basic ambulation skills, exhibiting high impact, stress, or energy levels, typical of the prosthetic demands of the child, active adult, or athlete
KM	Replacement of facial prosthesis including new impression/moulage
KN	Replacement of facial prosthesis using previous master model

 LET'S CODE IT! SCENARIO

Sam Tanner, a 29-year-old male, returned home after being in a rehabilitation center for 3 months. He had a below-knee amputation (BKA) after he was hurt in a rescue mission following a major hurricane. Alice Conner fitted him for an initial, below-knee patellar tendon bearing (PTB) type socket prosthesis because he has the ability to walk on and even maneuver over such low obstacles as sidewalk curbs and stairs.

Let's Code It!

Alice Conner ordered and supplied an *initial, below-knee PTB type socket prosthesis*. In the HCPCS Level II Alphabetic Index, you find

Prosthesis
  Fitting, L5400–L5460, L6380–L6388

The notes did say that Alice fitted him, so this should provide a good lead. When you get to this section, beginning with L5400, you find a code whose description matches the notes very well:

L5500   **Initial, below knee PTB type socket, non-alignable system, pylon, no cover, SACH foot, plaster socket, direct formed**

(*NOTE:* SACH stands for solid ankle, cushioned heel.)
  You also have to support the service with a modifier to explain Sam's abilities:

K2   **Lower extremity prosthesis functional level 2—has the ability or potential for ambulation with the ability to traverse low-level environmental barriers such as curbs, stairs, or uneven surfaces. Typical of the limited community ambulator**

And report this as

L5500-K2   **Initial, below knee PTB type socket, non-alignable system, pylon, no cover, SACH foot, plaster socket, direct formed, lower extremity prosthesis functional level 2**

Durable Medical Equipment

When the services relate to the provision of or adjustments to a piece of durable medical equipment (DME), a modifier from Table 22-16 may be needed to clarify a certain condition or circumstance.

TABLE 22-16 DME Modifiers

KA	Add on option/accessory for wheelchair
KC	Replacement of special power wheelchair interface
KF	Item designated by FDA as Class III device
NB	Nebulizer system, any type, FDA-cleared for use with specific drug
NR	New when rented
NU	New equipment
RA	Replacement of a DME, orthotic, or prosthetic item
RB	Replacement of a part of a DME, orthotic, or prosthetic item furnished as part of a repair
TW	Backup equipment
UE	Used durable medical equipment (DME)

YOU CODE IT! CASE STUDY

On January 5, a respiratory suction pump was provided to Teresa Christley, who was diagnosed with emphysema. On January 6, another suction pump was delivered to Teresa. The first unit had to be replaced because of a defective piece.

You Code It!

Go through the steps, and determine the HCPCS Level II code or codes that should be reported for these services for Teresa Christley.

Step #1: Read the case carefully and completely.

Step #2: Abstract the scenario. Which key words or terms describe what service the physician provided to the patient during this encounter?

Step #3: Are there any details missing or incomplete for which you would need to query the physician? [If so, ask your instructor.]

Step #4: Determine the correct CPT procedure code or codes to explain the details about what was provided to the patient during this encounter.

Step #5: Check for any relevant guidance, including reading all of the symbols and notations.

Step #6: Do you need to append any modifiers to ensure complete and accurate information is provided?

Step #7: Double-check your work.

Answer:

The code for the provision of the pump is E0600. Did you determine the correct modifier for the second claim?

Jan 5:	E0600	Respiratory suction pump, home model, portable or stationary, electric
Jan 6:	E0600-RA	Respiratory suction pump, home model, portable or stationary, electric; replacement of DME

Location

The following modifiers describe situations when you will need to clarify the location at which services were provided:

PN Non-excepted service provided at an off-campus, outpatient, provider-based department of a hospital

PO Expected services provided at off-campus, outpatient, provider-based department of a hospital

SG	Ambulatory surgical center (ASC) facility service
SU	Procedure performed in physician's office (i.e., to denote use of facility and equipment)
TN	Rural/outside providers' customary service area

Podiatric Care

There are times when particular services are recategorized, determined by certain signs and/or symptoms that the patient may be exhibiting. The following list identifies modifiers used to indicate some of these circumstances when a podiatrist provides treatment to a patient:

Q7	One **class A finding**
Q8	Two **class B findings**
Q9	One class B and two **class C findings**

Recording

The following modifiers indicate the use of recording equipment as a part of the service, treatment, or procedure provided to the patient:

QC	Single-channel monitoring
QD	Recording and storage in solid-state memory by a digital recorder
QT	Recording and storage on tape by an analog tape recorder

Other Services

The modifiers shown in Table 22-17 do not seem to fit into any of the other categories we have established. Review all the modifiers in the list, and see if you can come up with examples of how and when they would be used.

Class A Finding
Nontraumatic amputation of a foot or an integral skeletal portion.

Class B Finding
Absence of a posterior tibial pulse; absence or decrease of hair growth; thickening of the nail, discoloration of the skin, and/or thinning of the skin texture; and/or absence of a posterior pedal pulse.

Class C Finding
Edema, burning sensation, temperature change (cold feet), abnormal spontaneous sensations in the feet, and/or limping.

TABLE 22-17 Other Services Modifiers

AT	Acute treatment (to be used only with 98940, 98941, 98942)
EJ	Subsequent claims for a defined course of therapy
ET	Emergency services
GQ	Via asynchronous telecommunications system
GT	Via interactive audio and video telecommunication systems
GW	Service not related to the hospice patient's terminal condition
Q2	HCFA/ORD demonstration project procedure/service
Q3	Live kidney donor surgery and related services
QJ	Services/items provided to a prisoner or patient in state or local custody, however the state or local government, as applicable, meets the requirements in 42 CFR 411.4(b)
SK	Member of high-risk population (use only with immunization codes)
ST	Related to trauma or injury
SY	Persons who are in close contact with member of high-risk population (use with immunization codes only)
TC	Technical component
TG	Complex/high-tech level of care
TH	Obstetrical treatment/services, prenatal or postpartum
TS	Follow-up service
UF	Services provided in the morning
UG	Services provided in the afternoon
UH	Services provided in the evening
UJ	Services provided at night
UK	Services provided on behalf of the client to someone other than the client (collateral relationship)

TABLE 22-18 Medicaid Services Modifiers

U1	Medicaid level of care 1, as defined by each state
U2	Medicaid level of care 2, as defined by each state
U3	Medicaid level of care 3, as defined by each state
U4	Medicaid level of care 4, as defined by each state
U5	Medicaid level of care 5, as defined by each state
U6	Medicaid level of care 6, as defined by each state
U7	Medicaid level of care 7, as defined by each state
U8	Medicaid level of care 8, as defined by each state
U9	Medicaid level of care 9, as defined by each state
UA	Medicaid level of care 10, as defined by each state
UB	Medicaid level of care 11, as defined by each state
UC	Medicaid level of care 12, as defined by each state
UD	Medicaid level of care 13, as defined by each state

Medicaid Services

Each state administers its own version of the federal Medicaid program and determines its own specific descriptions of the different levels of care. To maintain consistency, HCPCS Level II has the modifiers shown in Table 22-18 that can be used nationwide—even though the description of each modifier will change, as defined by each state.

Special Rates

The following two modifiers are used to indicate that a service or procedure was provided to a patient during an unusual time frame, that is, not during regular working hours:

TU   Special payment rate, overtime
TV   Special payment rates, holidays/weekends

22.7 Sequencing Multiple Modifiers

There may be circumstances where one case is so complex, unusual, or special that you need more than one modifier to explain the whole scenario.

Two or Three Modifiers Needed

There are occasions when a particular procedure code will require the amendment of more than one modifier. In these cases, you must place the modifiers in a particular order depending upon what each modifier represents. Let's review a few different situations.

Generally, the CPT modifier that most directly changes, or modifies, the specific code description will be placed closest to the procedure code. These are called **service-related modifiers** because they change, or alter, the description of the service (such as 23 Unusual Anesthesia or 32 Mandated services), rather than those modifiers that explain personnel in attendance (such as 62 Two Surgeons) or an event (such as 57 Decision for Surgery).

Service-Related Modifier
A modifier relating to a change or adjustment of a procedure or service provided.

> ### EXAMPLE
> Dr. Weaver, and his surgical team, began the pancreatic transplantation procedure on Kenneth. Once the incision had been made, the patient's heartbeat became erratic and could not be brought back under control, so the procedure was discontinued. The procedure code reported requires two modifiers: 48554-53-66.
>
> *(continued)*

Modifier 53 explains that the procedure was discontinued. This modifier relates the fact that everyone involved, including the facility, prepared for the surgery and began the procedure but had to stop. This will explain why, sometime down the road, this same patient may again go through a pancreatic transplantation. In addition, this modifier will enable the health care professionals and the facility to get some reimbursement to cover the cost of the services they did provide.

Modifier 66, on the other hand, explains that a surgical team was participating in the surgery. This does not affect the specific code description of the procedure. It explains why the third-party payer will need to reimburse more than one surgeon. This modifier also may help to prevent the claim for each of those additional team members from being denied, or placed into determination, slowing the reimbursement process and avoiding an audit.

When an HCPCS Level II modifier is used in addition to a CPT modifier, the CPT modifier is placed closest to the procedure code, and the HCPCS Level II modifier follows.

EXAMPLE

24201-76-LT   Removal of foreign body, upper arm or elbow area; deep, repeat procedure by same physician, left side

There is an exception to this rule when reporting anesthesia services. The Physical Status Modifier always is reported closest to the anesthesia procedure code.

EXAMPLE

Dr. Cowles administered the general anesthesia when Dr. Dean had to take the patient back into the surgery unexpectedly to attend to a problem with the replantation procedure for the patient's index finger of his right hand. For Dr. Cowles, the code is 01810-P1-76.

 LET'S CODE IT! SCENARIO

Dr. Tuders performed a bilateral osteotomy on the shaft of Arlis Richardson's femur. Another surgeon performed the same procedure on Arlis 2 weeks ago but was unsuccessful, so Dr. Tuders repeated the procedure. As an expert in this procedure, he was brought in to perform the surgery only and will not be involved in any preoperative or postoperative care of the patient.

Let's Code It!

To accurately report Dr. Tuders's surgical services to Arlis Richardson, you would need the following:

27448 **Osteotomy, femur, shaft, or supracondylar; without fixation**
-50 **Modifier to report that it was a bilateral procedure**
-54 **Modifier to report Dr. Tuders was providing surgical care only**
-77 **Modifier to report that this is a repeat procedure by another physician**

Therefore, the code you report will look like this:

27448-50-54-77

More Than Three Modifiers Needed

The outpatient claim form, upon which you will record your chosen codes and other information to request reimbursement from the third-party payer, has a limited amount of space in which to place the necessary information, particularly when it comes to the inclusion of modifiers. Some third-party payers do not permit multiple modifiers to be listed on the same line as the CPT code. Therefore, should your case require three or more modifiers to completely explain all of the circumstances involved, you can use modifier 99.

> **99**   **Multiple Modifiers:** Under certain circumstances two or more modifiers may be necessary to completely delineate a service. In such situations modifier 99 should be added to the basic procedure, and other applicable modifiers may be listed as part of the description of the service.

Sequencing Multiple Modifiers

When you need more than one modifier with a procedure or service code, you must place the modifiers in order of specificity, with the most important, most precise modifier closest to the main code.

 YOU CODE IT! CASE STUDY

Dr. Cabbot drained an abscess on Mark Swanson's left thumb and another on his second finger. Both were simple procedures.

You Code It!

Go through the steps of coding, and determine the code or codes that should be reported for this encounter between Dr. Cabbot and Mark Swanson.

Step #1: Read the case carefully and completely.

Step #2: Abstract the scenario. Which key words or terms describe what service the physician provided to the patient during this encounter?

Step #3: Are there any details missing or incomplete for which you would need to query the physician? [If so, ask your instructor.]

Step #4: Determine the correct CPT procedure code or codes to explain the details about what was provided to the patient during this encounter.

Step #5: Check for any relevant guidance, including reading all of the symbols and notations.

Step #6: Do you need to append any modifiers to ensure complete and accurate information is provided?

Step #7: Double-check your work.

Answer:

The correct procedure code for the I&D of the abscess is 10060. Did you determine the correct modifiers?

> **10060-FA**   Incision and drainage of abscess, simple or single; left hand, thumb
> **10060-F1-59**   Incision and drainage of abscess, simple or single; left hand, second digit; separate procedure

Without the modifiers *FA* for left hand, thumb; *F1* for left hand, second digit; and *59* for distinct procedural service, the claim form could not clearly communicate that Dr. Cabbot did work on two different fingers.

22.8 Supplemental Reports

Remember, *documentation* is your watchword. It is the backbone of the health information management industry. In many situations when a modifier is used, a **supplemental report** is needed for additional clarification.

Generally, the modifier itself provides a certain amount of explanation; however, the insurance carrier wants more details. You can be efficient and send the specific information along with the claim, or you can wait until the carrier requests additional information. Either way, you will have to supply all the facts. However, if you wait to be asked, you will be delaying payment to your facility.

You will need to use your judgment, so as you look at the modifiers you include to tell the whole story, review the codes and modifiers to evaluate if there are any unanswered questions so you can use a supplemental report to answer them.

Supplemental Report
A letter or report written by the attending physician or other health care professional to provide additional clarification or explanation.

EXAMPLES

Here a just a few of the modifiers that might need a supplemental report to ensure complete communications.

22	**Increased Procedural Services** . . . *what was it that required the additional time and effort?*
23	**Unusual Anesthesia** . . . *why was this necessary?*
52	**Reduced Services** . . . *why couldn't the physician complete the planned procedure in full?*
53	**Discontinued Procedure** . . . *why did the physician have to stop?*

 LET'S CODE IT! SCENARIO

Aden Carrington, a 9-year-old boy, had a superficial cut, about 3.3 cm, on his left cheek, after being in a car accident and hit by broken glass. Dr. Kern is ready to perform a simple repair of the wound, but she is very concerned. Aden has Tourette's syndrome, which causes him to jerk or move abruptly, especially when nervous. Although anesthesia is not typically used for a simple repair of a superficial wound, Dr. Kern administers general anesthesia. Sharon Haverty, a CRNA, assists Dr. Kern with monitoring Aden during the procedure.

Let's Code It!

Dr. Kern performed a *simple repair* of Aden's *superficial wound* on his *face*. Go to the Alphabetic Index in your CPT code book and look up *Repair*. As you look down the list of anatomical sites, you do not see face or cheek listed. You know that the repair was simple, and when you look at that listing, you note the direction "*See* Integumentary System, Repair, Simple." Once you go to that listing, you find the suggested codes 12001–12021. Let's take a look at the complete description in the numeric listing.

12011 **Simple repair of superficial wounds of face, ears, eyelids, nose, lips and/or mucous membranes; 2.5 cm or less**

The basic description matches the notes exactly. However, several choices are determined by the size of the wound. The notes state that Aden's wound was 3.3 cm. This brings you to the correct code:

12013 **Simple repair of superficial wounds of face, ears, eyelids, nose, lips and/or mucous membranes; 2.6 cm to 5.0 cm**

Great! Now, you have to address the fact that Dr. Kern gave Aden *general anesthesia*. This was done for a very valid medical reason, and Dr. Kern (and her facility) should be properly reimbursed for the service. Anesthesia is not included with code 12013 because it is not normally required. Aden's case is unusual. Unusual circumstances often require modifiers, so let's look at the CPT code book's ***Appendix A*** to see if there is an applicable modifier. Modifier 23 seems to fit.

(continued)

23   **Unusual Anesthesia:** *Occasionally, a procedure, which usually requires either no anesthesia or local anesthesia, because of unusual circumstances must be done under general anesthesia. This circumstance may be reported by adding modifier 23 to the procedure code of the basic service.*

So modifier 23 should be appended, or attached, to the procedure code.

12013-23

You know that you have to code the anesthesia service as well.

00300   **Anesthesia for all procedures on the integumentary system, muscles and nerves of head, neck, and posterior trunk, not otherwise specified**

Let's look to see if there is an applicable CPT modifier to explain that an anesthesiologist was not involved. Modifier 47 seems to fit.

47   **Anesthesia by Surgeon:** *Regional or general anesthesia provided by the surgeon may be reported by adding modifier 47 to the basic service. (This does not include local anesthesia.) Note: Modifier 47 would not be used as a modifier for the anesthesia procedures.*

Well, the note within the description of modifier 47 tells you that this modifier is necessary but that it cannot be used with code 00300. You have to attach the modifier to the procedure code. Therefore, you submit the claim with one CPT code and two modifiers: 12013-23-47. In addition, it is smart to include a supplemental report with the claim to explain the use of general anesthesia. You are aware that the insurance company needs to know the details before paying the claim.

Chapter Summary

Modifiers provide additional explanation to the third-party payer so that it can fully appreciate any special circumstances that affected the procedures and services provided to the patient. In health care, as well as in so many other instances of our lives, most things do not fit neatly into predetermined descriptions. By using modifiers correctly, you provide an additional explanation and promote the efficient and more accurate reimbursement of your facility.

CODING BITES

CPT MODIFIER REFERENCES:

Inside the front cover of your CPT code book: CPT modifiers and short descriptions

Appendix A: CPT modifiers, some Level II (HCPCS/National) Modifiers, and full descriptions

HCPCS LEVEL II MODIFIER REFERENCE:

Appendix 2: Modifiers

[*NOTE*: Different publishers may place the Modifier listing in different locations of the HCPCS Level II code book.]

CHAPTER 22 REVIEW
CPT and HCPCS Level II Modifiers

Enhance your learning by completing these exercises and more at mcgrawhillconnect.com!

Let's Check It! Terminology

Match each key term to the appropriate definition.

Part I

1. LO 22.1 Containing both letters and numbers.

2. LO 22.1 A two-character alphabetic or alphanumeric code that may be appended to a code from the main portion of the CPT book or a code from the HCPCS Level II book.

3. LO 22.8 A letter or report written by the attending physician or other health care professional to provide additional clarification or explanation.

4. LO 22.1 A modifier relating to a change or adjustment of a procedure or service provided.

5. LO 22.2 A nurse practitioner, certified registered nurse anesthetist, certified registered nurse, clinical nurse specialist, or physician assistant.

6. LO 22.1 A two-character code that affects the meaning of another code; a code addendum that provides more meaning to the original code.

7. LO 22.1 A facility specially designed to provide surgical treatments without an overnight stay; also known as a same-day surgery center.

8. LO 22.2 A modifier adding information about the professional(s) attending to the provision of this procedure or treatment to the patient during this encounter.

9. LO 22.1 A two-character code that may be appended to a code from the main portion of the CPT book to provide additional information.

10. LO 22.1 A two-character alphanumeric code used to describe the condition of the patient at the time anesthesia services are administered.

A. Alphanumeric
B. Ambulatory Surgery Center (ASC)
C. CPT Code Modifier
D. HCPCS Level II Modifier
E. Modifier
F. Nonphysician
G. Personnel Modifier
H. Physical Status Modifier
I. Service-Related Modifier
J. Supplemental Report

Part II

1. LO 22.6 Nontraumatic amputation of a foot or an integral skeletal portion.

2. LO 22.6 A Medicaid preventive health program for children under 21.

3. LO 22.6 Nourishment delivered using a combination of means other than the gastrointestinal tract (such as IV) in addition to via the gastrointestinal tract.

4. LO 22.6 Edema, burning sensation, temperature change (cold feet), abnormal spontaneous sensations in the feet, and/or limping.

5. LO 22.6 Chronic, irreversible kidney disease requiring regular treatments.

6. LO 22.6 Absence of a posterior tibial pulse; absence or decrease of hair growth; thickening of the nail, discoloration of the skin, and/or thinning of the skin texture; and/or absence of a posterior pedal pulse.

7. LO 22.6 The measurement of how many liters of a drug or chemical are provided to the patient in 60 seconds.

8. LO 22.2 A physician who fills in, temporarily, for another physician.

A. Automated Multi-Channel Chemistry (AMCC)
B. Class A Finding
C. Class B Finding
D. Class C Finding
E. Clinical Laboratory Improvement Amendment (CLIA)
F. Early and Periodic Screening, Diagnostic, and Treatment (EPSDT)
G. End-stage renal disease (ESRD)
H. Locum Tenens Physician

9. LO 22.6 Federal legislation created for the monitoring and regulation of clinical laboratory procedures.

10. LO 22.6 A formula to determine the effectiveness of hemodialysis treatment.

11. LO 22.6 Automated organ disease panel tests performed on the same patient, by the same provider, on the same day.

I. Liters per Minute (LPM)

J. Parenteral Enteral Nutrition (PEN)

K. Urea Reduction Ratio (URR)

  ## Let's Check It! Concepts

Choose the most appropriate answer for each of the following questions.

Part I

1. LO 22.1 A modifier explains

   a. the reason a procedure was performed.

   b. an unusual circumstance.

   c. the date of service.

   d. the level of education of the physician.

2. LO 22.1 CPT code modifiers are appended to

   a. policy numbers.   **b.** diagnosis codes.   **c.** procedure codes.   **d.** pharmaceutical codes.

3. LO 22.2 Service performed by a resident without the presence of a teaching physician under the primary care exception is identified with modifier

   a. AG   **b.** AK   **c.** GC   **d.** GE

4. LO 22.3 A Physical Status Modifier may only be appended to

   a. surgical codes.   **b.** radiology codes.

   c. anesthesia codes.   **d.** evaluation and management codes.

5. LO 22.1 An example of an HCPCS Level II modifier is

   a. 23   **b.** LT   **c.** P4   **d.** 99

6. LO 22.2 An example of a personnel modifier is

   a. 81   **b.** 47   **c.** LC   **d.** 57

7. LO 22.7 If a third-party payer limits your use of multiple modifiers, you should use

   a. no modifiers   **b.** 91   **c.** 51   **d.** 99

8. LO 22.3 P5 is an example of a(n)

   a. HCPCS Level II modifier.

   b. CPT modifier.

   c. Physical Status Modifier.

   d. personnel modifier.

9. LO 22.7 When appending both a CPT modifier and an HCPCS Level II modifier to a procedure code,

   a. the HCPCS Level II modifier comes first.

   b. the CPT modifier comes first.

   c. it doesn't matter which comes first.

   d. use neither—they cancel each other out.

10. LO 22.8 A(n) _____ is a letter or report written by the attending physician or other health care professional to provide additional clarification or explanation.

    a. supplemental report   **b.** service-related report

    c. ambulatory surgery report   **d.** personnel report

Part II

1. LO 22.6 Appending modifier A7 identifies a(n)

   a. aphakic patient.

   b. most recent URR reading of 65 to 69.9

   c. state-supplied vaccine.

   d. dressing for seven wounds.

2. LO 22.4 Discontinued outpatient hospital/ambulatory surgery center (ASC) procedure prior to the administration of anesthesia is identified with modifier

   a. 27   b. 73   c. 74   d. AJ

3. LO 22.6 LPM stands for

   a. local procedure modality.

   b. licensed practical medicine.

   c. local patient median.

   d. liters per minute.

4. LO 22.4 Multiple outpatient hospital E/M encounters on the same date are identified by modifier

   a. 27   b. 73   c. 74   d. 82

5. LO 22.6 An example of DME is

   a. an aspirin.

   b. the administration of a vaccination.

   c. a wheelchair.

   d. the removal of a cyst.

6. LO 22.6 CLIA is identified with modifier

   a. BL   b. QW   c. SQ   d. AV

7. LO 22.6 EPSDT for school-based individualized education program (IEP) services provided outside the public school district responsible for the student is identified by

   a. TR   b. EP   c. G7   d. TM

8. LO 22.5 Dr. Fullmark repairs a laceration on Johnny's left lower eyelid. What modifier would be appended?

   a. E4   b. E3   c. E2   d. E1

9. LO 22.5 Which of the following modifiers identifies the right foot, third digit?

   a. T2   b. T7   c. T8   d. T9

10. LO 22.8 Which of the following modifiers may need a supplemental report?

   a. 50   b. 57   c. 66   d. 53

Let's Check It! Rules and Regulations

Please answer the following questions from the knowledge you have gained after reading this chapter.

1. LO 22.1 Why are modifiers used?

2. LO 22.3 Explain what an anesthesia Physical Status Modifier is and why it is used.

3. LO 22.2 Explain what an anesthesia personnel modifier is and why it is important to use them. Include an example.

4. LO 22.8 What is a supplemental report? Why would a supplemental report be needed, and when do you submit it?

5. LO 22.6 Explain the difference between a Class A finding, a Class B finding, and a Class C finding.

YOU CODE IT! Practice

Using the techniques described in this chapter, carefully read through the case studies and determine the most accurate modifier(s) for each case study. NOTE: All insurance carriers and third-party payers for the patients accept HCPCS Level II codes and modifiers.

Part I

1. Dr. Clayton removed Ricky Pujara's gallbladder 10 days ago. Today, he comes to see Dr. Clayton because of a problem with his knee. Which modifier should be appended to the encounter's E/M code?

2. Dr. Smyth performed an appendectomy on Lynda Lyman. However, the operation took twice as long as usual because Lynda weighs 356 pounds.

3. Dr. Julienne performed a biopsy on the left external ear of Ben Maas, a 69-year-old male.

4. Christopher Slice, a 17-year-old male, was brought into the OR in the Bracker ASC to have a programmable pump inserted into his spine for pain control. After the anesthesia was administered and Chris was fully unconscious, Dr. Sutton made the first incision. Chris began to hemorrhage. The bleeding was stopped, the incision was closed, and the procedure was discontinued.

5. Glenda Roberts, a 61-year-old female, goes to see Dr. Zentz at the referral of her family physician, Dr. Younts, for his opinion as to whether or not she should have surgery. After the evaluation and Glenda's agreement, Dr. Zentz schedules surgery for Thursday. Which modifier should be appended to Dr. Zentz's consultation code for today's evaluation?

6. Patricia Harris, an 82-year-old female, is having Dr. Harmon remove a cyst from her left ring finger.

7. Charles McBroom, a 4-week-old male, was rushed into surgery for repair of a septal defect. If the repair is not completed successfully, he may not survive. What is the correct anesthesia Physical Status Modifier?

8. Dr. Shull is preparing to perform open-heart surgery on Fred Faulkner. Dr. Lowell is asked to assist because a surgical resident is not available. Which modifier should be appended to the procedure code on Dr. Lowell's claim for services?

9. Carolyn Lovett, a 37-year-old female, comes to see Dr. Richardson for a complete physical examination, required by her insurance carrier.

10. George Carlos, a 9-week-old male, was born prematurely and weighs 3.8 kg. Dr. Wilson performs a cardiac catheterization on George.

11. Dr. Kelley excised an abscess on Clyde Hawken's great toe, right foot.

12. Annie Mathewson, a 12-year-old female, has been complaining of hearing a constant ringing in her right ear. Dr. Burwell performs an assessment for tinnitus in the right ear only.

13. Dr. Maxwell performed a percutaneous transluminal coronary atherectomy, by mechanical method, on Ronald Yates's left circumflex artery.

14. John Davis, a 25-year-old male, came to Dr. Browne to have corrective surgery on both of his eyes.

15. Tamara Connelly, a 16-year-old female, hurt her shoulder while camping. The clinic in the area took an x-ray but did not have a radiologist, so Tamara brought the films to Dr. Evely for interpretation and evaluation. Which modifier should Dr. Evely's coder append to the code for the x-rays?

Part II

1. Dr. White performed a blepharotomy on Vanetta Regis, draining the abscess on her upper left eyelid.

2. Stacey Maxell, a nurse midwife, helped Janise Edge deliver her first baby, a girl.

3. Wilfred Edmonds, a 67-year-old male diagnosed with terminal bone cancer, has been in the hospice facility for 3 weeks and is showing signs of an ear infection. Dr. Johns was called in to attend Wilfred's ear problem.

4. Blake Gamble, an EMT, answered a call, with his partner, to Bracker Nursing Home. There was a small fire in the laundry room, and two patients were overcome by smoke enough to require hospitalization. Blake transported both patients at the same time in his ambulance and made one trip to the hospital.

5. Donnie Hentschell, a licensed psychotherapist, began the first of a series of court-ordered therapy sessions with Sonia Jacobs.

6. Dr. Rodriguez was called in to provide monitored anesthesia care for a procedure that will be performed on Malaka Kinlaw. Malaka has a history of acute cardiopulmonary problems.

7. Doon Jung, a registered nurse, works at the Bracker Nursing Facility. He changed the dressing on three wounds that Sang Killingsworth had on her leg.

8. Frank Wenami is the coding specialist for Bracker Dialysis Center. He is preparing the claim for services provided to Jenny Fortner, a patient with ESRD, who moved to the area just last week. Bracker Dialysis provided four dialysis treatments for Jenny during the month.

9. Cindy Kidman, one of the coding specialists at Weston Hospital, discovered that a claim had been submitted with an incorrect code. She has corrected the procedure code and is resubmitting the claim.

10. Nancy Nemeir works at Bracker Medical Equipment Inc. She meets with Earl Hillier, who was recently prescribed an electric wheelchair by Dr. Franks. Nancy explains the options of purchasing and renting the chair, and Earl decides to purchase the wheelchair.

11. Dr. Ott excised a lesion from Oliver Olden's right thumb.

12. Gwen Osby gave Frances Volkesberg, a 72-year-old female, a flu shot.

13. Dr. Parker saw Barbara Gillins and provided service defined as level 3 by Medicaid in her state.

14. Keren Haynes is a certified diabetic educator. She met with Bonnie Haversat to provide services.

15. The peer review organization (PRO) ordered Dr. Dumont to provide a second opinion on the surgical options for Maxine Nevradi.

 ## YOU CODE IT! Application

The following exercises provide practice in abstracting the physician's notes and learning to work with physician documentation for various types of situations that might require a modifier. These case studies are modeled on real patient encounters. Using the techniques described in this chapter, carefully read through the case studies and determine the most accurate CPT code(s) and modifiers, if appropriate, to report the physician's services for each case study. NOTE: All insurance carriers and third-party payers for the patients accept HCPCS Level II codes and modifiers.

GREGORY SAME DAY SURGERY

955 East Healthcare Boulevard • SOMEWHERE, FL 32811 • 407-555-1597

PATIENT: RISHER, BELVA

ACCOUNT/EHR #: RISHBE001

DATE: 10/03/19

Diagnosis: Fecal incontinence, diarrhea, constipation

Procedure: Total colonoscopy with hot biopsy destruction of sessile 3-mm mid-sigmoid colon polyp and multiple cold biopsies taken randomly throughout the colon

Physician: Marion M. March, MD

Anesthesia: Demerol 50 mg and Versed 3 mg, both given IV

(continued)

PROCEDURE: Pt is a 43-year-old female. Patient was placed into position. Digital examination revealed no masses. The pediatric variable flexion Olympus colonoscope was introduced into the rectum and advanced to the cecum. A picture was taken of the appendiceal orifice and the ileocecal valve.

The scope was then carefully extubated. The mucosa looked normal. Random biopsies were taken from the ascending colon, the transverse colon, the descending colon, the sigmoid colon, and the rectum. There was a 3-mm sessile polyp in the mid-sigmoid colon that a hot biopsy destroyed.

IMPRESSION: Sigmoid colon polyp destroyed by hot biopsy
RECOMMENDATIONS: Follow-up in 7 days for biopsy results.

MMM/mg   D: 10/03/19 09:50:16   T: 10/05/19 12:55:01

Determine the most accurate CPT code(s) and necessary modifier(s) for the colonoscopy.

GREGORY SAME DAY SURGERY

955 East Healthcare Boulevard • SOMEWHERE, FL 32811 • 407-555-1597

PATIENT: GILMORE, STEVEN

ACCOUNT/EHR #: GILMST001

DATE: 09/13/19

Diagnosis: Family history of colon cancer

Procedure: Colonoscopy

Physician: Marion M. March, MD

Anesthesia: Versed 4 mg, Demerol 75 mg

PROCEDURE: Pt is a 59-year-old male presenting for a colonoscopy. Pt receives educational material and is informed of the risks. He acknowledges he understands the nature of the procedure, the risks, and the consequences, and consents to the procedure.

The patient is placed in the left lateral decubitus position. The rectal exam reveals normal sphincter tone and no masses. A colonoscope is introduced into the rectum and advanced to the distal sigmoid colon. Further advancement is impossible due to the marked fixation and severe angulation of the rectosigmoid colon. Procedure is discontinued.

On withdrawal, no masses or polyps are noted, and the mucosa is normal throughout. Rectal vault is unremarkable. The patient tolerates the procedure without difficulty.

IMPRESSION: Normal colonoscopy, only to the distal sigmoid colon
PLAN: Strong recommendation for a barium enema

MMM/mg   D: 09/13/19 09:50:16   T: 09/13/19 12:55:01

Determine the most accurate CPT code(s) and necessary modifier(s) for the colonoscopy.

WESTON HOSPITAL

591 Chester Road • Masters, FL 33955

PATIENT: SCHERINI, STEPHANIE

ACCOUNT/EHR #: SCHEST001

DATE: 11/09/19

Diagnosis: Chronic obstructive lung disease

Procedure: Lung transplant, single, with cardiopulmonary bypass

Surgical Team: Marion M. March, MD, primary; Fredrick Avatar, MD; Gene Lavelle, MD

Anesthesia: General

PROCEDURE: Pt is a 37-year-old female brought into the OR, placed on the table, and draped in sterile fashion. Anesthesia was administered. At thoracotomy, the left lung was removed by dividing the left main stem bronchus at the level of the left upper lobe. The two pulmonary veins and single pulmonary artery were divided distally. An allograft left lung was inserted. The recipient left main stem bronchus and pulmonary artery were re-resected to accommodate the transplant. The recipient pulmonary veins were opened into the left atrium. An end-to-end anastomosis of the recipient's respective structures (pulmonary artery, main stem bronchus, and left atrial cuffs) was made to the similar donor structures. Two chest tubes were inserted. Bronchoscopy was performed in the OR. Cardiopulmonary bypass was successfully completed.

Patient tolerated the procedure well and was taken to the recovery room.

MMM/mg   D: 11/09/19 09:50:16   T: 11/13/19 12:55:01

Determine the most accurate CPT code(s) and necessary modifier(s) for the transplantation.

PRADER, BRACKER, & ASSOCIATES

A Complete Health Care Facility

159 Healthcare Way • SOMEWHERE, FL 32811 • 407-555-6789

PATIENT: WILBORN, AMANDA

ACCOUNT/EHR #: WILBAM001

DATE: 11/21/19

Attending Physician: Renee O. Bracker, MD

Referring Physician: Valerie R. Reymond, MD

S: Pt is a 41-year-old female who was injured in a car accident. She presents today at the recommendation of Dr. Reymond for a fitting for a prosthetic spectacle.

O: HEENT is unremarkable. Monofocal measurements are taken, and data for the creation of an appropriate prosthesis are recorded.

A: Aphakia, left eye

P: Return in 2 weeks for final fitting

ROB/mg   D: 11/21/19 09:50:16   T: 11/23/19 12:55:01

Determine the most accurate CPT code(s) and necessary modifier(s) for the fitting of the prosthetic spectacle.

PRADER, BRACKER, & ASSOCIATES

A Complete Health Care Facility

159 Healthcare Way • SOMEWHERE, FL 32811 • 407-555-6789

PATIENT: HOLDER, ANDREW

ACCOUNT/EHR #: HOLDAN001

DATE: 12/10/19

Procedure Performed: CT brain w/o contrast

Radiologist: Michael B. Hawkins, MD

Clinical Information: Evaluation for VP shunt, postsurgical

Attending Physician: Renee O. Bracker, MD

TECHNICAL INFORMATION: Contiguous 3-mm-thick axial images were obtained through the skull base and posterior fossa structures followed by 7-mm-thick axial images through the remainder of the brain. The examination was performed without the use of intravenous contrast material.

The scan was performed at an independent imaging center and sent to me via secured PACS system, so I could interpret.

INTERPRETATION: Evaluation of the posterior fossa demonstrates bilateral vertebral artery calcification. No abnormal intra- or extra-axial collections are noted. There is no evidence of midline shift.

Analysis of the region of the sella turcica demonstrates calcification, likely atherosclerotic involving the cavernous carotid arteries bilaterally seen on series 2 image 7.

Supratentorially, the lateral ventricles are prominent in size. A ventriculostomy catheter is seen coursing from the region of the postcentral sulcus with its distal tip terminating within the frontal horn of the right lateral ventricle abutting the septum pellucidum. Hypodensity is seen within the periventricular white matter particularly abutting the frontal horns of the lateral ventricles bilaterally. There is a mild degree of cerebral volume loss. No abnormal intra- or extra-axial collections are noted.

Evaluation of the visualized skull and paranasal sinuses demonstrates a right parietal burr hole defect for placement of the patient's ventriculostomy catheter. A subcutaneous ventriculostomy valve is seen on series 3 image 26.

RECOMMENDATIONS: There is mild prominence of the lateral ventricles bilaterally without evidence of dilation of the cerebral aqueduct or fourth ventricle.

MBH/mg   D: 12/10/19 09:50:16   T: 12/12/19 12:55:01

Determine the most accurate CPT code(s) and necessary modifier(s) for the x-ray. *TIP:* Don't forget your HCPCS transportation code with modifier.

CPT Evaluation and Management Coding

23

Learning Outcomes

After completing this chapter, the student should be able to:

LO 23.1 Explain the purpose of E/M codes.

LO 23.2 Abstract the details for determining the location of the encounter.

LO 23.3 Interpret the relationship between physician and patient.

LO 23.4 Analyze the documentation to accurately determine the type of E/M service provided.

LO 23.5 Ascertain the correct code for preventive care (annual physicals).

LO 23.6 Cull the appropriate information from the documentation related to E/M services.

LO 23.7 Apply the rules of the global surgical package.

LO 23.8 Assign E/M modifiers and add-on codes accurately.

LO 23.9 Determine the most accurate way to report special evaluation services.

LO 23.10 Validate and report the provision of coordination and management services.

Key Terms

Anticipatory Guidance
Basic Personal Services
Care Plan Oversight Services
Chief Complaint (CC)
Consultation
Critical Care Services
End-Stage Renal Disease (ESRD)
Established Patient
Evaluation and Management (E/M)
Global Surgical Package
History of Present Illness (HPI)
Hospice
Interval
Level of Patient History
Level of Physical Examination
Medical Decision Making (MDM)
New Patient
Nursing Facility
Past, Family, and Social History (PFSH)
Preventive
Problem-Pertinent System Review
Relationship
Risk Factor Reduction Intervention
Transfer of Care

 STOP! Remember, you need to follow along in your CPT code book for an optimal learning experience.

23.1 What Are E/M Codes?

Evaluation and Management (E/M) is the first section in the CPT book and lists codes numbered 99201–99499. These codes are used to report and reimburse physicians for their expertise and thought processes involved in diagnosing and treating patients, such as

• Talking with the patient and his or her family.

• Reviewing data such as complaints, signs, symptoms, and examination results.

• Doing research in medical books and journals.

• Consulting with other health care professionals.

All these elements, including the training and education that this health care professional has had, go into the decision of what to do next for the patient—what advice, what prescription, what test, what treatment, what procedure. E/M codes provide a way to reimburse the health care professional for his or her assessment and supervision of the patient and the determination of the best course for his or her care.

Preventive
A type of action or service that stops something from happening or from getting worse.

GUIDANCE CONNECTION

When a specific code is approved for use in reporting services provided using synchronous, audiovisual, telecommunications equipment [indicated by a star (★) symbol to the left of the code], face-to-face may also occur electronically. Refer to the chapter *CPT and HCPCS Level II Modifiers,* where you will find a section on *Service-Related Modifiers,* specifically modifier 95.

GUIDANCE CONNECTION

Read the additional explanations in the **Evaluation and Management (E/M) Services Guidelines,** subhead **Time,** paragraphs **Face-to-face . . .** and **Unit/floor time . . . ,** in your CPT book directly in front of the E/M section that lists all the codes.

Evaluation and management (E/M) services go beyond those included in the typical office or hospital visit. **Preventive** medicine assessments—more commonly called annual physicals or wellness visits, evaluations of patients in short-term and long-term care facilities, counseling, and critical care—are just some of the areas of focus that might be required of the attending physician. This chapter reviews these subcategories of E/M codes.

As you just read, E/M codes are used to describe specifically the physician's expertise and assessment that was provided during an encounter between him or her and a patient. There are many different types of E/M codes, as you will learn throughout this and the next chapter. Let's begin by reviewing the pieces of information you will need to abstract from the physician's documentation to code the E/M portion of the encounter properly.

Face-to-Face (Office and Other Outpatient Visits)

You may have noticed the phrase *face-to-face* in the code description qualification about time. CPT is very specific about what is included in this element of E/M services provided by a physician to a patient, such as the time it takes to collect health care–related history, perform the physical examination, and counsel the patient (as discussed previously).

Everyone understands that most physicians will spend time, before and after their encounters with patients, reviewing records, going over test results, conferencing with other professionals and the patients by writing letters and reports, making phone calls, and performing other non-face-to-face tasks. Officially, these are <u>not</u> included in the time component of the E/M codes.

Unit/Floor Time (Hospital and Other Inpatient Visits)

When a physician attends to a patient in a facility, such as a hospital or nursing home, the measure of time, for purposes of E/M coding, is described a bit differently than for outpatient encounters.

In outpatient encounters, time is measured by face-to-face—the number of minutes spent with the patient. With inpatient services, in addition to the face-to-face time that the physician may spend at bedside examining the patient, there are additional components included in the measure of time. These additional components are known as *unit/floor time,* which include

- Meeting with nursing staff and other health care professionals.
- Speaking with family members.
- Time the physician spends going over the patient's chart and reviewing notes by other professionals caring for the patient while the physician is still physically present in the hospital unit.

23.2 Location Where the E/M Services Were Provided

The first element you must identify when coding E/M services is the location of the encounter between the health care professional (physician) and the patient. Exactly where did the provider see the patient: in an outpatient location (such as a physician's office), in the hospital, in a skilled nursing facility? Did they just speak on the phone, or did the provider see the patient somewhere else?

Unlike when you are coding other procedures, it can be more efficient to go directly to the E/M section of CPT rather than beginning with the Alphabetic Index. Knowing where this encounter took place between the provider and the patient will enable you to narrow down the range of possible codes and get to the accurate one more effectively.

In addition, going to the location subsection of the E/M section will let you know what additional information you need to determine the right code.

For example, when the encounter occurs at the physician's office, you will need to know the level of history taken, the level of examination performed, and the complexity of medical decision making (MDM). However, when the encounter occurs on the telephone, you will need to know how long the physician was on the phone and the date of the most recent face-to-face E/M service. You will learn more about non-face-to-face encounters, such as telephone calls, later in this chapter and in the next chapter.

Take out your copy of the *Current Procedural Terminology* (CPT) code book so we can go through this together. Go to the **Evaluation and Management (E/M)** section of the CPT book. Look at the first subheading on the first page: **Office or Other Outpatient Services**.

This header, like many others throughout the section, identifies the location of the encounter—where the physician met with the patient.

Once you are in the subsection that identifies where the encounter happened, you can see what additional information you will need to gather from the physician's notes to determine the correct code. For example, in the **Office or Other Outpatient Services** subsection, you can see that the next piece of data you need to know is the relationship between this provider and this patient—whether this patient is a *new patient* or an *established patient*. However, under the **Hospital Inpatient Services** subsection, the next piece of information you will need to cull from the documentation is whether this is the *initial* hospital care visit or a *subsequent* hospital care visit.

Evaluation and Management (E/M)
Specific components of a meeting between a health care professional and a patient.

EXAMPLES

Nicholas Marrin, a 59-year-old male, was brought into the emergency department (ED) with sharp pain in his chest radiating downward into his left arm. The best, most appropriate E/M code will be found in the 99281–99288 range of codes, under **Emergency Department Services.**

Dr. Harman goes to the Sother Nursing Home to see his patient Robin Farber, a 93-year-old female. The best, most appropriate E/M code will be found in the 99304–99318 range of codes, under **Nursing Facility Services.**

Armani Belez, a 35-year-old female, comes to see Dr. Abrahams at his office. The best, most appropriate E/M code will be found in the 99201–99215 range of codes, under **Office or Other Outpatient Services.**

Location-Specific Headings in the E/M Section

The location-specific headings in the E/M section:

Office or Other Outpatient Services

Hospital Observation Services

Hospital Inpatient Services

Office or Other Outpatient Consultations

Inpatient Consultations

Emergency Department Services

Nursing Facility Services

Domiciliary, Rest Home (e.g., Boarding Home), or Custodial Care Services

Domiciliary, Rest Home (e.g., Assisted Living Facility), or Home Care Plan Oversight Services

Home Services

Non-Face-to-Face Services

Nursing Facility
A facility that provides skilled nursing treatment and attention along with limited medical care for its (usually long-term) residents, who do not require acute care services (hospitalization).

LET'S CODE IT! SCENARIO

Suzette Kabole, an 87-year-old female, broke her hip 1 month ago. She has been a patient of Dr. Okine for several years. Since her release from the hospital, Suzette has been homebound until her hip completely heals. Therefore, Dr. Okine went to her home to check on her progress.

Let's Code It!

Read the notes again, and look for the key words that tell you the location of the encounter and the relationship between patient and physician.

The notes state that the doctor went to "*her home.*" That phrase tells us the location of the encounter. Look through the E/M section of the CPT book, and find the group of E/M codes that report this location: **Home Services** . . . codes 99341–99350.

YOU INTERPRET IT!

Match the E/M subsection code range for each of these locations:

1. Preventive medicine services	**a.** 99201–99205
2. Telephone with patient	**b.** 99217–99226
3. Emergency Department	**c.** 99381–99429
4. Hospital observation	**d.** 99441–99443
5. Walk-in clinic	**e.** 99281–99288

Relationship
The level of familiarity between provider and patient.

New Patient
A person who has not received any professional services within the past 3 years from either the provider or another provider of the same specialty who belongs to the same group practice.

Established Patient
A person who has received professional services within the last 3 years from either this provider or another provider of the same specialty belonging to the same group practice.

Consultation
An encounter for purposes of a second physician's opinion or advice, requested by another physician, regarding the management of a patient's specific health concern. A consultation is planned to be a short-term relationship between a health care professional and a patient.

23.3 Relationship between Provider and Patient

Throughout the E/M section of the CPT book, subheadings identify the **relationship** between the provider and the individual. E/M codes use different types of relationship for determining the best, most appropriate code. You may have to identify, from the documentation, if the relationship between the physician and patient is as a **new patient** or **established patient**; if this is initial care or subsequent care; or if this qualifies as a temporary relationship—a **consultation**.

New or Established Patient

In many cases, you must know the relationship between the patient and the provider so that you can communicate an understanding of how familiar the physician is with the patient; the patient's personal history, social history, and family history; and other elements that may affect the physician's decisions regarding the patient's health. Certainly you can understand that the first time they meet, the physician knows absolutely nothing about the patient. He or she must spend time asking questions to help collect the information that will be critical to determining the correct diagnosis and course of treatment. When the physician sees the patient again, however, all the doctor will need to do is quickly read through the patient's file to refresh his or her memory of past conditions and issues.

New Patient

The CPT code set defines a new patient as "*one who has not received any professional services from the physician within the past three years.*" This includes not only this specific physician but also any other group practice member who belongs to the exact same specialty or subspecialty, whether they are a physician or another health care professional.

Established Patient

It is logical, then, to understand that an established patient is one who *has* received professional services from this physician *or* another physician or health care professional in this same group practice who has the exact same specialty credentials, within the last 3 years.

Some location subsections have different codes for a new patient and an established patient, and others do not. You must read the descriptions at the beginning of each subsection to be certain whether this is a criterion for a particular E/M code. For example, the subheading **Emergency Department Services** offers the same codes whether the individual is a new or an established patient.

GUIDANCE CONNECTION

Read the additional explanations in the **Evaluation and Management (E/M) Services Guidelines,** subhead **Definitions of Commonly Used Terms— New and Established Patient,** in your CPT book directly in front of the E/M section that lists all the codes.

EXAMPLE

Leonora Lopez, a 25-year-old female, comes to see Dr. Poker at his office and complains of severe pain in her right wrist and forearm. She just moved to the area, and this is the first time Dr. Poker has seen her.

"... *at his office* ..." identifies the LOCATION of the encounter.

"... *this is the first time Dr. Poker has seen her*" identifies the RELATIONSHIP for this professional and this patient.

Therefore, the E/M codes applicable for this encounter are now in the smaller range of 99201–99205, **Office or Other Outpatient Services, New Patient.**

Initial or Subsequent Care

For services located in hospitals, nursing facilities, intensive neonatal and pediatric critical care departments, and intensive care locations, you will need to identify whether the encounter is the initial or a subsequent visit rather than if the relationship is new or established. This distinction is similar to the *new* or *established* concept, as these two terms describe how up-to-date the physician is on the current condition of this patient.

Initial care visits are reported for the first time a physician, the one for whom you are coding, sees a patient *at a location* for a specific course of treatment or care.

Subsequent care visits are reported for the second time and all visits thereafter that a physician sees a patient *at a location* during the course of the same treatment or care.

EXAMPLE

Barry Balmer is admitted to the hospital on Saturday after having a myocardial infarction (MI) while playing tennis. His regular cardiologist, Dr. Hamilton, is out of town for the weekend, so Dr. Zenbar admits Barry to the hospital on Saturday and checks in on his care on Sunday. Monday, when Dr. Hamilton returns, she goes to see Barry in the hospital and takes charge of his care.

- On Saturday, an *initial* hospital care visit is reported for Dr. Zenbar because this is his first time seeing Barry during this course of treatment at the hospital.

- On Sunday, a *subsequent* hospital care visit is reported for Dr. Zenbar because this is his second time seeing Barry during this course of treatment at the hospital.

- On Monday, an *initial* hospital care visit is reported for Dr. Hamilton because this is her first time seeing Barry during this course of treatment at the hospital, even though it is Barry's third day in the hospital.

- On Tuesday, a *subsequent* hospital care visit is reported for Dr. Hamilton because this is her second time seeing Barry during this course of treatment at the hospital.

Consultations

There are times when the relationship between a patient and a health care provider is expected to be temporary, typically lasting only one visit. In such cases, one physician or health care professional will ask another physician to meet with a patient and evaluate a patient's condition only to offer his or her own professional opinion about the patient's diagnosis and/or treatment options. This temporary relationship is known as a consultation.

When a patient goes to a physician for a *consultation* because the first physician is merely seeking a *second opinion* from the consulting physician regarding diagnosis and/or treatment of the patient, it will be reported from the **Consultations** subsection of E/M. Different from other subsections, the consultation codes 99241–99255 are separated into two parts on the basis of the location of where the consultation took place: **Office and Other Outpatient Consultations** and **Inpatient Consultations**.

GUIDANCE CONNECTION

Read the additional explanations in the in-section guidelines located within the **Evaluation and Management (E/M)** section, subhead **Consultations,** directly above code 99241 in your CPT book.

If the second opinion is requested by the patient or a family member instead of another health care professional, this is *not* reported as a Consultation. It would be reported as a New Patient encounter.

EXAMPLE

Dr. Gail reviews Derita Beck's lab tests and notices that her lipase level is very high. This may indicate a problem with the patient's pancreas. While Derita is healthy overall, Dr. Gail does not want to take any chances, so he refers Derita to Dr. Keith, a gastroenterologist, for a second opinion. Derita goes to see Dr. Keith, who examines her, reviews the test results, and writes a letter to Dr. Gail agreeing with his assessment. Derita goes back to Dr. Gail and does not see Dr. Keith again.

The relationship between Dr. Keith and Derita Beck is not defined as new or established but as a consultation—a second opinion requested by another physician. Therefore, Dr. Keith's coder will report this one encounter from the **Consultations** subsection, codes 99241–99255.

 LET'S CODE IT! SCENARIO

Denny Rossman, a 49-year-old male, was having pain in his lower abdomen, especially when going to the bathroom. His primary care physician, Dr. Lein, did a PSA and was not very concerned, so he told Denny to come back in 6–8 months for a follow-up. Denny did not feel comfortable about Dr. Lein's decision and made an appointment for a second opinion with Dr. Ellis, a urologist.

Let's Code It!

The notes indicate that it was Denny, "the patient," who "requested the consultation" with Dr. Ellis. Therefore, it is coded as a new patient office visit, and you will find the correct code in the 99201–99205 range.

Referral or Consultation?

Referral and consultation are two terms that are commonly used and confused. When one physician *transfers* the care and treatment for a patient (in total or for one particular issue) to another physician, this is a *referral*. The patient is merely being recommended to see another physician and is expected to become a patient of the other physician. These visits are reported using the regular E/M codes, based on the location of the encounter between the new physician (the specialist) and the patient—for example, physician's office 99201–99205, etc.

If the patient goes back to see the "consultant" again, this second E/M encounter will be reported as an established patient encounter because this means that the "consultant" has accepted this individual as a patient for continued care. This is the same as when the first physician may refer the patient to another physician for continuing care and not just a second opinion. More commonly known as a referral, the industry term for this is **transfer of care**. Transfer of the care of a patient can be complete, such as when a physician is retiring, or just for one particular portion of a patient's care, such as a primary care physician sending a patient to a specialist for care of just the one issue.

Transfer of Care
When a physician gives up responsibility for caring for a patient, in whole or with regard to one specific condition, and another physician accepts responsibility for the care of that patient.

EXAMPLE

Dr. Sanger has been Penny Condrel's primary care physician for many years. Today, Penny comes in complaining of a rash all over her legs. Dr. Sanger refers Penny to Dr. Arias, a dermatologist, so that he can take over the diagnosis and treatment of this skin condition. Dr. Arias agrees to take Penny on as his patient to treat this rash. In this case, there has been a transfer of care for Penny's rash from Dr. Sanger to Dr. Arias.

For that first visit, the relationship between Dr. Arias and Penny is one of a new patient, not a consultation, because Dr. Arias has accepted Penny as a patient and the relationship is not a temporary one. This relationship will be ongoing until Penny's problem is resolved. However, Dr. Sanger will remain Penny's primary care physician.

23.4 Types of E/M Services

As you read through the documentation, you also will need to identify the specific *type of service* provided by the physician. This detail will contribute to your ability to determine which subsection of the E/M codes will provide you with accurate code descriptions related to this specific encounter.

- Active Care
- Observation
- Critical Care
- Case Management
- Care Plan Oversight
- Preventive Medicine
- Non-Face-to-Face
- Special Services
- Newborn Care
- Delivery/Birthing Room
- Care Management Services

Level of Service

While accurately reporting the level of expertise and knowledge used by the physician during a visit may seem intangible, the ***Evaluation and Management (E/M) Services Guidelines*** provide you with a checklist type of criteria—very specific and tangible measurements to help you determine the appropriate level of service based on the documentation for the encounter. Let's begin this step of E/M by discussing the elements you need to determine what level of each component has been provided:

- Patient history taken.
- Physical examination performed.
- Medical decision making required to determine a diagnosis, or possible diagnoses, and a treatment plan or next step.

Level of Patient History

As you look at the codes shown in the E/M Section of CPT, under the header **Office or Other Outpatient Services**, you can see that included in the code description is a list with three bullets. Notice that the first key component (bullet) describes the **level of patient history** taken during this encounter by the physician.

There are four levels of patient history. You can measure the level of patient history taken by the physician by reading the notes and matching the documentation to this list. Gathering information from the patient is an important part of the evaluation process for the physician to complete. This is the portion of the visit where the physician asks the patient questions about his or her health and the situations surrounding the health concern that brought him or her to see this doctor.

Problem-Focused History

a. A discussion of the patient's **chief complaint (CC)**.

b. A brief **history of present illness (HPI)** or concern.

Taking a problem-focused history from the patient is going to gather information about only the reason the patient came to this physician today. The physician and patient are not discussing anything else—no other concern, just this one aspect.

> ### EXAMPLE
>
> **Antonio 1**
>
> Antonio goes to Dr. Grace because he has a cough. *[Antonio's chief complaint (CC)]*
>   Dr. Grace documents that Antonio explained what type of cough (dry or wet), how long he has been coughing, whether the cough is worse when lying down, and the color of any mucus that may be coughed up. *[Documentation of the history of Antonio's present illness (HPI)]*

Expanded Problem-Focused History

a. A discussion of the patient's chief complaint.

b. A brief history of this present illness or concern.

c. A **problem-pertinent system review**.

This means that the physician will expand the scope of the information he or she is gathering to extend through all of the systems throughout the entire body directly related to the chief complaint. The systems included in the CPT definition of a review of systems (ROS):

1. Constitutional symptoms, such as fever, weight loss, etc.
2. Eyes
3. Ears, mouth, nose, and throat
4. Cardiovascular
5. Respiratory
6. Gastrointestinal
7. Genitourinary
8. Musculoskeletal
9. Integumentary (skin and/or breast)
10. Neurologic
11. Psychiatric
12. Endocrine
13. Hematologic/lymphatic
14. Allergic/immunologic

Level of Patient History
The amount of detail involved in the documentation of patient history.

Chief Complaint (CC)
The primary reasons why the patient has come for this encounter, in the patient's own words.

History of Present Illness (HPI)
The collection of details about the patient's chief complaint, the current issue that prompted this encounter: duration, specific signs and symptoms, etc.

Problem-Pertinent System Review
The physician's collection of details of signs and symptoms, as per the patient, affecting only those body systems connected to the chief complaint.

Detailed History

a. A discussion of the patient's chief complaint.

b. An extended history of this present illness or concern.

c. A problem-pertinent system review extended to include some additional systems.

d. A pertinent **past, family, and social history (PFSH)**.

Past, Family, and Social History (PFSH)
Collection of details, related to the chief complaint, regarding possible signs, symptoms, behaviors, genetic connection, etc.

> before; whether he has a history of sinus problems, heart problems, respiratory problems, and/or throat problems; whether anyone in his family ever suffered a cough like this; whether he smokes or lives/works/socializes with anyone who smokes; and in what type of environment he works. *[Dr. Grace is now asking more questions, seeking a potential connection to a chronic problem (had this in the past), genetics (anyone in the family have this), and social (behaviors that are known to contribute to the chief complaint).]*

Comprehensive History

a. A discussion of the patient's chief complaint.

b. An extended history of this present illness or concern.

c. A review of systems related to the problem.

d. A review of all additional body systems.

e. A complete PFSH.

EXAMPLE

Antonio 4

In addition to the previous questions, the documentation for the visit between Antonio and Dr. Grace may show information about Antonio's complete medical history beyond those issues related to the respiratory system, to include his entire body; about his allergies, vaccinations, vacations or other travel, general health, weight gain or loss, history of hypertension, diabetes; about the health of his parents, siblings, etc. *[Dr. Grace is now asking more questions, to get specific knowledge about Antonio's overall health as well as the health of his family. This broader understanding of Antonio's health can provide important clues to his current diagnosis.]*

Table 23-1 may provide you with help to determine what level of history is documented.

Level of Physical Examination

The second key component (bullet) describes the **level of physical examination** that was performed during an encounter with the physician. There are four levels of physical examination. You can measure the level of examination performed by the physician by reading the notes and matching the documentation to the following list.

Problem-Focused Examination

a. A limited examination of the affected body area or organ system.

Level of Physical Examination
The extent of a physician's clinical assessment and inspection of a patient.

TABLE 23-1 Determine Level of History Documented

	Problem-Focused (PF)	Expanded PF	Detailed	Comprehensive
Chief complaint	✓	✓	✓	✓
HPI (history of present illness)	Brief	Extended	Extended	Extended
System review	None	Problem-pertinent	Extended problem-pertinent	Complete
PFSH (past, family, and social history)	None	None	Pertinent	Complete

Expanded Problem-Focused Examination

a. A limited examination of the affected body area or organ system.

b. An examination of any *other* symptomatic or related body area(s) or organ system(s).

Detailed Examination

a. An extended examination of the affected body area(s) or organ system(s).

b. An examination of any *other* symptomatic or related body area(s) or organ system(s).

The CPT book categorizes 7 body areas and 11 organ systems in its determination of the best, most appropriate level of physical examination. The CPT definitions of each body area and each recognized organ system are a bit different than you learned in anatomy class:

BODY AREAS

1. Head, including the face
2. Neck
3. Chest, including breasts and axilla
4. Abdomen
5. Genitalia, groin, buttocks
6. Back
7. Each extremity (arms and legs)

ORGAN SYSTEMS

1. Eyes
2. Ears, mouth, nose, and throat
3. Cardiovascular

GUIDANCE CONNECTION

Read the additional explanations in the **Evaluation and Management (E/M) Services Guidelines,** subhead **Determine the Extent of Examination Performed,** in your CPT book directly in front of the E/M section that lists all the codes.

4. Respiratory
5. Gastrointestinal
6. Genitourinary
7. Musculoskeletal
8. Skin
9. Neurologic
10. Psychiatric
11. Hematologic/lymphatic/immunologic

Comprehensive Examination

a. A general, multisystem examination—*or*—

b. A complete examination of a single organ system

Table 23-2 may provide you with help to determine what level of physical examination is documented.

> **EXAMPLE**
>
> **Antonio 8**
>
> In addition to all of the above, Dr. Grace may have taken a chest x-ray, done a respiratory efficiency test, and taken a sputum culture and/or throat cultures.

Level of Medical Decision Making

Medical Decision Making (MDM)
The level of knowledge and experience needed by the provider to determine the diagnosis and/or what to do next.

The third bullet describes the level of **medical decision making (MDM)** provided by the physician during this encounter. This can be the most challenging component because, in essence, you need to determine from the documentation how hard the physician had to think to determine what to do next to help this patient with this concern. It may be that the physician writes a prescription, recommends a treatment or surgery, or orders some diagnostic tests to provide further information. Your understanding of anatomy and physiology will help you with this portion of determining the most accurate code. There are four levels of MDM.

Straightforward MDM

a. A small number of possible diagnoses.

b. A small number of treatment or management options.

c. A low to no risk for complications.

d. Little to no data or research to be reviewed.

> **EXAMPLE**
>
> **Antonio 9**
>
> If when Dr. Grace looked down Antonio's throat he observed inflammation of his tonsils, and if Antonio has no problematic history, then Dr. Grace's decision making may be very straightforward. Dr. Grace was trained to recognize tonsillitis and knows exactly what to prescribe to help Antonio heal.

TABLE 23-2 Determine Level of Physical Examination Documented

	Problem-Focused (PF)	Expanded PF	Detailed	Comprehensive
Affected body area or organ system	Limited	Limited	Extended	Complete
Other symptomatic or related organ system	None	✓	✓	Complete

Low-Complexity MDM

a. A limited number of possible diagnoses.

b. A limited number of treatment or management options.

c. A limited amount of data to be reviewed.

d. A low risk for complications.

EXAMPLE

Antonio 10

If Dr. Grace observed Antonio had a different type of inflammation (other than tonsillitis), such as some indication that his condition might be strep throat or pharyngitis, the process of determining what is best to do is slightly more complex. If so, then a culture would need to be taken for a lab test.

Moderate-Complexity MDM

a. A multiple number of possible diagnoses.

b. A multiple number of treatment or management options.

c. A moderate amount of data to be reviewed.

d. A moderate level of risk for complications, possibly due to other existing diagnoses or medications currently being taken.

EXAMPLE

Antonio 11

In addition to the inflammation Dr. Grace observed, he also noted worrisome sounds in Antonio's lungs. This complicates matters because the diagnosis possibilities now extend from tonsillitis to strep throat to asthma, bronchitis, or pneumonia. Or perhaps Antonio has a history of asthma or previous bouts with pneumonia. Or perhaps Antonio has other known current illnesses, such as hypertension or diabetes, which may make diagnosing and treating this condition much more complicated.

CODING BITES

Certain terms in the physician's notes may indicate a more complex process of MDM on the physician's part. Orders for several tests with terms such as *rule out, possible,* and *likely* might indicate the physician is looking for evidence of several possible diagnoses.

High-Complexity MDM

a. A large number of possible diagnoses.

b. A large number of treatment or management options.

c. A large amount of data and/or research to be reviewed.

d. A high level of risk for complications, possibly due to other existing diagnoses and/or medications currently being taken.

EXAMPLE

Antonio 12

In highly complex cases, the documentation will show issues such as multiple co-morbidities (other conditions or diseases), current multiple medications that may make determining the best treatment for a problem more dangerous for fear of adverse interactions, perhaps allergies to medications under consideration, or other factors that make the determination of the best course of treatment for the patient incredibly complicated.

TABLE 23-3 Determine Level of Medical Decision Making Documented

	Straightforward	Low Complexity	Moderate Complexity	High Complexity
Number of possible diagnoses	1 or 2	Few	Several	Many
Number of management options	1 or 2	Few	Several	Many
Quantity of information to be obtained, reviewed, analyzed (test results, records, etc.)	None, 1, or 2	Few	Several	Many
Risk of significant complications (morbidity, mortality, interactions, allergies, co-morbidities, systemic underlying conditions, etc.)	None, 1, or 2	Few	Several	Many

Table 23-3 may provide you with help to determine what level of MDM is documented.

EXAMPLE

Bernard Clinton comes in to his physician's office with a large shard of glass in his hand. You can see that the number of potential diagnoses is very small: a foreign body in his hand. There are a small number of treatment options: remove the shard. There are no real health complications, and the physician should not have to research Bernard's condition before deciding what to do. This is a straightforward level of MDM.

EXAMPLE

Karen Potts comes to see her family physician, Dr. Seridan, and complains of malaise and fatigue. She denies any major changes in her diet or lifestyle prior to the onset of her symptoms. This is a complex situation that will take a lot of investigation and knowledge on the part of the physician to determine Karen's underlying condition. There are numerous possible diagnoses and, therefore, a large number of management options. Dr. Seridan may have to perform several diagnostic tests to help him determine the problem. This is a highly complex case.

GUIDANCE CONNECTION

Read the additional explanations in the **Evaluation and Management (E/M) Services Guidelines,** subhead **Determine the Complexity of Medical Decision Making,** in your CPT book directly in front of the E/M section that lists all the codes.

 YOU CODE IT! CASE STUDY

Dr. Sternan was asked by Dr. MacAndrews to provide a second opinion on Arthur Jankowski, a 17-year-old male. Arthur's pulmonary specialist, Dr. MacAndrews, wants to perform a lung transplant because of his diagnosis of cystic fibrosis. Dr. Sternan examined Arthur's respiratory system in his hospital room, reviewed the x-rays ordered by Dr. MacAndrews, and wrote a report agreeing that Dr. MacAndrews should perform the surgery.

You Code It!

Go through the steps of E/M coding, and determine the E/M code that should be reported for this encounter between Dr. Sternan and Arthur Jankowski.

Step #1: Read the case completely.

Step #2: Abstract the notes: Which key words can you identify relating to the E/M service performed?

(continued)

Step #3: What is the location?

Step #4: What is the relationship?

Step #5: What level of patient history was taken?

Step #6: What level of physical examination was performed?

Step #7: What level of MDM was required?

Step #8: What is the most accurate E/M code for this encounter?

Step #9: Double-check your work.

Answer:

Did you determine this to be the correct code?

99252   Inpatient consultation, expanded problem-focused

Good work!

Combining Multiple Levels into One E/M Code

Now that you have determined what level of history was taken, what level of physician exam was performed, and what level of MDM was provided by this physician, this all needs to be put together into one code. When all three key components point to the same code, this is a piece of cake.

GUIDANCE CONNECTION

Read the additional explanations in the **Evaluation and Management (E/M) Services Guidelines,** subhead **Instructions for Selecting a Level of E/M Serivce,** in your CPT book directly in front of the E/M section that lists all the codes.

EXAMPLE

Antonio 13

Antonio came to see Dr. Grace in Dr. Grace's office because he had a cough. He had not ever seen Dr. Grace before. After carefully reviewing the documentation, you determine that Dr. Grace took an expanded problem-focused history, he performed an expanded problem-focused physical exam, and the level of MDM was straightforward. All three of these levels of key components point directly to code 99202.

CODING BITES

When the patient history, examination, and MDM are not performed at the same level, the guidelines instruct you to choose the one code that identifies the required key components that have been *met or exceeded* by the physician's documentation.

But what about when the three levels point toward different E/M codes? How do you mesh them all into one code? The CPT guidelines state, ". . . must meet or exceed the stated requirements to qualify for a particular level of E/M service." Let's use a scenario to figure this out together.

 LET'S CODE IT! SCENARIO

Sadie Adanson, an 89-year-old female, was admitted today into McGraw Skilled Nursing Facility (SNF) by Dr. Domino for rehabilitation and care. She suffered a stroke 2 weeks ago and was just discharged from the hospital. Dr. Domino documented a comprehensive level of history. She performed a detailed level of physical exam. Due to the patient's advanced age, co-morbidities, and long list of current medications, as well as the late effects of the stroke, Dr. Domino's MDM was of high complexity.

(continued)

First, identify the location where the encounter between Dr. Domino and Sadie Adanson occurred. The notes state, "*admitted into McGraw Skilled Nursing Facility.*" Turn in the CPT book, E/M section, to **Nursing Facility Services.** This subsection of E/M is divided into two parts: **Initial Nursing Facility Care** and **Subsequent Nursing Facility Care.**

The documentation states that Sadie was admitted today, so this must be the first time Dr. Domino is caring for Sadie at this nursing home. Now you know that the correct code for Dr. Domino's evaluation of Sadie for this visit must be within the **Initial Nursing Facility Care 99304–99306** range.

Next, you need to check the requirements for this range of codes. The code descriptions tell you that ALL THREE key components—level of history, exam, and MDM—must be met or exceeded to qualify. In a full case, you will go back and read through the physician's notes to determine the level provided for each of the three components, as you learned earlier in this chapter. This scenario is provided with a shortcut, indicating the levels for you: "*comprehensive history . . . detailed exam . . . MDM high complexity.*"

> *Comprehensive* history meets the descriptions for 99304, 99305, and 99306.

> *Detailed* exam only meets the description of 99304. Codes 99305 and 99306 both require a comprehensive exam to have been performed.

> MDM *high* complexity meets the description of 99306 and exceeds (a higher level was actually documented) that for codes 99304 and 99305.

You must find the one code that is satisfied by ALL THREE levels of care.

99304:
> You have documentation that is equal to this level of history.
> You have documentation that is equal to this level of exam.
> You have documentation that is greater than this level of MDM.

99305:
> You have documentation that is equal to this level of history.
> You do **NOT** have documentation that is equal to this level of exam.
> You have documentation that is greater than this level of MDM.

99306:
> You have documentation that is equal to this level of history.
> You do **NOT** have documentation that is equal to this level of exam.
> You have documentation that is equal to this level of MDM.

The only code that has ALL THREE levels equal to or greater than its requirements is **99304,** so this is the code that must be reported.

Now, let's take a look at another scenario that requires only two of the three components.

 LET'S CODE IT! SCENARIO

Patrick Chapman, a 77-year old male, has been living at Northside Assisted Living Facility for 6 months. Dr. Colon, his primary physician since he moved in, comes in today to see Patrick because of a complaint of leg pain. Dr. Colon documents a problem-focused interval history, an expanded problem-focused exam, and MDM of moderate complexity.

Read through the scenario, and identify the location where Dr. Colon provided his evaluation and management services: "*assisted living facility.*"

(continued)

Let's turn to the **Domiciliary, Rest Home or Custodial Care Services** subsection of E/M. Why? In the first paragraph under this heading, you will see that CPT directs you to use this category of E/M codes "to report evaluation and management services in an assisted living facility."

This subsection is divided into **New Patient** and **Established Patient,** so go back to the scenario. It states, "*Dr. Colon, his primary physician since he moved in,*" meaning that Patrick qualifies as an established patient. This narrows down the choices to **Established Patient 99334–99337.**

These codes require TWO of the THREE key components. In a full case, you will go back and read through the physician's notes to determine the level provided for each of the three components, as you learned earlier in this chapter. As we did before, this scenario is provided with a shortcut, indicating the levels for you:

> **Problem-focused interval history meets the requirement for 99334.**
>
> **Expanded problem-focused exam meets the requirement for 99335 and exceeds the requirement for 99334.**
>
> **MDM moderate complexity meets the requirement for 99336 and exceeds the requirements for 99334 and 99335.**

You must find the one level that is satisfied by at least TWO of the THREE levels of care.

> **99334:**
>> You have documentation that is equal to this level of history.
>> You have documentation that is greater than this level of exam.
>> You have documentation that is greater than this level of MDM.
>
> **99335:**
>> You have documentation that is NOT equal to this level of history.
>> You have documentation that is equal to this level of exam.
>> You have documentation that is greater than this level of MDM.
>
> **99336:**
>> You have documentation that is NOT equal to this level of history.
>> You have documentation that is NOT equal to this level of exam.
>> You have documentation that is equal to this level of MDM.

Now, you must report the highest level of code that has at least TWO levels equal to or greater than its requirements. The only choice is **99335.**

 GUIDANCE CONNECTION

Read the list of these elements, body areas, and organ systems found in the **Evaluation and Management (E/M) Services Guidelines,** subhead **Select the Appropriate Level of E/M Services Based on the Following,** in your CPT book directly in front of the E/M section that lists all the codes.

 YOU CODE IT! CASE STUDY

Daman Cordero, a 41-year-old male, came to see Dr. Decklin in her office for the first time because of a cough, fever, excessive sputum production, and difficulty in breathing. He had been reasonably well until now. Dr. Decklin did an expanded problem-focused exam of the patient's respiratory system and took Daman's personal, family, and social history in detail. After a chest x-ray was taken to rule out pneumonia, Dr. Decklin's straightforward MDM led her to diagnose him with bronchitis and prescribe an antibiotic and a steroid.

(continued)

Go through the steps of E/M coding, and determine the E/M code that should be reported for this encounter between Dr. Decklin and Daman Cordero.

Step #1: Read the case completely.

Step #2: Abstract the notes: Which key words can you identify relating to the E/M service performed?

Step #3: What is the location?

Step #4: What is the relationship?

Step #5: What level of patient history was taken?

Step #6: What level of physical examination was performed?

Step #7: What level of MDM was required?

Step #8: What is the most accurate E/M code for this encounter?

Step #9: Double-check your work.

Answer:

Did you determine the correct code to be **99202**? Good work!

You know, from the notes, that Daman saw the doctor "in her office." This tells you the location. You also can detect that Daman is a new patient because Dr. Decklin is seeing him "for the first time."

You would need to use code 99203 because the physician documented "history in detail." However, the level of physical examination performed would better match code 99202 because she performed only "an expanded problem-focused exam." Code 99202 also is supported by the "straightforward medical decision making." So when you examine the requirements to meet or exceed the key components of code 99202, you consider the following:

- **Expanded problem-focused history:** *Exceeded.*
- **Expanded problem-focused exam:** *Met.*
- **Straightforward decision making:** *Met.*

The correct E/M code for this scenario is **99202**.

Critical Care and Intensive Care Services

Critical Care Services
Care services for an acutely ill or injured patient with a high risk for life-threatening developments.

GUIDANCE CONNECTION

Read the additional explanations in the in-section guidelines located within the **Evaluation and Management (E/M)** section, subhead **Critical Care Services,** directly above code 99291 in your CPT book.

Critical care services include the management and care of severely ill patients, and this takes a great deal of skill, knowledge, and time. Critically ill or injured patients have a high likelihood of developing a deteriorating life-threatening condition. E/M services reported include

- Highly complex decision making to assess, manipulate, and support vital system function.
- Treatment of single or multiple vital organ system failure.
- Efforts to avoid additional life-threatening decline of the patient's condition.
- Interpretation of various vital function factors.
- Evaluation of advantages and disadvantages of using advanced technology.

The health care provider must document the amount of time spent so that you will know how to code the encounter. The physician may spend his or her time

- Reviewing test results and films at the nurses' station.
- Discussing the patient's treatment and care with the other members of the medical team.
- Charting (writing in the patient's chart).
- Attending to the patient at bedside.

All such activities are a part of the time spent providing critical care.

Critical care services can be, but do not have to be, provided in a coronary care unit (CCU), an intensive care unit (ICU), a respiratory care unit (RCU), or an emergency care facility.

The codes you choose to report critical care services are determined by the services provided for the critically ill or injured patient and the total length of unit/floor time of the encounter. Use the following for coding physician services for the critically ill or injured patient:

99291   **Critical care, evaluation and management of a critically ill or critically injured patient; first 30–74 minutes**

+99292   **each additional 30 minutes**

(*NOTE:* If the physician spends *less than 30 minutes* of unit/floor E/M time with a critically ill or critically injured patient, regular E/M inpatient codes should be reported. Critical care codes do not become applicable until the 30th minute.)

CODING BITES

If a physician goes to see a patient who is currently in the hospital and given a bed in the CCU but who is not critically ill, you are not permitted to use the critical care codes 99291–99292. You have to code it as a regular hospital visit.

LET'S CODE IT! SCENARIO

Rafael Soriano, a 17-year-old male, was brought into the ED by ambulance after being involved in a motorcycle accident. He was not wearing a helmet, and his head hit a brick wall. After initial evaluation and testing by the ED physician, Rafael was sent to the CCU and Dr. Haung spent 2 hours reviewing test results, performing a complete physical exam of Rafael, and discussing a care management plan with the rest of the medical team.

Let's Code It!

Dr. Haung spent "*2 hours*" managing the care of Rafael Soriano in the "*critical care unit.*" Turn to the Critical Care codes, and let's look at the chart. Two hours *equals* 2 *times* 60 minutes, or 120 minutes. When you look at the chart, you will see that 105–134 minutes (120 minutes is right in the middle of this range) is coded with 99291×1 and 99292×2 (read ×2 as reported twice). Look at the following complete description:

99291   **Critical care, evaluation and management of the critically ill or critically injured patient; first 30–74 minutes**

+99292   **each additional 30 minutes**

You know that Dr. Haung spent 120 minutes and that 120 minutes *minus* 74 minutes (which is represented by code 99291) leaves 46 minutes unreported. Therefore, you must add 99292 to report an additional 30 minutes. However, 16 minutes still remains. So you must include 99292 again to account for the leftover minutes. The claim form that you complete will show **99291, 99292, 99292** *or* **99291, 99292×2.** Great job!

Inpatient Neonatal and Pediatric Critical Care

These services will most often be provided in sections of a hospital known as a neonatal intensive care unit (NICU) or pediatric intensive care unit (PICU), but these codes are not exclusive to those designated areas. The guidelines included in the CPT directly above code 99468 contain a great deal of detail on the specific services that are included in these codes and not reported separately.

Determining the most accurate code in this subsection will require you to have two essential pieces of information:

- Age: Is the patient 28 days or younger, 29 days to 24 months, or 2 to 5 years of age?

- Initial or subsequent: Was this the first day of care for this baby or second/additional day of care by this physician for this newborn?

CODING BITES

If the same physician provides critical care services to the same patient on the same date as other E/M services, codes from both subheadings may be reported.

GUIDANCE CONNECTION

Read the additional explanations in the in-section guidelines located within the **Evaluation and Management (E/M)** section, subhead **Initial and Continuing Intensive Care Services,** directly above code 99477 in your CPT book.

GUIDANCE CONNECTION

Read the additional explanations of these elements used to determine the most accurate E/M code involving the measurement of time spent with the patient in the **Evaluation and Management (E/M) Services Guidelines,** subhead **Time,** in your CPT book directly in front of the E/M section that lists all the codes.

Note that these code descriptions report a day of E/M service, not just history/exam/MDM or even time spent.

Intensive Care Services—Child

There is a difference between a patient who is critically ill and one who requires intensive care services, such as intensive observation, cardiac and respiratory monitoring, vital sign monitoring, and other services detailed in the guidelines for this subsection (shown above code 99477).

Determining the most accurate code in this subsection will require you to have two essential pieces of information:

- 99477 reports the initial hospital care for a neonate, 28 days of age or younger, who requires intensive care, as per those services identified in the guidelines.
- Subsequent intensive care codes 99478–99480 are distinguished by the present weight of the neonate.

Note that these code descriptions report a day of E/M service, not just history/exam/MDM or even time spent.

Time

Under certain circumstances, the correct E/M code is not determined by the key components of history, physical exam, and MDM but is based on the amount of time the physician spent evaluating the patient's condition and managing his or her care. In these cases, the time shown in the last paragraph of the E/M code description is used as a guide. This detail can be found following the three bullets for the key components. You will see that the last sentence reads something like *Typically, 20 minutes are spent face-to-face with the patient and/or family* (found in the last portion of the code 99202 description). This gives you an approximate time frame that may be used instead of the other key components to determine the appropriate level. In order to use this guideline to choose a code, the documentation must contain the appropriate specific information.

Counseling between Physician and Patient

If the physician spends more than half (51% or more) of the total time *counseling* the patient, then time spent shall be used as the key element in determining the best, most appropriate E/M code. This is not psychological counseling with a therapist (reported with codes 90804–90857) but the physician's discussing diagnosis and treatment with the patient. It might be to review test results or to go over care options with a family member. The CPT guidelines specify the following:

- The results of recommendations for diagnostic tests and/or the review of the results of tests and impressions already gathered.

> **EXAMPLE**
>
> The doctor writes, "*I discussed with the patient that the MRI shows an area of concern. . . .*"

- The options of multiple treatments, including risks and benefits.

> **EXAMPLE**
>
> The doctor writes, "*I explained to the patient that his condition can be treated with medication or surgery. The research shows that this new drug has been quite effective; however, there are some side effects. . . .*"

- Directions to the patient for treatment and/or follow-up.

- Emphasis on the importance of compliance with the agreed-upon treatment plan.

- Risk factor reduction.

- Patient and family education.

GUIDANCE CONNECTION

Read the additional explanations in the **Evaluation and Management (E/M) Services Guidelines,** subhead **Counseling,** in your CPT book directly in front of the E/M section that lists all the codes.

Counseling and/or Risk Factor Reduction Intervention

A physician may see a patient at a visit, separate from the annual preventive medicine evaluation, for the purposes of helping the patient learn about, understand, and/or adopt better health practices, including

- Preventing injury or illness, such as the proper way to lift or the importance of testing one's blood glucose levels regularly.
- Encouraging good health, such as nutritional counseling or a new exercise regime.

Services such as these are reported with codes from

99401–99404	Preventive medicine, individual counseling
99411–99412	Preventive medicine, group counseling
99429	Unlisted preventive medicine services

GUIDANCE CONNECTION

Read the additional explanations in the in-section guidelines located within the **Evaluation and Management (E/M)** section, subhead **Counseling Risk Factor Reduction and Behavior Change Intervention,** directly above code 99401 in your CPT book.

Long-Term Care Services

Specific codes are used to report E/M services provided to patients in residential care facilities.

Use 99304–99318 and 99379–99380 for reporting services to patients in the following places:

- Skilled nursing facilities (SNF).
- Intermediate care facilities (ICF).
- Long-term care facilities (LTCF).
- Psychiatric residential treatment centers.

Use 99324–99340 for reporting services to patients in locations where room, meals, and **basic personal services** are provided, but medical services are not included:

- Assisted living facilities
- Domiciliaries
- Rest homes
- Custodial care settings
- Alzheimer's facilities

EXAMPLE

Dr. Banks goes to see Peter Lister at the halfway house where he resides. Peter is autistic, and Dr. Banks wants to examine him and adjust his medication for asthma. You should report Dr. Banks's visit to Peter with code 99334.

Care Plan Oversight Services

When a physician provides **care plan oversight services**, you have to use the appropriate code determined by the length of time involved and the type of facility in which the patient is located.

99339–99340	for patients in assisted living or domiciliary facility
99374–99375	for home health care patients
99377–99378	for hospice patients
99379–99380	for residents in a nursing facility—but only if the management of the patient involves repeated direction of therapy by the attending physician

Admission to a Nursing Facility

When a patient is admitted into a nursing facility as a continued part of an encounter at the physician's office or the emergency department (ED) (on the same day by the same physician), you report only one code (from the **Nursing Facility** section of the E/M codes) that will include all the services provided from all the locations on that day. The admission to the hospital from the physician's office or ED is reported all in the one hospital admission E/M code. The same rule also applies to admission to a nursing facility.

However, if the patient has been discharged from inpatient status on the same day as being admitted to a nursing facility, you code the physician's discharge services separately from the admission.

Three key components, similar to other E/M codes, are used to determine the appropriate level of E/M service provided by the attending physician to a patient on the first day at a nursing facility. There is no differentiation made in this section of codes between a new patient and an established patient.

Physicians use different methods and tools to assess a patient's status and to create and/or update an appropriate treatment plan for the ongoing care of the individual. Such methods and tools include

- Resident assessment instrument (RAI)
- Minimum data set (MDS)
- Resident assessment protocols (RAP)

Subsequent Nursing Facility Care

Once the patient is in the facility, it is expected that the physician will continue to review the patient's chart, as well as assess test results and changes in the patient's health status. Notice that the code description for the history key component includes the term **interval**. The physician needs to evaluate the patient's history only back to the last visit to gain a complete, up-to-date picture of the individual's health. The continuing care type of assessment is reported with the most appropriate code from the 99307–99310 range.

If the physician does only an annual assessment of the patient in the nursing facility (typically in cases where the patient is stable, progressing as expected, or recovering), you use code

Interval
The time measured between one point and another, such as between physician visits.

> **99318**   Evaluation and management of a patient involving an annual nursing facility assessment

 LET'S CODE IT! SCENARIO

Mara Morietty, a 55-year-old female, was diagnosed with advanced pancreatic cancer and is being cared for at her home by her family, with the help of a home health agency. Dr. Clarke is providing care plan oversight services for the first month of care. The plan includes home oxygen, IV medications for pain control management, and diuretics for edema and ascites control. Dr. Clarke also discusses end-of-life issues, living will directive, and other concerns with the family, the nurse, and the social worker. Dr. Clarke includes documentation of his 45-minute assessment, as well as notes on modifications to the care plan. Certifications of care from the nursing staff, the social worker, the pharmacy, and the company supplying the durable medical equipment for support are also in the record.

Let's Code It!

Dr. Clarke documented that he provided *"care plan oversight services"* for Mara Morietty. Turn to the Alphabetic Index, and look up *Care Plan Oversight Services*. The index instructs you to see *Physician Services*. Turn to *Physician Services,* and you will see *Care Plan Oversight Services*.

As you look at the indented list below that phrase, note that you have to identify the location at which the patient is being cared for. Mara is being cared for at home by a home health agency. This index entry suggests codes 99374 and 99375.

> **Physician services**
> Care Plan Oversight Services
>   Home Health Agency Care. 99374, 99375

Now, let's turn to code 99374 to read the entire code description:

> **99374**   Physician supervision of a patient under care of home health agency (patient not present) in home, domiciliary or equivalent environment requiring complex and multidisciplinary care modalities involving regular physician development and/or revision of care plans; 15–29 minutes
>
> **99375**   30 minutes or more

Dr. Clarke's notes report that he spent 45 minutes. Therefore, the correct code is **99375.**

GUIDANCE CONNECTION

Read the additional explanations in the in-section guidelines located within the **Evaluation and Management (E/M)** section, subhead **Case Management Services,** including **Medical Team Conferences,** directly above code 99366, in your CPT book.

Case Management Services

If a patient has several or complex health issues or diagnoses, a team of health care professionals may have to work together to provide proper management and treatment. The team may involve several physicians or the attending physician and a physical therapist, for example, conferencing together. To properly reimburse the health care professional for the time and expertise spent on the patient's behalf with other professionals, you report such services using codes from ranges

99366–99368	**Medical Team Conferences**
99441–99443	**Telephone Services**
99444	**On-Line Medical Evaluation**
99446–99452	**Interprofessional Telephone/Internet/ Electronic Health Record Consultations**
99453–99454, 99091	**Digitally Stored Data Services/Remote Physiologic Monitoring**
99457	**Remote Physiologic Monitoring Treatment Management Services**

YOU CODE IT! CASE STUDY

Scott Germain, an 81-year-old male, is still having pain and swelling in his hands. Dr. Daniels, an orthopedist, came in to evaluate Scott 2 weeks ago, and Ira Hansrani's last physical therapy session with Scott was yesterday.

Dr. Rubine, the gerontologist and primary care physician for Scott, reads the up-to-date notes and test results, and sets up a meeting in the conference room with Ira Hansrani, the physical therapist, and Dr. Daniels to discuss adjusting Scott's therapy plan, based on current test results. The meeting lasts 45 minutes.

You Code It!

Go through the steps of coding, and determine the E/M code that should be reported for the encounter between Dr. Rubine, Dr. Daniels, and Ira Hansrani.

Step #1: Read the case completely.

Step #2: Abstract the notes: Which key words can you identify relating to the E/M service performed?

Step #3: What is the location?

Step #4: Is this an "interdisciplinary team"?

Step #5: Is the patient or patient's family present (in the meeting)?

Step #6: How long did the meeting last?

Step #7: Double-check your work.

Answer:

Did you determine these to be the correct codes?

Reported for Dr. Rubine:
99367   **Medical team conference with interdisciplinary team, 30 minutes or more; participation by physician**

Reported for Dr. Daniels:
99367   **Medical team conference with interdisciplinary team, 30 minutes or more; participation by physician**

Reported for Ira Hansrani, PT:
99368   **Medical team conference with interdisciplinary team, 30 minutes or more; participation by nonphysician qualified health care professional**

Great work!

Newborn and Pediatric E/M Care

The E/M for a newborn or child may be performed by a neonatologist, pediatrician, or other physician. This portion of the E/M section is divided into several parts:

Newborn Care

Determining the most accurate code in this subsection will require you to have two essential pieces of information:

- Location: Hospital or birthing center, or other location.
- Initial or subsequent: Was this the first day of care for this newborn or the second/additional day of care by this physician for this newborn?

Note that these code descriptions report a day of E/M service, not just history/exam/MDM or even time spent.

Delivery/Birthing Room Attendance and Resuscitation

When requested by the delivering physician (most often the obstetrician), a neonatologist or pediatrician may need to be there in the delivery room to resuscitate and/or stabilize a baby immediately upon his or her birth.

CODING BITES

A newborn is described as a baby aged 28 days old or younger.

CODING BITES

When a physician sees a newborn at an office visit after seeing the baby initially at the hospital or other birth location, the visit is coded as an established patient visit (as long as it is within 3 years, of course).

> **EXAMPLE**
>
> Dr. Baldwin is a neonatologist. Dr. Matthews, an obstetrician, asked Dr. Baldwin to be in attendance during the delivery of Anita Mescale's baby because of a concern over her excessive alcohol consumption during pregnancy. Dr. Baldwin was there and stabilized the baby after birth. You would report Dr. Baldwin's service with code 99464.

Home Services

If a physician provides E/M services to a patient at his or her private residence, use codes 99341–99350. Determine the most appropriate code by using the same key components as those for E/M services provided in the physician's office.

Some home health agencies employ physicians, some physicians may volunteer to see homebound patients, while others visit only established patients who are homebound.

When a health care professional other than the physician—such as a nurse or respiratory therapist—cares for a patient at the patient's home, report these services with a code from the range 99500–99602 in the *Medicine* section of CPT.

 LET'S CODE IT! SCENARIO

Jules Paganto, a 39-year-old male, suffers from agoraphobia and cannot leave his home. Dr. Volente went to the house to examine Jules because he was complaining of chest congestion. Dr. Volente took a problem-focused history, as this was the first time he had seen Jules. The doctor examined Jules's HEENT and chest and concluded that Jules had a chest cold. He told Jules to get some over-the-counter cold medicine and to call if the symptoms did not go away within a week.

(continued)

You need to find the appropriate code to reimburse Dr. Volente for his E/M services to Jules Paganto. You know that "*Dr. Volente went to the house,*" so the location section is titled **Home Services.** The notes say that "*this was the first time he had seen Jules,*" meaning that Jules is a new patient, narrowing the choices to codes 99341–99345. The book tells us that a new patient home visit requires three key components: history, examination, and MDM. According to the notes, Dr. Volente

1. Took a *problem-focused history.*
2. Examined the patient's head, ears, eyes, nose, throat (HEENT), and chest: *expanded problem-focused* because the doctor examined the affected body system and other related organ systems.
3. Concluded, without tests or additional resources: *straightforward.*

When you assess the levels and use the meet or exceed rule, the most accurate code for the visit is **99341.** Good job!

Non-Face-to-Face: Telephone Services and Online Medical Evaluation

Everyone is trying to work more efficiently by using the telephone or the Internet to communicate with an established patient and/or the patient's family, coordinate care, discuss test results, or answer a question. This makes good sense.

To report E/M services provided by the physician over the telephone, a code from the range 99441–99443 should be used. The different codes are distinguished by the length of time of the call. However, before you report one of these codes, there are restrictions. If the phone call is a follow-up to an E/M service provided for a related problem or concern that occurred within the previous 7 days, none of these codes can be reported because the phone call is considered part of that service. In the same light, if the phone call results in the decision for the patient to come in to see the physician as soon as possible, this phone call is considered a part of that future E/M service, so one of these codes would not be used, either.

Code 99444 is used to report an online E/M service to an established patient, a guardian, or a health care provider as a response to a patient's question. Similar to the restriction on the reporting of a telephone call, code 99444 should not be reported when this e-mail or Internet communication is connected to an E/M service provided for a related concern that occurred within the previous 7 days or within a surgical procedure's postoperative period.

GUIDANCE CONNECTION

Read additional explanations in the in-section guidelines within the **Evaluation and Management (E/M) Services** section, subhead **Non-Face-to-Face Services,** related to codes 99441–99457 in your CPT book.

YOU CODE IT! CASE STUDY

Renay Miller, a 47-year-old female, had just seen the doctor during her annual physical 2 weeks earlier. Today she phoned Dr. Reese to ask if she could travel out of the country, due to her condition. They spoke for about 7 minutes regarding recommended precautions.

Go through the steps of coding, and determine the E/M code that should be reported for the encounter between Dr. Reese and Renay Miller.

Step #1: Read the case completely.

Step #2: Abstract the notes: Which key words can you identify relating to the E/M service performed?

Step #3: What is the location?

(continued)

Step #4: Is this a "face-to-face" or "non-face-to-face" call?

Step #5: How long did the call last?

Step #6: Double-check your work.

Answer:

Did you determine this to be the correct code?

> **99441**   Telephone evaluation and management service by a physician . . . provided to an established patient . . . ; 5–10 minutes of medical discussion

23.5 Preventive Medicine Services

CODING BITES

Online Digital Evaluation and Management Services codes:
99421–99423
NEW for 2020
Check your 2020 CPT coding manual for details.

There may be times when the physician's notes do not clearly identify all the individual components (for instance, history, exam, and medical decision making [MDM]) of an encounter, such as when a patient comes in for an annual physical. In these cases, you should be careful not to force the components or make them up. Instead, you should look at other areas of the E/M section. For example, the *Preventive Medicine* section, codes 99381–99429, may be more appropriate.

When provided at the same time as a comprehensive preventive medical examination, preventive medicine service codes 99381–99397 include

- Counseling
- **Anticipatory guidance**
- **Risk factor reduction interventions**

In regard to these preventive evaluations, the term *counseling* does not refer to a formalized relationship between a mental health counselor, psychologist, or psychiatrist but to the advice and guidance provided by a health care professional to his or her patient. From your own personal experience, you may be familiar with discussions with your physician during your annual physical. The talks cover everything from quitting smoking to exercising more and perhaps having a better diet. These are all examples of counseling.

Anticipatory Guidance
Recommendations for behavior modification and/or other preventive measures.

Risk Factor Reduction Intervention
Action taken by the attending physician to stop or reduce a behavior or lifestyle that is predicted to have a negative effect on the individual's health.

Anticipatory guidance refers to the physician's offering suggestions for behavior modification or other preventive measures related to a patient's high risk for a condition. The concern may be based on specifics in a patient's condition or history (or perhaps a family history or an occupational hazard).

EXAMPLE

Dr. Herbert provides anticipatory guidance to Kenneth Simons with regard to being careful about protecting his respiratory health. Kenneth works at an automobile paint shop, and the fumes are very dangerous if a breathing mask is not worn.

A physician prescribing a patch to help a patient quit smoking or referring a patient to a registered dietitian to help him or her with a new diet—each of these is considered a risk factor reduction intervention. It means the physician is taking action to intervene with, or help stop, patient behaviors that put the patient at a higher risk for certain illnesses or conditions.

Specific **Preventive Medicine** codes are determined first by New Patient or Established Patient, and second by the patient's age:

- Infant (age younger than 1 year).
- Early childhood (age 1 through 4 years).
- Late childhood (age 5 through 11 years).
- Adolescent (age 12 through 17 years).
- 18–39 years.
- 40–64 years.
- 65 years and older.

You may be familiar with the standards of care that have physicians check different parts of the body in different ways, determined by the patient's age, such as:

- Behavioral assessments for children ages 0 to 11 months, 1 to 4 years, 5 to 10 years, 11 to 14 years, and 15 to 17 years.
- Hearing screening for all newborns.
- Diabetes (type 2) screening for adults with high blood pressure.

If elements such as risk factor reduction intervention or counseling occur during a separate visit (not at the same time as the physical examination), you have to code them separately with a code from the 99401–99412 range.

If, during the course of the preventive medicine examination, the physician finds something of concern that warrants special and extra attention involving the key components of a problem-oriented E/M service, the extra work should be coded with a separate E/M code appended with modifier 25. It is applicable only when the same physician does the extra service on the same date.

 LET'S CODE IT! SCENARIO

Kensie Hamilton, a 47-year-old female, comes to see her regular physician, Dr. Granger, for her annual physical. During the examination, Dr. Granger finds a mass in her abdomen that concerns him. After the exam, he sits and talks with Kensie about past or current problems with her abdomen, including pain, discomfort, and other details regarding her abdominal issue. He asks whether any family members have had problems in that area, as well as about her alcohol consumption and sexual history as they relate to this concern. Dr. Granger then goes into his office to analyze the multiple possibilities of diagnoses, evaluates the information in Kensie's chart, and reviews the moderate risk of complications that might occur due to her current list of medications. He orders an abdominal CT scan, blood work, and a UA for further input.

Let's Code It!

According to the notes, *Dr. Granger* performed an "*annual physical exam,*" also known as a preventive medicine exam, on Kensie, a "*47-year-old.*" Go to the Alphabetic Index and look up *Evaluation and Management, Preventive Services,* or go directly to the E/M section and look for the **Preventive Medicine Services** subheading. The phrase "*her regular physician*" reveals that Kensie is an established patient, helping you to determine to report code

99396   Periodic comprehensive preventive medicine, established patient, 40–64 years

Dr. Granger's notes also reveal that during the exam he found a mass in Kensie's abdomen that he felt needed further investigation. He spent additional time getting details about her personal, family, and social history regarding abdominal problems; he reviewed concerns about multiple possible diagnoses, complications, and treatments. As per the guidelines, this is extra work done on Dr. Granger's part, and, therefore, he is entitled to additional reimbursement, reported with a separate E/M code. As you review the notes, you should be able

(continued)

to determine the best, most appropriate E/M code for the additional service. Dr. Granger did a comprehensive examination, and his MDM was certainly at a high level of complexity, leading you to the code

99215   Office or other outpatient visit with comprehensive exam and medical decision making of high complexity

plus this modifier:

-25   Significant, separately identifiable evaluation and management service

The claim form for Dr. Granger's encounter with Kensie will show **99396** and **99215-25**. Good job!

Code 99396 will reimburse Dr. Granger for his time and services for the annual physical, and code 99215 will reimburse him for the extra work he did regarding the abdominal mass. The modifier −25 explains that, while unusual, Dr. Granger did both of these services at the same encounter.

(*NOTE:* More information on E/M modifiers is provided later in this chapter.)

23.6 Abstracting the Physician's Notes

You learned about abstracting clinical documentation in the chapter *Abstracting Clinical Documentation*. Abstracting for details regarding evaluation and management (E/M) is a bit different because you have to cull out details about the physician's thought processes, in addition to specifically *what* was done and *why*. Very rarely will physicians actually identify the level of MDM in their notes with a statement such as "MDM was low complexity." So, you really need to hone your interpretative skills.

GUIDANCE CONNECTION

Read additional explanations in the in-section guidelines located within the **Evaluation and Management (E/M)** section, subhead **Preventive Medicine Services,** directly above code 99381 in your CPT book.

 YOU CODE IT! CASE STUDY

Gloria Merro, a 33-year-old female, comes to see Dr. Feldner at his office with complaints of severe pain in her right wrist and forearm. She just moved to the area, and this is the first time Dr. Feldner has seen her. Gloria sees Dr. Feldner for a very specific concern. The doctor asks Gloria about any medical history she may have related to her arm (diagnosed osteoporosis, previous broken bones, etc.). Next, Dr. Feldner examines Gloria's arm. He suspects that the arm is broken and orders an x-ray to be taken.

You Code It!

Go through the steps to determine the E/M code that should be reported for this encounter between Dr. Feldner and Gloria Merro.

Step #1: Read the case completely.

Step #2: Abstract the notes: Which key words can you identify relating to the E/M service performed?

Step #3: What is the location?

Step #4: What is the relationship?

Step #5: What level of patient history was taken?

Step #6: What level of physical examination was performed?

(continued)

Step #7: What level of MDM was required?

Step #8: What is the most accurate E/M code for this encounter?

Step #9: Double-check your work.

Answer:

Did you determine this to be the correct code?

99201   Office or other outpatient visit, new patient

Let's carefully review the physician's notes.

- Where did the encounter occur? Gloria went *"to see Dr. Feldner at his office."* This will lead us to the first sub-heading in the E/M section, **Office or Other Outpatient Services.**

- What is the relationship? The notes state, *"She just moved to the area, and this is the first time Dr. Feldner has seen her."* This brings us to the category of **New Patient,** and the code range 99201–99205.

- What is the level of history? The notes state, "*The doctor asks Gloria about any medical history she may have related to her arm,*" meaning that all the history he took was *problem-focused.*

- What is the level of exam? You will see that "*Dr. Feldner examines Gloria's arm.*" This means only one body area (each extremity) or one organ system (musculoskeletal) was examined. That's *problem-focused.*

- What is the level of MDM? In this case, did you analyze the situation and determine that the MDM was *straight-forward*? However, you can see that the documentation supports the definition of this level: There is only one diagnosis, the management options are limited (put a cast on it), there are very few complications, and Dr. Feldner didn't really have to do any research to recommend a course of treatment.

This brings you to the best, most appropriate E/M code: **99201.**

Please understand that the physicians will not come right out and use the same words as the code descriptions to describe what occurred during the encounter. Let's inspect various statements from patients' charts and identify the key words that lead to the correct E/M code.

1. George Semple, a 57-year-old male, was seen for the first time by Dr. Brieo in the office for a contusion of his hand. Dr. Brieo asked questions about the bruise on George's hand and examined his hand thoroughly.

    a. Location: *Office* tells us where the encounter took place.

    b. Relationship: *First time* tells us this is a new patient.

    c. Key components: *History–problem-focused, physical examination–problem-focused, medical decision making–straightforward.* Therefore, the correct code is **99201.**

2. Dr. Fein performed an initial observation at the hospital of Lois Martin, a 31-year-old female. After asking about her personal medical history, including pertinent history of stomach problems, digestive problems, and pertinent family and social history directly relating to her complaints, he examined Lois's abdomen, chest, neck, and back, which revealed lower right quadrant pain accompanied by nausea, vomiting, and a low-grade fever. Dr. Fein made the straightforward decision to admit Lois overnight to the hospital to rule out appendicitis.

    a. Location: *Initial observation at the hospital* tells us this code is in the **Hospital Observation Services** section.

    b. Relationship: *Observation at the hospital* codes are the same for both new and established patients.

    c. Key components: *History–detailed, physical examination–detailed, medical decision making–straightforward,* and *overnight admission to the hospital* all lead us to the correct code of **99218.**

3. Dr. Murphy, a general surgeon, saw Teena Harrison, a 46-year-old female, in her office for a second opinion requested by Teena's gynecologist, Dr. Enterez, regarding a lump in her right breast. Dr. Murphy took a brief history of Teena's present illness and a personal and family medical history relating to her hematologic and lymphatic system, which was positive for breast cancer on her maternal side. After reviewing the mammogram and performing a limited physical exam of her breasts and chest area, the physician made the straightforward decision to advise a lumpectomy.

   a. Location: *In her office* tells us where the encounter took place.

   b. Relationship: *Second opinion requested by a physician* tells us this is a consultation.

   c. Key components: *History—expanded problem-focused, physical examination—expanded problem-focused,* and *medical decision making—straightforward* lead us directly to the correct code of **99242.**

4. David Emerson, a 17-year-old male, presented at the ED with a painful, swollen wrist. The patient stated he had been hurt at a softball game. Dr. Lubner took a brief history and asked some key questions about David's arm/hand. He then examined David's wrist and arm, checked his musculoskeletal system, and ordered x-rays to be taken. It was rather simple to determine that David's diagnosis was a sprained wrist.

   a. Location: *ED* tells you the location.

   b. Relationship: Codes in the **Emergency Department Services** section do not differentiate between new and established patients.

   c. Key components: *History—expanded problem-focused, physical examination—expanded problem-focused,* and *medical decision making—low complexity* tell us the extent of the encounter. The correct code is **99282.**

23.7 E/M in the Global Surgical Package

As a part of the standard of care, there are certain E/M encounters that are already included in the code for a surgical procedure. This is called the **global surgical package**. Specific details about this will be included in the *CPT Surgery Section* chapter. For now, let's skip to the time frame, after the procedure is over and the patient is discharged.

Global Surgical Package
A group of services already included in the code for the operation and not reported separately.

You are probably familiar with this: A patient is being discharged after a procedure, and the physician says, "I want to see you in my office in a week." A physician gets paid for performing surgery *and* for the time spent checking on the patient after the surgery to make certain the body is healing correctly. When the follow-up visit in the office (or wherever) occurs, you will not report this by using a regular E/M code because the physician will not be paid separately. However, you do need to report that this encounter occurred. Therefore, you will report a *special services* code from the *Medicine* section of the CPT book. Take a look at this code:

    99024   **Postoperative follow-up visit, normally included in the surgical package to indicate that an evaluation and management service was performed during a postoperative period for a reason(s) related to the original procedure**

YOU CODE IT! CASE STUDY

Ten days after Dr. Rollins performed a carpal tunnel revision on Nicole Letchin's left hand, Nicole, a 23-year-old female, came to see him in his office, as instructed when he discharged her. He asked how she was feeling, checked the flexibility of the wrist, removed the stitches, and checked the healing of the incision. She was doing fine, so Dr. Rollins told her to come in only if she needed anything.

You Code It!

Go through the steps of coding, and determine the E/M code that should be reported for the encounter between Dr. Rollins and Nicole Letchin.

Step #1: Read the case completely.

Step #2: Abstract the notes: Which key words can you identify relating to the E/M service performed?

Step #3: What is the location?

Step #4: What is the relationship?

Step #5: Is this E/M service already included in the global surgical package?

Step #6: What is the most accurate E/M code for this encounter?

Step #7: Double-check your work.

Answer:

Did you determine this to be the correct code?

> **99024**   **Postoperative follow-up visit, normally included in the surgical package . . .**

I knew you could do it!

23.8 E/M Modifiers and Add-On Codes

Several modifiers may be used in conjunction with an E/M code to provide additional information about an encounter. Each modifier specifically explains an unusual circumstance that may justify the payment to the provider and helps you avoid having to appeal a denied claim later on. CPT Level I modifiers are two-digit codes that are listed in *Appendix A* of the CPT book. You first learned about these modifiers in the chapter *CPT and HCPCS Level II Modifiers* in this textbook.

Open your CPT book to *Appendix A* and read along as we review some of these modifiers.

> **24 Unrelated Evaluation and Management Service by the Same Physician or Other Qualified Health Care Professional During a Postoperative Period:** The physician or other qualified health care professional may need to indicate that an evaluation and management service was performed during a postoperative period for a reason(s) unrelated to the original procedure. This circumstance may be reported by adding modifier 24 to the appropriate level of E/M service.

As a part of the standard of care and the global surgical package, a physician gets paid for performing surgery and for the time spent checking on the patient after the surgery to make certain the body is healing correctly. Modifier 24 would explain that the physician had to see the patient about a *totally different concern* during this time period.

YOU CODE IT! CASE STUDY

Dr. Marple removed Christen Ellison's gallbladder (cholecystectomy) on February 27. The global period for this surgical procedure is 90 days. On March 15, Christen came to see Dr. Marple because he had been out in his garden and developed a rash on his arms. The physician examined Christen's arms and gave him an ointment for the rash.

You Code It!

Go through the steps of coding, and determine the E/M code that should be reported for the encounter between Dr. Marple and Christen Ellison.

Step #1: Read the case completely.

Step #2: Abstract the notes: Which key words can you identify relating to the E/M service performed?

Step #3: What is the location?

Step #4: What is the relationship?

Step #5: What level of patient history was taken?

Step #6: What level of physical examination was performed?

Step #7: What level of MDM was required?

Step #8: What is the most accurate E/M code for this encounter?

Step #9: Do you need to clarify any detail or explain something with a modifier?

Step #10: Double-check your work.

Answer:

Did you determine the correct code to be **99212-24**? Good for you!

Christen came to see Dr. Marple, meaning the encounter happened at the doctor's office. Considering that *Dr. Marple just performed surgery on Christen* 2 weeks ago, it is very reasonable to consider Christen an established patient. Dr. Marple did a *problem-focused examination* (limited exam of the problem area), and his *decision making was straightforward.* This directs us to code 99212.

Ninety days from February 27 goes all the way to May 27. That means the visit for the rash, which is a concern totally unrelated to the gallbladder surgery, occurred within the 90-day period. We must explain that Dr. Marple should be compensated separately for the encounter because it has nothing to do with the surgery. So our code will be 99212-24.

25 **Significant, Separately Identifiable Evaluation and Management Service by the Same Physician or Other Qualified Health Care Professional on the Same Day of the Procedure or Other Service:** It may be necessary to indicate that on the day a procedure or service identified by a CPT code was performed, the patient's condition required a significant, separately identifiable E/M service above and beyond the other service provided or beyond the usual preoperative and postoperative care associated with the procedure that was performed. A significant, separately identifiable E/M service is defined or substantiated by documentation that satisfies the relevant criteria for the respective E/M service to be reported. The E/M service may be prompted by the symptom or condition for which the procedure and/or service was provided. As such, different diagnoses are not required for reporting of the E/M services on the same date. This circumstance may be reported by adding modifier 25 to the appropriate level of E/M service. **Note:** This modifier is not used to report an E/M service that resulted in a decision to perform surgery. See modifier 57. For significant, separately identifiable non-E/M services, see modifier 59.

Certainly this happens quite frequently: A patient goes to see the doctor for a minor procedure in the office. Then the patient says, "*Oh, Doc, while I'm here, I want to talk to you about. . . .*" Should that happen, you have to append the E/M code with modifier 25 to explain that there were two visits in one at this encounter.

 LET'S CODE IT! SCENARIO

Gladys Topfer goes to see her dermatologist for a scheduled appointment to have a 1.5-cm mole removed from her cheek. Once Dr. Assanti completes the procedure, Gladys asks the doctor to look at a cyst that has developed under her arm. Dr. Assanti discusses the presence of the cyst with her (How long has it been there? Does it hurt? etc.), and then he examines her underarm area and determines that the best course of action is to wait and see what happens with the cyst. He advises Gladys to keep the area clean and to come back in 3 weeks if the cyst has not gone away.

Let's Code It!

Gladys met with *her dermatologist* (documenting that she is an established patient), Dr. Assanti, at his office (identifying an outpatient location). The notes document that Dr. Assanti did a *problem-focused history* (because they discussed nothing else other than the cyst) and a *problem-focused examination* (because Dr. Assanti examined only the area where the cyst is located), and his *decision making was straightforward* (because he is very knowledgeable about cysts and Gladys has no other conditions or medications that would cause more evaluation). This directs you to code 99212.

But wait! The claim for this encounter is going to include the code for the surgical removal of the mole—a totally different concern from the reason prompting the E/M of the patient. In essence, there were two encounters in one: the first for the removal of the mole and the second for the concern about the cyst. Therefore, the correct code would be **99212-25** (plus the procedure code for the excision of the mole: CPT code 11312).

32   **Mandated Services:** Services related to *mandated* consultation and/or related services (e.g., third-party payer, governmental, legislative, or regulatory requirement) may be identified by adding modifier 32 to the basic procedure.

Modifier 32 indicates that a third-party payer, a governmental agency, or other regulatory or legislative action required the encounter, consultation, and/or procedure(s).

 LET'S CODE IT! SCENARIO

Alene Morgen, a 49-year-old female, went to see Dr. Blume for a comprehensive physical assessment, as a requirement for her special coverage application. The insurance carrier would not consider the policy without the examination. She had never seen Dr. Blume before today's visit.

(continued)

Alene met with the physician at his office and had never seen Dr. Blume before, meaning that she is a new patient. According to the notes, Dr. Blume did an initial comprehensive preventive medicine E/M of a 49-year-old female. That directs you to code 99386.

Notice that the insurance carrier, a third-party payer, mandated the evaluation. Therefore, you must add the modifier to the E/M code to get **99386-32** to explain this fact.

| 57 | **Decision for Surgery:** An evaluation and management service that resulted in the initial decision to perform the surgery may be identified by adding modifier 57 to the appropriate level of E/M service. |

Documentation of an encounter may start off with the discussion between physician and patient about test results and treatment options. If the two (physician and patient) agree that a surgical procedure should be scheduled, then the E/M code should be appended with modifier 57.

 LET'S CODE IT! SCENARIO

Dr. Richards referred Timothy Dunne, a 67-year-old male, to Dr. Eliot for a consultation to determine whether he needs a prostatectomy. After taking a comprehensive history, performing a comprehensive examination, and reviewing all the previous test results, Dr. Eliot informs Timothy that he recommends the procedure. Timothy agrees, and they select a date the following week for the surgery to be performed.

Timothy met with Dr. Eliot at his office at the request of *Dr. Richards* for a *consultation*. According to the documentation, Dr. Eliot did a *comprehensive history* and a *comprehensive examination*. His medical decision making was of moderate complexity. This directs you to code 99244. BUT this encounter ended in Timothy's decision to have Dr. Eliot perform the surgery. As you learned earlier in this chapter, this means there has been a transfer of care in addition to the decision for surgery. Therefore, you must add the modifier 57 to the E/M code for a new patient office visit: **99204-57.**

Prolonged Services: 99354–99359

In some cases, patients require greater than the usual amount of attention from a physician, more time than would regularly be spent—either face-to-face or without direct contact—over the course of 1 day.

Prolonged service codes report E/M services that are at least 30 minutes longer than the amount of time represented by standard E/M codes. These codes may be reported in addition to standard E/M codes at any level, as appropriate.

To determine the best, most appropriate code from this subcategory, you have to calculate the total number of minutes that the physician spent with, or on behalf of, the patient, during one date of service. The codes will be calculated as follows:

- The first code would be the standard evaluation and management code (such as 99213).

- Then, depending upon how long the physician spent with the patient, you would also report code . . .

  + 99354 or 99356 for the time spent lasting at least 30 minutes over the standard evaluation and management service and includes time spent up to 74 minutes.

  + 99355 or 99357 for each 30 minutes additionally spent, over the 74 minutes reported by 99354 or 99356, until the total amount of time spent by the physician is represented.

 GUIDANCE CONNECTION

Read the additional explanations in the in-section guidelines located within the **Evaluation and Management (E/M)** section, subhead **Prolonged Services,** directly above code 99354 in your CPT book.

EXAMPLE

Dr. Alfredo spent a total of 2 hours, in his office, with Mona Catzer working with her to stabilize her diabetes mellitus. The codes used to report this E/M encounter are

99214	Office visit, established patient, detailed	25 min.
+99354	Prolonged physician service in the office; first hour	60 min.
+99355	additional 30 minutes	30 min.
	TOTAL	**115 min**

23.9 Special Evaluation Services

In cases when a patient is about to have a life insurance or disability certificate issued, the insurer often requires the attending physician to provide an evaluation to establish a baseline of data. The visit does not involve any actual treatment or management of the patient's condition—it accounts for the time to create the appropriate documentation. The codes in range 99450–99456 apply to both new and established patients.

The three codes within this subsection are very specific as to which services are included:

99450 **Basic life and/or disability examination that** includes:
- Measurement of height, weight, and blood pressure;
- Completion of a medical history following a life insurance pro forma;
- Collection of blood sample and/or urinalysis complying with "chain of custody" protocols; and
- Completion of necessary documentation/certificates.

99455 **Work related or medical disability examination** by the treating physician that includes:
- Completion of a medical history commensurate with the patient's condition;
- Performance of an examination commensurate with the patient's condition;
- Formulation of a diagnosis, assessment of capabilities and stability, and calculation of impairment;
- Development of future medical treatment plan; and
- Completion of necessary documentation/certificate and report.

99456 **Work related or medical disability examination** by other than the treating physician that includes:
- Completion of a medical history commensurate with the patient's condition;
- Performance of an examination commensurate with the patient's condition;
- Formulation of a diagnosis, assessment of capabilities and stability, and calculation of impairment;
- Development of future medical treatment plan; and
- Completion of necessary documentation/certificate and report.

Be aware of the notation beneath code 99456:

(Do not report 99455, 99456 in conjunction with 99080 for the completion of Workman's Compensation forms)

99080 **Special reports such as insurance forms, more than the information conveyed in the usual medical communications or standard reporting form**

23.10 Coordination and Management Services

Complex Chronic Care Coordination Services

Patients with chronic illnesses, such as diabetes mellitus or hypertension, need more attention from their health care team. Code 99487 represents the first hour of clinical staff time for complex chronic care coordination directed by a physician or other qualified health care professional with no face-to-face time. Code 99487 is used for a face-to-face visit, and code 99489 is an add-on code for each additional 30 minutes of complex chronic care coordination.

Numerous studies have proven that patients with chronic illnesses and conditions benefit from coordinated care across the many disciplines of physicians and other members of the clinical staff in addition to community service agencies. This specific subset of E/M codes focuses on support services and management of care provided to patients who are living in their own homes, domiciliaries, rest homes, or assisted living facilities.

These services are provided to patients who

- Require repeated hospital admissions or ED visits.
- Are diagnosed with one or more chronic continuous or episodic medical and/or psychiatric conditions lasting at least 1 year (12 months).
- Are at significant risk of death, acute exacerbation, decompensation, and/or functional decline.
- Require continuing care from multiple health care specialties that need to be coordinated for efficacy and efficiency of medical conditions, psychosocial conditions, and activities of daily living (ADLs).
- Require moderate or highly complex medical decision making during treatment.

Physicians and other qualified health care professionals must implement a documented care plan to coordinate multiple disciplines and agencies, which is shared with the patient and/or family or caregiver.

With all of the services and activities involved with the care of a chronically ill patient, CPT has specifically identified those services characteristically reported by these codes, including

- Developing and maintaining a comprehensive care plan.
- Facilitating access to care and services needed by the patient and/or family.
- Assessing and supporting patient compliance with the treatment plan, including schedule of medication.
- Educating the patient, family, and/or caregiver to enable and support self-management, independent living, and ADLs.
- Identifying community and health care resources available to the patient and/or family.
- Communicating with home health agencies and other community services available and used by the patient.
- Communicating aspects of care to the patient, family, and/or caregiver.
- Collecting health outcomes data and registry documentation.

Services identified by code 99487 overlap long-standing E/M codes. Therefore, when reporting 99487 (to set off clause), do not separately report the following:

- Care plan oversight services (CPT codes 99339, 99340, 99374–99378).
- Prolonged services without direct patient contact (99358, 99359).
- Anticoagulant management (99363, 99364).
- Medical team conferences (99366–99368).
- Education and training (98966–98968, 99441–99443).
- Online medical evaluation (98969, 99444).

GUIDANCE CONNECTION

Read the additional explanations in the in-section guidelines located within the **Evaluation and Management (E/M)** section, subhead **Complex Chronic Care Management Services,** directly above code 99487 in your CPT book.

- Preparation of special reports (99080).
- Analysis of data (99090, 99091).
- Transitional care management services (99495, 99496).
- Medication therapy management services (99605–99607).

Codes 99487 and 99489 should not be reported separately, nor should they include the time spent when reporting the following:

- End-stage renal disease services (ESRD) (90951–90970) during the same month.
- Postoperative care services during the global period.
- E/M services (99211–99215, 99334–99337, 99347–99350).
- E/M services while patient is an inpatient or in observation (99217–99239, 99241–99255, 99291–99318).
- Transitional care management services (99495, 99496).

As you can see, 99487 would be reported only once per month by the physician or health care professional who has taken on the role of coordinator for this patient for the first 60–89 minutes of services.

Add-on code 99489 can be reported in conjunction with 99487 to represent time greater than 89 minutes during the month.

Transitional Care Management Services

GUIDANCE CONNECTION

Read the additional explanations in the in-section guidelines located within the **Evaluation and Management (E/M)** section, subhead **Transitional Care Management Services,** directly above code 99495 in your CPT book.

It can be a complex event to transfer the care and management of a patient's ongoing condition from one facility to another, especially when the new location will involve a new care team. Code 99495 (transitional care management services) requires the physician to document the following elements:

- Communication (direct contact, telephone, electronic) with the patient and/or caregiver within 2 business days of discharge.
- Medical decision making of at least moderate complexity during the service period.
- Face-to-face visit within 14 calendar days of discharge.

Code 99496 (transitional care management services) requires the following elements:

- Communication (direct contact, telephone, electronic) with the patient and/or caregiver within 2 business days of discharge.
- Medical decision making of high complexity during the service period.
- Face-to-face visit within 7 calendar days of discharge.

Providers are often concerned that patients with multiple medical and/or psychosocial issues may "slip through the cracks" when transferred from inpatient status to the care of an assisted living facility, a domiciliary, or the patient's own home. These two codes provide an effective way to report the provision of these services to an established patient by the physician or other qualified health care professional or licensed clinical staff member under direction of the physician.

Transitional care management (TCM) includes one episode of face-to-face contact along with non-face-to-face services provided by the physician and clinical staff. The period of TCM service begins on the date of discharge and runs for 29 consecutive days.

Within 48 hours (2 days) after discharge, the first TCM interactive contact between the reporting physician and the patient must occur. This contact may be face-to-face, over the telephone, or by use of electronic communication. The contact must encompass the professional's ability to promptly act upon patient needs and go beyond simply scheduling follow-up care.

When the provider documents two or more attempted contacts within the prescribed time period and is unable to connect with the patient, family, and/or caregiver, the provider may still report TCM services as long as the other transitional care management criteria have been met.

Reporting either of the two TCM codes requires at least one face-to-face visit, as well as reconciliation of prescribed medication, with the patient. For patients requiring highly complex medical decision-making services, the provider must meet with the patient face-to-face within the first 7 calendar days after the patient is discharged from inpatient status.

For patients requiring a moderate level of medical decision making, the first face-to-face visit must occur during the first 14 calendar days of discharge. This first patient contact is included in the TCM code and not reported separately. However, any additional E/M services provided afterwards may be reported with a separate E/M code accordingly.

The CPT guidelines include specific services by the physician or other health care professional included in TCM, as well as services provided by clinical staff under the direction of that physician.

Services provided by the physician or other qualified health care professional include

- Obtaining and reviewing the discharge information.
- Reviewing the need for or follow-up on pending diagnostic tests and treatments.
- Educating the patient, family, and/or caregiver.
- Establishing (or reestablishing) referrals.
- Arranging for required community resources.
- Assisting in scheduling any required follow-up with community providers and services.
- Interacting with other qualified health care professionals who will assume (or reassume) care of the patient's system-specific problems.

Services provided by clinical staff under the direction of the physician include

- Communicating about various aspects of care with the patient, family, caregiver, and/or other professionals.
- Identifying available community and health resources.
- Assessing and supporting compliance with the treatment plan, including medication management.
- Communicating with home health agencies and other community services used by the patient.
- Educating the patient, family, and/or caregiver to support self-management, independent living, and ADL.
- Facilitating access to care and services required by the patient, family, and/or caregiver.

When reporting 99495 or 99496, do *not* separately report the following:

- Care plan oversight services (CPT codes 99339, 99340, 99374–99380).
- Prolonged services without direct patient contact (99358, 99359).
- Medical team conferences (99366–99368).
- Education and training (98960–98962, 99071, 99078).
- Telephone services (98966–98968, 99441–99443).
- **ESRD** services (90951–90970).
- Online medical evaluation (98969, 99444).
- Preparation of special reports (99080).
- Analysis of data (99090, 99091).
- Complex chronic care coordination services (99487–99489).
- Medication therapy management services (99605–99607).

End-Stage Renal Disease (ESRD)
Chronic, irreversible kidney disease requiring regular treatments.

TCM may be reported only once within 30 days of discharge by only one health care professional, even if there is a subsequent discharge within that time. This professional is permitted to report hospital or observation discharge services concurrently with TCM services, but not within the global period of postoperative care.

Cognitive Assessment, Psychiatric Collaborative, and General Behavioral Health Integration Care Management Services

Health care professionals have gained greater understanding about those who may benefit from cognitive, mental, or behavioral support. These are some of the codes available for reporting these services from the appropriate professionals:

99483	Assessment of and care planning for a patient with cognitive impairment
99492	Initial psychiatric collaborative care management
99493	Subsequent psychiatric collaborative care management
+99494	Initial or subsequent psychiatric collaborative care management, each add'l 30 mins
99484	Care management services for behavioral health conditions

Chapter Summary

Evaluation and management (E/M) codes report the energy and knowledge a health care professional puts into gathering information, reviewing data, and determining the best course of treatment for the patient's current condition. Many health information management professionals find these difficult to correctly determine due to the complex formula of such codes. Don't become overwhelmed. Once you get a job, you will find that a particular portion of this section will become your main focus.

> **EXAMPLE**
> - If you work for a provider in a private medical office, most of your E/M codes will be found under the **Office** heading on the first two pages of the section.
> - If you work for a physician who cares for patients at a skilled nursing facility, you will use codes from under the **Nursing Facility Services** heading.

So in the real world, most of the time, you will be using the same small set of codes over and over again. But because you don't know where you will be working in the future, you should learn the entire section.

In this chapter you learned that, for the key components of coding for services rendered in a nursing home, a long-term care facility, or the patient's home, you use a different set of codes from those reporting physician services in an office or a hospital.

Understand that the elements of the distinct types of encounters, such as annual physicals (preventive medical assessments) and case management services, also use varying sets of parameters.

Your job as a professional coding specialist is to understand the variety of essentials involved in coding E/M services properly and to report those services accurately.

You Interpret It! Answers

1. c (99381–99429), **2.** d (99441–99443), **3.** e (99281–99288), **4.** b (99217–99226), **5.** a (99201–99205)

CHAPTER 23 REVIEW
CPT Evaluation and Management Coding

Let's Check It! Terminology

Match each key term to the appropriate definition.

Part I

1. LO 23.3 The level of familiarity between provider and patient.

2. LO 23.3 An encounter for purposes of a second physician's opinion or advice, requested by another physician, regarding the management of a patient's specific health concern.

3. LO 23.4 The extent of a physician's clinical assessment and inspection of a patient.

4. LO 23.4 The collection of details about the patient's chief complaint, the current issue that prompted this encounter: duration, specific signs and symptoms, etc.

5. LO 23.4 The level of knowledge and experience needed by the provider to determine the diagnosis and/or what to do next.

6. LO 23.4 The amount of detail involved in the documentation of patient history.

7. LO 23.4 Collection of details, related to the chief complaint, regarding possible signs, symptoms, behaviors, genetic connection, etc.

8. LO 23.3 A person who has received professional services within the last 3 years from either this provider or another provider of the same specialty belonging to the same group practice.

9. LO 23.3 A person who has not received any professional services within the past 3 years from either the provider or another provider of the same specialty who belongs to the same group practice.

A. Chief Complaint

B. Consultation

C. Established Patient

D. Evaluation and Management (E/M)

E. History of Present Illness

F. Level of Patient History

G. Level of Physical Examination

H. Medical Decision Making (MDM)

I. New Patient

10. LO 23.2 Specific characteristics of a face-to-face meeting between a health care professional and a patient.

11. LO 23.4 The primary reasons why the patient has come for this encounter, in the patient's own words.

12. LO 23.4 The physician's collection of details of signs and symptoms, as per the patient, affecting only those body systems connected to the chief complaint.

J. PFSH

K. Problem-Pertinent System Review

L. Relationship

Part II

1. LO 23.7 A group of services already included in the code for the operation and not reported separately.

2. LO 23.5 Action taken by the attending physician to stop or reduce a behavior or lifestyle that is predicted to have a negative effect on the individual's health.

3. LO 23.4 An organization that provides services to terminally ill patients and their families.

4. LO 23.4 Services that include washing/bathing, dressing and undressing, assistance in taking medications, and getting in and out of bed.

5. LO 23.1 A type of action or service that stops something from happening or from getting worse.

6. LO 23.2 A facility that provides skilled nursing treatment and attention along with limited medical care for its (usually long-term) residents, who do not require acute care services (hospitalization).

7. LO 23.4 The time measured between one point and another, such as between physician visits.

8. LO 23.4 Services for a patient who has a life-threatening condition expected to worsen.

9. LO 23.10 Chronic, irreversible kidney disease requiring regular treatments.

10. LO 23.4 E/M of a patient, reported in 30-day periods, including infrequent supervision along with pre-encounter and post-encounter work, such as reading test results and assessment of notes.

11. LO 23.5 Recommendations for behavior modification and/or other preventive measures.

12. LO 23.3 When a physician gives up responsibility for caring for a patient, in whole or with regard to one specific condition, and another physician accepts responsibility for the care of that patient.

A. Anticipatory Guidance

B. Basic Personal Services

C. Care Plan Oversight Services

D. Critical Care Services

E. ESRD

F. Global Surgical Package

G. Hospice

H. Interval

I. Nursing Facility

J. Preventive

K. Risk Factor Reduction Intervention

L. Transfer of Care

 ## Let's Check It! Concepts

Choose the most appropriate answer for each of the following questions.

Part I

1. LO 23.1 E/M codes enable the physician to be reimbursed for all of these services except
   a. talking with the patient and his or her family.
   b. taking continuing education classes.
   c. consulting with other health care professionals.
   d. reviewing data such as test results.

2. LO 23.2 Often, finding the correct E/M code begins with knowing
   a. where the patient met with the physician.
   b. which credential is held by the provider.

c. what type of insurance policy is held by the patient.

d. what the patient does for an occupation.

3. LO 23.3 A patient who has not seen a particular physician in the last 3 years is categorized as

   a. an established patient.   **b.** a referral.

   c. a consultation.   **d.** a new patient.

4. LO 23.4 The three key components of many E/M codes include all of these *except*

   a. history.   **b.** exam.   **c.** chief complaint.   **d.** MDM.

5. LO 23.4 Levels of patient history include all *except*

   a. expanded problem-focused.   **b.** comprehensive.

   c. detailed.   **d.** high complexity.

6. LO 23.4 Body areas that might be included in a physical examination include

   a. eyes.   **b.** each extremity.   **c.** respiratory.   **d.** neurologic.

7. LO 23.4 When services are provided at different levels, the guidelines state you should code to a level of

   a. at least one of three key components achieved.   **b.** all key components met or exceeded.

   c. the number of minutes face-to-face.   **d.** the number of diagnosis codes.

8. LO 23.4 If _____ of the time with the patient is spent counseling, you should use time rather than key components to determine the level of service code.

   a. 51% or more   **b.** 45% or more   **c.** 50% or less   **d.** 25% or more

9. LO 23.3 A consultation is expected to be a(n) _____ relationship with the patient.

   a. extended   **b.** transferred   **c.** temporary   **d.** continuing

10. LO 23.3 A patient seen in the office and then admitted to the hospital the same day should be coded with E/M codes from subsection(s)

   a. Office Visit only.   **b.** Office Visit and Initial Hospital Care.

   c. Initial Hospital Care only.   **d.** Emergency Department.

Part II

1. LO 23.5 A preventive medical E/M encounter may include any of these services *except*

   a. counseling.   **b.** admission into the hospital.

   c. anticipatory guidance.   **d.** risk factor reduction intervention.

2. LO 23.8 If the physician finds a health concern during a preventive medicine examination requiring additional E/M services and the extra service is performed by the same physician on the same day, then the extra service should be coded with

   a. the preventive medicine code only.   **b.** the additional E/M code.

   c. whichever code is reimbursable at a higher rate.   **d.** a separate E/M code appended with modifier 25.

3. LO 23.4 E/M services provided to a patient in an assisted living facility are reported from the subsection

   a. Nursing Facility.

   b. Home Services.

   c. Domiciliary, Rest Homes, and Custodial Care Settings.

   d. Care Plan Oversight Services.

4. LO 23.4 If a patient is discharged from the hospital and admitted into a skilled nursing facility (SNF) on the same day by the same physician, report the E/M services with

   a. an admission to the nursing facility E/M code only.

   b. a hospital discharge code and an admission to the nursing facility code.

    c. one outpatient E/M services code.

    d. a subsequent nursing facility E/M code.

5. LO 23.4 Care plan oversight services provided for a patient in a hospice setting are coded from the

    a. 99339-99340 range.   **b.** 99374-99375 range.   **c.** 99377-99378 range.   **d.** 99379-99380 range.

6. LO 23.4 Frank Brookshire goes to Dr. Corriher's office for an appointment. After a full history, an exam, and comprehensive MDM, Dr. Corriher recommends that he be admitted into a psychiatric residential treatment center. He takes him over and admits him into the facility that afternoon. You will code the E/M services with

    a. one office visit code.

    b. an admission to nursing facility code.

    c. both an office visit code and an admission to nursing facility code.

    d. a domiciliary, rest home, custodial care center code only.

7. LO 23.4 Arlen Flowers, a 5-day-old male, was admitted into the NICU for complications of his low birthweight status. Dr. Hohman saw him yesterday and is in again today. You will code today's E/M services from the

    a. 99468-99469 range.   **b.** 99478-99479 range.

    c. 99307-99310 range.   **d.** 99210-99215 range.

8. LO 23.4 Critical care codes are determined by

    a. length of time.   **b.** inpatient or outpatient status.

    c. level of history, exam, and MDM.   **d.** new or established patient.

9. LO 23.4 Conferencing with other health care professionals regarding management and/or treatment of a patient is

    a. included in all E/M codes.   **b.** coded as a consultation E/M code.

    c. coded from 99366-99368.   **d.** coded from 99201-99205.

10. LO 23.8 A modifier

    a. explains an unusual circumstance.   **b.** has five digits.

    c. begins with the letter *M*.   **d.** explains how a patient became injured.

Let's Check It! Guidelines

Refer to the Official Evaluation and Management (E/M) Services Guidelines and fill in the blanks accordingly.

not	history	subspecialty
counseling	Medical decision making	hospital
face-to-face	chief complaint	office
outpatient	exact	examination
five	inpatient	Concurrent care
coordination	emergency department	time

1. Solely for the purposes of distinguishing between new and established patients, professional services are those _____ services rendered by physicians and other qualified health care professionals who may report evaluation and management services reported by a specific CPT code(s).

2. An established patient is one who has received professional services from the physician/qualified health care professional or another physician/qualified health care professional of the _____ same specialty and _____ who belongs to the same group practice, within the past 3 years.

3. A _____ is a concise statement describing the symptom, problem, condition, diagnosis, or other factor that is the reason for the encounter, usually stated in the patient's words.

4. _____ is the provision of similar services (e.g., hospital visits) to the same patient by more than one physician or other qualified health care professional on the same day.

5. Levels of E/M services are _____ interchangeable among the different categories or subcategories of service.

6. The E/M codes recognize _____ types of presenting problems.

7. Time is not a descriptive component for the _____ levels of E/M services because emergency department services are typically provided on a variable intensity basis, often involving multiple encounters with several patients over an extended period of time. Therefore, it is often difficult to provide accurate estimates of the time spent face-to-face with the patient.

8. Intraservice times are defined as face-to-face time for _____ and other _____ visits and as unit/floor time for _____ and other _____ visits.

9. The extent of the _____ is dependent upon clinical judgment and on the nature of the presenting problem(s).

10. The extent of the _____ performed is dependent on clinical judgment and on the nature of the presenting problem(s).

11. _____ refers to the complexity of establishing a diagnosis and/or selecting a management option.

12. When _____ and/or _____ of care dominates (more than 50%) the encounter with the patient and/or family (face-to-face time in the office or other outpatient setting or floor/unit time in the hospital or nursing facility), then _____ shall be considered the key or controlling factor to qualify for a particular level of E/M services.

Let's Check It! Rules and Regulations

Please answer the following questions from the knowledge you have gained after reading this chapter.

1. LO 23.2 List the location-specific headings in the E/M section.

2. LO 23.4 List the three components of an E/M code.

3. LO 23.5 Explain anticipatory guidelines.

4. LO 23.7 Explain a global surgical package.

5. LO 23.10 When transferring care and management of a patient to another facility, code 99495 requires the physician to document what elements?

 YOU CODE IT! Basics

Using the techniques described in this chapter, carefully read through the case studies and determine the most accurate E/M code(s) for each case study.

1. Makayla Sorensen, a 4-year-old female, sees Dr. Pitassin, a pediatrician, for the first time with itchy spots all over her body. After a detailed history and a detailed examination, his MDM is of a low complexity. Dr. Pitassin diagnoses her with chickenpox.

2. Loretta Stabler, an 81-year-old female, comes to see Dr. Gilman for her semi-annual checkup. Dr. Gilman notes he last saw the patient 6 months ago for a regular checkup. Dr. Gilman completes a detailed interval history with a comprehensive head-to-toe physical exam. He reviews and affirms the present medical plan of care. Loretta's condition is stable, her hypertension and diabetes (type 2) are in good control, and she has no new problems. There are minimal data for Dr. Gilman to review and several diagnoses to consider. The MDM is moderate.

3. George Terazzo, an 81-year-old male, collapsed at church during services and was brought to the ED. Dr. Horatio took a comprehensive history, performed a comprehensive examination, and made the decision to admit George into the observation unit of the hospital due to an irregular heartbeat with an unknown cause. MDM is of moderate complexity.

4. Sue Appleton, a 46-year-old female, was admitted this morning for observation after an MVA. Dr. Rhodes documents a detailed history and a comprehensive exam with a straightforward MDM. Sue is doing fine; all test results are within normal range. Dr. Rhodes discharges Sue the same afternoon.

5. Reisa Haven, a 39-year-old female, was sent by Dr. Alfaya to Dr. Avery, an OB-GYN, for an office consultation. She had been suffering with moderate pelvic pain, a heavy sensation in her lower pelvis, and marked discomfort during sexual intercourse. In a detailed history, Dr. Avery noted the location, severity, and duration of her pelvic pain and related symptoms. In the review of systems, Reisa had positive findings related to her gastrointestinal, genitourinary, and endocrine body systems. Dr. Avery noted that her past medical history was noncontributory to the present problem. The detailed physical examination centered on her gastrointestinal and genitourinary systems with a complete pelvic exam. Dr. Avery ordered lab tests and a pelvic ultrasound in order to consider uterine fibroids, endometritis, or other internal gynecologic pathology. MDM complexity was moderate.

6. Catalina King came into the ED with what appeared to be a wrist sprain that she sustained during a baseball game when she slid into home base. She was in obvious pain, and the wrist was swollen and too painful upon attempts to flex. Dr. Ervin performed an expanded problem-focused history and exam before he ordered x-rays. Reports confirmed a simple fracture of the distal radius. MDM was low.

7. George Carter was discharged today from the Bracker Nursing Center after Dr. Mintz spent 25 minutes performing a final examination, discussing George's stay, and providing instructions to George's wife for continuing care.

8. Heather Swann, a 68-year-old female, in good health, is a new patient at Victors Boarding Home. Dr. Cannon comes by to complete Heather's evaluation and documents an expanded problem-focused history and exam with an MDM of low complexity.

9. Marla Olden, a 38-year-old female, G2 P1, was admitted to Weston Hospital to deliver. Marla is considered a high-risk delivery. Dr. Kucherin was on standby for 30 minutes in the event a c-section was necessary. Marla delivered vaginally. Marla and baby are doing well. Code Dr. Kucherin's services.

10. Loretta Reubens, an 18-month-old female, is admitted today by Dr. Smallerman into the pediatric critical care unit because of severe respiratory distress.

 ## YOU CODE IT! Practice

Using the techniques described in this chapter, carefully read through the case studies and determine the most accurate E/M code(s) and modifier(s), if appropriate, for each case study.

1. Zena Awtrey, a 58-year-old female, sees Dr. Lunden for the first time for a variety of medical problems. She was diagnosed 5 years ago with insulin-dependent diabetes mellitus with complicating eye and renal problems. In addition, she suffers from hypertensive heart disease with episodes of congestive heart failure. Her peripheral vascular disease has worsened, and she can walk only a block before being crippled with extreme leg pain. The patient reports that a new problem has surfaced: throbbing headaches with radiating neck pain. Dr. Lunden and Zena thoroughly discuss her health concerns and issues. In order to manage and investigate the multiplicity of problems, Dr. Lunden takes a complete PFSH. A complete review of systems (ROS) is performed and comprehensive physical exam is completed. Dr. Lunden has to take a multitude of factors into consideration, as the patient's problems are highly complex.

2. Jamie Farmer, a 32-year-old male, goes to his family physician, Dr. Mitchell, for a tetanus shot after stepping on a rusty nail at the beach. While there, he asks Dr. Mitchell to look at a cut on his left hand. Dr. Mitchell examines the wound and tells him to keep the wound clean and bandaged. Dr. Mitchell documents a brief HPI and performs a limited exam of the left hand, MDM straightforward. Code only the E/M.

3. Owen Unger, a 19-month-old male, is admitted to the hospital by his pediatrician, Dr. Curtis, after a chest x-ray confirmed the child has pneumonia. Dr. Curtis and Mrs. Unger, Owen's mother, discuss the child's fever, cough, and diarrhea. Mrs. Unger provides a pertinent PFSH. An extended problem-focused ROS is completed and an extended examination of the cardiovascular and respiratory systems is performed. The course of treatment planned by Dr. Curtis is straightforward as the child's condition is of low severity.

4. Raymond Johnston, a 3-year-old male, showed no sign of improvement after 5 days of antibiotic therapy, so Dr. Servina admits Raymond into the hospital with a diagnosis of bacterial pneumonia. At Raymond's admittance, his vitals showed a temperature of 38.3°C (101°F), with a mild rash on his torso. The following day, Dr. Servina performed a problem-focused history and examination with MDM of low complexity. Code Dr. Servina's visit on the second day.

5. Tom Seihill, a 23-year-old male, was admitted into the hospital 2 days ago for bronchitis. While in the hospital, Tom requested that his family physician, Dr. Selbiger, perform a circumcision, so Dr. Selbiger called in Dr. Wacker, a urologist, for a consultation. Dr. Wacker discussed the request with Tom and took a brief history and performed a limited genitalia examination. Afterward, Dr. Wacker made a straightforward decision and recommended that Raymond have the surgical procedure done at a later date as an outpatient procedure. Code for Dr. Wacker's services.

6. Dr. Modesta spent 2½ hours administering critical care services and evaluating Carolina Tanner upon her admission into the ICU.

7. Howard Shires, a 78-year-old male, was diagnosed with advanced Alzheimer's disease about 1 year ago and has been in this facility for approximately 10 months. He was seen today by the nursing facility's physician, Dr. Bowyer, over concern of the development of urinary and fecal incontinence, as well as a number of other medical problems that have appeared to increase in severity. In addition to the detailed interval history, the physician spoke with family members and the nursing staff. Then, Dr. Bowyer reviewed the patient's record to create an extended history necessary for an extended review of systems (ROS). Dr. Bowyer performed a comprehensive physical exam to assess all body systems. Afterward, he wrote all new orders due to the dramatic change in the patient's physical and mental condition. A new complex treatment plan was created.

8. Royce Onoton's legs have finally healed to the point that he can be discharged from the nursing facility, where he has been for the last 6 weeks. Before he can go home, Dr. Zandi comes in for the final examination and to provide continuing care instructions to Royce's wife, who will be caring for Royce at home. Dr. Zandi prepares the discharge records and writes a prescription for Royce for pain. This whole process takes Dr. Zani about 45 minutes to complete.

9. Bernard Kristenson moved into the Prader Assisted Living Center today. Dr. Ramada, the center's resident physician, introduced himself to Bernard and then took an extended HPI and pertinent PFSH. Dr. Ramada performed a comprehensive examination. After reviewing the results of the examination, Dr. Ramada found management of Barnard's case to be moderate complexity.

10. Dr. Harrington provided care plan oversight services for Verniece Dantini, one of her patients at the Bracker Assisted Living Center. It took her 20 minutes.

11. Dr. Kaminsky spends approximately 1 hour in a meeting with an oncologist in Texas and a reconstructive surgeon in California. The three professionals discussed treatments and options for Karyn Cassey, a 41-year-old female, who was recently diagnosed with parosteal osteogenic sarcoma. Code the conference.

12. Raymond Catertell, a 23-year-old male, is the son of two alcoholics. Dr. Lowen spends 40 minutes with him providing risk factor reduction behavior modification techniques to help him avoid becoming an alcoholic himself.

13. Premier Life & Health Insurance Company required David Harrison, a 39-year-old male, to get Dr. Dijohn, his regular physician, to complete a certificate confirming that David's current disability prevents him from working at his regular job and makes him eligible for disability insurance.

14. Dr. Anderson works in a very small town in Ohio and travels up to 200 miles to see his patients in the surrounding rural areas. His patient Brenda Viard gave birth at her home the previous day to a 6-lb 3-oz baby girl, Alice Rose. Dr. Anderson sees Alice Rose for the first time today, does a complete history and exam, and prepares her medical chart. Alice Rose is a healthy newborn.

15. Petula Carter, a 4-day-old female, currently weighs 2,000 grams and requires intensive cardiac and respiratory monitoring. This is her third day in the NICU, and Dr. Wadhwa comes in to do his E/M of her condition.

YOU CODE IT! Application

The following exercises provide practice in the application of abstracting the physicians' notes and learning to work with documentation from our health care facility, Prader, Bracker, & Associates. These case studies are modeled on real patient encounters. Using the techniques described in this chapter, carefully read through the case studies and determine the most accurate E/M code(s) and modifier(s), if appropriate, for each case study.

WESTON HOSPITAL

629 Healthcare Way • SOMEWHERE, FL 32811 • 407-555-6541

PATIENT: TURNER, CHARLES

ACCOUNT/EHR #: TURNCH001

DATE: 10/01/19

Attending Physician: Renee O. Bracker, MD

S: This 27-year-old male was brought to the ED by ambulance after he was found unconscious on the living room floor. He regained consciousness within several minutes but complained of a severe headache and nausea. Pt states that the last thing he remembers he was on a ladder, changing a light bulb. He believes he lost his balance trying to reach too far and fell, hitting his head on the end-table.

O: Ht 5′10″, Wt 195 lb., R 16. Head: Scalp laceration on the right posterior parietal bone. Bruise indicates trauma to this area. Eyes: PERRLA. Neck: Neck muscles are tense; there is minor pain upon rotation of the head. Musculoskeletal: All other aspects of the shoulders, arms, and legs are unremarkable. X-rays of skull, two views, and soft tissue of the neck are all benign.

A: Concussion

P: 1. MRI to rule out subdural hematoma

   2. Repair laceration and bandage

ROB/mg   D: 10/01/19 09:50:16   T: 10/05/19 12:55:01

Determine the most accurate E/M code(s).

PRADER, BRACKER, & ASSOCIATES

A Complete Health Care Facility

159 Healthcare Way • SOMEWHERE, FL 32811 • 407-555-6789

PATIENT: BROMWELL, BRANDON

ACCOUNT/EHR #: BROMBR001

DATE: 10/18/19

Attending Physician: Oscar R. Prader, MD

(continued)

S: Brandon is a 9-month-old male brought in today by his mother. I last saw this patient at his regular 6-month checkup. He has been irritable lately and is tugging at his right ear. Brandon has been running a low-grade fever since yesterday. There has been no cough. Pt has a history of problems with his ears and sinuses.

O: Ht 25″, Wt 26 lb., R 20, T 101.3. HEENT: Purulent nasal discharge, yellow-green in color, is noted. Right TM is erythematous unilaterally, bulging, and with purulent effusions. Oropharynx is nonerythematous without lesions. One tooth on the bottom. Tonsils are unremarkable. Neck: Neck is supple with good range of motion (ROM). Positive cervical adenopathy. Lungs: Clear. Heart: Regular rate and rhythm without murmurs.

A: Acute suppurative otitis media, right side

P: 1. Rx Augmentin 40 mg/kg divided tid 10 days

    2. Bed rest, lots of fluids

    3. Follow-up prn or if no improvement in 10 days

ORP/mg   D: 10/18/19 09:50:16   T: 10/23/19 12:55:01

Determine the most accurate E/M code(s).

PRADER, BRACKER, & ASSOCIATES

A Complete Health Care Facility

159 Healthcare Way • SOMEWHERE, FL 32811 • 407-555-6789

PATIENT: HENSLEY, ERNEST

ACCOUNT/EHR #: HENSER001

DATE: 09/29/19

Attending Physician: Benjamin L. Johnston, MD

Referring Physician: Oscar R. Prader, MD

S: Pt is a 35-year-old male, referred by Dr. Prader for a consultation regarding a sore on his left temple, at the hairline. Pt states he is very involved in water sports. He knows the importance of sunscreen; however, he does not always remember to put it on. He has not had any dermatologic concerns prior to this. Patient states that his skin is occasionally dry and that he has adult onset acne.

O: Ht 6′1″, Wt 225 lb., R 17, T 98.6. After an examination of the skin along the hairline, as well as the rest of the face and neck, a culture is taken of the lesion. The pathology report confirms a malignant melanoma of the skin of the scalp.

A: Malignant melanoma, scalp

P: 1. Discuss surgical and pharmaceutical options for treatment

    2. Report sent to Dr. Prader

ORP/mg   D: 09/29/19 09:50:16   T: 10/01/19 12:55:01

Determine the most accurate E/M code(s).

PRADER, BRACKER, & ASSOCIATES

A Complete Health Care Facility

159 Healthcare Way • SOMEWHERE, FL 32811 • 407-555-6789

PATIENT: SARGENT, ALEXANDER

ACCOUNT/EHR #: SARGAL001

DATE: 10/25/19

Attending Physician: Renee O. Bracker, MD

S: This 85-year-old male is seen today at Northside Assisted Living Center, where he has been living for the last 6 months. The last time I saw this patient was right before he moved into the center. Nurse Thomas states that he has been complaining of mild abdominal pain and some discomfort upon urination. Other than this issue, he has been well and stable.

O: Ht 5'6.5", Wt 145 lb., R 18, P 73, BP 137/81. Abdomen is unremarkable. No masses or rigidity noted.

A: Suspected bladder infection

P: Order written for UA to rule out bladder infection.

ROB/mg   D: 10/25/19 09:50:16   T: 10/28/19 12:55:01

Determine the most accurate E/M code(s) and modifier(s), if appropriate.

WESTON HOSPITAL

629 Healthcare Way • SOMEWHERE, FL 32811 • 407-555-6541

PATIENT: LEAMAN, HESTER

ACCOUNT/EHR #: LEAMHE001

DATE: 10/01/19

Attending Physician: Renee O. Bracker, MD

This 18-month-old female is being admitted to the pediatric critical care. Mother claims onset of symptoms was sudden. She states that she rushed the child to the ED immediately.

Child is unresponsive. Respiration is shallow. B/P 85/60 mmHg, T 102.

Complete blood workup ordered: CBC with diff, tox screen, bilirubin, and basic metabolic panel. IV fluids to keep hydrated.

Await test results.

ROB/mg   D: 10/01/19 09:50:16   T: 10/03/19 12:55:01

Determine the most accurate E/M code(s) and modifier(s), if appropriate.

Design elements: ©McGraw-Hill

CPT Anesthesia Section

24

Learning Outcomes

After completing this chapter, the student should be able to:

LO 24.1 Interpret the types of anesthesia provided.

LO 24.2 Determine the accurate code and physical status modifier for the administration of anesthesia.

LO 24.3 Incorporate the Official Guidelines for reporting.

LO 24.4 Apply the formula for using time to report anesthesia services.

LO 24.5 Select the accurate qualifying circumstances add-on codes.

LO 24.6 Identify special circumstances requiring a CPT modifier.

LO 24.7 Abstract the notes to append HCPCS Level II modifiers.

Key Terms

Anesthesia
Anesthesiologists
Certified Registered Nurse Anesthetist (CRNA)
Conscious Sedation
General Anesthesia
Local Anesthesia
Monitored Anesthesia Care (MAC)
Regional Anesthesia
Topical Anesthesia

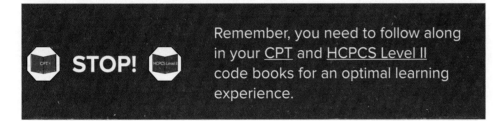

STOP! Remember, you need to follow along in your <u>CPT</u> and <u>HCPCS Level II</u> code books for an optimal learning experience.

24.1 Types of Anesthesia

Anesthesia is defined as the suppression of nerve sensations to relieve or prevent the feeling of pain, usually by the use of pharmaceuticals. Essentially, it is more commonly described as the administration of drugs to enable a patient to avoid the feeling of pain. While there are many types of anesthesia, they are all primarily divided into three preliminary categories: topical/local, regional, and general.

Topical and/or Local Anesthesia

Topical anesthesia refers to the numbing of surface nerves, whereas **local anesthesia** refers to the dulling of feeling in a limited area of the body.

Topical anesthesia is applied directly to the skin or mucous membranes, using a liquid or gel form. Typically, this is administered prior to very minor procedures on the epidural layer of the skin, or the eye, anus, vagina, mouth, gums, eardrum, or nose. Local anesthetics are most often administered by injection, directly into the anatomical site that is the object or target of the procedure. Lidocaine is one of the frequently used anesthetics.

EXAMPLE

Dr. Victors, a general dentist, rubbed a *topical anesthetic* onto Walter's gum to prevent him from feeling any pain from the injection of the *local anesthetic*. The local anesthetic will prevent him from feeling pain while the doctor drills the cavity that Walter has in his left, lower molar.

Anesthesia
The loss of sensation, with or without consciousness, generally induced by the administration of a particular drug.

Topical Anesthesia
The application of a drug to the skin to reduce or prevent sensation in a specific area temporarily.

Local Anesthesia
The injection of a drug to prevent sensation in a specific portion of the body; includes local infiltration anesthesia, digital blocks, and pudendal blocks.

Regional Anesthesia

The administration of a drug in order to interrupt the nerve impulses without loss of consciousness.

Regional Anesthesia

Regional anesthesia prevents a section of the body from transmitting pain and includes epidural, caudal, spinal, axillary, stellate ganglion blocks, regional blocks, and brachial anesthesia.

Regional anesthesia is most often used when the procedure

- Is focused on a specific region of the body.
- Involves a larger area of the body than could be treated with a local injection.
- Does not require general anesthesia.

In these cases, the chosen anesthetic is injected directly into a nerve, nerve plexus, or the spinal cord. There are two types of regional anesthesia:

- Peripheral nerve blocks, which are typically used for procedures performed on the extremities: arms or legs, or the groin, or the face.
- Epidural and spinal anesthesia, which employs an anesthetic injected into the spinal cord, most often to numb the lower abdomen, pelvic area, or the lower extremities.

EXAMPLE

Dr. Carloni, an anesthesiologist, was paged to come to the maternity ward to administer *epidural anesthesia* for Kimberly Saunders. After the epidural was given, Kimberly was able to proceed with the birth of her baby without the pain of childbirth. The loss of sensation was only from the waist down. She was otherwise awake and alert.

General Anesthesia

The administration of a drug in order to induce a loss of consciousness in the patient, who is unable to be aroused even by painful stimulation.

General Anesthesia

General anesthesia, also called *surgical anesthesia,* creates a total loss of consciousness and sensation. General anesthesia is given to the patient by inhalation, intravenous (IV) injection, or, on rare occasions, intramuscular (IM) injection.

Propofol is the drug most commonly used, administered by slow intravenous infusion. In some cases, a slow inhalation of anesthetic vapors is administered using a face mask.

EXAMPLE

Dr. Carver, an anesthesiologist, administered general anesthesia to Darnell Liberty after he was brought into the operating room (OR) and positioned on the table. Dr. Mendosa was preparing to remove Darnell's gallbladder because of the collection of stones in that organ, and everyone wanted to be certain that Darnell would not feel anything during the surgical procedure.

Conscious Sedation

The use of a drug to reduce stress and/or anxiety.

Moderate (Conscious) Sedation

One additional type of anesthesia that you should know about when coding anesthetic and surgical services is called **conscious sedation**. It is a form of ultralight general anesthesia that affects the entire body.

With conscious sedation, the physician gives the patient medication to reduce anxiety and stress. A short-acting benzodiazepine, such as midazolam (Versed), either alone or in combination with an opioid analgesic, such as fentanyl, is most often used for this purpose. The patient remains awake and aware of his or her surroundings and what is going on. He or she can answer questions and respond to verbal commands.

Most often, conscious sedation is used for procedures that will not typically cause pain but may be worrisome to patients, causing them to be nervous and frightened. The services of an anesthesiologist are not required for the provision of conscious sedation, so the physician performing the procedure, or a member of the nursing staff, may administer this before the patient goes into the procedure room. This is one of the reasons the codes for this service are not found in the *Anesthesia* section of CPT, but in the *Medicine* section.

Codes 99151–99157 report the administration of moderate (conscious) sedation and include

- Assessing the patient.
- Establishing IV access and fluids to maintain patency, when performed.
- Administering the drug.
- Maintaining the sedated level.
- Monitoring oxygen saturation, heart rate, and blood pressure.
- Observing and assessing the patient during recovery.

Coding for the administration of conscious sedation also has a few guidelines to help you determine the best, most appropriate code:

1. Who is administering the sedation?
   a. If the physician performing the procedure also administers the conscious sedation, use a code from the 99151–99153 range (located in the *Medicine* section of the CPT book).
   b. If a different physician or other health care professional, other than the professional performing the procedure, administers the conscious sedation, use a code from the 99155–99157 range (located in the *Medicine* section of the CPT book).
   c. If an **anesthesiologist** administers the moderate sedation, this is known as **Monitored Anesthesia Care (MAC)**, which is reported from the *Anesthesia* section of CPT (codes 00100-01999).
2. The time spent with the patient under conscious sedation helps to determine the correct code or codes. Intraservice work is measured in an initial 15-minute segment, followed by 15-minute segments. The clock starts when the physician administers the sedative and stops when the patient is discharged and the physician is no longer required to supervise the patient. Total time is calculated only for the minutes the physician continuously spends face-to-face with the patient.
3. The patient's age is the other factor that will lead you to the correct code.
4. Codes 99151–99153 require the presence of an independent qualified observer to monitor the patient's conscious status during the procedure. This is the sole responsibility for this individual.

Anesthesiologists
Physicians specializing in the administration of anesthesia.

Monitored Anesthesia Care (MAC)
The administration of sedatives, anesthetic agents, or other medications to relax but not render the patient unconscious while under the constant observation of a trained anesthesiologist; also known as "twilight" sedation.

EXAMPLES

99151	Moderate sedation services provided by the same physician or other qualified health care professional performing the diagnostic or therapeutic service that the sedation supports, requiring the presence of an independent trained observer to assist in the monitoring of the patient's level of consciousness and physiological status; initial 15 minutes of intraservice time, patient younger than 5 years of age
99152	initial 15 minutes of intraservice time, patient age 5 years or older
+99153	each additional 15 minutes intraservice time (List separately in addition to code for primary service)

GUIDANCE CONNECTION

Read the additional explanations in the in-section guidelines located within the **Medicine** section, subhead **Moderate (Conscious) Sedation**, directly above code 99151 in your CPT book.

LET'S CODE IT! SCENARIO

*Caterina Zingler, a 41-year-old female, came into the same day surgery center to have Dr. Freeman perform a hemorrhoidopexy by stapling. She was very nervous because she had never had this procedure before. Raymond Elvers, a **certified registered nurse anesthetist (CRNA)**, administered Versed, IV, a sedative to relieve her anxiety. The procedure is not really painful, so there was no need for a full anesthetic or painkiller. Raymond sat with Caterina throughout the procedure to ensure her safety and comfort level. Dr. Freeman accomplished the procedure in one stage, taking 30 minutes.*

> **Certified Registered Nurse Anesthetist (CRNA)**
>
> A registered nurse (RN) who has taken additional, specialized training in the administration of anesthesia.

Let's Code It!

Raymond Elvers, a CRNA, administered Versed, a mild "sedative," to Caterina before Dr. Freeman performed the procedure. Read the complete description for the procedure code used to report the performing of a *"hemorrhoidopexy by stapling"* (46947). This includes all of the details about the procedure, except the administration of the moderate sedation. Let's go to the Alphabetic Index and find *moderate sedation.*

> **Moderate Sedation**
>
> *See* Sedation

Turn to *Sedation,* where you find:

> **Sedation**
>
> Moderate 99151–99153, 99155–99157
>
>   with independent observation 99151–99153

Read, carefully, the complete descriptions of all of these codes in the *Main Section* of the CPT book and analyze the details within each.

Code 99151 requires the physician who performed the procedure to administer the moderate sedation, whereas 99155 requires another physician or health care professional. Which is correct? Go back to the documentation, which states, *"Raymond Elvers, a certified registered nurse anesthetist (CRNA), administered Versed, IV, a sedative to relieve her anxiety."* This would lead you to 99155.

You will see that code 99155 is the more accurate. This identifies **moderate sedation,** administered by a **different health care professional** [Raymond Elvers, CRNA] **than the professional who performed the procedure** [Dr. Freeman]**, initial 15 minutes intraservice, patient younger than 5 years of age**.

Wait a minute; the documentation states the patient is *"a 41-year-old female."* Take a look at code **99156 initial 15 minutes intraservice time, patient age 5 years or older**. That's more accurate.

Are you done? Not yet. Code 99156 only reports 15 minutes. The documentation states, *"taking 30 minutes."* You will need to also report code 99157 for the next 15 minutes, so Dr. Freeman and Raymond Elvers can be accurately reimbursed for all of the time they spent.

So, in addition to the code for the *hemorrhoidopexy* (46947), you need to include two additional codes for the *moderate sedation* (99156 and 99157) on the report and claim form.

Good job!

24.2 Coding Anesthesia Services

When coding anesthesia services, you should follow these steps to find the best, most appropriate code.

1. *Confirm* that the physician who performed the procedure for which the anesthesia was required is a different professional from the person who administered the anesthesia.

On those occasions when the same physician who performs the procedure also administers regional or general anesthesia, you must append modifier 47 Anesthesia by Surgeon to the appropriate procedure code. The modifier is *not* attached to an anesthesia procedure code; it is added to the basic procedure code. No additional code from the **Anesthesia** section will be used. See the subsection *Special Circumstances* later in this chapter to learn more about using modifier 47.

2. *Identify* the anatomical site of the patient's body upon which the surgical procedure was performed.

3. *Confirm* the exact surgical procedure performed, as documented in the physician's notes (also known as the *operative report*).

4. *Consult* the Alphabetic Index of the CPT book, look under the heading of **Anesthesia**, and read down the list to find the anatomical site shown below that heading. Identify the suggested code or codes for this site.

EXAMPLE

Anesthesia
Skull 00190

---

5. *Turn* to the *Main Section* of the CPT book, **Anesthesia** section, and find the subsection identifying that anatomical site.

EXAMPLES

| 00212 | Anesthesia for intracranial procedures; subdural taps |
| 00216 | vascular procedures |

---

6. *Read* the descriptions written next to each code option suggested in the Alphabetic Index carefully. Then compare them with the terms used by the physician in his or her notes documenting the procedure. This will lead you to the best, most appropriate code available.

 LET'S CODE IT! SCENARIO

Dr. Fonda is called in to administer general anesthesia to Morgan Saffire, a 6-month-old female, diagnosed with congenital tracheal stenosis. Dr. Caudwell performs a surgical repair of her trachea.

Let's Code It!

The notes indicate that Dr. Fonda administered the anesthesia and Dr. Caudwell performed a "*surgical repair of her trachea.*" Remember, this means that an anesthesia code will be used, not a modifier appended to the procedure code. So let's go ahead and find the best code for the anesthesia service.

Turn to the Alphabetic Index and look up *anesthesia*. Going down the alphabetic listing of the sites beneath this heading, look for more than a page until you get to the correct anatomical site: *Trachea.*

Trachea 00320, 00326, 00542
    Reconstruction 00539

The physician's notes state that Dr. Caudwell performed a "*repair,*" not a reconstruction, so focus on the codes shown next to *Trachea*. Turn to the *Main Section* of the CPT book to find the codes 00320, 00326, and 00542.

(continued)

Read the descriptions written next to each code, as well as the others found in the subsection, in order to determine the best, most appropriate code available.

Neck

00320	Anesthesia for all procedures on esophagus, thyroid, larynx, trachea and lymphatic system of neck; not otherwise specified, age 1 year or older
00322	Anesthesia for all procedures on esophagus, thyroid, larynx, trachea and lymphatic system of neck; needle biopsy of thyroid
00326	Anesthesia for all procedures on the larynx and trachea in children less than 1 year of age
00542	Anesthesia for thoracotomy procedures involving lungs, pleura, diaphragm, and mediastinum (including surgical thoracoscopy); decortication

As you review the code descriptions, you can identify which terms or words are most important in matching the code to the physician's documentation of the procedure. Look at the physician's notes one more time and identify the key terms.

Dr. Fonda is called in to administer general anesthesia to Morgan Saffire, a 6-month-old female, diagnosed with congenital tracheal stenosis. Dr. Caudwell performs a surgical repair of her trachea.

The combination of all these terms matches only one of our available code descriptions, doesn't it?

00326	Anesthesia for all procedures on the larynx and <u>trachea</u> in children <u>younger than 1 year</u> of age

You found the best, most appropriate code for the administration of general anesthesia for Morgan's surgery.

GUIDANCE CONNECTION

Read the additional explanations in the **Anesthesia Guidelines** in your CPT book directly before the **Anesthesia** section that lists all the codes.

Physical Status Modifiers

The American Society of Anesthesiologists (ASA) established six levels of measuring the physical condition of a patient with regard to the administration of anesthesia. Each level, identified by the letter *P* and a number from 1 to 6, denotes issues that may increase the complexity of delivering anesthetic services and is measured at the time the anesthetic is about to be administered. The anesthesiologist is the professional who determines the correct Physical Status Modifier. However, you, as the coding specialist, must be certain to look for the information and include it on the claim form.

Physical Status Modifiers are mandatory with every code from the *Anesthesia* section of the CPT book and are placed directly after the five-digit CPT code (with a hyphen between the two). For example: 00000-P1. (*NOTE:* Physical Status Modifiers are different from the regular CPT and HCPCS modifiers.)

Following are the Physical Status Modifiers that are to be used only with anesthesia codes:

P1 (*a normal healthy patient*). Modifier P1 indicates that the patient to whom the anesthetic was given had no medical concerns that would interfere with the anesthesiologist's responsibilities for keeping the patient sedated and safe.

EXAMPLE

Dr. Tristan administered general anesthesia to Austin Berger, a 15-year-old otherwise healthy female gymnast, before Dr. Armaden performed an arthroscopic extensive debridement of her shoulder joint. The correct code is 01630-P1.

P2 (*a patient with mild systemic disease*). When a patient has a disease that may affect the general workings of his or her body, it must be taken into consideration with regard to administering anesthesia. However, if the disease is under control, then its involvement is less of a concern.

> ### EXAMPLE
> Dr. Steiner administered general anesthesia to Venice Binle, a 41-year-old female with controlled type 1 diabetes mellitus, for her radical mastectomy with internal mammary node dissection, to be performed by Dr. Cabara. The correct code is 00406-P2.

P3 (*a patient with severe systemic disease*). In this case, the patient's disease is serious throughout his or her body and is an important factor for the anesthesiologist to contend with, in addition to the reason for the procedure.

> ### EXAMPLE
> Dr. Jeffries administered general anesthesia to Wilson Meyers, a 62-year-old male with benign hypertension due to Cushing's disease. Wilson came today for Dr. Ephron to perform a laparoscopic cholecystectomy with cholangiography for acute cholecystitis. The correct code is 00790-P3.

P4 (*a patient with severe systemic disease that is a constant threat to life*). Modifier P4 describes any patient having medical problems that have invaded or affected multiple systems of the body. The large number of issues regarding the effects of the disease, along with existing medications and treatments that have been ongoing in the patient's system, and the potential interactions with the anesthetic make it a very complex case.

> ### EXAMPLE
> Dr. Rockenbach administers general anesthesia to Ethan Vox, a 71-year-old male. Ethan has advanced esophageal cancer that has metastasized throughout his body. Dr. Glasser will be performing a partial esophagectomy. The correct code is 00500-P4.

P5 (*a moribund patient who is not expected to survive without the operation*). This is a life or death situation, but not necessarily an emergency. In such cases, the patient is in critical condition, and there are serious medical complications that make administering anesthesia more challenging.

> ### EXAMPLE
> Dr. Jeppapi administered general anesthesia to Zena Afronski, a 31-year-old female with acute arteriosclerosis. Dr. Able was called back in from vacation to perform a heart/lung transplant this morning. The correct code is 00580-P5.

P6 (*a declared brain-dead patient whose organs are being removed for donor purposes*). This modifier is provided by the ASA for use with brain-dead patients. Individuals in this condition need to have anesthesia administered to slow bodily functions and give the transplant team time to harvest the viable organs.

GUIDANCE CONNECTION

Read the additional explanations in the **Anesthesia Guidelines,** subsection **Anesthesia Modifiers,** in your CPT book directly in front of the **Anesthesia** section that lists all the codes, and read the entire descriptions in **Appendix A,** subsection **Anesthesia Physical Status Modifiers,** in your CPT book.

Determine which Physical Status Modifier is most accurate from the descriptions below of the patients' conditions.

1. Uma Koslozki, a 53-year-old female, with controlled hypertension. _____

2. Zachery Gregson is brought into the OR to have knee replacement surgery. He has acute COPD. _____

3. Tyler Madison is brought in to have his tonsils out. He is a healthy 12-year-old male. _____

24.3 Anesthesia Guidelines

Anesthesia Guidelines

The Official Guidelines specifically intended for coding anesthesia services (general and regional anesthesia) are shown at length on the pages at the beginning of the *Anesthesia* section of the CPT book. Go through these guidelines and review how they might help you determine the best, most appropriate anesthesia code.

- *Time Reporting:* You will learn more about this method sometimes used to report anesthesia services provided. Guidelines for this are included in this front part of the section.

- *Supplied Materials:* You might have questions if the anesthesiologist's documentation includes the use of special drugs or equipment such as a surgical tray. These guidelines include some direction.

- *Separate or Multiple Procedures:* When multiple procedures are performed during the same operative session, but the anesthesia is continuous, the anesthesia should be coded for the most complicated procedure only. These guidelines will provide you with the correct way to report these situations on behalf of the anesthesiologist.

- *Special Report:* There are times when something unusual occurs, or a situation where a less-than-common procedure is performed. How will this affect your reporting for the anesthesiologist? Check these guidelines.

- *Anesthesia Modifiers:* You learned about these in the previous chapter on *CPT and HCPCS Level II Modifiers.* They are repeated here for your convenience.

- *Qualifying Circumstances:* Later in this chapter, you will learn about these add-on codes that are used to explain when an anesthesiologist has an additional challenge keeping the patient sedated and safe. These are listed here, for your ease of reference.

  YOU CODE IT! CASE STUDY

Gerald Chang, a healthy 19-year-old male, was in a motorcycle accident. Today, Dr. Oliver, an anesthesiologist, was called in to administer general anesthesia so Dr. Joshua could insert internal fixation on Gerald's compound fracture of the right distal ulna and radius, as well as complete an arthroscopic repair of the right rotator cuff.

You Code It!

You need to determine the correct code or codes to report Dr. Oliver's work during this surgical event. He administered general anesthesia while Dr. Joshua performed two procedures: insertion of internal fixation on a compound fracture (01830) + repair of a rotator cuff injury (01630). Identify which Official Guideline will guide you in how to accurately code Dr. Oliver's work in this case.

(continued)

Step #1: Read the case carefully and completely.

Step #2: Abstract the scenario. Which key words or terms describe what service the physician provided to the patient during this encounter?

Step #3: Are there any details missing or incomplete for which you would need to query the physician? [If so, ask your instructor.]

Step #4: Determine the correct CPT procedure code or codes to explain the details about what was provided to the patient during this encounter.

Step #5: Check for any relevant guidance, including reading all of the symbols and notations.

Step #6: Do you need to append any modifiers to ensure complete and accurate information is provided?

Step #7: Double-check your work.

Answer:

Did you determine this to be the correct code to report, and which Official Guideline did you use?

01830-P1-AA   **Anesthesia for open or surgical arthroscopic/endoscopic procedures on distal radius, distal ulna, wrist, or hand joints; not otherwise specified, healthy patient, anesthesia administered by anesthesiologist**

Two procedures were performed during this one anesthetic administration: the compound fracture is more complex and severe than a rotator cuff injury. Therefore, in accordance with the Official Guidelines titled *Separate or Multiple Procedures,* you will only report the one code for the "most complex procedure."
   Good work!

Anesthesia Code Package

All the codes within the *Anesthesia* section of the CPT book include activities that are most often performed by **anesthesiologists** when they are preparing to administer anesthesia to a patient. The following services are included in the *anesthesia code package* and are not coded separately.

Anesthesiologists
Physicians specializing in the administration of anesthesia.

1. *Usual preoperative visits.* Most of the time, the anesthesiologist will stop in to interview the patient, in addition to taking the time to thoroughly read the chart and patient history, before administering the anesthesia. It gives the physician the opportunity to discuss any potential reactions or other considerations with the patient.

2. *Anesthesia care during the procedure.* The time and expertise the anesthesiologist spends in addition to administering the actual anesthetic, including observing the patient throughout the procedure, are very important parts of his or her job responsibilities.

3. *Administration of fluids.* The anesthesiologist gives the patient fluids as well as analgesics (liquid form) as needed during the procedure.

4. *Usual monitoring services* (such as ECG [electrocardiogram], temperature, BP [blood pressure]). As a part of the natural course of the anesthesiologist's duties, he or she must monitor the patient's vital signs throughout the procedure and make certain that there are no unexpected effects from the anesthesia.

5. *Usual postoperative visits.* The anesthesiologist normally visits the patient while he or she is in recovery to ensure that there are no lingering effects of the anesthesia and there are no other concerns as a result of the anesthesia.

YOU CODE IT! CASE STUDY

PATIENT: Darlena Eskine

DATE OF OPERATION: 02/17/2019

PREOPERATIVE DIAGNOSIS: Avascular necrosis, right hip.

POSTOPERATIVE DIAGNOSIS: Avascular necrosis, right hip.

OPERATION PERFORMED: Right total hip arthroplasty.

SURGEON: Arthur Hunter, MD

ANESTHESIOLOGIST: Samuel Samahdi, MD

INDICATIONS FOR OPERATION: The patient is an overall healthy 39-year-old former athlete who presents for hip arthroplasty having failed nonoperative treatment options. The risks, benefits, and treatment alternatives were discussed including, but not limited to, infection, bleeding, blood clots, nerve injury, dislocation, leg length inequality, prosthetic wear, loosening, need for further surgery, failure to relieve pain, etc. The patient's questions were answered, and the surgical plan was approved.

DESCRIPTION OF OPERATION: The patient was taken into the operating room, the appropriate extremity was identified, and the patient was positioned with appropriate padding to all pressure areas. After sterile skin preparation and draping, a posterior incision was performed. The skin and subcutaneous tissues were divided to the level of the fascia, which was then incised along the course of its fibers for a posterior approach. Leg lengths were measured prior to dislocation and then the hip capsule was excised, and a femoral neck cut was made. The acetabulum was then exposed and examined. No significant osteophytes were found. No significant acetabular defect was found.

The acetabulum was prepared. The last reamer used was 51 mm. No bone graft was used to reconstruct the acetabular defect. The acetabular component, 52 mm Pinnacle, was positioned appropriately and impacted into position, and mechanical stability was achieved. Supplemental screw fixation was not used. A neutral 36 liner was then appropriately chosen and positioned and the device assembled. Femoral exposure was obtained and the femoral canal was prepared. A trial reduction was performed and hip stability was assessed.

After the appropriate component position was determined, final canal preparation was completed. The component was then impacted into position, and mechanical stability was achieved. A trial reduction was performed, leg length and hip stability were assessed, the appropriate neck length was chosen, and a +8.5 ceramic head was impacted into position. The final reduction was performed, and hip stability was assessed. The hip was stable to 90 degrees of internal rotation, 20 degrees of abduction, 20 degrees of extension, 20 degrees of adduction, and 60 degrees of external rotation really with no tendency to dislocate.

The wound was irrigated profusely, a final inspection was performed, and bleeding was controlled and the wound was closed in layers. The hip capsule was not sutured. A drain was not placed. Sterile dressings were applied, and a radiograph was ordered. The components were found to be in appropriate alignment. The plan is for a routine postoperative course with weightbearing as tolerated and ambulation. Sciatic nerve was explored at the end of the procedure and found to be intact.

You Code It!

Read this operative report and determine what code or codes should be reported for Dr. Samadhi's services.

Step #1: Read the case carefully and completely.

Step #2: Abstract the scenario. Which key words or terms describe what service the physician provided to the patient during this encounter?

Step #3: Are there any details missing or incomplete for which you would need to query the physician? [If so, ask your instructor.]

Step #4: Determine the correct CPT procedure code or codes to explain the details about what was provided to the patient during this encounter.

Step #5: Check for any relevant guidance, including reading all of the symbols and notations.

(continued)

Step #6: Do you need to append any modifiers to ensure complete and accurate information is provided?

Step #7: Double-check your work.

Answer:

Did you determine this to be the correct code to report?

01214-P1-AA   **Anesthesia for open procedures involving hip joint; total hip arthoplasty, healthy patient, anesthesia administered by anesthesiologist**

24.4 Time Reporting

Time reporting may be used for billing general anesthesia services in certain areas or by certain third-party payers instead of CPT codes. If this is the custom in your local area, the clock begins when the anesthesiologist starts to prepare the patient for the administration of the anesthetic drug in the OR and is typically measured in 15-minute increments. The time ends when the anesthesiologist is no longer required to be present, once the patient has been safely transferred to postoperative supervision. When multiple procedures are completed during the same operative session, the time calculated should be the total time for all the procedures performed. A formula is used to calculate the amount of compensation the anesthesiologist will receive. The formula is

$$\text{Compensation} = (B + T + M) \times CF$$

where

B = base unit
T = time spent by the anesthesiologist with the patient
M = modifying factors
CF = conversion factor

The base unit is assigned by the American Society of Anesthesiologists (ASA), as published in the annual *Relative Value Guide*. The unit includes reimbursement for the usual time and services performed by the anesthesiologist preoperatively and postoperatively. Modifying factors are any adjustments made to allow for the additional challenges presented by the physical status of the patient at the time anesthesia is administered. The conversion factor is the number used to translate units into dollars.

Figure 24-1 is an example of an anesthesiologist's sedation record showing the time log of service.

GUIDANCE CONNECTION

Read the additional explanations in the **Anesthesia Guidelines,** subhead **Time Reporting,** in your CPT book directly before the **Anesthesia** section that lists all the codes.

YOU INTERPRET IT!

Here are the facts as reported by Dr. Haverall's sedation record of general anesthesia administered to Allen Dagmar for his perineal prostatectomy, performed by Dr. Kessler.

Base unit(s): 6

Time: 60 minutes [15 minutes × 4]

Modifying factors: None

Conversion factor: 21.9935

4. Determine the compensation the anesthesiologist should receive.

Remember . . . (*B* + *T* + *M*) × *CF* = Compensation

Monitoring	Time	*Level of Sedation	Pulse	Resp	B/P	O₂ sat	**Skin	ecg/rhythm as ordered	Medications
Pre Sedation	1300	I	51	17	142/43	98	WD	SR	
During Sedation Procedure	1400	I	61	18	149/72	92	WD	SR	Demerol 25mg Versed 2
	1403	II	66	17	109/53	97	WD	SR	TEE Probe in
	1406	II	70	19	156/64	100	WD	SR	
	1409	II	72	18	154/72	100	WD	SR	
	1412	II	73	18	146/44	100	WD	SR	10cc NSXI contrast
	1415	II	72	18	152/45	100	WD	SR	TEE done
Post Sedation	1420	I	59	18	153/59	97	WD	SR	
	1425	I	57	18	143/58	96	WD	SR	
	1430	I	56	15	124/50	96	WD	SB	
	1435	I	5	16	115/48	96	WD	SR	

Notify physician immediately if any symptomatic change in heart rate, resp status or O2 sat. < 92%
(if patient had a baseline O2 sat < 92% physician must set acceptable post sedation O2 sat. level)

** Skin W/D = Warm/Dry, D = Diaphoretic, C - Cool	Color 1 - Pink 2 - Pale 3 - Cyanotic 4 - Mottled
Level 1 Awake, verbalizes, cooperative	Observe & record Q 15 min: level of sedation.
Level 2 Drowsy but awake, eyes closed or open, verbalizes	Observe & record Q 15 min: level of sedation, cont pulse ox, resp, pulse, BP.
Level 3 Eyes closed, mimics sleep, arouses with minimal to moderate stimulation.	Continuous observation. Record Q5 min: Level of sedation, cont pulse oximeter, resp, pulse, BP.
Level 4 Sleep, arousable with moderate to intense stimulation May have potential for loss of protective reflexes.	Continuous observation. Record Q5 min: Level of sedation, cont Level of sedation, cont pulse oximeter, resp, pulse, BP.

* CAUTION: Asleep and nonarousable, temporary loss of protective reflexes: patient has progressed beyond Level IV and now falls under the guidelines of anesthesia.

NARRATIVE NOTES NPO until 1700. check gag reflex before feed. Pt. tole. well. No c/o of sz. throat, pt. alert x 3. Trans. to room. Report given to

Signature: RN

FIGURE 24-1 Anesthesiologist's sedation record

24.5 Qualifying Circumstances

Sometimes special circumstances, also called qualifying circumstances, cause the anesthetic process to be more complicated than usual. In these cases, a second—or add-on—code is used to identify that circumstance.

The available add-on codes for qualifying circumstances are

+99100 *Patient of extreme age . . . younger than 1 year or older than 70 years*
—This add-on code is not to be used when the code description already includes an age definition, such as code 00326, 00834, or 00836.

+99116 *Anesthesia complicated by total body hypothermia*
—Hypothermia is defined as *extremely low body temperature,* below 36.1°C (97°F). Because monitoring vital signs, including body temperature, is an important part of the anesthesia process, a very low body temperature would make the safe administration of anesthesia more complex.

+99135 *Anesthesia complicated by controlled hypotension*
—Hypotension is defined as *abnormally low blood pressure.* The critical connection between blood pressure and heart rate makes this situation

very intricate for the anesthesiologist. Controlled hypotension is utilized during surgical procedures to reduce bleeding and the need for blood transfusions. This has become more popular, as it contributes to a satisfactory bloodless surgical field.

+99140   *Anesthesia complicated by emergency conditions*
        —An emergency is characterized as a situation in which the patient's life, or an individual body part, would be threatened if there were any delay in providing treatment. In such a case, the anesthesiologist may not have the time to get the patient history or other information necessary to do his or her job most efficiently or effectively.

GUIDANCE CONNECTION

Read the additional explanations in the **Anesthesia Guidelines,** subsection **Qualifying Circumstances,** in your CPT book directly in front of the **Anesthesia** section that lists all the codes.

 YOU CODE IT! CASE STUDY

Arlena Smithson, a 77-year-old female, comes to see Dr. Beele for a total knee arthroplasty due to acute arthritis. Dr. Knight is called in to administer the general anesthesia for the procedure. Arlena is in otherwise good health.

You Code It!

Go through the steps, and determine the code(s) that should be reported for the anesthesia provided by Dr. Knight to Arlena.

Step #1: Read the case carefully and completely.

Step #2: Abstract the scenario. Which key words or terms describe what service the physician provided to the patient during this encounter?

Step #3: Are there any details missing or incomplete for which you would need to query the physician? [If so, ask your instructor.]

Step #4: Determine the correct CPT procedure code or codes to explain the details about what was provided to the patient during this encounter.

Step #5: Check for any relevant guidance, including reading all of the symbols and notations.

Step #6: Do you need to append any modifiers to ensure complete and accurate information is provided?

Step #7: Double-check your work.

Answer:

Did you determine these to be the correct codes?

    01402-P1   **Anesthesia for open or surgical arthroscopic procedures on knee joint; total knee arthroplasty; a normal healthy patient**

    99100   **Anesthesia for patient of extreme age, younger than 1 year and older than 70**

24.6 Special Circumstances

Unusual Anesthesia

Unusual circumstances might require the administration of general anesthesia for a procedure that typically requires either local anesthesia or no anesthesia. In these cases, the modifier 23 Unusual Anesthesia must be appended to the procedure code for that basic service (not to the anesthesia code); you will not assign a code from the *Anesthesia* section of CPT.

Turn to the CPT code book's *Appendix A* and read the CPT modifier description:

23   **Unusual Anesthesia:** Occasionally, a procedure, which usually requires either no anesthesia or local anesthesia, because of unusual circumstances must be done under general anesthesia. This circumstance may be reported by adding modifier 23 to the procedure code of the basic service.

 ## LET'S CODE IT! SCENARIO

Louisa Cabaña, a 61-year-old female, arrived for the insertion of a permanent pacemaker, atrial with transvenous electrodes. Dr. Snyder, knowing that Louisa has been diagnosed with Parkinson's disease, causing her to have uncontrollable tremors, decided that conscious sedation (which is the standard of care) was insufficient to ensure the patient's safety. He called Dr. Corman to administer general anesthesia.

Let's Code It!

Dr. Snyder decided that Louisa needed general anesthesia for this procedure, even though it is not the standard, because her Parkinson's disease made the procedure unsafe without it. He was inserting *a permanent pacemaker, atrial with transvenous electrodes.* Dr. Corman, an anesthesiologist, administered the anesthesia.

The Alphabetic Index shows

Insertion
Pacemaker, Heart 33206–33208
    Pulse Generator Only. 33212, 33213, 3221

Look through the descriptions for the codes in the first range, 33206–33208. Do any of the descriptions match the notes?

33206   **Insertion of new or replacement of permanent pacemaker with transvenous electrode(s); atrial**

Before you move on to the next section, remember that Dr. Snyder administered general anesthesia. You will learn from experience that conscious sedation is the standard of care for this procedure. Generally, there is no need for general anesthesia—the cost or the risk. General anesthesia is unusual. How will you ensure Dr. Snyder and Dr. Corman get properly reimbursed for the administration of the anesthesia? This is what modifiers do—identify unusual circumstances. Modifier 23 is specifically for a case when unusual anesthesia is used.

In this case, the correct code is **33206-23.**

You also would include a Supplemental Report to explain the medical necessity for providing this patient with general anesthesia, so the third-party payer and anyone else will understand this was the right thing to do for this patient.

 ## GUIDANCE CONNECTION

Read the additional explanations in the **Anesthesia Guidelines,** first column, last paragraph, in your CPT book directly before the **Anesthesia** section that lists all the codes, and read the entire description of modifier 47 in **Appendix A,** subsection **Modifiers,** in your CPT book.

Same Physician Administering Anesthesia and Performing the Procedure

If the physician performing the procedure also administers either regional or general anesthesia, the modifier 47 Anesthesia by Surgeon must be appended to the procedure code for that basic service (not to the anesthesia code). In such cases, an anesthesia code would *not* be reported. However, it is permissible to report a code for the injection of the anesthetic drug.

Turn to the CPT code book's *Appendix A* and read the CPT modifier description:

47   **Anesthesia by Surgeon:** Regional or general anesthesia provided by the surgeon may be reported by adding modifier 47 to the basic service. (This does not include local anesthesia.) NOTE: Modifier 47 would not be used as a modifier for the anesthesia procedures.

YOU CODE IT! CASE STUDY

Hallie Van Masters, a 27-year-old female, came to see Dr. Knowles for a repair of her extensor tendon in her right wrist. Dr. Knowles administered a regional nerve block and then performed the repair.

You Code It!

Go through the steps, and determine the procedure code(s) that should be reported for this encounter between Dr. Knowles and Hallie Van Masters.

Step #1: Read the case carefully and completely.

Step #2: Abstract the scenario. Which key words or terms describe what service the physician provided to the patient during this encounter?

Step #3: Are there any details missing or incomplete for which you would need to query the physician? [If so, ask your instructor.]

Step #4: Determine the correct CPT procedure code or codes to explain the details about what was provided to the patient during this encounter.

Step #5: Check for any relevant guidance, including reading all of the symbols and notations.

Step #6: Do you need to append any modifiers to ensure complete and accurate information is provided?

Step #7: Double-check your work.

Answer:

Did you determine these to be the correct codes?

25270-47	**Repair, tendon or muscle, extensor, forearm and/or wrist; primary, single, each tendon or muscle, regional anesthesia administered by surgeon**
64450	**Injection, anesthetic agent; other peripheral nerve or branch**

Excellent!

24.7 HCPCS Level II Modifiers

Specific HCPCS Level II modifiers are designated for use with anesthesia service codes (see Table 24-1). These modifiers are used only if the insurance carrier, such as Medicare, accepts HCPCS Level II codes and modifiers. It is your responsibility, as a

TABLE 24-1 HCPCS Level II Anesthesia-Related Modifiers

AA	Anesthesia services performed personally by the anesthesiologist
AD	Medical supervision by a physician: *more than 4 concurrent anesthesia procedures*
G8	Monitored anesthesia care (MAC) for deep complex, complicated, or markedly invasive surgical procedure
G9	Monitored anesthesia care (MAC) for a patient who has a history of a severe cardiopulmonary condition
QK	Medical direction of *2, 3, or 4 concurrent anesthesia procedures involving qualified individuals*
QS	Monitored anesthesiology care services (can be billed by a qualified nonphysician anesthetist or a physician)
QX	Qualified nonphysician anesthetist with medical direction by a physician
QY	Medical direction of one qualified nonphysician anesthetist by an anesthesiologist
QZ	CRNA without medical direction by a physician

GUIDANCE CONNECTION

Read the HCPCS Level II code book, subsection **Level II National Modifiers**.

professional coder, to know the rules for the different third-party payers with which you will work.

The QY modifier would be used to indicate that an anesthesiologist was available and oversaw the administration of anesthesia services provided by someone else, such as a CRNA. The QY modifier is for the supervision of one case at a time. QK is used for two to four cases at one time, and AD is for more than four cases at one time.

  LET'S CODE IT! SCENARIO

PATIENT: Randolph Butterman

PREOPERATIVE DIAGNOSIS: Caries and tooth eruption disturbance.

POSTOPERATIVE DIAGNOSIS: Caries and tooth eruption disturbance.

SURGICAL PROCEDURE: Extraction of tooth and alveoplasty

#6, 7, 8, 9, 10, 11, 14, 18, 19, 20, 21, 22, 23, 24, 25, 26, 27, 28, 29, 30, 31, 32

IV FLUIDS: 1200 mL of normal saline.

ESTIMATED BLOOD LOSS: 20 cc.

INDICATIONS FOR PROCEDURE: Extractions of remaining teeth under general anesthesia due to severe periodontal disease.

PROCEDURE IN DETAIL: The patient was identified in the preoperative holding area, at which time informed consent was given by the patient after addressing risks, benefits, and alternatives, and answering all questions. The patient was then transferred to the operating room. The patient was prepped and draped in a normal fashion.

The patient was anesthetized using general anesthesia due to the extensive nature of the procedure. Dr. Kendale, an anesthesiologist, personally cared for this patient due to the patient's uncontrolled type 2 diabetes mellitus.

A bite block was placed, a throat pack was placed, and attention was addressed to teeth #6, 7, 8, 9, 10, 11, 14, 18, 19, 20, 21, 22, 23, 24, 25, 26, 27, 28, 29, 30, 31, 32. These teeth were extracted using elevators and forceps. A mucoperiosteal buccal flap was elevated along the maxilla and mandibular alveolus. The alveolus of the maxilla and mandible (upper left, right, lower left, right) was trimmed and carved using ronguer forceps and bone files to appropriately remove undercuts and sharp points. Specimens were sent to pathology. The surgical sites were irrigated thoroughly with normal saline. Gel foam was packed into the extraction sockets for hemostasis. The tissue was closed with 3-0 chromic gut sutures.

Dentures were fitted and found to have adequate retention and occlusion. Gauze was then packed over dentures for pressure hemostasis.

Let's Code It!

You are going to report Dr. Kendale's services as the anesthesiologist during this surgery. First, the anesthesia code. Turn to the Alphabetic Index in your CPT book, and find:

Anesthesia

There is a very long list beneath this main term. Look for teeth—no listing, extraction—no listing, . . . try . . .

Mouth 00170, 00172

Turn to the **Anesthesia** section in the *Main Part* of CPT, and take a look:

00170 Anesthesia for intraoral procedures, including biopsy; not otherwise specified
00172 Anesthesia for intraoral procedures, including biopsy; repair of cleft palate

(continued)

There is no documentation that Randolph had a cleft palate, so 00172 cannot be reported. What about 00170? Intraoral means within the oral cavity. That's accurate. But what about the biopsy? There is no indication a biopsy was performed during these extractions, or was it. Read again, the sentence "*Specimens were sent to pathology.*" That supports the biopsy, so you now can confirm 00170 as the correct code.

Do you need any modifiers? You have already learned that every anesthesia code requires a Physical Status Modifier. Is there anything in the documentation that will help you? Look at "*the patient's uncontrolled type 2 diabetes mellitus.*" This sentence will lead you to Physical Status Modifier P3.

Do you need to report any other modifiers? Dr. Kendale is an anesthesiologist, and he personally administered the anesthesia for this procedure. Is there a modifier that can report this? Check the list. Modifier AA explains this perfectly.

Now, you can report this code with these modifiers to clearly communicate Dr. Kendale's work during this procedure.

00170-P3-AA **Anesthesia for intraoral procedures, including biopsy; not otherwise specified, patient with severe systemic disease, anesthesia services performed personally by the anesthesiologist**

Good work!

Chapter Summary

For the most part, anesthesia coding is for the purposes of submitting health insurance claim forms on behalf of the anesthesiologist or a member of his or her staff, such as a CRNA.

To find the best, most appropriate code that accurately represents the anesthesia services administered, you first must know which type of anesthesia was used. Then you must determine the anatomical site upon which the procedure was performed and exactly which procedure was provided to the patient. In addition, you must know who administered the anesthesia to the patient: Was it the physician who also performed that procedure, or was it a different health care professional? When using HCPCS Level II modifiers, you also need to know whether the physician who administered the anesthetic was an anesthesiologist.

Once you determine the best, most appropriate code for the dispensation of the anesthesia, you also have to append the correct modifiers, when applicable.

CODING BITES

Physical Status Modifiers

P1 *A normal healthy patient*

P2 *A patient with mild systemic disease*

P3 *A patient with severe systemic disease*

P4 *A patient with severe systemic disease that is a constant threat to life*

P5 *A moribund patient who is not expected to survive without the operation*

P6 *A declared brain-dead patient whose organs are being removed for donor purposes*

(continued)

Qualifying Circumstances Add-On Codes	
+99100	Patient of extreme age
+99116	Anesthesia complicated by total body hypothermia
+99135	Anesthesia complicated by controlled hypotension
+99140	Anesthesia complicated by emergency conditions

You Interpret It! Answers

1. P2, **2.** P4, **3.** P1, **4.** $527.84

CHAPTER 24 REVIEW
CPT Anesthesia Section

Mc Graw Hill **connect**

Enhance your learning by completing these exercises and more at mcgrawhillconnect.com!

Let's Check It! Terminology

Match each key term to the appropriate definition.

1. **LO 24.1** The administration of sedatives, anesthetic agents, or other medications to relax but not render the patient unconscious while under the constant observation of a trained anesthesiologist; also known as "twilight" sedation.

2. **LO 24.1** The loss of sensation, with or without consciousness, generally induced by the administration of a particular drug.

3. **LO 24.1** The application of a drug to the skin to reduce or prevent sensation in a specific area temporarily.

4. **LO 24.1** The administration of a drug in order to interrupt the nerve impulses without loss of consciousness.

5. **LO 24.1** The administration of a drug in order to induce a loss of consciousness in the patient, who is unable to be aroused even by painful stimulation.

6. **LO 24.1** The use of a drug to reduce stress and/or anxiety.

7. **LO 24.3** Physicians specializing in the administration of anesthesia.

8. **LO 24.1** A registered nurse (RN) who has taken additional, specialized training in the administration of anesthesia.

9. **LO 24.1** The injection of a drug to prevent sensation in a specific portion of the body; includes local infiltration anesthesia, digital blocks, and pudendal blocks.

A. Anesthesia
B. Anesthesiologists
C. Certified Registered Nurse Anesthetist (CRNA)
D. Conscious Sedation
E. General Anesthesia
F. Local Anesthesia
G. Monitored Anesthesia Care (MAC)
H. Regional Anesthesia
I. Topical Anesthesia

Let's Check It! Concepts

Choose the most appropriate answer for each of the following questions.

1. **LO 24.1** The categories of anesthesia include all *except*

   a. topical/local.   **b.** moderate sedation.   **c.** regional.   **d.** general.

2. **LO 24.2** A normally healthy patient presents today for lens surgery. What would be the correct anesthesia code for this procedure?

   a. 00140-P1   **b.** 00142-P2   **c.** 00142-P1   **d.** 00144-P3

3. **LO 24.6** Unusual circumstances might require the administration of general anesthesia for a procedure that typically requires either local anesthesia or no anesthesia. What modifier would be appended to the procedure code in these circumstances?

   a. 23   **b.** QZ   **c.** 47   **d.** G9

4. **LO 24.1** MAC is an acronym that stands for

   a. medically administered care.

   b. mutually accessible care.

   c. monitored anesthesia care.

   d. medical anesthetic characters.

5. **LO 24.7** All of the following are HCPCS Level II modifiers *except*

   a. AD   **b.** G8   **c.** 57   **d.** QX

6. **LO 24.2** When the physician performing the procedure also administers regional or general anesthesia, modifier 47 should

   a. be appended to the correct anesthesia code.

   b. be appended to the correct procedure code.

   c. be appended to either the correct anesthesia code or the correct procedure code.

   d. not be used in this circumstance.

7. **LO 24.3** The anesthesia code package includes all *except*

   a. preoperative visits.

   b. postoperative visits.

   c. usual monitoring services.

   d. home health follow-up.

8. **LO 24.4** When reporting anesthesia services using time reporting, the formula used is

   a. $(B + T + M) \times CF$ **b.** $(B + Q + CF) \times T$ **c.** $(Q + T + CF) \times B$ **d.** $(CF + B + T) \times M$

9. **LO 24.5** Qualifying circumstances are conditions that might require more work on the part of the anesthesiologist, including all *except*

   a. extreme age.

   b. emergency conditions.

   c. severe systemic disease.

   d. total body hypothermia.

10. **LO 24.2** A Physical Status Modifier describes issues that may increase the complexity of delivering anesthetic services, including

    a. emergency situations.

    b. mild systemic disease.

    c. extreme age.

    d. controlled hypotension.

Let's Check It! Guidelines

Refer to the Anesthesia Guidelines and fill in the blanks accordingly.

five-digit	over	99155, 99156, 99157	safely	Medicine
minimal	second	All	complex	moderate
multiple	ends	anesthesia	99070	physical status modifier
plus	total	not	facility	deep
99151, 99152, 99153	nonfacility	single	above	"P"
time	separately	monitored	1 to 6	

1. Services involving administration of _____ are reported by the use of the anesthesia _____ procedure code plus modifier codes.

2. To report _____ (conscious) sedation provided by a physician also performing the service for which conscious sedation is being provided, see codes _____.

3. When a second physician other than the health care professional performing the diagnostic or therapeutic services provides moderate (conscious) sedation in the _____ setting, the second physician reports the associated moderate sedation procedure/service _____; when these services are performed by the second physician in the _____ setting, codes 99155, 99156, 99157 would _____ be reported.

4. Moderate sedation does not include _____ sedation (anxiolysis), _____ sedation, or _____ anesthesia care.

5. Anesthesia _____ begins when the anesthesiologist begins to prepare the patient for the induction of anesthesia in the operating room and _____ when the anesthesiologist is no longer in personal attendance, that is, when the patient may be _____ placed under postoperative supervision.

6. "Special Services and Reporting" are listed in the _____ section.

7. Supplies and materials provided _____ and _____ those usually included in the office visit or other services rendered may be listed _____. Drugs, tray supplies, and materials provided should be listed and identified with _____ or the appropriate supply code.

8. When _____ surgical procedures are performed during a _____ anesthetic administration, the anesthesia code representing the most _____ procedure is reported. The time reported is the combined _____ for all procedures.

9. _____ anesthesia services are reported by use of the anesthesia five-digit procedure code _____ the addition of a _____.

10. Physical Status Modifiers are represented by the initial letter _____ followed by a single digit from _____.

Let's Check It! Rules and Regulations

Please answer the following questions from the knowledge you have gained after reading this chapter.

1. LO 24.2 List the six steps to coding anesthesia.
2. LO 24.3 What is included in the anesthesia code package?
3. LO 24.4 Why is time important to coding anesthesia? When does the clock start and stop?
4. LO 24.5 List the qualifying circumstance add-on codes with their description.
5. LO 24.7 Explain the difference between HCPCS Level II modifiers QX, QY, and QZ.

YOU CODE IT! Basics

Using the techniques described in this chapter, carefully read through the case studies and determine the most accurate anesthesia code(s) and modifier(s), if appropriate, for each case study.

1. Dr. Carey administers general anesthesia so Dr. Tucker can perform a transconjunctival blepharoplasty. Patient has a diagnosis of controlled hypertension.

2. Dr. Tumbokon administers anesthesia and performs a biopsy to rule out salivary duct carcinoma. Patient is otherwise healthy.

3. Dr. Lynn administers anesthesia before performing a bone marrow aspiration on Mayra Magazine's posterior iliac crest. Mayra is a 36-year-old female who has been diagnosed with anemia and congestive heart failure.

4. Tierra, a healthy 29-year-old female, is taken to the OR, where Dr. Denmark administers spinal anesthesia and performs a tubal ligation by the bipolar coagulation method.

5. Geoffrey Foulks, an otherwise healthy 11-week-old male, is taken to the OR to repair his congenital cleft lip. Geoffrey weights 12 lbs. and has a 10 g/dL hemoglobin. Dr. Fairbanks administers general anesthesia, and Dr. Olafson successfully performs the Millar procedure.

6. Paulette Milling, a 51-year-old female, has been diagnosed with a thyroid cyst. She presents today for a needle biopsy of the thyroid cyst. Dr. Singletary administers general anesthesia because of her epilepsy. Otherwise, she is healthy.

7. Brian, a healthy 13-month-old male, is brought to the OR, where Dr. Thomas administers general anesthesia so Dr. Richardson, a pediatric urologist, can perform a laparoscopic orchipexy.

8. Jessica Hamilton, an otherwise healthy 12-year-old female, was playing in a treehouse when she fell approximately 6 feet, causing a tracheobronchial injury (TBI). Jessica was taken to the OR on an emergency basis, where Dr. Mortimer administers general anesthesia so Dr. Skipper can perform the tracheobronchial reconstruction.

9. The patient is taken to the OR, where Dr. Sidney administers the general anesthesia so Dr. Weigle, an orthopedic surgeon, can perform an ankle arthroplasty. Patient has an implanted pacemaker.

10. Dr. Benefield administers anesthesia and performs a vasectomy. Patient is otherwise healthy.

11. Dr. Simmons administers anesthesia and performs a thoracentesis, no imaging guidance.

12. Dr. Coleman administers anesthesia for Dr. Cho to harvest a liver from a brain-dead patient for transplantation.

13. Dr. Caulkins administers anesthesia for pelvic body cast application revision. The patient is otherwise healthy.

14. Dr. Jones administers anesthesia for osteotomy of the humerus. Patient has been diagnosed with ongoing cardiac ischemia.

15. Dr. Payne administers anesthesia for third-degree burn debridement; total body surface 5%. Patient has been diagnosed with well-controlled DM/HTN.

 YOU CODE IT! Practice

Using the techniques described in this chapter, carefully read through the case studies and determine the most accurate anesthesia code(s) and modifier(s), if appropriate, for each case study.

1. Connie Huffman, a healthy 28-year-old female, received anesthesia before delivering her son at the hospital. It was a vaginal delivery. Patient is otherwise healthy.

2. Dr. Masters administered general anesthesia to Ashton Hopkins, an otherwise healthy 32-year-old firefighter. Dr. Woody performed a third-degree burn excision, followed by a skin grafting on Ashton's chest, where 9% of his body surface was burned while he was rescuing a little girl from a house fire.

3. David Wolff, a 53-year-old male, was previously diagnosed with benign hypertension due to morbid obesity. Dr. Adams administers general anesthesia so that Dr. McKnight can perform a direct venous thrombectomy on his lower left leg.

4. Dr. Carroll administered anesthesia to Margaret Lindler, a 41-year-old female, diagnosed with a malignant neoplasm of the uterus. Her gynecologist, Dr. Ramage, performed a vaginal hysterectomy.

5. Dr. Billingsworth administered anesthesia to Ralph Skipper, a 7-month-old male requiring a hernia repair in the lower abdomen. Dr. Sims, the neonatologist, noted that, without the surgery, Ralph was not expected to survive.

6. Martha Gantt, a 76-year-old female with a history of hypertension and diabetes mellitus, is brought into the OR for Dr. Brunson to perform a corneal transplant. Dr. Williams, the anesthesiologist, administers the anesthesia.

7. Dr. Elliston is preparing to perform a ventriculography with burr holes on Daniel Ewing, a 12-year-old male, who fell off the monkey bars onto a cement floor yesterday. Dr. Hallbeck administers the anesthesia. Daniel is otherwise healthy.

8. Dr. Hanh administers anesthesia so that Dr. Lindholm can perform a diagnostic lumbar puncture on Keith Franklin, a 56-year-old male. Over the course of the last year, Keith, a construction worker, has developed

essential hypertension, which is currently controlled by diet. This lumbar puncture is to confirm the suspected diagnosis of bacterial meningitis.

9. Gerry Sherman, a healthy 28-year-old male, plays professional basketball and is given anesthesia by Dr. Wallace before having a diagnostic arthroscopy of his right knee by Dr. Hook.

10. Carlton Dazquez, a 17-year-old male, was in a go-kart accident and fractured his upper arm 3 months ago. Today, Dr. Hytower operated on him to repair the malunion of his humerus. Dr. Murphy administered the anesthesia. Carl is otherwise healthy.

11. Trisha Moultrie brought her 3-year-old daughter, Tamara, into the emergency room with a deep laceration of her scalp above her right ear, measuring 2.25 cm. Tamara was distraught, crying, and combative, kicking at the physician and the nurse as they attempted to clean the wound. At the recommendation of Dr. White, Trisha held Tamara in her lap, while the physician administered 1 mg of Versed, IM. Once the sedation took effect, Dr. White was able to perform a layered repair of the laceration while the nurse monitored Tamara's vital signs. The entire procedure took 25 minutes. Code the moderate sedation only.

12. Regina Weyeneth, a healthy 23-year-old female, was given an epidural during labor, with the expectations of a vaginal delivery. After a time, Dr. Bedenbaugh, her obstetrician, determined that the labor was obstructed and notified the hospital staff that they would have to do a cesarean (c-section).

13. Dr. Anderson administered anesthesia to Barbara Brooks, a 52-year-old female, in preparation of the breast reconstruction with TRAM flap to be performed by Dr. Mocase. Barbara has a history of breast cancer and is postmastectomy; she is otherwise healthy.

14. Dr. Solington brought Howard Chen, a 10-month-old male, into the OR for repair of his complete transposition of the great arteries under cardiopulmonary bypass. Pump oxygenation was used. Howard was not expected to survive without the surgery. Dr. Misher, the anesthesiologist, administered the anesthesia.

15. Meredith Susswell, a 79-year-old female, was given anesthesia by Dr. Yabsley, the anesthesiologist, in preparation for the repair of her ventral hernia in her lower abdomen, to be performed by Dr. Carrouth. Meredith has uncontrolled diabetes mellitus and essential hypertension.

 YOU CODE IT! Application

The following exercises provide practice in the application of abstracting the physicians' notes and learning to work with documentation from our health care facility, Anytown Anesthesiology Associates. These case studies are modeled on real patient encounters. Using the techniques described in this chapter, carefully read through the case studies and determine the most accurate anesthesia code(s) and modifier(s), if appropriate, for each case study.

ANYTOWN ANESTHESIOLOGY ASSOCIATES

241 MAIN STREET • ANYTOWN, FL 32711 • 407-555-1234

PATIENT: PERSILE, LORRAINE

ACCOUNT/EHR #: PERSLO001

DATE: 10/15/19

Preoperative DX: Locked right knee, rule out medial meniscus tear

Postoperative DX: 1. Grade 2 tear, anterior, cruciate ligament

2. Medial meniscus tear, anterior, horn

3. Grade 2 chondrosis, medial femoral condyle

(continued)

Procedure: 1. Arthroscopy

2. Partial anterior cruciate ligament debridement

3. Partial medial meniscectomy

Attending Physician: Renee O. Bracker, MD

Anesthesia: General

Anesthesiologist: Lawrence Miller, MD

INDICATIONS: The patient is a 33-year-old female who was in her usual state of good health until about 10 days ago when she sustained a twisting injury to the right knee with inability to fully extend the knee, with pain and swelling.

PROCEDURE: Estimated blood loss: None. Complications: None. Tourniquet time: See anesthesia notes. Specimens: None. Drains: None. Disposition: To the recovery room in stable condition.

Pt was taken to surgery and placed on the OR table in the supine position. After adequate general anesthesia was administered, she received a gram of intravenous Kefzol preoperatively. A proximal thigh tourniquet was applied. Examination revealed no significant Lachman or drawer and a moderate effusion. No varus or valgus instability. Distal pulses intact. The right lower extremity was placed in the arthroscopic leg holder; shaved, prepped, and draped in the usual meticulously sterile fashion for lower extremity surgery. Esmarch exsanguinations of the limb were performed, and the tourniquet was inflated. Proximal medial, anteromedial, and anterolateral portals were fashioned. A systematic evaluation of the knee was performed. The undersurface of the patella demonstrated normal tracking with no chondrosis.

The suprapatellar pouch, medial, and lateral gutters were well within normal limits, and in the notch a grade 2 tear of the anterior cruciate ligament was identified. There were some bloody fragments of the ACL that seemed to be impinging in the medial compartment. This was meticulously debrided. Approximately 50% of the ACL appeared to be intact. Attention was turned to the lateral compartment. The articular surface of the meniscus was normal. On the medial side, a grade 2 lesion in medial femoral condyle, lateral side, was noted. This was not debrided. Also, an anterior tear of the medial meniscus, which was frayed and torn, was another potential source of impingement. This was meticulously debrided to a smooth, stable mechanical limb, and the wound was irrigated and closed with 4-0 nylon simple interrupted sutures. Xeroform, 4 × 4s, Webril and Ace bandage from the tips of the toes to the groin completed the sterile dressing. There were no intraoperative or immediate postoperative complications.
The prognosis is good, although it may be limited by potential for arthritis and instability in the future.

LM/mg   D: 10/15/19 09:50:16   T: 10/23/19 12:55:01

Determine the most accurate anesthesia code(s) and modifier(s), if appropriate.

ANYTOWN ANESTHESIOLOGY ASSOCIATES

241 MAIN STREET • ANYTOWN, FL 32711 • 407-555-1234

PATIENT: HAMMOND, NEIL

ACCOUNT/EHR #: HAMMNE001

DATE: 10/21/19

Preoperative DX: C5–C6 and C6–C7 herniated nucleus pulposus

Postoperative DX: Same

Procedure: C5–C6 and C6–C7 anterior cervical diskectomy and fusion with cadaver bone and plate

(continued)

Attending Physician: Oscar R. Prader, MD

Anesthesia: General endotracheal

Anesthesiologist: Eric Keist, MD

INDICATIONS: The patient is a 35-year-old male with a history of neck and arm pain. MRI scan showed disk herniation at C5–C6 and C6–C7. The patient failed conservative measures and was subsequently set up for surgery. Patient has been diagnosed with DM/HTN, which is well under control.

PROCEDURE: The patient was taken to the OR. The patient was induced, and an endotracheal tube was placed. A Foley catheter was placed. The patient was given preoperative antibiotics. The patient was placed in slight extension. The left neck was prepped and draped in the usual manner. A linear incision was made above the C6 vertebral body. The platysma was divided. Dissection was continued medial to the sternocleidomastoid to the prevertebral fascia. The longus colli were cauterized and elevated. The C5–C6 disk space was addressed first. A retractor was placed. A large anterior osteophyte was removed with a large Leksell and drill. Distraction pins were then placed. The disk space was drilled out. Large bone spurs were drilled posteriorly. The posterior longitudinal ligament was removed. A free fragment was removed from beneath the ligament. The dura was visualized. A piece of bank bone was measured and slightly countersunk. The C6–C7 disk space was then addressed. Distraction pins were placed. A large anterior osteophyte was removed with a large Leksell and drill. The disk space was drilled out. Large bone spurs were drilled posteriorly. The Kerrison punch was used to remove the posterior longitudinal ligament. The dura was visualized. One piece of bank bone was in the C5, one in the C6, and two in the C7 vertebral bodies. The locking screws were tightened. The wound was irrigated. A drain was placed. The platysma was approximated with simple interrupted Vicryl. The dressing was applied. The patient was placed in a soft collar. The patient tolerated the procedure without difficulty. All counts were correct at the end of the case. The patient was extubated and transferred to recovery.

EK/mg   D: 10/21/19 09:50:16   T: 10/23/19 12:55:01

Determine the most accurate anesthesia code(s) and modifier(s), if appropriate.

ANYTOWN ANESTHESIOLOGY ASSOCIATES

241 MAIN STREET • ANYTOWN, FL 32711 • 407-555-1234

PATIENT: WAYMEN, MARK

ACCOUNT/EHR #: WAYMMA001

DATE: 11/07/19

Preoperative DX: Inguinal hernia, right

Postoperative DX: Inguinal hernia, right, direct and indirect

Procedure: Repair of right inguinal hernia with mesh

Attending Physician: Oscar R. Prader, MD

Anesthesia: General

Anesthesiologist: Lawrence Miller, MD

PROCEDURE: The patient is a 41-year-old male who was taken to the OR and prepped in the usual sterile fashion. After satisfactory anesthesia, a transverse incision was made above the inguinal ligament and carried down to the fascia of the external oblique, which was then opened, and the cord was mobilized. The ilioinguinal nerve was identified and protected. A relatively large indirect hernia was found. However, there

(continued)

was an extension of the hernia, such that one could definitely tell there had been a long-standing hernia here that probably had enlarged fairly recently. The posterior wall, however, was quite dilated and without a great deal of tone and bulging as well, and probably fit the criteria for a hernia by itself. Nonetheless, the hernia sac was separated from the cord structures, and a high ligation was done with a purse string suture of 2-0 silk and a suture ligature of the same material prior to amputating the sac. The posterior wall was repaired with Marlex mesh, which was sewn in place in the usual manner, anchoring two sutures at the pubic tubercle tissue, taking one lateral up the rectus sheath and one lateral along the shelving border of Poupart's ligament past the internal ring. The mesh had been incised laterally to accommodate the internal ring. Several sutures were used to tack the mesh down superiorly and laterally to the transversalis fascia. Then the two limbs of the mesh were brought together lateral to the internal ring and secured to the shelving border of Poupart's ligament. The mesh was irrigated with Gentamicin solution. The subcutaneous tissue was closed with fine Vicryl, as was the internal oblique. Marcaine was infiltrated in the subcutaneous tissue and skin. The wound was closed with fine nylon. The patient tolerated the procedure well.

LM/mg   D: 11/07/19 09:50:16   T: 11/11/19 12:55:01

Determine the most accurate anesthesia code(s) and modifier(s), if appropriate.

ANYTOWN ANESTHESIOLOGY ASSOCIATES

241 MAIN STREET • ANYTOWN, FL 32711 • 407-555-1234

PATIENT: DRESSLER, SIMONE

ACCOUNT/EHR #: DRESSI001

DATE: 11/15/19

Preoperative DX: Chronic cholelithiasis

Postoperative DX: Chronic cholelithiasis; subacute cholecystitis

Procedure: Laparoscopic cholecystectomy; intraoperative cholangiogram

Attending Physician: Renee O. Bracker, MD

Anesthesia: General endotracheal

Anesthesiologist: Melinda Abruzzo, MD

PROCEDURE: The patient, a 57-year-old female, was taken to the OR. The patient was induced and an endotracheal tube was placed. The patient was then placed in the supine position. The abdomen was prepped and draped in the usual fashion. The patient had several previous lower midline incisions and right flank incision; therefore, the pneumoperitoneum was created via epigastric incision to the left of the midline with a Verres needle. After adequate pneumoperitoneum, the 11-mm trocar was placed through the extended incision in the left epigastrium just to the left of the midline, and the laparoscope and camera were in place. Inspection of the peritoneal cavity revealed it to be free of adhesions, and another 11-mm trocar was then placed under direct vision through a small infraumbilical incision. The scope and camera were then moved to this position, and the gallbladder was easily visualized. The gallbladder was elevated, and Hartmann's pouch was grasped. Using a combination of sharp and blunt dissection, the cystic artery was identified. The gallbladder was somewhat tense and subacutely inflamed. Therefore, a needle was passed through the abdominal wall into the gallbladder, and the gallbladder was aspirated free until it collapsed. One of the graspers was held over this region to prevent any further leakage of bile. Again, direction was turned to the area of the triangle of Calot. The cystic duct was dissected free with sharp and blunt dissection. A small opening was made in the duct, and the cholangiogram catheter was passed. The cholangiogram revealed no stones or filling defects in the bile duct system. The biliary

(continued)

tree was normal. There was good flow into the duodenum, and the catheter was definitely in the cystic duct. The catheter was removed, and the cystic duct was ligated between clips, as was the cystic artery. The gallbladder was then dissected free from the hepatic bed using electrocautery dissection, and it was removed from the abdomen through the umbilical port. Inspection of the hepatic bed noted that hemostasis was meticulous. The region of dissection was irrigated and aspirated dry. The trocars were removed, and the pneumoperitoneum was released. The incisions were closed with Steri-Strips, and the umbilical fascial incision was closed with 2-0 Maxon. The patient tolerated the procedure well; there were no complications. She was returned to the recovery room awake and alert.

MA/mg   D: 11/15/19 09:50:16   T: 11/19/19 12:55:01

Determine the most accurate anesthesia code(s) and modifier(s), if appropriate.

ANYTOWN ANESTHESIOLOGY ASSOCIATES

241 MAIN STREET • ANYTOWN, FL 32711 • 407-555-1234

PATIENT: LYNDON, JAMES

ACCOUNT/EHR #: LYNDJA001

DATE: 12/01/19

Preoperative DX: Sensory deficit of common digital nerve; tendon laceration

Postoperative DX: Same

Procedure: Repair of digital nerve, right hand; repair of tendon laceration

Attending Physician: Renee O. Bracker, MD

Anesthesia: General

Anesthesiologist: Eric Keist, MD

INDICATIONS: The patient is a 23-year-old male who was stabbed in the right hand during a street fight. Examination showed a sensory deficit of the thumb and index finger due to an injury to the common digital nerve and a tendon laceration involving the abductor pollicis and first dorsal interosseous. He was taken immediately to the OR for repair.

PROCEDURE: The patient was taken to the OR. General anesthesia was administered, a tourniquet was applied, and the wound was explored. The common digital nerve to the thumb was identified and found to be divided at the level just proximal to the first metacarpal. The digital nerve to the radial aspect of the index finger was also divided. The abductor pollicis and the first dorsal interosseous tendons were then repaired with 3-0 Vicryl to the fascia.

Following this, both digital nerves were repaired by using interrupted 9-0 Nylon, suturing epineurium to epineurium. When completed, the wound was thoroughly irrigated with saline solution and the skin was closed with interrupted Ethilon. A dorsal splint was applied to the thumb and remains in IP flexion at about 30 degrees and slight adduction. Tourniquet time totaled 190 minutes.

EK/mg   D: 12/01/19 09:50:16   T: 12/04/19 12:55:01

Determine the most accurate anesthesia code(s) and modifier(s), if appropriate.

Design elements: ©McGraw-Hill

CPT Surgery Section

Learning Outcomes

After completing this chapter, the student should be able to:

LO 25.1 Distinguish among the types of surgical procedures.

LO 25.2 Determine which services are included in the global surgical package.

LO 25.3 Interpret the impact on coding of the global time frames.

LO 25.4 Identify unusual services and treatments and report them accurately.

LO 25.5 Abstract physician documentation of procedures on the integumentary system.

LO 25.6 Apply the guidelines, accurately, for coding procedures on the musculoskeletal system.

LO 25.7 Recognize the details required to accurately report procedures on the respiratory system.

LO 25.8 Identify guidelines to correctly report services to the cardiovascular system.

LO 25.9 Distinguish the various procedures on the digestive system.

LO 25.10 Ascertain the elements of coding services to the urinary system.

LO 25.11 Determine how to accurately report procedures on the genital systems: male and female.

LO 25.12 Interpret documentation to accurately report procedures on the nervous system.

LO 25.13 Recognize the necessary details to report procedures on the eye, ocular adnexa, and auditory system.

LO 25.14 Report accurately the different services provided during an organ transplant.

LO 25.15 Demonstrate the proper way to report the use of an operating microscope with a CPT code.

Key Terms

Allotransplantation
Arthrodesis
Closed Treatment
Complex Closure
Donor Area (Site)
Excision
Fornix
Full-Thickness
Global Period
Harvesting
Intermediate Closure
Laminectomy
Manipulation
Open Treatment
Percutaneous Skeletal Fixation
Recipient Area
Saphenous Vein
Simple Closure
Standard of Care
Surgical Approach
Transplantation

 STOP! Remember, you need to follow along in your CPT code book for an optimal learning experience.

25.1 Types of Surgical Procedures

Typically, a surgical procedure can be performed in any one of several locations: the physician's office, an ambulatory care center, or a hospital. Of course, the location will most often be determined by the intensity or complexity of the procedure. You certainly would not expect an entire operating room (OR) at the hospital to be used for a physician repairing a simple laceration (cut), and no one could imagine agreeing to have a heart transplant performed in a physician's office. As a coding specialist, your responsibilities will vary, depending upon where you work, when it comes to coding surgical procedures. In addition, there may be more than one coding specialist involved with reporting one procedure.

EXAMPLE

For a surgical procedure performed in a hospital operating room (OR), there may be as many as three coders involved:

1. The hospital's coder codes for the support personnel, facilities, and supplies.
2. The surgeon's coder codes for his or her professional services.
3. The anesthesiologist's coder codes for his or her professional services.

Coding operative reports and procedure notes becomes easier with experience because the longer you work for a physician or facility, the more you will learn about the procedures and services he or she performs. Experience will train you to decipher which services are included in procedures and which are not. Throughout this chapter and the next, the guidelines and specifications for coding the various types of surgical and nonsurgical procedures are reviewed.

In CPT, the term *surgery* is not limited to only those services and treatments performed in an OR or even in a hospital. Within this section of the CPT book, codes are listed that report

- Incision and drainage of a cyst.
- Debridement.
- Simple repair of a superficial wound.

All these services can easily be performed in a physician's office. In addition, many procedures are now performed at an ambulatory surgical center or outpatient department.

When hearing the word *surgery,* most people picture an all-white room with health care professionals dressed in masks, gowns, and gloves and a patient under general anesthesia. However, this is a very narrow perspective on surgical procedures. You, as a professional coding specialist, need to understand the various types of surgical processes because this detail may be important for determining the most accurate code.

Prophylactic, Diagnostic, and Therapeutic Procedures

Under certain circumstances, the purpose of a procedure will affect the code you use to report the service. Three key terms to watch for are *prophylactic, diagnostic,* and *therapeutic.*

- A *prophylactic* treatment is one that is performed to prevent a condition from developing. This may be a surgical procedure, a series of injections, or a prescription.

- A *diagnostic* procedure or test is performed so that the physician can gather more details about a condition or concern at issue. In other words, the reason for performing the test or procedure is to get closer to an accurate diagnosis.

- A *therapeutic* procedure is provided, most often, to correct or fix a problem.

Surgical Approach
The methodology or technique used by the physician to perform the procedure, service, or treatment.

There are times when, for the safety of the patient, a procedure begins as a diagnostic examination and turns into a therapeutic procedure. Generally, a therapeutic or surgical procedure will include the diagnostic portion, thereby requiring only one code when both are done during the same encounter.

Above, in both of the two laparoscopic codes (49320 and 50541), CPT includes the guideline "*Surgical laparoscopy always includes diagnostic laparoscopy.*" Therefore, if the physician performed a diagnostic laparoscopy solely to determine what was wrong with the patient, the correct code might be 49320. However, if while the physician was performing the diagnostic laparoscopy, he observed a renal cyst and decided to ablate the cyst at the same time, this would mean that a diagnostic procedure (to discover the cyst) and a therapeutic procedure (ablation of the cyst) were done at the same time. In that case, only 50541 might be reported, as it is one code that includes both the diagnostic and therapeutic portions of the procedure.

Surgical Approaches

Procedure coding requires that you understand the various **surgical approaches** a physician can take to provide care for a patient:

- A *noninvasive,* or *external,* procedure is one that does not enter the patient's body; these are procedures that are applied or performed directly to the skin without physical entry into the visceral (internal) part of the body. An example of a noninvasive procedure is a shave biopsy, a technique to acquire pathology specimens of an elevated growth on the skin by razor.

- *Minimally invasive* procedures are becoming more and more available as health care researchers continue to find methods to diagnose and correct problems with the least amount of trauma to the patient. Although there is a big difference in our perception between a patient being stabbed by a mugger and a patient being cut open by a physician during a surgical procedure, the human body knows only that it is being invaded by a sharp piece of metal. It is traumatic, and healing must occur at the point of the incision as well as to whatever was done to internal organs.

- The *percutaneous approach* uses instruments inserted into the body by way of a puncture or small incision to access the intended anatomical site. Example: needle biopsy.

- The *percutaneous endoscopic approach* uses instruments inserted into the body by way of a puncture or small incision to access and visualize the intended anatomical site. Example: diagnostic anoscopy.

- The *via natural or artificial opening approach* involves instrumentation entered into the body through a natural opening (such as the vagina) or an artificial opening (such as a stoma) to visualize the intended anatomical site. Example: flexible esophagoscopy.

- The *via natural or artificial opening endoscopic approach* involves insertion of a scope through a natural opening (such as the mouth) or an artificial opening (such as a stoma) to visualize and aid in the performance of a procedure on the intended anatomical site. Example: colonoscopy with polyp removal.

🢒 GUIDANCE CONNECTION

Read additional explanations in the **Surgery Guidelines,** subheads **Follow-Up Care for Diagnostic Procedures** and **Follow-Up Care for Therapeutic Surgical Procedures,** in your CPT book directly in front of the Surgery section that lists all the codes.

Follow-Up Care for Diagnostic Procedures

When a diagnostic procedure is performed, the code includes only that care related to the recovery from this procedure, not any treatment for the condition identified. Care for the condition (therapeutic services) is not included.

Follow-Up Care for Therapeutic Surgical Procedures

The code reporting the provision of a therapeutic procedure only includes the care related to that procedure. Complications, exacerbations, recurrence, or the presence of other diseases or injuries requiring additional services should be reported separately.

- *Open approach* procedures are fully invasive, as the surgeon cuts the body open to enable access to internal tissues and organs. These procedures involve using a scalpel or laser to cut through the skin, membranes, and body layers to access the intended anatomical site.

EXAMPLES

Surgical procedures on a woman's uterus can be performed using

- The vaginal canal as the entry point (endoscopic using a natural opening) to avoid surgical entry through the abdomen, reported with

    58262   Vaginal hysterectomy, for uterus 250g or less; with removal of tube(s) and/or ovary(s)

- Laparoscopy (a minimally invasive procedure through the abdominal cavity) via small incisions into the patient's skin and muscle, reported with

    58542   Laparoscopy, surgical, supracervical hysterectomy, for uterus 250g or less; with removal of tube(s) and/or ovary(s)

- Open procedure with a longer incision through the abdominal wall, reported with

    58150   Total abdominal hysterectomy (corpus and cervix), with or without removal of tube(s), with or without removal of ovary(s)

You can see that all three of these codes accurately report a hysterectomy (the surgical removal of the uterus) with the removal of the fallopian tubes and ovaries. The difference between these codes is the surgical technique reported: 58150 reports an open abdominal procedure using an incision through the patient's abdominal wall, 58262 reports a procedure using a natural orifice (the vagina) so that no surgical incision was required, and 58542 reports a laparoscopic procedure that uses three tiny incisions in the patient's abdomen. The information provided by the reporting of these different versions of this procedure includes not only the level of work required by the physician to perform the procedure but also the level of postoperative care that the patient will require.

YOU INTERPRET IT!

Interpret each of these procedural statements to determine the type of procedure being documented: Diagnostic, Prophylactic, or Therapeutic.
1. Biopsy was performed to determine if mass is benign or malignant. _____
2. Lithotripsy to destroy kidney stones. _____
3. Cholecystectomy. _____
4. Pneumonia vaccine administered. _____

Interpret each of these procedural statements to determine the type of surgical approach being documented: Open, Percutaneous, or Endoscopic/Laparoscopic.
5. A 7-cm incision was made. _____
6. A needle-biopsy was performed. _____
7. The scope was passed through the patient's mouth into the stomach. _____

25.2 The Surgical Package

One of the trickiest portions of coding surgical events is distinguishing between which services and procedures are included in the code and which services and procedures might need to be coded separately for additional reimbursement. Whereas the services included in each surgical protocol may vary with the procedure itself, some elements are already integrated in most CPT codes.

Services Always Included

Let's begin by reviewing services that are *always included* in CPT surgical procedure codes.

Once the physician and patient agree to move forward with the operation or procedure, the surgical package includes the following elements:

1. *Evaluation and management (E/M) encounters provided after the decision to have surgery.* These visits may begin the day before the surgical procedure (for more complex procedures) or the day of the procedure (for minor procedures), as needed.

2. *Local infiltration, metacarpal/metatarsal/digital block, or topical anesthesia.* You learned about the different types of anesthesia in the chapter *CPT Anesthesia Section.* The surgical package includes specific types of local and regional anesthesia services only when they are provided by the surgeon (the same professional who will be performing the procedure).

3. *The operation itself, along with any services normally considered a part of the procedure being performed.* This would include supplies, as well as applying sutures, bandages, casts, and so on to enable the patient to leave the OR safely after the procedure.

4. *Immediate postoperative care.* This includes assessing the patient in the recovery area; attending to any complications exhibited by the patient (not including any additional trips to the OR); dictating or writing the operative notes; talking with the patient, the patient's family, and other health care professionals; and writing orders.

5. *Follow-up care.* This care includes postoperative visits; care for typical complications following surgery; pain management; dressing changes; removal of sutures, staples, tubes, casts, and so on; and any other services considered to be the **standard of care** during the **global period** for the specific surgical procedure. However, be careful. Some procedures may require a longer period of postoperative care by the surgeon. The period is determined by the accepted standard of care guidelines for each specific procedure and the details regarding the particular patient's health. More about this in the section *Global Period Time Frames.*

6. *Supplies provided in a physician's office.* With a few specific exceptions, included supplies are determined by the insurance carrier.

Services Not Included

Some functions that are commonly performed when a patient is going to have, or has had, surgery are *not included* in the surgical package. When such services and/or procedures are performed, you must code them separately.

1. *Diagnostic tests and procedures.* Tests or procedures that the physician needs to confirm the medical necessity for the surgery or investigate other issues related to the surgery are coded separately.

> **EXAMPLE**
> Diagnostic tests and procedures, such as biopsies, blood tests, and x-rays.

2. *Postoperative therapies.* Examples of postoperative therapies include immunosuppressive therapy after an organ transplant and chemotherapy after surgery to remove a malignancy.

GUIDANCE CONNECTION

Read additional explanations in the **Surgery Guidelines,** subhead **CPT Surgical Package Definition,** in your CPT book directly in front of the Surgery section that lists all the codes.

CODING BITES

Remember that an encounter that ends with an agreement to have surgery is reported with an E/M code appended with modifier **57 Decision for Surgery.** This is a notification of a surgical package that will soon begin.

Standard of Care
The accepted principles of conduct, services, or treatments that are established as the expected behavior.

Global Period
The length of time allotted for postoperative care included in the surgical package, which is generally accepted to be 90 days for major surgical procedures and up to 10 days for minor procedures.

3. *A more comprehensive version of the original procedure.* If the physician attempted to use a less extensive procedure first that was not sufficient to treat the patient, the second, more extensive procedure would be coded separately, with its own surgical package; it is not an extension of the first procedure. Also, the CPT code for the second event would be appended with modifier 58.

EXAMPLE

Dr. Keystone performed a lumpectomy on Joan Calcanne's left breast. The biopsy of the tissue removed during the lumpectomy showed that the malignancy had spread farther through the breast. Dr. Keystone had to take Joan back into the OR 1 week later for a simple, complete mastectomy. The code for the mastectomy is appended with modifier 58.

19301	Mastectomy, partial (e.g., lumpectomy, tylectomy, quadrantectomy, segmentectomy)
19303-58	Mastectomy, simple, complete, more extensive procedure

4. *Staged or multipart procedures.* Each stage or operation has its own surgical package and global period for aftercare. You must add modifier 58 to the second procedure code and all additional procedure codes reported for the same encounter.

> **58** **Staged or Related Procedure or Service by the Same Physician During the Postoperative Period.** It may be necessary to indicate that the performance of a procedure or service during the postoperative period was: (a) planned or anticipated (staged); (b) more extensive than the original procedure; or (c) for therapy following a surgical procedure. This circumstance may be reported by adding modifier 58 to the staged or related procedure.

EXAMPLE

Albert Rodgers, a 31-year-old male, suffered a fracture to his upper arm that severely damaged the shaft of his right humerus. Dr. Curran decides to first do a bone graft to support the healing process of the fracture and to follow that with a second surgical procedure—an osteotomy—in about 4 weeks. This is a staged, or multipart, surgical procedure.

24516	Treatment of humeral shaft fracture, with insertion of intramedullary implant, with or without cerclage and/or locking screws
24400-58	Osteotomy, humerus, with or without internal fixation, staged procedure by the same physician during the postoperative period

5. *Management of postoperative complications that require additional surgery.* As you may remember about the surgical package from *Services Always Included* (earlier in this section), the physician's attention to any postoperative complications is included in the original package *unless* those complications require the patient to return to the operating room. In such cases, you must use a modifier with the CPT code for the procedure performed.

> **76** **Repeat Procedure by the Same Physician.** It may be necessary to indicate that a procedure or service was repeated subsequent to the original procedure or service. This circumstance may be reported by adding modifier 76 to the repeated procedure or service.

> **78** **Unplanned Return to the Operating/Procedure Room by the Same Physician Following Initial Procedure for a Related Procedure During the Postoperative Period.** It may be necessary to indicate that another procedure was performed during the postoperative period of the initial procedure

(unplanned procedure following initial procedure). When this procedure is related to the first, and requires the use of an operating/procedure room, it may be reported by adding modifier 78 to the related procedure.

> **EXAMPLE**
>
> Lilly Drummond, a 14-year-old female, was burned on her left forearm when she missed catching a flaming baton during cheerleading practice. Five days ago, Dr. Cheng applied a skin allograft to the burned area. Lilly is admitted today because the graft is not healing properly, and Dr. Cheng is going to apply a new allograft of 20 sq. cm.
>
> 15271-76   Application of skin substitute graft to trunk, arms, legs, total wound surface area up to 100 sq. cm; first 25 sq. cm or less wound surface area; repeat procedures by the same physician

77   **Repeat Procedure by Another Physician.** The physician may need to indicate that a basic procedure or service performed by another physician had to be repeated. This situation may be reported by adding modifier 77 to the repeated procedure/service.

> **EXAMPLE**
>
> Ray DeVilldus, an 18-year-old male, was stabbed in the chest during a fight. Dr. Swartz performed a complex repair of a 6-cm laceration of the chest. The next day, Dr. Swartz left for a medical conference. The guy who stabbed Ray showed up at the hospital, and Ray got out of bed, against doctor's orders, and engaged in another fight, ripping open his stitches. Dr. Tyson, filling in for Dr. Swartz, had to take Ray back into the OR and redo the repair. Dr. Tyson will send the claim with the following code:
>
> 13101-77   Repair, complex, trunk; 2.6 cm to 7.5 cm; repeat procedure by another physician

6. *Unrelated surgical procedure during the postoperative period.* If the same physician must perform an unrelated surgical procedure during the postoperative period, you have to include a modifier to explain that this procedure has nothing to do with the first.

   79   **Unrelated Procedure or Service by the Same Physician During the Postoperative Period.** The physician may need to indicate that the performance of a procedure or service during the postoperative period was unrelated to the original procedure. This circumstance may be reported by using modifier 79.

> **EXAMPLE**
>
> Judith Conchran, a 41-year-old female, had a gastric bypass performed by Dr. Fellowes 10 days ago. She comes to see him today because she has a fever and pain radiating across her abdomen. Dr. Fellowes examines her, calls an ambulance, and takes her to the hospital and up to the operating room, where he performs an appendectomy to remove her ruptured appendix. The global postoperative period for a gastric bypass is 90 days. Dr. Fellowes performed Judith's appendectomy during the postoperative period for the bypass, and it had nothing to do with the first procedure. Therefore, our correct code would be
>
> 44960-79   Appendectomy; for ruptured appendix with abscess or generalized peritonitis; unrelated procedure or service by the same physician during the postoperative period

7. *Supplies.* In certain cases, for certain procedures performed in a physician's office, a separate code is permitted for supplies, such as a surgical tray, casting supplies, splints, and drugs. You have to check the reimbursement rules for the specific third-party payer.

EXAMPLE

Illea Beurus was prepped and ready for the procedure to begin. Dr. Hernandez performed the closed manipulation of the fracture. Instead of the usual plaster cast, fiberglass was used.

99070   Supplies and materials (except spectacles), provided by the physician or other qualified health care professional over and above those usually included with the office visit or other services rendered (list drugs, trays, supplies, or materials provided)

YOU INTERPRET IT!

Determine if the service or procedure provided in these statements is Included in the Surgical code (package) *or* Reported with a separate code.

8. Jeanine came to see Dr. Kidmon in his office 1 week after he performed her hysterectomy, as he instructed her to do. He wanted to check her sutures and healing progress. _____

9. While at Dr. Kidmon's office, Jeanine asked him to check her left breast because she felt a lump. He was concerned and performed a biopsy on the lump. _____

10. After Dr. Kidmon performed a mastectomy on Jeanine's left breast, he explained to her that they would need to complete a series of skin grafts. One graft would be done each month for 3 months. All are part of the postoperative care for mastectomy patients. Jeanine agreed. _____

25.3 Global Period Time Frames

Essentially, all procedures have assigned global period time frames based on the standard of care for a treatment or service. These range from 0 (zero) for a very simple procedure to 10 days for a minor procedure to 90 days for major surgery.

Zero-Day Postoperative Period

For procedures such as endoscopies and some minor procedures:

- No preoperative period.
- No postoperative days.
- Visit on day of procedure is generally not payable as a separate service.

10-Day Postoperative Period

For other minor procedures, 10 days following the day of the surgery:

- No preoperative period.
- Visit on day of the procedure is generally not payable as a separate service.

90-Day Postoperative Period

For major procedures, the total global period is actually 92 days: 1 day before the day of the surgery plus the day of surgery plus 90 days immediately following the day of surgery.

- One day preoperative included.
- Day of the procedure is generally not payable as a separate service.

YOU INTERPRET IT!

Use your resources and good critical thinking to determine the global surgery period for these procedures.

11. Metacarpal osteotomy [CPT code 26565] _____

12. Initial pericardiocentesis [CPT code 33010] _____

13. Cervical lymphadenectomy [CPT code 38724] _____

14. Placement of seton [CPT code 46020] _____

15. Cystourethroscopy, with biopsy [CPT code 52204] _____

25.4 Unusual Services and Treatments

Treatment Plan Provided by More Than One Physician

It is expected that the same physician will provide all of the surgical package's elements. This is an umbrella that covers only one health care professional.

Occasionally, however, more than one physician will be involved in providing all the necessary services for one patient having one operation. In such cases, modifiers explain to the third-party payer who did what and when.

54 **Surgical Care Only.** You must add this modifier to the correct CPT surgical procedure code when your physician is only going to perform the procedure itself, and not provide or be involved in any preoperative or postoperative care of the patient.

55 **Postoperative Management Only.** This modifier is added to the CPT code for the surgical procedure included on a claim from the physician who only cares for the patient after the operation.

GUIDANCE CONNECTION

Refer to the *Global Surgery Booklet* from CMS:

https://www.cms.gov/ Outreach-and-Education/Medicare-Learning-Network-MLN/MLNProducts/ downloads/ GlobalSurgery-ICN907166.pdf

To find the official Global Surgery Period for each CPT code, use the Physician Fee Schedule Look-Up Tool:

https://www.cms.gov/ Medicare/Medicare-Fee-for-Service-Payment/PFSlookup/ index.html

Scroll all the way down the page to ACCEPT. This will bring you to the next screen, where you will specify the parameters about the code for which you are seeking information. Remember, CPT is also known as HCPCS Level I, so in that field, you can enter the CPT code. Click SUBMIT.

On the next screen, be certain to click "Show All Columns."

56 **Preoperative Management Only.** When a physician, other than the surgeon who performed the procedure, cares for the patient from the decision to have surgery up to but not including the operation itself, modifier 56 is appended to the CPT code for the procedure.

 ## LET'S CODE IT! SCENARIO

Nadia Forrester, a 37-year-old female, was on vacation, hiking through the mountains, when she fell over a log and wrenched her knee very badly. She was flown to the nearest hospital and placed under the care of Dr. Petrone. After the diagnostic tests were completed, Dr. Petrone recommended arthroscopic surgery to treat the knee. Dr. Petrone called in Dr. Wellington, an orthopedic surgeon, to perform the procedure. Dr. Wellington performed a surgical arthroscopy and repaired the medial meniscus. Immediately after the surgery, Nadia flew home, and she went to her family physician, Dr. Shields, for the follow-up appointments.

Let's Code It!

The notes indicate that Dr. Petrone, Dr. Wellington, and Dr. Shields were all involved, to some extent, in caring for Nadia during the procedure—*surgical arthroscopy* and *repair of the medial meniscus*. Let's go to the Alphabetic Index and look up the procedure.

Find *arthroscopy*. As you go down the list, you will see the subcategories *Diagnostic* and *Surgical*. You know from the notes that this was surgical. Continue down and find the anatomical site for this procedure: **Knee . . . 29871–29889**. Indented under knee, you will find additional listings that don't really match, so let's look at the suggested codes:

29871 **Arthroscopy, knee, surgical; for infection, lavage and drainage**

The description is correct, up to the semicolon. So continue down the page to find any additional information that might be applicable to the case, according to our documentation. (Remember: Read up to the semicolon on the code because it is at the margin, and then finish the description with each indented description.)

Continue reading until you see

29882 **with meniscus repair (medial OR lateral)**

The complete description of this code is

29882 **Arthroscopy, knee, surgical; with meniscus repair (medial OR lateral)**

This matches the notes exactly, doesn't it? It does! Good job!

As you have learned, the surgical package for this procedure includes all the services and treatments that Nadia received. However, instead of just one physician, Nadia actually had three doctors caring for her throughout. Each physician will send his or her own claim form in an effort to get paid for the services he or she provided. You need to supply some explanation to the third-party payer so that it can understand receiving three claim forms for one procedure provided to the one patient.

Dr. Petrone will have the 29882-56 code with modifier to indicate he only provided the preoperative care.
Dr. Wellington will have the 29882-54 code with modifier to indicate he only performed the surgery.
Dr. Shields will have the 29882-55 code with modifier to indicate she only provided the postoperative care.

Increased Procedural Services

Every service and treatment or procedure has an industry standard of care. Included in the assessment of each service is a calculation of how much work is involved and how long it will take to complete the procedure. It is all part of the formula used by third-party payers to determine how much to pay the health care professional. As you might expect, though, particularly in health care, things do not always go exactly as planned. There may be an issue with a patient that requires more work on the physician's part.

When this happens, the physician should receive additional compensation. Therefore, you have to attach the modifier 22 to the procedure code to identify an unusual circumstance. You also have to attach documentation that fully explains the circumstances.

> **22**   **Increased Procedural Services.** When the work required to provide a service is substantially greater than typically required, it may be identified by adding modifier 22 to the usual procedure code. Documentation must support the substantial additional work and the reason for the additional work (i.e., increased intensity, time, technical difficulty of procedure, severity of patient's condition, physical and mental effort required). Note: The modifier should not be appended to an E/M service.

 ## YOU CODE IT! CASE STUDY

Frederick Stiner, a 15-year-old male, is 5 ft. 6 in., 365 lb. Dr. Girst performs a partial colectomy with anastomosis. The procedure, however, takes several hours longer than usual due to the fact that Frederick is morbidly obese.

You Code It!

Go through the steps, and determine the procedure code(s) that should be reported for this encounter between Dr. Girst and Frederick Stiner.

Step #1: Read the case carefully and completely.

Step #2: Abstract the scenario. Which key words or terms describe what service the physician provided to the patient during this encounter?

Step #3: Are there any details missing or incomplete for which you would need to query the physician? [If so, ask your instructor.]

Step #4: Determine the correct CPT procedure code or codes to explain the details about what was provided to the patient during this encounter.

Step #5: Check for any relevant guidance, including reading all of the symbols and notations.

Step #6: Do you need to append any modifiers to ensure complete and accurate information is provided?

Step #7: Double-check your work.

Answer:

Did you determine this to be the correct code?

44140-22   Colectomy, partial; with anastomosis, increased procedural service

In addition to the code, you should attach a letter with the claim to explain the circumstance that complicated the procedure.

 ## GUIDANCE CONNECTION

Read the additional explanations in the **Surgery Guidelines**, subhead **Separate Procedure**, in your CPT book directly in front of the Surgery section that lists all the codes.

CODING BITES

Read the entire description of these modifiers, and all others, in your **CPT book, Appendix A.**

Separate Procedure

Throughout the CPT book, you will see code descriptions that include the notation "separate procedure." Such services and treatments are generally performed along with a group of other procedures. When this happens, you will be able to find a combination, or bundled, code that includes all the treatments together. However, this particular procedure also can be performed alone. If so, you would use the code for the "separate procedure."

 LET'S CODE IT! SCENARIO

Dr. Capella performed a repair of the secondary tendon flexor in Bruce Roden's right foot. He first performed an open tenotomy and then did the repair with a free graft.

Let's Code It!

The *repair* that Dr. Capella performed on Bruce Roden actually includes the *tenotomy.* Therefore, we will use the one combination code for the entire procedure.

Go to the Alphabetic Index, and look up the procedure: *repair.* Under *Repair,* let's find the anatomical site: *foot.* Under *foot,* let's find the part of the foot that was treated: *tendon.* The Alphabetic Index suggests the code range 28200–28226, 28238. Let's go to the first one.

| 28200 | Repair, tendon, flexor, foot; primary or secondary, without free graft, each tendon |
| 28202 | secondary with free graft, each tendon (includes obtaining graft) |

It seems we have found the code description that matches the physician's notes.

| 28202 | Repair, tendon, flexor, foot; secondary with free graft, each tendon (includes obtaining graft) |

Great job!

Had Dr. Capella performed the tenotomy only, the correct code would be

| 28230 | Tenotomy, open, tendon flexor; foot, single or multiple tendon(s) (separate procedure) |

On occasion, you may find that the "separate procedure" is performed along with other procedures, not those in the bundle. Should this be the situation, you have to add the modifier 59 to the "separate procedure" code. Documentation must support these facts, as always.

| 59 | **Distinct Procedural Service.** When the physician performs a procedure or service that is not normally performed with the other procedures or services, modifier 59 should be added to the second procedure. |

25.5 Integumentary System

The largest organ of the human body, the skin, is the main component of the integumentary system, along with the hair and nails. Most people take this for granted. Yet this is the body's protective layer, the first line of defense for the anatomical organs and systems within.

Incision and Drainage (I&D)

A cyst, an abscess, a furuncle (boil), or a paronychia (infected skin around a fingernail or toenail) can harbor infection. When this happens, most often a physician will perform an incision (cut into the tissue) and drainage (I&D) to extract the infectious material.

Debridement

The process of carefully cleaning out a wound to encourage the healing process is called *debridement.* The basis of this term comes from the word *debris,* meaning wreckage or rubble, and relates to the process of taking away necrotic (dead or dying) tissue that can impede the creation of new, healthy tissue. This may be necessary for burn patients, for victims of penetrating wounds, and sometimes for patients with complex wounds such as an open, penetrating fracture.

CODING BITES

Remember: There is a difference between *incision* and *excision.*

Incision means *cut into,* while excision means *cut out.*

You can see, from the descriptions of the codes in this subsection, that you will need to identify the total body surface area (TBSA) that was debrided, in order to determine an accurate code.

Biopsies

Biopsies are performed, most often, for diagnostic purposes. These procedures are done to obtain a sampling of cells or piece of tissue from the body that can then be pathologically analyzed. Although a specimen of tissue may be excised, shave removed, or lased and then sent to pathology for testing, this does not automatically indicate the need for a separate biopsy code. The guidelines state that you should use a biopsy procedure code only when the procedure is conducted individually, or distinctly separate, from any other procedure or service performed at the same time.

There are many different types of biopsies, and you will need to know the details (from the documentation) to help you determine the correct code:

- *Fine-needle aspiration biopsy:* The physician uses a thin needle to draw out—or drain—a specimen (some fluid or gas) to be used for pathology testing.

- *Core-needle biopsy:* The physician uses a hollow needle, a bit larger than the needle used during a fine-needle biopsy, to extract a cylindrical section of tissue to be analyzed.

- *Excisional biopsies* and *incisional biopsies:* A sampling of tissue of the abnormal area; an entire organ or tumor is taken during the procedure and sent to the pathology lab. These can include tangential biopsy, punch biopsy, and incisional biopsy.

- *Endoscopic biopsy:* During a percutaneous endoscopy or via a natural or artificial opening endoscopic procedure, a specimen of an abnormal or suspicious tissue is obtained and sent to the lab.

GUIDANCE CONNECTION

Read the additional explanations in the in-section guidelines located within the **Surgery** section, subhead **Biopsy,** directly above code 11102 in your CPT book.

LET'S CODE IT! SCENARIO

Seth Berensen, a 69-year-old male, came to see Dr. Tyner to get rid of some skin tags on his left cheek. After applying a local anesthetic, Dr. Tyner removed nine tags and sent them to the lab.

Let's Code It!

Let's go to the Alphabetic Index and find the key term for the procedure: *removal.* Now, what did the physician remove? *Skin tags.* Find the term "skin tags" indented under *Removal . . . skin tags . . . :* The codes suggested

(continued)

are 11200–11201. Turn to the numeric listing of the book, in the *Surgery* section, and look for those codes. You will see

11200   **Removal of skin tags, multiple fibrocutaneous tags, any area; up to and including 15 lesions**
+11201   **each additional 10 lesions or part thereof (list separately in addition to code for primary procedure)**
          (Use 11201 in conjunction with 11200)

The next question is . . . How many skin tags (lesions) did the physician remove from Seth's face? When you reread the notes, you will see that he removed *nine tags*. This confirms the correct code is 11200.

     The notes also indicate that the lesions were sent to pathology, meaning a biopsy. Should we add another code for the biopsy? Remember that the guidelines state that a separate code for the biopsy is used only when the biopsy is a procedure distinctly separate from other procedures and not a part of another service. In this case, the biopsy is a part of the removal of the skin tags and does not require a second code.

Excisions

Excision

The full-thickness removal of a lesion, including margins; includes (for coding purposes) a simple closure.

Full-Thickness

A measure that extends from the epidermis to the connective tissue layer of the skin.

Simple Closure

A method of sealing an opening in the skin (epidermis or dermis), involving only one layer. It includes the administration of local anesthesia and/or chemical or electrocauterization of a wound not closed.

GUIDANCE CONNECTION

Read the additional explanations in the in-section guidelines within the **Surgery** section, subheads **Excision—Benign Lesions,** directly above code 11400; **Excision—Malignant Lesions,** directly above code 11600; and **Excision,** directly above code 19081, in your CPT book.

When the physician removes a lesion from a patient, you must code the **excision** of each lesion separately. Codes for the excision, or **full-thickness** removal (Figure 25-1), of a lesion are determined first by the anatomical site from where the lesion was removed and then by the size of the lesion removed. The code for the excision includes the administration of a local anesthetic and a **simple closure** of the excision site, as mentioned in the definition.

     To correctly measure what was excised, you must look at the dimensions of the lesion itself *plus* a proper margin around the lesion. That will give you the total amount actually excised by the physician and lead you to the correct code. In order to find the correct size of the lesion excised, we must do the following: Add the size of the lesion to the size of the margin doubled (margins *all around* means that the diameter will have a margin on each side).

     The formula is

Coded size of lesion = size of lesion + (size of margins × 2)

     As always, you must read carefully. Some surgeons include the measurement of the margins in their operative notes. In other cases, you may need to review the pathologist's report to determine an accurate measurement. And, typically, the measurements will be presented in centimeters (cm). Just in case:

1 centimeter (cm) = 10 millimeters (mm) = 0.4 inch (in.)

1 millimeter (mm) = 0.1 centimeter (cm) = 0.04 inch (in.)

1 inch (in.) = 2.54 cm

FIGURE 25-1 This illustration shows how you will determine the size of the lesion for coding

LET'S CODE IT! SCENARIO

Dr. Lanahan excised a lesion that measured 2.0 cm by 1.0 cm, with 0.2-cm margins all around, from Anson Hillam's neck. The pathology report confirmed that the lesion was benign.

Let's Code It!

Let's go to the Alphabetic Index and find the suggested code or codes. Look up *excision* for the procedure and then *neck* for the anatomical site, right? Well, you will see that there is no listing for *neck* under *excision*. What should you do now? Analyze what you see in the physician's notes. Where exactly is the lesion? It isn't really on his *neck;* it is on his *skin*. So look at *excision, skin*. Aha! Under *skin,* you will see *lesion*. Good. And now, look for *benign,* as per the notes, to find suggested codes 11400–11471.

When you go to the numeric listing, you will see the description for the first code in our range:

11400   **Excision, benign lesion including margins, except skin tag (unless listed elsewhere), trunk, arms or legs; excised diameter 0.5 cm or less**

The description for code 11400 matches our physician's notes except for the mention of the anatomical sites: trunk, arms, or legs. Our patient had the lesion on her neck. Continue looking down the listings, and take a look at the description for code 11420.

11420   **Excision, benign lesion including margins, except skin tag (unless listed elsewhere), scalp, neck, hands, feet, genitalia; excised diameter 0.5 cm or less**

This matches our physician's notes! Next, you must determine the size of the lesion. Remember the formula:

Coded size of lesion = size of lesion + (size of margins × 2)

To the size of the lesion (2.0 cm, which is its largest measurement), we add the size of the margin (0.2 cm) times 2 (margins *all around* mean that the diameter will have a margin on each side). With the figures in place, our formula becomes

Coded size of lesion = 2.0 cm + (0.2 cm × 2) = 2.4 cm

Therefore, the total size of the lesion excised is 2.4 cm. Now find the descriptions indented underneath 11420.

11423   **Excision, benign lesion including margins, except skin tag (unless listed elsewhere), scalp, neck, hands, feet, genitalia; excised diameter 2.1 to 3.0 cm**

This matches exactly. You have found the code: 11423. Good work!

You may find that the physician's notes indicate that the excision of the lesion was complicated or unusual in some way. Should this be the situation, remember to add modifier 22 Increased Procedural Services to the procedure code. The difficulty is related to the process of excising the lesion, not the closure.

 ## LET'S CODE IT! SCENARIO

Dr. Samsune excised a lesion that measured 2.1 by 3.0 cm, with 0.5-cm margins on each side, from Sally Hardy's abdomen. Sally is diagnosed clinically obese and the excess fatty tissue around the lesion required a complex closure of the excision site. The pathology report confirmed that the lesion was malignant.

Let's Code It!

The Alphabetic Index will direct you to a slightly different group of codes—*excision, skin, lesion, malignant*—suggesting a code within the range of 11600–11646. Just as before, you will need to find the code in this range that identifies the correct anatomical location of the lesion:

(continued)

11600   Excision, malignant lesion including margins, trunk, arms or legs; excised diameter 0.5 cm or less

The abdomen is a part of the trunk, so this code is OK. Next, you will need to add up the size of the lesion.

Coded size of lesion = 3.0 cm + (0.5 cm × 2) = 4.0 cm

The answer 4.0 cm leads to the code

11604   Excision, malignant lesion including margins, trunk, arms or legs; excised diameter 3.1 to 4.0 cm

Excellent! Sally's case was not as complicated as Anson's, so modifier 22 will not be required. However, Dr. Samsune did note that Sally's procedure "required a complex closure of the excision site." The guidelines tell you that only a simple closure is included in the excision code. A complex closure, just like an intermediate closure, is coded in addition to the code for the excision. So let's code it!

Let's go back to the Alphabetic Index and find the key term *closure*. None of the indented descriptors seem to match, so you should investigate the code range shown next to the word *closure*: 12001–13160.

You will notice the heading immediately above the first code in the range: 12001. It reads "Repair—Simple." But you are looking for a complex closure, so continue down the page. The next section, above code 12031, is "Repair—Intermediate." This is closer to what you need, but not exactly. Above code 13100 you find the heading you have been looking for: "Repair—Complex."

Remember that Sally's lesion was located on her abdomen (trunk). Look at the codes in this section, and find the best code for the *complex closure* of her excision site.

13100   Repair, complex, trunk; 1.1 cm to 2.5 cm

Excellent! You have found the correct level of closure (repair) for the correct anatomical site (trunk). Now, you must find the correct size of the excision site. Your calculation totaled 4.0 cm, which brings you to the correct code:

13101   Repair, complex, trunk; 2.6 cm to 7.5 cm

Excellent! You now know that, for this one procedure on Sally, the claim form will include these codes:

11604   Excision, malignant lesion including margins, trunk, arms or legs; excised diameter 3.1 to 4.0 cm
13101   Repair, complex, trunk; 2.6 cm to 7.5 cm

Good job!

Intermediate Closure
A multilevel method of sealing an opening in the skin involving one or more of the deeper layers of the skin. Single-layer closure of heavily contaminated wounds that required extensive cleaning or removal of particulate matter also constitutes intermediate closure.

Complex Closure
A method of sealing an opening in the skin involving a multilayered closure and a reconstructive procedure such as scar revision, debridement, or retention sutures.

Reexcision

When the pathology report indicates that the physician did not excise around the lesion (the margins) widely enough to get all the malignancy, an additional excision procedure may be needed.

If the reexcision is performed during the same operative session, adjust the total size of the lesion being coded to include the new total measurement. Report just the one code, with the largest measurement shown in the operative or procedure notes.

If the reexcision is performed during a subsequent encounter during the postoperative period, you should attach modifier 58 Staged Procedure to the procedure code for that second excision. The reexcision to remove additional tissue around the original site during the postoperative period would directly apply to modifier 58's description: (b) more extensive than the original procedure.

Repair (Closures)

Simple closure is included in the excision code. However, if the closure of the excision site becomes more involved and is described as an **intermediate closure** or a **complex closure**, the repair is no longer included in the code for the excision procedure. You need to report an additional code.

As you read the procedure notes or operative report, pay close attention to the description documented as to how deep into the skin the physician worked. When you see a layered closure that involves the deeper layers of the subcutaneous tissue, the superficial fascia, and the epidermal and dermal layers of the skin, you will report an intermediate repair. Also reported as an intermediate repair is a single-layer closure that first requires extensive cleaning or particulate matter removal before closing.

When a complex repair has been performed, the documentation will include more than just a layered enclosure: Scar revision, traumatic laceration debridement, avulsions, extensive undermining, stent insertion, or retention suture(s) all describe this more involved level of repair.

When multiple wounds are repaired with the same complexity on the same anatomical site(s) as indicated by the code descriptor, add all the lengths together to use one code for the total repair. You may sometimes have more than one code to report repairs performed at this encounter. In these cases, the codes should be listed in order from the most complex to the simplest, then from head to toe. All procedure codes, after the first, should have the modifier 59 Distinct Procedural Service appended.

GUIDANCE CONNECTION

Read the additional explanations in the in-section guidelines located within the **Surgery** section, subhead **Repair (Closure),** directly above code 12001 in your CPT book.

 GUIDANCE CONNECTION

In-Section Guidelines (above code 12001 in the Surgery section)

The multiple wound repair guideline is <u>different</u> from the guideline for multiple lesions. Remember that, with lesions, each lesion is coded separately. With wounds, you will *report one code for the total length of all wounds being repaired on the same anatomical site with the same level of repair (simple, intermediate, complex).*

When more than one level of wound repair is used during the same encounter for the same patient, list the more complicated as the primary procedure and the less complicated as the secondary procedures, using modifier 59.

CODING BITES

Modifier 59 is used to report multiple procedures that are performed at the same encounter by the same provider. This modifier is appended to the codes reporting the second and additional services, not the primary procedure code.

Debridement or decontamination of a wound is included in the code for the repair of that wound. However, if the contamination is so extensive that it requires extra time and effort, it should be coded separately. Also, if the debridement is performed and the wound is not closed or repaired during the same session, code the debridement separately.

LET'S CODE IT! SCENARIO

Fiona Curtis, a 27-year-old female, got into a bar fight and sustained multiple wounds to her hand and arm. Dr. Rockville performed intermediate repair of a 5- by 2-cm wound and a 3.1- by 1-cm wound on Fiona's right hand and a simple repair to a 3.2- by 1-cm wound to her right forearm.

Let's Code It!

You can see by Dr. Rockville's notes that Fiona had two wounds treated with intermediate closures, both on her right hand, and one wound with a simple repair, on her right forearm. Let's go to the Alphabetic Index and find *repair, wound, intermediate* (suggesting code range 12031–12057) and *repair, wound, simple* (suggesting code range 12001–12021).

The intermediate repairs were done to the right *hand,* so let's turn to the numeric listing for the code range 12031–12057 and find the best code for this anatomical site.

12041   Repair, intermediate, wounds of neck, hands, feet and/or external genitalia; 2.5 cm or less

(continued)

There were two wounds on Fiona's right hand (the first is 5 × 2 cm and the second 3.1 × 1 cm). The guidelines state that, because the wounds are on the same anatomical site as per the code description (*hands*) and received the same level of repair (*intermediate*), you must add them together. Let's add the two longest measurements together (5 cm + 3.1 cm) for a total of 8.1 cm. This brings us to the correct code:

12044   **Repair, intermediate, wounds of neck, hands, feet and/or external genitalia; 7.6 cm to 12.5 cm**

Good job! Now, the last wound on Fiona's forearm is different. It is a simple repair rather than an intermediate repair, and the wound is on her arm, not her hand. Therefore, this wound repair will have its own code. Follow the code descriptions and see if you can come up with the most accurate code. Did you determine this to be the correct code?

12002   **Simple repair of superficial wounds of scalp, neck, axillae, external genitalia, trunk and/or extremities (including hands and feet); 2.6 cm to 7.5 cm**

Now that you know the guideline regarding multiple wound repairs, do you think any adjustments should be made to the claim form you are preparing for Dr. Rockville to be reimbursed for his work on Fiona? You need to report them in the correct sequence and append a modifier:

12044   **(The intermediate repair tells us this was the more severe or complicated procedure. Therefore, this code is reported first.)**

12002-59   **(This was the simple repair of a smaller wound. This was less complicated and, therefore, the code is listed second and appended with the modifier 59.)**

That's great! You did excellent work!

 YOU CODE IT! CASE STUDY

A woman was screaming in a parking lot and calling for help. She had accidentally locked her keys in the car, along with her infant son. It was a hot day, and she was quite concerned about her child. Alex Franklin came along and used a rock to break a window on the other side of the car, reached in through the broken glass, and unlocked the door. Without question, Alex is a hero, but he also cut his wrist on the broken glass. At the ED, Dr. Zander discovered that the subcutaneous tissue at the laceration site was littered with tiny shards of glass. Dr. Zander administered a local anesthetic. It took Dr. Zander quite a long time to debride the 5.3- by 1.6-cm wound of all the glass before he was able to suture it.

You Code It!

Go through the steps, and determine the procedure code(s) that should be reported for this encounter between Dr. Zander and Alex Franklin.

Step #1: Read the case carefully and completely.

Step #2: Abstract the scenario. Which key words or terms describe what service the physician provided to the patient during this encounter?

Step #3: Are there any details missing or incomplete for which you would need to query the physician? [If so, ask your instructor.]

Step #4: Determine the correct CPT procedure code or codes to explain the details about what was provided to the patient during this encounter.

Step #5: Check for any relevant guidance, including reading all of the symbols and notations.

Step #6: Do you need to append any modifiers to ensure complete and accurate information is provided?

Step #7: Double-check your work.

(continued)

Adjacent Tissue Transfer and/or Rearrangement

When an excision is repaired with an adjacent tissue transfer or rearrangement, you will see several terms in the procedure notes that are included in this code subcategory.

- Z-plasty is a double transposition flap, most often used to correct a skin web or perform a scar revision.
- W-plasty uses several small, triangular-shaped flaps, alternating inversion, just like the letter "W," to break up a long scar.
- V-Y plasty uses a V-shaped flap that is next to the defect with surrounding skin raised up and brought into the wound.
- Rotation flap is a raised subdermal plane, semicircular in shape, pivoted around into the defect.
- Random island flap is a section of skin moved into the defect with its blood supply.
- Advancement flap involves a subdermal place of skin, longitudinally moved to the defect.

The correct code to report a tissue transfer or rearrangement requires two elements from the physician's notes:

- Anatomical site: The anatomical location of the primary defect—the skin opening that needs to be repaired—as well as the location of the secondary defect—the skin area from where the surgeon took the skin being transferred.
- Size of the defect: Add together the sizes of the primary defect and the secondary defect.
- For all defects over 30 sq. cm, all anatomical sites are reported with the same codes—code 14301 with code 14302, depending upon the total size.

GUIDANCE CONNECTION

Read additional explanations in the in-section guidelines located within the **Surgery** section, subhead **Adjacent Tissue Transfer or Rearrangement,** directly above code 14000 in your CPT book.

 LET'S CODE IT! SCENARIO

Larissa Cheek had a 2.5 cm × 1 cm contracted scar on the back of her hand, making it difficult to use her fingers completely. Dr. Villa performed a Z-plasty tissue transfer to disrupt the scar tissue and elongate the transferred tissues. He notes that the secondary defect was 3 sq. cm.

Let's Code It!

Dr. Villa did a "*Z-plasty tissue transfer*" on Larissa. However, when you look in the CPT Alphabetic Index for *Z-plasty,* you will find nothing. Take a look at the Alphabetic Index for *transfer.* There are a few items listed below, but none of these seem to relate to the procedure on Larissa. So let's take a look at the CPT Alphabetic Index listings for *tissue.* Below this you will see:

Tissue
Transfer

(continued)

Adjacent
Skin 14000–14350

As you review the guidelines in this subsection, shown above code 14000, you can see that Z-plasty is included in this section, confirming that you are in the right area. Next, you can see that the code descriptions require you to know the anatomical location of the procedure.

14000	**Adjacent tissue transfer or rearrangement, trunk**
14020	**Adjacent tissue transfer or rearrangement, scalp, arms, and/or legs**
14040	**Adjacent tissue transfer or rearrangement, forehead, cheeks, chin, mouth, neck, axillae, genitalia, hands and/or feet**
14060	**Adjacent tissue transfer or rearrangement, eyelids, nose, ears, and/or lips**

Go back to the scenario and identify the anatomical site: "*on the back of her hand.*" This leads you to code 14040. You must now choose between the following two codes, determined by the size of the defects:

14040	**Adjacent tissue transfer or rearrangement, forehead, cheeks, chin, mouth, neck, axillae, genitalia, hands and/or feet; defect 10 sq. cm or less**
14041	**defect 10.1 sq. cm to 30.0 sq. cm**

How big was the defect? In the guidelines above code 14000, it says, "*The primary defect resulting from the excision and the secondary defect resulting from flap design to perform the reconstruction are measured together to determine the code.*"

Larissa's original scar—the primary defect—is noted to be 2.5 cm × 1. Multiply these two numbers to get 2.5 sq. cm. The secondary defect, the source of the tissue transfer, is noted to be 3 sq. cm. Add 2.5 sq. cm to 3 sq. cm and get a total of 5.5 sq. cm. Compare this measurement to the measurements included in the code descriptions for tissue transfers done on the hands. This confirms the correct code for the procedure Dr. Villa did for Larissa:

14040	**Adjacent tissue transfer or rearrangement, forehead, cheeks, chin, mouth, neck, axillae, genitalia, hands and/or feet; defect 10 sq. cm or less**

Good job!

Skin Replacement Surgery and Flaps

The codes for skin grafts are determined by three things:

1. The size of the **recipient area** (the size of the wound to be grafted).
2. The location of the recipient area (the anatomical site).
3. The type of graft (pinch graft, split graft, full-thickness graft, and so on).

Recipient Area
The area, or site, of the body receiving a graft of skin or tissue.

The codes include a simple debridement, or avulsion, of the recipient site. Through **harvesting**, grafts can be taken from another part of the patient's body, another body (a live donor), a cadaver (a deceased person), skin substitutes (such as neodermis, synthetic skin), or another species (for instance, a porcine graft). You have to know where the graft came from in order to determine the best, most appropriate code.

Harvesting
The process of taking skin or tissue (on the same body or another).

It is not uncommon for skin grafts to be planned, from the beginning, to be done in stages. When this is the case, the second and subsequent portions of the staged procedure should be appended with modifier 58. This is directly described in CPT's modifier 58 description: (a) planned or anticipated (staged).

Donor Area (Site)
The area or part of the body from which skin or tissue is removed with the intention of placing that skin or tissue in another area or body.

If the **donor area (site)** requires a skin graft or a local flap to repair it, it should be coded as an additional procedure. When evaluating the size of the wound that has been grafted, the measurement of *100 sq. cm* is used with patients aged 10 and older. The code descriptor referring to a *percentage of the body area* applies only to patients under the age of 10.

EXAMPLE

15002   Surgical preparation or creation of recipient site by excision of open wounds, burn eschar, or scar (including subcutaneous tissues), or incisional release of scar contracture, trunk, arms, legs; first *100 sq cm or 1% of body area of infants and children*

GUIDANCE CONNECTION

Read additional explanations in the in-section guidelines located within the **Surgery** section, subhead **Skin Replacement Surgery,** directly above code 15002 in your CPT book.

In the subheading relating to flaps and grafts, when the physician attaches a flap, either in transfer or to the final site, the anatomical site identified in the code's description is the *recipient* site, not the donor site.

EXAMPLE

15733   Muscle, myocutaneous, or fasciocutaneous flap; head and neck with named vascular pedicle (ie, buccinators, genioglossus, temoralis)

GUIDANCE CONNECTION

Read the additional explanations in the in-section guidelines located within the **Surgery** section, subhead **Flaps (Skin and/or Deep Tissues),** directly above code 15570 in your CPT book.

When a tube is formed to be used later, or when "delay" of flap is done before the transfer, the anatomical sites indicated in the code description refer to the *donor* site, not the recipient site.

EXAMPLE

15620   Delay of flap or sectioning of flap (division and inset); at forehead, cheeks, chin, mouth, neck, axillae, genitalia, hands or feet

When extensive immobilization is performed, such as large plaster casts or traction, the application of the immobilization device should be coded as a separate procedure. However, make note that the procedure codes in the range 15570–15738 already include small or standard immobilization, such as a sling or splint.

 YOU CODE IT! CASE STUDY

Evan Riggs, an 11-year-old male, had burn eschar on his face from an accident. Dr. Charne performed a surgical preparation of the area. Two days later, Dr. Charne applied a dermal autograft to the 30-sq.-cm area.

You Code It!

Based on the notes, find the best, most appropriate procedure code(s) to report all of Dr. Charne's work for Evan's injury.

Step #1: Read the case carefully and completely.

Step #2: Abstract the scenario. Which key words or terms describe what service the physician provided to the patient during this encounter?

Step #3: Are there any details missing or incomplete for which you would need to query the physician? [If so, ask your instructor.]

Step #4: Determine the correct CPT procedure code or codes to explain the details about what was provided to the patient during this encounter.

Step #5: Check for any relevant guidance, including reading all of the symbols and notations.

Step #6: Do you need to append any modifiers to ensure complete and accurate information is provided?

Step #7: Double-check your work.

(continued)

Answer:

Did you determine the following codes?

15004   **Surgical preparation or creation of recipient site by excision of open wounds, burn eschar, or scar (including subcutaneous tissues), or incisional release of scar contracture, face, scalp, eyelids, mouth, neck, ears, orbits, genitalia, hands, feet, and/or multiple digits; first 100 sq cm or 1% of body area of infants and children**

15135-58   **Dermal autograft, face, scalp, eyelids, mouth, neck, ears, orbits, genitalia, hands, feet, and/or multiple digits; first 100 sq cm or less, or 1% of body area of infants and children; staged procedure**

Great work!

GUIDANCE CONNECTION

Read additional explanations in the in-section guidelines located within the **Surgery** section, subhead **Destruction,** directly above code 17000 in your CPT book.

Destruction

Destruction is the term used for the removal of diseased or unwanted tissue from the body by surgical or other means, such as surgical curettement (also known as curettage), laser treatment, electrosurgery, chemical treatment, or cryosurgery. Ablation is the surgical destruction of tissue or a body part. When the tissue is destroyed rather than excised, there is nothing left. Therefore, there will be no specimens sent to pathology for analysis. The codes in the destruction subheading of the surgical section include the administration of local anesthesia.

There are several methods that a physician can use to destroy tissue.

- *Cauterization* is the process of destroying tissue with the use of a chemical or electricity to seal a wound and stop bleeding. Some cauterizations can be accomplished with extreme heat or cold. For example, you might see physician's notes document the removal of an internal polyp with the use of hot forceps.

- *Cryosurgical* or *cryotherapy* techniques use liquid nitrogen or freezing carbon dioxide to destroy the tissue of concern.

- *Curettage* is the method of using a special surgical tool, called a curette, to scrape an organ, a muscle, or other anatomical site.

- *Electrosurgical* methods use high-frequency electrical current instead of a scalpel to separate and destroy tissue. One example of this is electrolysis, which removes hair by using electricity to destroy the hair follicle.

- *Laser* surgery uses light to cut, separate, or destroy tissue. The term *laser* is actually an acronym for "light amplification by stimulated emission of radiation."

 LET'S CODE IT! SCENARIO

Derrick Franks, a 54-year-old male, came to see Dr. Johnston, his podiatrist, for the removal of a benign plantar wart from the sole of his left foot. Dr. Johnston administered a local anesthetic and then destroyed the wart using a chemosurgical technique. A protective bandage was applied to the foot, and Frank was sent home with an appointment to return in 1 week for a follow-up check.

Let's Code It!

The notes indicate that Derrick had a *benign plantar wart* that Dr. Johnston *destroyed* using *chemosurgery*. Let's go to the Alphabetic Index and look up *destruction*.

(continued)

Under *destruction,* you will see an alphabetical list that includes both anatomical sites as well as skin conditions, such as cysts and lesions. You know from the notes that Dr. Johnston destroyed a wart on Derrick's foot. There are no listings for foot or sole of foot. However, there is a listing for *Warts, flat . . . 17110–17111.* Do you know if a plantar wart is a flat wart? Because this is the only choice here, let's go to the codes suggested and see if the numeric listing can provide more information.

The code descriptions read

17110   **Destruction (e.g., laser surgery, electrosurgery, cryosurgery, chemosurgery, surgical curettement), of benign lesions other than skin tags or cutaneous vascular proliferative lesions; up to 14 lesions**

17111   **15 or more lesions**

These descriptions do not really answer our question about whether a plantar wart is a flat wart or a benign lesion. But before you query the doctor, go to the beginning of this subsection and read down.

Directly below the description for code 17111 is a notation:

(For destruction of extensive cutaneous neurofibroma over 50–100 lesions, see 0419T, 0420T)

Directly below the description for code 17003 is a notation:

(For destruction of common or plantar warts, see 17110, 17111.)

This is an excellent example of how you must investigate all possibilities and really give the CPT book a chance to point you toward the correct code.

Dr. Johnston destroyed with chemosurgery Derrick's benign lesion that was not a skin tag or a cutaneous vascular proliferative lesion, and he only had one. Code 17110 is perfect!

Mohs Micrographic Surgery

The group of codes for Mohs micrographic surgery (17311–17315) will be used only when you are coding for a physician who is specially trained in this type of procedure because it requires one doctor to act as *both* surgeon and pathologist. If two different professionals perform these functions, these codes cannot be used.

If a repair is performed during the same session, the repair, flap, or graft procedures should be coded separately.

If a biopsy is performed on the same day as the Mohs surgery because the physician suspects that the patient has skin cancer, it should be reported separately as well, appended with modifier 59 Distinct Procedural Service.

GUIDANCE CONNECTION

Read the additional explanations in the in-section guidelines located within the **Surgery** section, subhead **Mohs Micrographic Surgery,** directly above code 17311 in your CPT book.

25.6 Musculoskeletal System

The musculoskeletal system subsection of codes reports procedures and treatments performed on the bones, ligaments, cartilage, muscles, and tendons in the human body (Figure 25-2).

Cast Application

Earlier in this chapter, you learned about the surgical package, and all of the services it includes. In addition, codes in this subsection already include the application and removal of a cast or traction device as a part of the procedure performed.

So, when would you report a code from the subsection **Application of Casts and Strapping**, codes 29000 through 29799? There are times when no other procedure is performed. When the only service provided is the cast application, this will be reported from here.

FIGURE 25-2 These illustrations show some of the over 600 muscles and 206 bones in the human body

GUIDANCE CONNECTION

Read additional explanations in the in-section guidelines located within the **Surgery** section, subhead **Application of Casts and Strapping,** directly above code 29000 in your CPT book.

EXAMPLES

Dr. Philphot performed a closed realignment, manipulating the fractured calcaneal bone back together, and applied a foot-to-knee plaster cast.

- The application of this cast would be included in the code for the treatment of the fracture:

    28405   Closed treatment of calcaneal fracture; with manipulation

Justine had fractured her ulna and radius after falling off her skateboard. She got caught in an unexpected rainstorm that drenched her, and her cast. Dr. Keller replaced the long-arm cast.

- The application of this cast was the only service provided for the treatment of Justine's fracture; therefore, it would be reported separately.

    29065   Application, cast; shoulder to hand (long arm)

Fracture Reduction

A fracture reduction is the process of returning the bone fragments back to their original and correct location and configuration. The type of fracture will determine the specific components of this procedure. For example, a simple fracture might possibly be reduced with a closed treatment, while a multifragmentary fracture or one with bone loss may require an open treatment with additional work, such as a bone graft or internal fixation, to restore the bone to its previous length, alignment, and ability to rotate (such as with an articulation). Reduction or **manipulation** may be necessary to realign the bone pieces so that union can occur properly. This may be done externally (closed reduction, known as manipulation) or surgically (open reduction).

Details from the CPT Coding Guidelines, found at the beginning of the **Musculoskeletal System** section of the *Surgery* section of CPT, remind you that

Manipulation
The attempted return of a fracture or dislocation to its normal alignment manually by the physician.

Manipulation is used throughout the musculoskeletal fracture and dislocation subsections to specifically mean the attempted reduction or restoration of a fracture or joint dislocation to its normal anatomic alignment by the application of manually applied forces.

This will support your determination for the correct code as you see that the codes for treatment of either an open fracture or a closed fracture are categorized by the method of reduction (manipulation) and fixation/immobilization used to stabilize the realigned bone.

Certainly, you already know that the CPT procedure code will be determined, in part, by which specific bone is fractured and therefore needs treatment.

EXAMPLES

23525   Closed treatment of sternoclavicular dislocation; with manipulation
27178   Open treatment of slipped femoral epiphysis; closed manipulation with single or multiple pinning

The key terms you will need to identify from the documentation also will vary depending upon the particular fractured bone that is being treated. For example:

Open treatment and/or reduction of vertebral fracture(s) and/or dislocation(s), posterior approach, 1 fractured vertebra or dislocated segment;

Lumbar	22325
Cervical	22326
Thoracic	22327
Additional fractured vertebra	+22328

When the fractured bone is a segment of the spinal column, you will need to abstract three key important pieces of information: the location of the bone on the vertebral column (i.e., cervical, thoracic, lumbar), the number of fractured vertebrae reduced, and the approach—posterior or anterior. The codes shown above (22325–22328) are only to be reported when the physician used a posterior, or back, approach. When the approach used to visualize and reduce the fracture was from the front—an anterior approach—codes 63081–63091 are used instead.

Open or Closed Treatment

Procedures and services can be provided for various sites of the musculoskeletal system as an open treatment or a closed treatment. These two words, *open* and *closed,* are used for both the description of the fracture itself (in the diagnostic statement) and the description of the procedure. Be careful not to confuse these identifiers because they are NOT interrelated—that is, a compound (open) fracture is not automatically treated with an open procedure. Be certain to differentiate the description of the fracture from the description of the procedure. Let's begin with understanding what CPT means by open treatment or closed treatment.

Open Treatment

CPT defines **open treatment** as a procedure provided to treat a fractured bone that is either

Surgically opened, so that the fracture can be visualized and internal fixation may be applied.

or

Not opened surgically, but the fractured bone is opened remotely from the site to enable the surgeon to insert an intramedullary nail.

Open Treatment
Surgically opening the fracture site, or another site in the body nearby, in order to treat the fractured bone.

Closed Treatment

According to CPT, the **closed treatment** of a fracture is performed

- With or without manipulation.
- With or without traction.
- Without the fracture being opened and visualized.

Penetrating Trauma Wounds

The CPT book distinguishes between wounds and penetrating trauma wounds. A penetrating trauma wound requires

1. Surgery to explore the wound.
2. Determination of the depth and complexity of the wound.
3. Identification of any damage created by the penetrating object (such as the stabbing from a knife or the wound from a bullet).
4. Debridement of the wound to remove any particles, dirt, and foreign fragments.
5. Ligation or coagulation of minor subcutaneous tissue, muscle fascia, and/or muscle (not severe enough to require a thoracotomy or laparotomy).

You will use codes 20100–20103 to report the exploration of such wounds. Then, code whichever repair the physician actually performs, as documented in the notes.

Bone Grafts and Implants

Medical science and technology have progressed amazingly. Be certain to differentiate between skin grafts (reported from the Integumentary System subsection of CPT) and bone, cartilage, tendon, and fascia lata grafts that are coded from the Musculoskeletal System subsection.

If the code description does not specifically reference the harvesting of the graft or implant (for example, code 20936 "includes harvesting the graft"), then the procedure for obtaining autogenous bone, cartilage, tendon, fascia lata grafts, or other tissues should be reported separately.

Spine

As you may remember from anatomy class, the human spine is referred to in sections: cervical (at or near the neck), thoracic (the chest area), lumbar (at the waist and lower back), and sacral. References to the individual vertebrae are most often identified by their alphanumeric identifiers, such as C1 (cervical vertebra number 1), L5 (lumbar vertebra number 5), or S3 (sacral vertebra number 3), as you can see in Figure 25-3.

Laminotomy

A laminotomy is a partial laminectomy used to treat lumbar disc herniation. Removing a portion of the lamina is often sufficient to access the affected nerve root. Then, the disc herniation can be visualized and accessed from beneath the nerve root. This procedure should be reported with the most accurate code, based on the details in the documentation:

63020   Laminotomy (hemilaminectomy), with decompression of nerve root(s), including partial facetectomy, foraminotomy and/or excision of herniated intervertebral disc, including open or endoscopically-assisted approach; one interspace, cervical

63030   Laminotomy (hemilaminectomy), with decompression of nerve root(s), including partial facetectomy, foraminotomy and/or excision of herniated intervertebral disc, including open or endoscopically-assisted approach; one interspace, lumbar

+63035 each additional interspace, cervical or lumbar (List separately in additional to code for primary procedure.)

Compare these two different codes. What's the difference?

63020	63030
Laminotomy (hemilaminectomy)	Laminotomy (hemilaminectomy)
With decompression of nerve root(s)	With decompression of nerve root(s)
Including partial facetectomy, foraminotomy and/or excision of herniated intervertebral disc	Including partial facetectomy, foraminotomy and/or excision of herniated intervertebral disc
including open or endoscopically-assisted approach	including open or endoscopically-assisted approach
One interspace, cervical	One interspace, lumbar

You can see that the only difference between the two code descriptions is the location of the vertebra being treated. This is a piece of information you will need to determine the correct code.

Then, depending upon how many discs were involved, you might add

+63035 each additional interspace, cervical or lumbar

Arthrodesis

Arthrodesis is the surgical immobilization of a joint so that the bones can heal, or grow solidly, together. While this is most often performed on the spine, it also can be done on any joint in the body, including ankle, elbow, shoulder, etc.

When coding arthrodesis, you will need to identify the approach technique used by the physician, such as

- Lateral extracavitary technique.
- Anterior transoral or extraoral technique.
- Anterior interbody technique.
- Posterior technique: craniocervical or atlas-axis.
- Posterior or posterolateral technique.
- Posterior interbody technique with number of interspaces treated.

Arthrodesis can be performed alone or in combination with other procedures such as bone grafting, osteotomy, fracture care, vertebral corpectomy, or **laminectomy**. When arthrodesis is done at the same time as another procedure, modifier 51 Multiple Procedures should be appended to the code for the arthrodesis. This applies to almost all procedures, with the exception of bone grafting and instrumentation. Modifier 51 Multiple Procedures is not used in those cases because bone grafts and instrumentation are never performed without arthrodesis.

FIGURE 25-3 The vertebrae of the spinal column are numbered from the head to the coccyx

Source: www.boundless.com

Arthrodesis
The immobilization of a joint using a surgical technique.

Laminectomy
The surgical removal of a vertebral posterior arch.

 LET'S CODE IT! SCENARIO

Caryn Philips, a 51-year-old female, was diagnosed with degenerative disc disease 3 months ago. She is admitted today for Dr. Cheffer to perform a posterior arthrodesis of L5–S1 (transverse process), utilizing a morselized autogenous iliac bone graft harvested through a separate fascial incision. Caryn tolerates the procedure well and is returned to her hospital room after 2 hours in recovery.

(continued)

Pull out the description of the procedures that Dr. Cheffer performed. First, note the *"posterior arthrodesis of L5–S1"* and then the *"morselized autogenous iliac bone graft harvested through a separate fascial incision."*

Let's begin in the Alphabetic Index with the listing for *arthrodesis*. The designation of L5–S1 tells you this was done to Caryn's spine. However, *spine* isn't listed under arthrodesis. Keep reading and you will see *vertebra* listed, *lumbar* underneath that, and *posterior* beneath that. However, the physician noted "transverse process," which is listed here as well. Let's investigate code 22612, as suggested by the Alphabetic Index.

22612   **Arthrodesis, posterior or posterolateral technique, single level; lumbar (with or without lateral transverse technique)**

This matches the physician's notes.

Now, let's move to the next procedure performed. Look in the Alphabetic Index under *bone graft*. Read through the list until you reach the item that reflects what was done for Caryn: *spine surgery*. Indented below that you will see *autograft* (the same as *autogenous*) and then *morselized*. The index suggests code 20937. Turn to the numeric list and take a look at the code's description:

+20937   **Autograft for spine surgery only (includes harvesting the graft); morselized (through separate skin or fascial incision)**

Notice the symbol to the left of code 20937: **+**. The plus sign means this is an add-on code and it cannot be used alone. However, the notation below 20937 indicates that you are permitted to use this code along with 22612.

In addition, the guidelines state that when arthrodesis is performed with another procedure, you need to add modifier 51 to the arthrodesis code *except* when the other procedure is a bone graft. This is the case in Caryn's record, so the claim form for Caryn Phillip's surgery will show procedure codes 22612 and 20937—with no modifiers. Great job!

GUIDANCE CONNECTION

Read the additional explanations in the in-section guidelines within the **Surgery** section, subhead **Spine,** subsection **Arthrodesis,** directly above code 22532 in your CPT book.

Percutaneous Skeletal Fixation

The insertion of fixation instruments (such as pins) placed across the fracture site. It may be done under x-ray imaging for guidance purposes.

Skeletal Fixation

Whether the fracture is open or closed, it may require fixation. *Internal fixation* is the process of placing plates and screws, or pins, or other devices directly onto or around the bone, inside of the patient. When *external fixation* is used, a device—such as a brace, cast, or halo—prevents motion in a certain area of the body. The care for a fracture also may include the external application of traction.

It is not always necessary for the physician to visualize the specific fracture directly, yet some type of immobilization is required to ensure proper healing. X-ray imaging is used to provide guidance so pins or other fixation can be accurately applied. This is known as **percutaneous skeletal fixation** because the procedure is not an open procedure, yet it is not completely closed either.

EXAMPLE

25606   Percutaneous skeletal fixation of distal radial fracture or epiphyseal separation

External fixation, as the name implies, is the attachment of skeletal pins along with a device to provide stability and corrective action on either a permanent or temporary basis. This is only reported separately when this portion of the process is not already part of the procedure.

EXAMPLE

21454   Open treatment of mandibular fracture with external fixation

Internal fixation is, most often, applied directly to the bone during an open procedure or treatment.

EXAMPLE

29855   Arthroscopically aided treatment of tibial fracture, proximal (plateau); unicondylar, includes internal fixation, when performed (includes arthroscopy)

 GUIDANCE CONNECTION

Read the additional explanations in the in-section guidelines located within the **Surgery** section, subhead **Spine (Vertebral Column),** subsection **Fracture and/or Dislocation,** directly above code 22310 in your CPT book.

 LET'S CODE IT! CASE SCENARIO

Peter Kessler, a 17-year-old male, plays basketball on his high school team. While practicing in his driveway, he fell and fractured the shaft of his tibia. Dr. Warden, the orthopedist on duty at the emergency room, is able to use a percutaneous fixation using pins.

Let's Code It!

Let's turn to the Alphabetic Index. This time, we won't look up the procedure by the type of treatment (*percutaneous*), but we will look at the condition that was treated: *fracture.* Under *fracture,* find the anatomical site of the fracture—*tibia*—and then the *percutaneous fixation.* The index suggests code 27756. Let's check the description in the numeric listing:

27756   **Percutaneous skeletal fixation of tibial shaft fracture (with or without fibular fracture) (e.g., pins or screws)**

That's exactly what Dr. Warden did. Great job!

Spinal Procedures

There are several procedures often performed on patients with spinal concerns:

- *Arthrodesis* is the surgical immobilization of a joint.
- *Arthroplasty* is the insertion of an artificial disc.
- *Discectomy* is the surgical removal of an intervertebral disc, either a portion of the disc or the entire component.
- *Laminectomy* is the surgical removal of the lamina (posterior arch) of the vertebra.
- *Osteotomy* is performed to remove, or cut out, a portion of a bone.
- *Vertebroplasty* and *kyphoplasty* may be performed surgically or percutaneously for the purpose of repairing a vertebra that has been compromised by a compression fracture.

Spinal Fusion

Spinal fusion permanently locks two or more spinal vertebrae together so that they move as a single unit utilizing bone grafts, with or without screws, plates, cages, or other devices. The bone grafts are placed around the problem area of the spine during surgery. As the body heals itself, the graft helps join the bones together.

Performed under general anesthesia, fusion of lumbar vertebrae is generally done using a posterior lumbar approach, whereas cervical vertebrae are accessed using an anterior cervical approach. An anterior thoracic approach is normally used for fusion of thoracic vertebrae.

Spinal fusion is known to diminish mobility because of the connections made between the individual vertebrae involved in the procedure. This is one of the primary reasons health care technology has been working diligently on an artificial intervertebral disc that can continue to permit individual vertebral motion. Artificial discs have been evidenced to allow for six degrees of freedom.

After removing the ineffective or damaged disc, two metal plates are pressed into the bony endplates above and below the interspace and held into place by metal spikes. A plastic spacer, usually made of a polyethylene core, is inserted between the plates. The patient's own body weight compresses the spacer after the surgery is complete.

YOU CODE IT! CASE STUDY

Allyssa Erickson, an 83-year-old female, fell and sustained a fracture to the C4 vertebral body. Due to the position of the fracture, Dr. Rubbine was able to use a closed treatment without having to put her through a surgical procedure. Dr. Rubbine then put Allyssa into a brace.

You Code It!

Go through the steps, and determine what procedure code(s) should be reported for this encounter between Dr. Rubbine and Allyssa Erickson.

Step #1: Read the case carefully and completely.

Step #2: Abstract the scenario. Which key words or terms describe what service the physician provided to the patient during this encounter?

Step #3: Are there any details missing or incomplete for which you would need to query the physician? [If so, ask your instructor.]

Step #4: Determine the correct CPT procedure code or codes to explain the details about what was provided to the patient during this encounter.

Step #5: Check for any relevant guidance, including reading all of the symbols and notations.

Step #6: Do you need to append any modifiers to ensure complete and accurate information is provided?

Step #7: Double-check your work.

Answer:

Did you find this to be the correct code?

22310   **Closed treatment of vertebral body fracture(s), without manipulation, requiring and including casting or bracing**

Great job!

Lumbar Puncture (Spinal Tap)

When a patient exhibits certain signs and symptoms, the physician may decide to perform a lumbar puncture, commonly known as a spinal tap. In this procedure, a needle is inserted into the spinal canal between two lumbar vertebrae to collect cerebrospinal fluid (CSF).

The two key procedure codes are differentiated by the reason the procedure is performed—diagnostic or therapeutic.

62270	**Spinal puncture, lumbar, diagnostic;**
62272	**Spinal puncture, therapeutic, for drainage of cerebrospinal fluid (by needle or catheter);**

25.7 Respiratory System

The organs and tissues involved with bringing oxygen into the body and discharging gases make up the respiratory system. Procedures and treatments affecting this sector are coded from the **Respiratory System** subsection.

Sinus Endoscopy

The upper respiratory system includes the nasal passages and sinus cavities. The standard for a nasal/sinus endoscopic procedure, performed for diagnostic purposes, includes assessment of the interior nasal cavity, the middle and superior meatus, the turbinates, and the sphenoethmoid recess. Therefore, the inspection of all of these areas is included in the diagnostic sinus endoscopy procedure code.

When a surgical sinus endoscopy is provided, the code descriptions include both the sinusotomy and a diagnostic endoscopy.

GUIDANCE CONNECTION

Read the additional explanations in the in-section guidelines located within the **Surgery** section, subhead **Respiratory System,** subsection **Endoscopy,** directly above code 31231 in your CPT book.

 LET'S CODE IT! SCENARIO

Epharim Habbati, a 41-year-old male, had been diagnosed with chronic sinusitis many years ago and has tried everything. He told Dr. Tolber that no medication has worked and the inflammation just won't go away. Dr. Tolber performed a nasal/sinus diagnostic endoscopy via the inferior meatus, with a maxillary sinusoscopy.

Let's Code It!

The documentation explains that Dr. Tolber performed a "*diagnostic endoscopy via the inferior meatus, with a maxillary sinusoscopy,*" so let's turn to the CPT Alphabetic Index and find *endoscopy.* You can see a long list of anatomical sites beneath. On what anatomical site did Dr. Tolber perform this endoscopy? The notes state "*nasal/sinus.*" Find the term *nose* under *endoscopy* and you will see there are three choices: *Diagnostic, Surgical,* and *Unlisted Services and Procedures.* Let's go back to the notes and find out which of these is most appropriate. The notes state specifically "*diagnostic endoscopy.*" The Alphabetic Index suggests a range of codes: 31231–31235. Let's turn to the *Main Portion* of CPT to read the complete code descriptions.

31231	**Nasal endoscopy, diagnostic; unilateral or bilateral (separate procedure)**
31233	**Nasal/sinus endoscopy, diagnostic; with maxillary sinusoscopy (via inferior meatus or canine fossa puncture)**
31235	**Nasal/sinus endoscopy, diagnostic; with sphenoid sinusoscopy (via puncture of sphenoidal face or cannulation of ostium)**

Let's go back to the physician's notes to confirm exactly what was done for Mr. Habbati.

diagnostic endoscopy . . . all three code choices include this term
via the inferior meatus . . . only code 31233 mentions the inferior meatus specifically
with a maxillary sinusoscopy . . . only code 31233 mentions the maxillary sinusoscopy

The code description for 31233 matches the notes and is our most accurate code to report.

Pleural and Lung Biopsies

A biopsy of the pleural tissue or lung tissue may be accomplished in one of several different ways.

Percutaneous Needle

When a percutaneous needle biopsy is performed, a hollow needle is inserted through a tiny incision and directed toward the internal area, typically with the support of imaging guidance. Only local anesthesia is used, and with only tiny incisions to mend, getting back to normal daily activities is quick.

32400	Biopsy, pleura, percutaneous needle
32405	Biopsy, lung or mediastinum, percutaneous needle

Thoracotomy with Biopsy

When a thoracotomy is performed, along with a lung or pleural biopsy, the patient's chest is surgically opened (an open procedure rather than a percutaneous approach). You will need to abstract, from the documentation, if the biopsy is performed to establish a diagnosis (diagnostic biopsy) or for therapeutic purposes (to surgically remove the abnormal tissues).

32096	Thoracotomy, with diagnostic biopsy of lung infiltrate (e.g., wedge, incisional), unilateral
32097	Thoracotomy, with diagnostic biopsy of lung nodule or masses (e.g., wedge, incisional), unilateral
32098	Thoracotomy, with biopsy(ies) of pleura

NOTE: Other thoracotomy procedures can be reported with a code from the range of 32100–32160.

 YOU CODE IT! CASE STUDY

Harrison Matthews, a 37-year-old male, was having frequent nosebleeds. Finally, after all other methods failed to provide relief, Dr. French performed an endoscopic surgical procedure to control his nasal hemorrhages.

You Code It!

Review the details of what Dr. French did for Harrison Matthews, and determine the CPT code or codes.

Step #1: Read the case carefully and completely.

Step #2: Abstract the scenario. Which key words or terms describe what service the physician provided to the patient during this encounter?

Step #3: Are there any details missing or incomplete for which you would need to query the physician? [If so, ask your instructor.]

Step #4: Determine the correct CPT procedure code or codes to explain the details about what was provided to the patient during this encounter.

Step #5: Check for any relevant guidance, including reading all of the symbols and notations.

Step #6: Do you need to append any modifiers to ensure complete and accurate information is provided?

Step #7: Double-check your work.

Answer:

Did you determine this to be the procedure code?

31238	Nasal/sinus endoscopy, surgical; with control of nasal hemorrhage

25.8 Cardiovascular System

Treatments and procedures on the heart as well as the entire network of veins, arteries, and capillaries are coded from the **Cardiovascular System** subsection.

Pacemakers

When a physician inserts a standard pacemaker system (CPT codes 33202–33275), the procedure includes the placement of a pulse generator into a subcutaneous envelope that has been created beneath the abdominal muscles distally to the ribs or placement in a subclavicular site. The generator itself contains a battery and one or more leads (electrodes) that are inserted transvenously (through a vein) or epicardially (on the surface of the heart). (See Figure 25-4.)

When the epicardial placement is used, a thoracotomy or thoracoscopy is necessary to insert the electrodes accurately.

| 33202 | Insertion of epicardial electrode(s); open incision (e.g., thoracotomy, median sternotomy, subxiphoid approach) |
| 33203 | Insertion of epicardial electrode(s); endoscopic approach (e.g., thoracoscopy, pericardioscopy) |

When a physician inserts a single-chamber pacemaker system into a patient, it includes the pulse generator and one electrode inserted into *either* the atrium or the ventricle.

When a dual-chamber pacemaker system is placed, the system includes the pulse generator and one electrode into *both* the right atrium and the right ventricle.

When the pulse generator is inserted at the same encounter, report 33202 or 33203 in addition to

33212	Insertion of pacemaker pulse generator only; with existing single lead
33213	Insertion of pacemaker pulse generator only; with existing dual leads
33221	Insertion of pacemaker pulse generator only; with existing multiple leads

In addition to the insertion method (epicardial or transvenous), coders must abstract from the physician's documentation the specific chamber or chambers of the heart affected. These codes include the insertion of the pulse generator subcutaneously, the transvenous placement of the electrode or electrodes, and moderate (conscious)

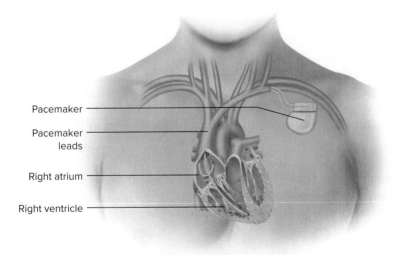

Pacemaker

Pacemaker leads

Right atrium

Right ventricle

FIGURE 25-4 An illustration showing the location of all of the components of an implanted dual-lead pacemaker sedation. If, during the insertion process, the skin pocket requires revision, this is also included in these codes (and all others from 33206 through 33249).

33206	**Insertion of new or replacement of permanent pacemaker with transvenous electrode(s); atrial**
33207	**Insertion of new or replacement of permanent pacemaker with transvenous electrode(s); ventricular**
33208	**Insertion of new or replacement of permanent pacemaker with transvenous electrode(s); atrial and ventricular**

You may notice that these code descriptions include the term *replacement,* insinuating that the patient already had a pacemaker in place. It is important to note that these codes do not include the work to remove a previous system, only the insertion of a new one. To report the physician's services to remove a previous system and insert a replacement system (pulse generator and transvenous electrode(s)) during the same encounter, you will report

33233	**Removal of permanent pacemaker pulse generator only**
✦	
33234	**Removal of transvenous pacemaker electrode(s); single lead system, atrial or ventricular**

or

33235	**Removal of transvenous pacemaker electrode(s); dual lead system**
	✦ One of these codes: 33206 or 33207 or 33208

When the physician documents that the patient has been upgraded from a single-chamber system to a dual-chamber system, the removal of the existing pulse generator and the insertion of the new dual-chamber system are reported with one code:

33214	**Upgrade of implanted pacemaker system, conversion of single chamber system to dual chamber system (includes removal of previously placed pulse generator, testing of existing lead, insertion of new lead, insertion of new pulse generator)**

For some patients, the physician determines that an additional lead (electrode) inserted into the left ventricle would be beneficial. This is known as *biventricular pacing.* When this additional electrode is inserted, it is separately reported:

33224	**Insertion of pacing electrode, cardiac venous system, for left ventricular pacing, with attachment to previously placed pacemaker or pacing cardioverter-defibrillator pulse generator (including revision of pocket, removal, insertion, and/or replacement of existing generator)**

or

✦33225	**Insertion of pacing electrode, cardiac venous system, for left ventricular pacing, at time of insertion of pacing cardioverter-defibrillator or pacemaker pulse generator (e.g., for upgrade to dual chamber system) (List separately in addition to code for primary procedure)**

Commonly referred to as replacing the battery in the pacemaker or cardioverter-defibrillator, this procedure involves the removal of the old pulse generator and the insertion of a new pulse generator. These two actions should be coded individually—one code for the removal of the old and another code for the insertion of the new. When this is documented, report the code determined by the number of leads (electrodes) already in place:

33227	**Removal of permanent pacemaker pulse generator with replacement of pacemaker pulse generator; single lead system**
33228	**Removal of permanent pacemaker pulse generator with replacement of pacemaker pulse generator; dual lead system**

33229   **Removal of permanent pacemaker pulse generator with replacement of pacemaker pulse generator; multiple lead system**

After a length of time, some patients may develop an erosion of the dermal and subcutaneous tissues, or an infection, at the location of the pulse generator. A situation of this nature may require the physician to relocate the "pocket." When this is documented, report the physician's services with this:

33222   **Relocation of skin pocket for pacemaker**

Reporting the insertion and replacement of a pacing cardioverter-defibrillator (ICD) system is very similar, but often does require different codes from within this subsection of CPT.

33249   **Insertion or replacement of permanent implantable defibrillator system, with transvenous lead(s), single or dual chamber**

33270   **Insertion or replacement of permanent subcutaneous implantable defibrillator system, with subcutaneous electrode, including defibrillation threshold evaluation, induction of arrhythmia, evaluation of sensing for arrhythmia termination, and programming or reprogramming of sensing or therapeutic parameters, when performed**

33271   **Insertion of subcutaneous implantable defibrillator electrode**

Implantable Defibrillators

Pacing cardioverter-defibrillator systems are similar to pacemaker systems. While they also consist of a pulse generator and electrodes, the units may use several leads inserted into a single chamber (ventricle) or into dual chambers (atrium and ventricle) (Figure 25-4). The system is actually a combination of antitachycardia pacing, low-energy cardioversion, and/or defibrillating shocks to address a patient's ventricular tachycardia or ventricular fibrillation.

In some cases, an additional electrode may be needed to regulate the pacing of the left ventricle, called *biventricular pacing*. When this occurs, the placement of the electrode transvenously should be coded separately, just as the pacemaker is coded, with either 33224 or 33225.

Leadless Pacemakers

An intracardiac pacemaker functions in much the same way as other pacemakers to regulate heart rate. However, these newly FDA-approved units are self-contained, one-inch-long devices that are implanted directly into the right ventricle chamber of the heart, and have _no_ leads and _no_ pockets. This pulse generator has an internal battery and electrode and is inserted into a cardiac chamber by transfemoral catheter (through an artery in the thigh). No incision or creation of a pocket reduces the opportunity for infection and eliminates unsightly scars. No leads avoid the repercussions of lead failure and result in no possible discomfort when moving, increasing mobility for the patient.

33274   **Transcatheter insertion or replacement of permanent leadless pacemaker, right ventricular, including imaging guidance (e.g., fluoroscopy, venous ultrasound, ventriculography, femoral venography) and device evaluation (e.g., interrogation or programming), when performed**

33275   **Transcatheter removal of permanent leadless pacemaker, right ventricular, including imaging guidance (eg, fluoroscopy, venous ultrasound, ventriculography, femoral venography), when performed**

Bypass Grafting

Venous Grafts

When a venous graft is performed, use codes from the range 33510–33516. All these codes include a **saphenous vein** graft.

GUIDANCE CONNECTION

Read the additional explanations in the in-section guidelines located within the **Surgery** section, subhead **Cardiovascular System,** subsection **Pacemaker or Implantable Defibrillator,** directly above code 33202 in your CPT book.

Saphenous Vein
Either of the two major veins in the leg that run from the foot to the thigh near the surface of the skin.

GUIDANCE CONNECTION

Read the additional explanations in the in-section guidelines within the **Surgery** section, subhead **Cardiovascular System,** subsection **Venous Grafting Only for Coronary Artery Bypass,** directly above code 33510 in your CPT book.

GUIDANCE CONNECTION

Read the additional explanations in the in-section guidelines within the **Surgery** section, subhead **Cardiovascular System,** subsection **Combined Arterial-Venous Grafting for Coronary Bypass,** directly above code 33517 in your CPT book.

However, if the graft is harvested from an upper extremity (arm) vein, you need to code this separately, using code 35500, in addition to the code for the bypass procedure itself.

+35500   Harvest of upper extremity vein, 1 segment, for lower extremity or coronary artery bypass procedure (List separately in addition to code for primary procedure.)

+35572   Harvest of femoropopliteal vein, one segment, for vascular reconstruction procedure (e.g., aortic, vena caval, coronary, peripheral artery) (List separately in addition to code for primary procedure.)

Combined Arterial-Venous Grafts

When both venous grafts and arterial grafts are used during the same procedure, you will use two codes. First, code the combined arterial-venous graft from the range 33517–33523. Just like the codes for the venous grafts, these include getting the graft from the saphenous vein. Second, code the appropriate arterial graft from the range 33533–33536. Harvesting the arterial vein section is included in those codes.

Arterial Grafts

When an arterial graft is performed, use codes from the range 33533–33536. All these codes include the use of grafts from the internal mammary artery, gastroepiploic artery, epigastric artery, radial artery, and arterial conduits harvested from other sites. For example, examine the following code descriptions:

33533   Coronary artery bypass, using arterial graft(s); single arterial graft

33534   Coronary artery bypass, using arterial graft(s); 2 coronary arterial grafts

33535   Coronary artery bypass, using arterial graft(s); 3 coronary arterial grafts

33536   Coronary artery bypass, using arterial graft(s); 4 or more coronary arterial grafts

Use one of the following codes (in addition to the code for the bypass procedure) if the graft is harvested from another site:

- From an upper extremity artery, add code 35600.
- From an upper extremity vein, add code 35500.
- From the femoropopliteal vein, use code 35572.

Composite Grafts

When two or more vein segments are harvested from a limb other than that part of the body undergoing the bypass, you must use the best, most appropriate code from the range 35681–35683 to report the harvesting and anastomosis of the multiple vein segments.

+35681   Bypass graft; composite, prosthetic and vein (List separately in addition to code for primary procedure.)

+35682   Bypass graft; autogenous composite, two segments of veins from two locations (List separately in addition to code for primary procedure.)

+35683   Bypass graft; autogenous composite, three or more segments of vein from two or more locations (List separately in addition to code for primary procedure.)

A little confusing? Hopefully, Table 25-1 will help you organize all the rules for coding bypass grafts.

TABLE 25-1 Bypass Grafts

Graft	Harvested from	Use Code(s)
Venous graft	Saphenous vein	Choose from 33510–33516
Venous graft	Upper extremity vein	Choose from 33510–33516; + 35500
Venous graft	Femoropopliteal vein	Choose from 33510–33516; + 35572
Arterial-venous	Saphenous vein	Choose from 33517–33523; + choose from 33533–33536
Arterial-venous	Upper extremity vein	Choose from 33510–33516; + choose from 33533–33536; + 35500
Arterial-venous	Upper extremity artery	Choose from 33510–33516; + choose from 33533–33536; + 35600
Arterial-venous	Femoropopliteal vein	Choose from 33510–33516; + choose from 33533–33536; + 35572
Arterial graft	Internal mammary artery Gastroepiploic artery Epigastric artery Radial artery Arterial conduits from other sites	Choose from 33533–33545
Arterial graft	Upper extremity vein	Choose from 33533–33545; + 35500
Arterial graft	Upper extremity artery	Choose from 33533–33545; + 35600
Arterial graft	Femoropopliteal vein	Choose from 33533–33545; + 35572
Composite graft	Two or more segments from another part of body	+ 35682 or 35683

Arteries and Veins

The primary vascular procedure codes 34001–37799 include

1. Ensuring both the inflow and the outflow of the arteries and/or veins involved (Figure 25-5).
2. The operative arteriogram that is performed by the surgeon during the procedure.
3. Sympathectomy for aortic procedures.

Endovascular Repair of Abdominal Aorta and/or Iliac Arteries

There are many therapeutic procedures available to treat conditions affecting the abdominal aorta and/or iliac arteries. Often, this involves the insertion, positioning, or deployment of a device known as a covered stent (see Figure 25-6). You may find the physician documentation may specify an endograft, endovascular graft, stentgraft, tube endograft, or endoprosthesis—all of which are variations of a stent.

CPT codes 34701 through 34834 provide the details of these various procedures from which you can determine the code that best reports where [which artery] as well as what specifically was done for this patient.

GUIDANCE CONNECTION

Read the additional explanations in the in-section guidelines within the **Surgery** section, subhead **Cardiovascular System,** subsection **Arterial Grafting for Coronary Artery Bypass,** directly above code 33533 in your CPT book.

Common carotid arteries

Brachiocephalic artery

Right subclavian artery

Right subclavian vein

Superior vena cava

Right axillary vein

Right atrium

Right ventricle

Hepatic veins

Inferior vena cava

Right internal iliac artery

Right external iliac artery

Internal jugular veins

Left subclavian artery

Left subclavian vein

Aortic arch

Pulmonary trunk

Left atrium

Ascending aorta

Left axillary vein

Left ventricle

Descending aorta

Arterial and venous branches in abdominal area

Common iliac arteries

Femoral veins

Femoral arteries

FIGURE 25-5 An illustration showing some of the arteries and veins of the body

YOU CODE IT! CASE STUDY

Jason Antone, a 54-year-old, was admitted to the hospital by Dr. Sabrina Jordan, for treatment of a chronic, contained rupture of an aneurysm of the infrarenal aorta. Jason was prepped and draped in the usual manner, and the procedure to deploy an aorto-bi-iliac endograft was performed.

You Code It!

Go through the steps, and determine the procedure code(s) that should be reported for this encounter between Dr. Jordan and Jason Antone.

Step #1: Read the case carefully and completely.

Step #2: Abstract the scenario. Which key words or terms describe what service the physician provided to the patient during this encounter?

Step #3: Are there any details missing or incomplete for which you would need to query the physician? [If so, ask your instructor.]

Step #4: Determine the correct CPT procedure code or codes to explain the details about what was provided to the patient during this encounter.

Step #5: Check for any relevant guidance, including reading all of the symbols and notations.

Step #6: Do you need to append any modifiers to ensure complete and accurate information is provided?

Step #7: Double-check your work.

(continued)

Narrowed artery with balloon catheter positioned.

Inflated balloon presses against arterial wall.

Blood vessel   Stent

FIGURE 25-6 Illustrations of a balloon catheterization and the placement of a stent

Catheterizations and Vascular Families

Understanding the vascular families can be useful to coders when reporting the provision of a catheterization. Tables 25-2, 25-3, and 25-4 show some examples of the vascular orders when reporting the catheterization of the aorta. The catheterization of the femoral or carotid arteries would each have their own families, of course. A full listing can be found in your CPT code book, *Appendix L, Vascular Families.*

A vascular family begins with the vessel that branches off from the aorta, femoral artery, or carotid artery and continues to track all vessels that branch from that. For example, in Table 25-2, in the first order (first column), you see the superior mesenteric, which is one of the arteries that branch off the aorta. The middle colic, interior

TABLE 25-2 Vascular Families: Superior Mesenteric

First Order	Second Order Branch	Third Order Branch
	Middle colic	
	Inferior pancreaticoduodenal	Posterior inferior pancreaticoduodenal
		Anterior inferior pancreaticoduodenal
	Jejunal	
Superior mesenteric	Ileocolic	
	Appendicular	
	Posterior cecal	
	Anterior cecal	
	Marginal	
	Right colic	

TABLE 25-3 Vascular Families: Left Common Carotid

First Order		Second Order Branch	Third Order Branch
Left common carotid		Left internal carotid	Left ophthalmic
			Left posterior communicating
			Left middle cerebral
			Left anterior cerebral
		Left external carotid	Left superior thyroid
			Left ascending pharyngeal
			Left facial
			Left lingual
			Left occipital
			Left posterior auricular
			Left superficial temporal
			Left internal maxillary

pancreaticoduodenal, jejunal, ileocolic, appendicular, posterior cecal, anterior cecal, marginal, and right colic arteries all branch off the superior mesenteric. From this point, only the interior pancreaticoduodenal has additional vessels branching off it—the posterior inferior pancreaticoduodenal and the anterior inferior pancreaticoduodenal.

LET'S CODE IT! SCENARIO

Lisa Westerly, an 11-week-old female, was diagnosed with ventricular septal defect (VSD) after her pediatrician, Dr. Harris, ordered an echocardiography. A large VSD was identified in the septum. Due to the size of the defect, Dr. Harris admitted Lisa into the hospital today to close the defect with a patch graft.

Let's Code It!

Review the notes and abstract the key terms. Let's go to the Alphabetic Index and look up *closure,* the procedure being performed. Under the word *closure,* you will find *septal defect,* ventricular which suggests three codes: 33776, 33780, 93581.

While we are in the Alphabetic Index, let's try one other way to look up the code. Let's go to *heart,* the anatomical site where the procedure is being performed. When you read the column below *heart,* you will see *septal defect,* which directs you to *See* Septal Defect. You also can look in the Alphabetic Index under the term *repair* (another word for the procedure being done). Under *repair,* find the anatomical site *heart,* then below that *septal defect,* which suggests 33545, 33608–33610, 33681–33688, 33692–33697, 33782, 33783. Indented below this adds *atrial and ventricular* with only one code suggestion—33647. *Ventricular septal defect septum* is a more specific match to the physician's notes than *septal defect,* but not exactly? Not certain? That's great because you need to let the actual code descriptions in the numeric listing give you more details before you make a decision. Therefore, you need to check them all.

This is where time and patience are important to the coding process. Read carefully through the description of each code suggested by the Alphabetic Index. You will probably agree that the best, most appropriate code is

33681   **Closure of single ventricular septal defect, with or without patch**

Great job!

TABLE 25-4 Vascular Families: Common Iliac

First Order	Second Order Branch	Third Order Branch	Beyond Third Order Branches
Common iliac	Internal iliac	Iliolumbar	
		Lateral sacral	
		Superior gluteal	
		Umbilical	
		Superior vesical	
		Obturator	
		Inferior vesical	
		Middle rectal	
		Inferior rectal	
		Internal pudendal	
		Inferior gluteal	
	External iliac	Inferior epigastric	Cremasteric
			Pubic
		Deep circumflex iliac	Ascending deep circumflex iliac
	Common femoral	Profunda femoris	Medial descending
			Perforating branches
			Lateral descending
			Lateral circumflex
		Deep external pudendal	
		Superficial external pudendal	
		Ascending lateral circumflex femoral	
		Descending lateral circumflex femoral	
		Transverse lateral circumflex femoral	
		Superficial femoral	Geniculate
			Popliteal
			Anterior tibial
			Peroneal
			Posterior tibial

Central Venous Access Procedures

Venous access devices (VADs) can be challenging to report because of the various types of procedures involved with their insertion as well as the multitude of purposes for the procedure itself. According to the CPT guidelines, the tip of the VAD or catheter must come to an end in the subclavian vein, brachiocephalic (innominate) vein, iliac vein, superior or inferior vena cava, or right atrium of the heart to be considered a *central* VAD or catheter.

Catheter or Device

A catheter is a tube that is used for various medical reasons. It may be inserted to withdraw bodily fluids, as a urinary catheter collects urine from the bladder. Catheters also can be used to deliver medications, such as an intravenous (IV) injection of drugs directly into the patient's veins. In addition, catheters can be used as a vehicle to enable the insertion of a device such as a stent.

In this usage, a device is most often a subcutaneous pump or a subcutaneous port designed to achieve ongoing access internally without the need to repeatedly obtain a new entry site.

Entry Site: Centrally Inserted or Peripherally Inserted

For these procedures, it is important to the coding process that you read the physician's notes carefully to determine exactly where on the patient's body the VAD or catheter was inserted. A centrally inserted device enters the body at the jugular, subclavian, or femoral vein or the inferior vena cava. A VAD or catheter that enters the body at either the basilic vein or the cephalic vein is called a peripherally inserted central catheter, often referred to by its initials—a PICC line.

Nontunneled or Tunneled

A tunneled catheter does exactly as its name describes—it tunnels under the skin. These tubes are more flexible; they are inserted into a vein at one location, such as the neck, chest, or groin, and wended through beneath the skin to emerge at a separate site in the body. A nontunneled catheter is inserted directly into the vein by venipuncture.

GUIDANCE CONNECTION

Read the additional explanations in the in-section guidelines within the **Surgery** section, subhead **Cardiovascular System,** subsection **Central Venous Access Procedures,** directly above code 36555 in your CPT book.

 YOU CODE IT! CASE STUDY

Elias McGynty is a 54-year-old male who has significant multivessel coronary artery disease. He has atypical anginal symptoms, which are probably secondary to his insulin-dependent (type 1) diabetes mellitus. Nonetheless, he is at risk for ischemia, and in order to reduce this risk, surgical myocardial revascularization is recommended.

PROCEDURE: A coronary artery bypass graft operation utilizing the left internal mammary artery as conduit to the left anterior descending. The remaining conduit will come from the greater saphenous veins. The risks and benefits of this procedure were explained to the patient. He signed the informed consent. The patient tolerated the procedure well and was brought into recovery conscious and aware.

Francis Lamiere, MD

You Code It!

Dr. Lamiere performed a coronary artery bypass graft on Elias McGynty. Determine the code or codes to report this work.

Step #1: Read the case carefully and completely.

Step #2: Abstract the scenario. Which key words or terms describe what service the physician provided to the patient during this encounter?

Step #3: Are there any details missing or incomplete for which you would need to query the physician? [If so, ask your instructor.]

Step #4: Determine the correct CPT procedure code or codes to explain the details about what was provided to the patient during this encounter.

Step #5: Check for any relevant guidance, including reading all of the symbols and notations.

Step #6: Do you need to append any modifiers to ensure complete and accurate information is provided?

Step #7: Double-check your work.

Answer:

Did you determine these to be the correct codes?

33533	Coronary artery bypass, using arterial graft(s); single coronary arterial grafts
+33517	Coronary artery bypass, using venous graft(s) and arterial graft(s); single venous graft

25.9 Digestive System

The digestive tract begins at the mouth and travels through the body all the way to the anus. The organs along the pathway process food and nourishment so cells can absorb nutrients and eliminate waste. The digestive tract also is referred to as the alimentary canal or the gastrointestinal (GI) tract.

Endoscopic Procedures

There are times when a physician needs to visually examine and/or obtain a specimen for pathological testing of the interior of an organ, such as the throat, stomach, or bladder, in order to make a more accurate diagnosis. In these cases, an endoscope may be used.

An esophagogastroduodenoscopy (EGD), more commonly known as an upper endoscopy, enables the physician to view the patient's esophagus, stomach, and duodenum without a surgical invasion of the body.

Endoscopic retrograde cholangiopancreatography (ERCP) uses a combination of x-rays and the endoscope to enable visualization of the patient's stomach, the duodenum, and the bile ducts in the biliary tree and pancreas.

Sigmoidoscopy and colonoscopy are endoscopic procedures used to examine the internal aspects of the lower digestive system. A sigmoidoscopy permits the physician to visually investigate a patient's anus, rectum, and sigmoid colon. A colonoscopy permits the physician to look at the entire large intestine: the anus, the rectum, the descending (sigmoid) colon, the transverse colon, the ascending colon, and the cecum.

Endoscopy can be used for therapeutic procedures as well, as when Dr. Sanger had to remove a penny (foreign body) from little Billy's esophagus after he tried to swallow the coin, code 43247 Esophagogastroduodenoscopy, flexible, transoral; with removal of foreign body(s).

Gastric Intubation

The insertion of a nasogastric (NG) tube may be done for many reasons. The stomach contents may need to be removed, presurgery, postsurgery, or to remove ingested substances (commonly known as "pumping the stomach"). In other cases, the tube may be required to deliver nutrition directly into the stomach. This may be done for a patient after a surgical procedure on the esophagus or the esophogastric junction. Alternately, the tube may be inserted through the mouth instead of the nose, known as oro-gastric tube placement, or percutaneously through the abdominal wall, known as a gastrostomy tube.

EXAMPLES

43752   Naso- or oro-gastric tube placement, requiring physician's skill and fluoroscopic guidance (includes fluoroscopy, image documentation, and report)

43753   Gastric intubation and aspiration(s), therapeutic, necessitating physician's skill (e.g., for gastrointestinal hemorrhage), including lavage if performed

---

Hernia Repair

A hernia is a situation where an organ pushes through an abnormal opening within a muscle or other structure that contains it. A hernia may occur in the inner groin (inguinal hernia), in the outer groin (femoral hernia), in the umbilicus (umbilical hernia), between the esophagus and stomach (hiatal hernia), and as the result of an incision (an incisional hernia).

Of course, the procedure will be different to repair a hernia, as determined by the anatomical location. As you can see by looking in the CPT Alphabetic Index, just knowing the physician performed a hernia repair is not enough detail to determine the code. You must identify, from the documentation, the specific anatomical site.

As with many other procedures, hernia repair can be done as an open procedure or laparoscopically. With some types of hernias, you also may need to know the patient's age. Diaphragmatic, inguinal, and umbilicus hernias are known to occur in neonates and children. And more specifics are needed about the hernia itself: initial or recurrent; incarcerated or strangulated. All of these details also will impact the determination of the code to report.

 YOU CODE IT! CASE STUDY

Thomas Mouldare, a 47-year-old male, was diagnosed with a diaphragmatic (hiatal) hernia that required surgery. Dr. Wallabee performed a Nissen fundoplication, laparoscopically. The upper area of the stomach (gastric fundus) is plicated (wrapped) around the distal portion of the esophagus. This is done to support and reinforce the effectiveness of the lower esophageal sphincter. Then, the esophageal hiatus is sutured to narrow the opening back to the correct width.

You Code It!

Review the details in this case study, and determine the code or codes required to accurately report Dr. Wallabee's surgical procedure on Thomas Mouldare.

Step #1: Read the case carefully and completely.

Step #2: Abstract the scenario. Which key words or terms describe what service the physician provided to the patient during this encounter?

Step #3: Are there any details missing or incomplete for which you would need to query the physician? [If so, ask your instructor.]

Step #4: Determine the correct CPT procedure code or codes to explain the details about what was provided to the patient during this encounter.

Step #5: Check for any relevant guidance, including reading all of the symbols and notations.

Step #6: Do you need to append any modifiers to ensure complete and accurate information is provided?

Step #7: Double-check your work.

Answer:

Did you determine this to be the correct code?

   43280   **Laparoscopy, surgical, esophagogastric fundoplasty (e.g., Nissen, Toupet procedures)**

Bariatric Surgery

Bariatric surgical procedures may be performed on the stomach, the duodenum, the jejunum, and/or the ileum and are most often provided to patients who have been diagnosed as morbidly obese. Consideration for performing this surgery may include the physician's evaluation of the candidate's eating behaviors as well as the patient's predisposition for serious obesity-related co-morbidities such as coronary heart disease, type 2 diabetes mellitus, and/or acute sleep apnea.

These surgeries may be performed as an open procedure or laparoscopically, and this detail will affect the determination of the correct code. The four most common versions of this surgery are

- *Adjustable gastric band (AGB).* See codes 43770–43774. AGB is a procedure that places a small, adjustable band to create a proximal pouch, thereby limiting the passage of food. The attending physician can increase or decrease the size of the passage using saline solution to inflate or deflate as needed for the patient's situation.

- *Roux-en-Y gastric bypass (RYGB).* See codes 43846, 43847, 43644. RYGB limits food intake by use of a small pouch that is similar in size to that created by the adjustable gastric band. In addition, absorption of food in the digestive tract is reduced by excluding most of the stomach, duodenum, and upper intestine from contact with food by routing food directly from the pouch into the small intestine.

- *Biliopancreatic diversion with a duodenal switch (BPD-DS).* See code 43845. BPD-DS, most often referred to as a "duodenal switch," includes transection of the stomach, a bypass to route digested material away from the small intestine, as well as re-routing bile and other digestive juices that impair digestion.

- *Vertical sleeve gastrectomy (VSG).* See code 43775. A VSG is performed and connected to a very short segment of the duodenum, which is then directly connected to a lower part of the small intestine. A small portion of the duodenum is untouched to provide passage for food and absorption of some vitamins and minerals. The distance between the stomach and colon is made much shorter after this operation, resulting in malabsorption.

A VSG procedure includes the resectioning of the stomach and is most often performed solely as the first stage of the multistaged BPD-DS on those patients determined to be unable to go through such a long procedure at one encounter. VSG is not without benefits, as research has shown that some VSG patients report significant weight loss. Should a second-stage procedure be performed, that second procedure and any others in the sequence would be reported with the appropriate procedure code appended by modifier 58 Staged Procedure.

During the postoperative period, adjustments of an adjustable gastric restrictive device are included in the global surgical package and therefore not coded separately.

GUIDANCE CONNECTION

Read the additional explanations in the in-section guidelines located within the **Surgery** section, subhead **Digestive System,** subsection **Bariatric Surgery,** directly above code 43770 in your CPT book.

 LET'S CODE IT! SCENARIO

Justin Abernathy, a 61-year-old male, was suffering from fecal incontinence, diarrhea, and constipation. He came to the Ambulatory Care Center so that his gastroenterologist, Dr. Minton, could perform a colonoscopy. First, Ellen Brennon, RN, administered Demerol and Versed by IV, and the patient was brought into the examination room. The variable flexion Olympus colonoscope was introduced into the rectum and advanced to the cecum. In the midsigmoid colon, a 3-mm sessile polyp was destroyed. The procedure took about 30 minutes, and Justin tolerated the procedure well.

Let's Code It!

We know that the main procedure was a *colonoscopy,* so let's look that up in the Alphabetic Index. When you refer to the notes, what else was done for Justin in conjunction with the colonoscopy? *A polyp was destroyed.*

Find *destruction* beneath *colonoscopy.* Do you know whether a polyp is a lesion or a tumor? It happens to be a lesion; however, you don't have to know this because the index suggests the same code for both: 45388. Let's look at the complete description in the numeric listing.

> **45388** **Colonoscopy, flexible; with ablation of tumor(s), polyp(s), or other lesion(s) (includes pre- and post-dilation and guide wire passage, when performed)**

(continued)

You also will need to code the administration of the moderate sedation that was given to Justin (the Demerol and Versed).

99156   **Moderate sedation services provided by a physician or other qualified health care professional other than the physician or other qualified health care professional performing the diagnostic or therapeutic service that the sedation supports; initial 15 minutes of intraservice time, patient age 5 years or older**

+99157   **each additional 15 minutes of intraservice time (List separately in addition to code for primary service.)**

You have three codes to report the whole story as to what Dr. Minton did for Justin during this encounter: **45388, 99156, 99157.** Great job!

25.10 Urinary System

The urinary system is responsible for maintaining the proper level and composition of fluids in the body.

Urinary Catheterization

There are many reasons why a urinary catheter might need to be inserted: patients with incontinence, especially those who are chronically bedridden or those with lower paralysis; those about to go through a surgical procedure, especially when general anesthesia is administered; as well as patients who suffer from reduced or blocked urine flow, such as male patients with enlarged prostates or female patients with uterine fibroid tumors. A patient with reduced renal function may require a catheterization so health care professionals can accurately monitor their urinary output.

The documentation may include details, such as the type of catheter used, including a Foley, a Robinson, a Carson, or a Tieman catheter. Each type performs differently with various features, determined by the specific issue being addressed.

GUIDANCE CONNECTION

Read the additional explanations in the in-section guidelines within the **Surgery** section, subhead **Urinary System,** subsection **Urodynamics,** directly above code 51725 in your CPT book.

Urodynamics

The codes listed for the procedures in the **Urodynamics** section, 51725–51798, include the services of the physician to perform the procedure (or directly supervise the performance of the procedure), as well as the use of all instruments, equipment, fluids, gases, probes, catheters, technician's fees, medications, gloves, trays, tubing, and other sterile supplies.

If the physician for whom you are coding did not actually perform the procedure but only interpreted the results, then the appropriate procedure code from this section should be appended with modifier 26 Professional Component.

 YOU CODE IT! CASE STUDY

Rachel Naviga, a 39-year-old female, G3 P3, states she has been dealing with stress incontinence increasingly over the last several years. She had three vaginal deliveries, with the largest infant weighing 7.5 lb. Rachel states that her leakage frequency, volume, timing, and associated symptoms (urgency, stress, urinary frequency, nocturia, enuresis, incomplete emptying, straining to empty, leakage without warning) have become bothersome and she wants to do something about it.

   Today she presents for a complex cystometrogram with voiding pressure study to confirm or deny the diagnosis of stress urinary incontinence prior to the scheduling of surgery.

(continued)

Go through the steps, and determine what procedure code(s) should be reported for the encounter with Rachel.

Step #1: Read the case carefully and completely.

Step #2: Abstract the scenario. Which key words or terms describe what service the physician provided to the patient during this encounter?

Step #3: Are there any details missing or incomplete for which you would need to query the physician? [If so, ask your instructor.]

Step #4: Determine the correct CPT procedure code or codes to explain the details about what was provided to the patient during this encounter.

Step #5: Check for any relevant guidance, including reading all of the symbols and notations.

Step #6: Do you need to append any modifiers to ensure complete and accurate information is provided?

Step #7: Double-check your work.

Answer:

Did you determine this to be the correct code?

> **51728**   **Complex cystometrogram (ie. calibrated electronic equipment); with voiding pressure studies (i.e., bladder voiding pressure), any technique**

Transurethral Surgery

When a diagnostic or therapeutic cystourethroscopic intervention is performed, the appropriate codes, 52204–52356, include the insertion and removal of a temporary stent. Therefore, those services are not reported separately—when done at the same time as the cystourethroscopy (Figure 25-7).

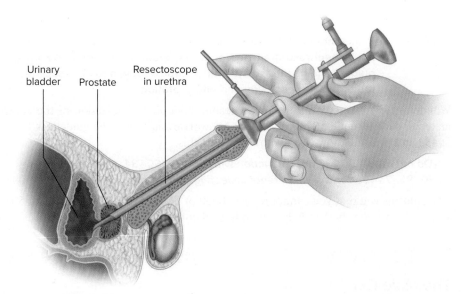

Urinary bladder   Prostate   Resectoscope in urethra

FIGURE 25-7 An illustration of a resectoscope inserted through the urethra of a male patient

If the physician, however, inserts a self-retaining, indwelling stent during the diagnostic or therapeutic cystourethroscopic intervention, use one of the following:

1. Code 52332 with the modifier 51, along with the code for the cystourethroscopy for a unilateral procedure.
2. Code 52332 with modifier 50 for a bilateral insertion of self-retaining, indwelling ureteral stents.

Note that when the physician removes the self-retaining, indwelling ureteral stent, use either 52310 or 52315 with modifier 58.

 LET'S CODE IT! SCENARIO

Ena Colby, a 41-year-old female, is admitted today for the surgical removal of a kidney stone. The stone was too big for her to pass, so Dr. Olympia decided to remove it surgically. The nephrolithotomy, with complete removal of the calculus, went as planned, and Ena tolerated the entire procedure well.

Let's Code It!

Dr. Olympia performed a *nephrolithotomy,* involving the *removal of a kidney stone,* also known as *calculus.* Let's try something direct and look up *nephrolithotomy* in the Alphabetic Index.

The Alphabetic Index suggests the code range 50060–50075. Let's go to the numeric listing and read the different code descriptions.

Do you agree that, according to the physician's notes, the best, most appropriate code available is the following?

50060   Nephrolithotomy; removal of calculus

You are getting very good at this.

Percutaneous Genitourinary Procedures

Diagnostic procedures, such as a nephrostogram or a ureterogram, are most often performed percutaneously, using some type of imaging to guide them. The most common are ultrasound and fluoroscopy.

A patient may have a nephrostomy catheter inserted due to ureter stenosis or obstruction preventing the flow of urine from the kidney to the bladder. A nephrostogram is done to confirm that the tube is positioned and working properly.

50432   Placement of nephrostomy catheter, percutaneous, including diagnostic nephrostogram and/or ureterogram when performed, imaging guidance (e.g., ultrasound and/or fluoroscopy) and all associated radiological supervision and interpretation

Wondering if you should also report a second code for the injection of the contrast material, such as code 50430 or 50431? No worries, just read the guidelines beneath 50432 and you will know exactly how to report this:

(Do not report 50432 in conjunction with 50430, 50431, 50432, 50694, 50695, 74425 for the same renal collecting system and/or associated ureter)

This informs you that you cannot report 50430 or 50431 at the same time with 50432. The guidelines are there to help you do this all correctly!

25.11 The Genital Systems: Male and Female

The Male Genital System

The male genital system is closely situated with the urinary bladder, so a urologist may be the specialist most often performing procedures on this area of the male anatomy.

 GUIDANCE CONNECTION

Read the additional explanations in the in-section guidelines within the **Surgery** section, subhead **Urinary System,** and throughout this subsection in your CPT book.

Penile Plaque

This type of plaque is a flat layer of scar tissue that can form on the inside of a thick membrane called the tunica albuginea, which envelops the erectile tissues, and is known as Peyronie disease. This is believed to begin as an inflammation, and the plaque is benign, not contagious, and not sexually transmitted. However, it can cause discomfort and pain in men with this condition. There are several ways to treat the problem.

Injections of steroids and chemotherapy agents, such as interferon, can be directly delivered to the site of the plaque to work to reduce the effect. These procedures may be reported with

54200   **Injection procedure for Peyronie disease**
54205   **Injection procedure for Peyronie disease; with surgical exposure of plaque**

The plaque can be surgically removed. This procedure may be performed just to excise the plaque, or it may include the grafting of material to replace tissue that was excised.

54110   **Excision of penile plaque (Peyronie disease)**
54111   **Excision of penile plaque (Peyronie disease); with graft to 5 cm in length**
54112   **Excision of penile plaque (Peyronie disease); with graft greater than 5 cm in length**

Severe cases may require more extensive reconstruction and will be reported with code

54360   **Plastic operation on penis to correct angulation**

 YOU CODE IT! CASE STUDY

Glenn Hagger, a 15-year-old male, came to see his regular physician, Dr. Carboni, for help. Glenn and his friends were fooling around at his father's construction company, and a staple gun went off, projecting a staple into his scrotum. Dr. Carboni carefully removed the staple and applied some antibiotic ointment to prevent infection until the two small wounds healed.

You Code It!

Go through the steps, and determine the procedure code(s) that should be reported for this encounter between Dr. Carboni and Glenn Hagger.

Step #1: Read the case carefully and completely.

Step #2: Abstract the scenario. Which key words or terms describe what service the physician provided to the patient during this encounter?

Step #3: Are there any details missing or incomplete for which you would need to query the physician? [If so, ask your instructor.]

Step #4: Determine the correct CPT procedure code or codes to explain the details about what was provided to the patient during this encounter.

Step #5: Check for any relevant guidance, including reading all of the symbols and notations.

Step #6: Do you need to append any modifiers to ensure complete and accurate information is provided?

Step #7: Double-check your work.

Answer:
Did you determine this to be the correct code?

    55120   **Removal of foreign body in scrotum**

This matches the physician's description perfectly!

The Female Genital System

Vulvectomy

Sometimes physicians use direct terms in their notes, such as *simple, partial, radical,* or *complete,* when describing vulvectomies. Such terms make finding the best code easier. However, other physicians may be more descriptive in their notes regarding the procedure. Therefore, you have to know what these terms mean. The CPT book defines them as follows:

- *Simple:* The removal of skin and *superficial* subcutaneous tissues.
- *Radical:* The removal of skin and *deep* subcutaneous tissues.
- *Partial:* The removal of *less than* 80% of the vulvar area.
- *Complete:* The removal of *more than* 80% of the vulvar area.

:: GUIDANCE CONNECTION

Read the additional explanations in the in-section guidelines within the **Surgery** section, subhead **Female Genital System,** subsection **Vulva, Perineum, and Introitus,** directly above code 56405 in your CPT book.

EXAMPLES

56620	Vulvectomy, simple; partial

The description of this code represents a physician's statement that he or she removed less than 80% of the skin and superficial subcutaneous tissues of the vulvar area.

56633	Vulvectomy, radical; complete

The description of this code represents a physician's statement that he or she removed more than 80% of the skin and deep subcutaneous tissues of the vulvar area.

Maternity Care and Delivery

The complete package of services provided to a woman for uncomplicated maternity care includes the antepartum (prenatal) care, the delivery of the baby, and the postpartum care of the mother. Similar to working with the services already provided in the global surgical package, you must know the components of the maternity care package. This is the only way you can determine what is already included and what services should be reported separately.

Antepartum Care

- Initial patient history.
- Subsequent patient history.
- Physical examinations.
- Documentation of weight, blood pressure, fetal heart tones, routine chemical urinalysis.
- Monthly visits from conception up to 28-weeks gestation.
- Biweekly visits from 28-weeks to 36-weeks gestation.
- Weekly visits from 36-weeks gestation to delivery.

Delivery Services

- Admission to the hospital.
- Admission history and physical examination (H&P).
- Management of uncomplicated labor.
- Delivery: vaginal (with or without episiotomy, with or without forceps) or cesarean section.

Postpartum Care

- Hospital and office visits following the delivery.

   Should a physician provide one portion of the services, but not all, this will affect the determination of the correct code.

EXAMPLES

Dr. Barber provided antepartum care for Nancy Trainer. While on vacation in Europe, Nancy suffered a miscarriage (spontaneous abortion) and lost the baby. Dr. Barber provided postpartum care for Nancy when she returned home. Therefore, instead of reporting

| 59400 | Routine obstetric care including antepartum care, vaginal delivery (with or without episiotomy, and/or forceps) and postpartum care |

or

| 59510 | Routine obstetric care including antepartum care, cesarean delivery, and postpartum care |

Dr. Barber's complete care for Nancy will be reported with two codes:

| 59425 | Antepartum care only; 4–6 visits |
| 59430 | Postpartum care only (separate procedure) |

GUIDANCE CONNECTION

Read the additional explanations in the in-section guidelines within the **Surgery** section, subhead **Maternity Care and Delivery,** directly above code 59000 in your CPT book.

 LET'S CODE IT! SCENARIO

PATIENT: Gloria Valdez

DATE OF DISCHARGE: 05/30/2019

ADMITTING DIAGNOSIS: Intrauterine pregnancy at 36 weeks and 5 days estimated gestational age. Presented with contractions and in latent labor.

DISCHARGE DIAGNOSIS: Status post normal spontaneous vaginal delivery at 36 weeks and 5 days estimated gestational age.

HISTORY OF PRESENT ILLNESS/HOSPITAL COURSE: This patient is a 31-year-old G4, P1-0-2-1 female for whom I have been attending through all prenatal care. She is at 36 weeks and 5 days estimated gestational age who presented with contractions and in latent labor. On vaginal examination, the patient was found to be 3 cm dilated, 70% effaced and −3 station. The fetal heart tracing at the time was in the 140s and reactive. The patient was admitted to Labor and Delivery for antibiotics and epidural. The patient continued to have a good labor pattern and proceeded to deliver a viable female infant weighing 5 pounds 7 ounces over an intact perineum with Apgars of 9 and 9 at 1 and 5 minutes. There were no nuchal cords, no true knots, and the number of vessels in the cord were three. Her postpartum course was uncomplicated and the patient was discharged to home in stable and satisfactory condition on postpartum day #2.

PROCEDURES PERFORMED: Normal spontaneous delivery and repair of midline episiotomy in the usual fashion.

COMPLICATIONS: None.

FINAL DIAGNOSIS: Status post normal spontaneous vaginal delivery at 36 weeks and 5 days estimated gestational age.

DISCHARGE INSTRUCTIONS: Call for increased pain, fever, or increased bleeding.

(continued)

CHAPTER 25 | CPT SURGERY SECTION   **769**

DIET: Advance as tolerated.

ACTIVITY: Pelvic rest for 6 weeks and nothing inserted into the vagina for 6 weeks, i.e., no tampons, douche, or sex.

MEDICATIONS AND FOLLOW-UP: Instructed patient to call me in the morning, or prn with any concerns. Then, I will see her in the office in 1 week.

Felicia Washington, MD

Let's Code It!

Dr. Washington has been caring for Gloria throughout this pregnancy and delivery. This is the big event, so turn to the CPT Alphabetic Index to

Table Cell
See Cesarean Delivery; Vaginal Delivery

Gloria has a vaginal delivery, so turn to

Vaginal Delivery. 59400, 59610-59614

Are there any items listed below this that match what Dr. Washington did for Gloria? Not exactly. So, turn to review the full descriptions of these codes.

59400   Routine obstetric care including antepartum care, vaginal delivery (with or without episiotomy, and/or forceps) and postpartum care

59610   Routine obstetric care including antepartum care, vaginal delivery (with or without episiotomy, and/or forceps) and postpartum care, after previous cesarean delivery

59612   Vaginal delivery only after previous cesarean delivery (with or without episiotomy and/or forceps);

59614   Vaginal delivery only after previous cesarean delivery (with or without episiotomy and/or forceps); including postpartum care

Do any of these codes accurately and completely report what Dr. Washington provided to Gloria for this pregnancy and delivery?

59400   Routine obstetric care including antepartum care, vaginal delivery (with or without episiotomy, and/or forceps) and postpartum care

Good work!

25.12 Nervous System

Procedures performed on the nervous system organs (the brain, spinal cord, nerves, and ganglia) and connective tissues are coded from the **Nervous System** subsection. These components of the human body are responsible for sensory, integrative, and motor activities.

Skull Surgery

The skull is, technically, the bone-shell that covers and protects the brain and organs within. To cushion the tissues, blood vessels, and nerves, the dura mater, arachnoid mater, and pia mater lie between the skull and these components (Figure 25-8).

The complexity of surgical treatment of skull base lesions often demands the skills of more than one surgeon during the same session. When one surgeon provides one portion of the procedure and another surgeon a different portion, each surgeon only uses the code for the surgical procedure he or she performed.

FIGURE 25-8 The internal components of the head

Typically, the segments of the procedure include the following:

1. The *approach* describes the tactic of the procedure, such as craniofacial, orbitocranial, or transcochlear:

   a. Anterior cranial fossa, 61580–61586

   b. Middle cranial fossa, 61590–61592

   c. Posterior cranial fossa, 61595–61598

2. The *definitive* describes the procedure itself, such as resection, excision, repair, biopsy, or transection:

   a. Base of anterior cranial fossa, 61600–61601

   b. Base of middle cranial fossa, 61605–61613

   c. Base of posterior cranial fossa, 61615–61616

3. The *repair/reconstruction* identifies a secondary repair, such as

   a. Extensive dural grafting

   b. Cranioplasty

   c. Local or regional myocutaneous pedicle flaps

   d. Extensive skin grafts

If one surgeon performs more than one of the procedures, each segment should be reported separately, with the second (and third, if applicable) appended with modifier 51 to indicate that multiple procedures were performed at the same session by the same physician.

When a surgeon embeds a neurostimulator electrode array and performs microelectrode recording, the recording is included in the implantation code and shouldn't be coded separately.

Code 62263 includes the following:

- Percutaneous insertion of an epidural catheter.
- Removal of the catheter several days later.
- Procedure injections.

GUIDANCE CONNECTION

Read the additional explanations in the in-section guidelines within the **Surgery** section, subhead **Nervous System,** subsection **Surgery of Skull Base,** directly above code 61580 in your CPT book.

CODING BITES

If multiple treatments are provided all in 1 calendar day, then use code 62264.

- Fluoroscopic guidance and localization.
- Multiple adhesiolysis sessions over the course of 2 or more days.

The code should be used only once to represent the entire series.

62263   **Percutaneous lysis of epidural adhesions using solution injection (e.g., hypertonic saline, enzyme) or mechanical means (e.g., catheter) including radiologic localization (includes contrast when administered), multiple adhesiolysis sessions; 2 or more days**

62264   **1 day**

Spinal Cord Injury Repair

Injury to the spinal cord is almost always the result of trauma. This damage can result in changes to the patient's strength, sensations, and other bodily functions that are regulated by these nerves, impacting virtually every aspect of life. The extent of the patient's ability to control his or her limbs will be determined by the location (specific site along the spine) and the severity of the damage. The location is identified by the lowest (most distal) segment of the spine that is unaffected by the injury.

At this time, treatments of spinal cord injuries are directed at pain control and stabilization of the spine to prevent additional irritation or damage to the nerves.

Methylprednisolone acetate (brand name Medrol) is an anti-inflammatory with immunosuppressive properties. Some spinal cord injury patients find that it can reduce the damage to the nerve cells as well as reduce inflammation near the site of the injury, decreasing pain and discomfort. This is an off-label use of this drug but has been found to be beneficial for these cases.

When the trauma causes something to press against the spinal cord, this compression can interfere with the transmission of impulses within the nerves. Surgical decompression of a nerve is typically provided by a neurosurgeon performing a procedure known as a neuroplasty. This procedure may be reported with, for example, CPT code 64713 Neuroplasty, major peripheral nerve, arm, or leg, open; brachial plexus or 64714 Neuroplasty, major peripheral nerve, arm, or leg, open; lumbar plexus.

Functional electrical stimulation (FES), also termed neuromuscular electric stimulation (NMES), may be used to support the restoration of neuromuscular function, sensory function, or autonomic function (e.g., bladder, bowel, or respiratory function) by employing electrical currents to activate damaged nerves within the spinal cord. Procedures focused on the use of spinal neurostimulator systems, reported with CPT codes 63650, 63655, and 63661–63664 (for insertion, revision, replacement, and/or removal), include the implanted neurostimulator, an external controller, an extension, and multiple contacts (also known as electrodes). These contacts may be located on a lead, similar to a catheter, or on a plate-shaped or paddle-like surface. Percutaneous stereotaxis (stereotactic surgery) may be used to stimulate the spinal cord by locating specific points in the brain that may be identified for additional therapy. This would be reported with CPT code 63610 Stereotactic stimulation of spinal cord, percutaneous, separate procedure not followed by other surgery.

Pain Management

Virtually everyone knows what pain feels like, and this is a very personal evaluation. Medically speaking, pain is an unpleasant sensation often initiated by tissue damage, resulting in impulses transmitted to the brain via specific nerve fibers. Most health care facilities use some type of pain scale from 0 to 10, with 0 indicating no pain at all and 10 representing excruciating, intolerable pain. In most instances, each number on the scale is accompanied by an illustration to help patients accurately communicate what they are feeling. This numeric scale (no illustrations), provided by the National Institutes of Health, can help improve communication with patients (Table 25-5).

TABLE 25-5 Numeric Rating Scale for Pain

0	= No pain
1–3	= Mild pain (nagging, annoying, interfering little with ADL*)
4–6	= Moderate pain (interferes significantly with ADL*)
7–10	= Severe pain (disabling; unable to perform ADL*)

*ADL = activities of daily living

Source: National Institute of Health.

When the documentation indicates that an encounter is prompted by a patient's need for pain management, especially when the pain is noted as acute and/or chronic, there are several options for treatment.

Electrical Reprocessing

Researchers are consistently searching for new ways to help patients manage their pain. Transcutaneous electrical modulation pain reprocessing (TEMPR), also referred to as scrambler therapy, administers electrical impulses designed to interrupt pain signals. Although this experimental procedure uses a type of transcutaneous electrical nerve stimulation (TENS), it is not the same procedure. Each session lasts about an hour, with the physician making adjustments approximately every 10 minutes. Each treatment session is reported with Category III code 0278T.

0278T Transcutaneous electrical modulation pain reprocessing (e.g., scrambler therapy), each treatment session (includes placement of electrodes)

Epidural/Intrathecal Medication Administration

Medication administered intrathecally (directly into the cerebrospinal fluid via the subarachnoid space in the spinal cord) may be used for chronic pain management. This methodology typically uses pumps, devices that can provide continual delivery of the drug, biologicals, or genetically engineered encapsulated cells. This route of administration has been found to be less invasive for the patient and enables treatment of a larger portion of the central nervous system utilizing the cerebrospinal fluid circulation pathways. Epidural administration tenders the medication into the dura mater of the spinal cord rather than the subarachnoid space.

EXAMPLES

62350	Implantation, revision, or repositioning of tunneled intrathecal or epidural catheter, for long-term medication administration via an external pump or implantable reservoir/infusion pump; without laminectomy
62360	Implantation or replacement of device for intrathecal or epidural drug infusion; subcutaneous reservoir
62362	Implantation or replacement of device for intrathecal or epidural drug infusion; programmable pump, including preparation of pump, with or without programming
99601	Home infusion/specialty drug administration, per visit (up to 2 hours)

Intravenous Therapy

This may be the administration route with which you are most familiar. The medication enters the body via the patient's vein, most often using a point inside the patient's antecubital fossa (elbow). If the condition is chronic, a peripherally inserted central catheter (PICC) line may be inserted and used for the administration of the medication for the duration of the therapy.

CODING BITES

Whenever you report the administration of a drug, you will need the code for the administration, such as implantation of a pump or infusion, as well as a code to report the specific drug that is administered. Most often, the codes used to report the specific drug come from the HCPCS Level II code set. See the chapter HCPCS Level II in this textbook for more information on these codes.

LET'S CODE IT! SCENARIO

Gerald Rosen, a 63-year-old male, was admitted for the implantation of a cerebral cortical neurostimulator. Dr. Grumman performed a craniotomy and then successfully implanted the electrodes.

Let's Code It!

Dr. Grumman first performed a *craniotomy.* Let's go to the Alphabetic Index and look. Below *craniotomy,* you will see the listing for *implant of neurostimulators.* That matches our notes, so let's go to the numeric listing and check the descriptions for 61850–61875, as suggested. Read through the codes and their descriptions in this section. Do you agree that the following matches our notes the best?

61860   Craniectomy or craniotomy for implantation of neurostimulator electrodes, cerebral, cortical

It does!

Endovascular Therapy

Included in this category of neurologic procedures are balloon angioplasties and intravascular stents. You learned about these types of procedures in the *Cardiovascular System* section of this chapter. However, the codes *here* report these procedures when done intracranially (within the skull) and not intracardially (within the heart).

An intra-arterial mechanical embolectomy or thrombectomy is most often performed to treat an acute ischemic stroke (when a thrombus or embolus blocks blood flow to the brain).

 LET'S CODE IT! SCENARIO

Alvin Bartholemew, a 71-year-old male, was admitted through the ED with signs of a stroke. He was taken into surgery immediately and Dr. Newton performed a percutaneous transluminal mechanical thrombectomy in the anterior parietal artery. Fluoroscopic guidance was used, and the thrombus was removed and Alteplase 0.9 mg/kg (a thrombolytic agent) was injected.

Let's Code It!

What did Dr. Newton do for Alvin? A *transluminal mechanical thrombectomy* was performed. Turn to the Alphabetic Index in your CPT code book to

Thrombectomy

There is a lengthy list below this term, so review them and read the scenario again and see if you can match any words in common . . .

(continued)

Thrombectomy
Percutaneous
        Intracranial artery. 61645
        Mechanical arterial 37184-37186

These both match but are in very different subsections of the **Surgery** section. Let's investigate these codes. Remember, you must review all of them before you can determine which is the most accurate.

61645   Percutaneous arterial transluminal mechanical thrombectomy and/or infusion for thrombolysis, intracranial, any method, including diagnostic angiography, fluoroscopic guidance, catheter placement, and intraprocedural pharmacological thrombolytic injection(s)

37184   Primary percutaneous transluminal mechanical thrombectomy, noncoronary, non-intracranial, arterial or arterial bypass graft, including fluoroscopic guidance and intraprocedural pharmacological thrombolytic injection(s); initial vessel
          [NOTE: Codes 37185 and 37186 are both add-on codes, so we can focus our analysis on this first code in this series. Then, if 37184 is the right code for this procedure, we can come back and analyze these add-on codes to determine if they are needed.]

Hmm. These two descriptions are very close. However, did you notice that code 61645 specifically states "intracranial," whereas code 37184 specifically states "non-intracranial."

Go back to the documentation. It does not state "intracranial" or "non-intracranial." It does state the thrombectomy was performed on the "*anterior parietal artery.*"

According to my medical dictionary, the *anterior parietal artery* is one of the branches of the middle cerebral artery, distributed to the front or forward part of the parietal lobe of the brain.

OK, so if the thrombectomy was performed to remove a thrombus from the anterior parietal artery, and you know that this artery is in the brain, this means that this procedure was "intracranial" [remember, the cranium is the skull].

Now you know exactly which code to report for this procedure:

61645   Percutaneous arterial transluminal mechanical thrombectomy and/or infusion for thrombolysis, intracranial, any method, including diagnostic angiography, fluoroscopic guidance, catheter placement, and intraprocedural pharmacological thrombolytic injection(s)

Good job!

25.13 The Optical and Auditory Systems

Optical System

Loss of sight, or even the reduction of vision, has both a social and an economic impact on a patient and his or her family. In the United States, it is estimated that 14 million people aged 12 and over have some type of visual impairment, and about 61 million adults are believed to be at high risk for acute vision loss.

There are two recesses in the human skull, each known as an orbit, or eye socket. Within this bony conical orbit sits the contents of the eye and its ancillary parts (muscles, nerves, blood vessels). The optical system is the most complex organ system of the human body (Figure 25-9).

Ophthalmologists diagnose and treat problems and concerns of the eye and ocular adnexa (anatomical parts and sites adjacent to an organ). Most commonly, cataracts are corrected and foreign materials are removed.

Glaucoma Surgery

Glaucoma is a malfunction of the fluid pressure within the eye; the pressure rises to a level that can cause damage to the optic disc and nerve. Treatment can successfully

Sclera

Vitreous humor

Iris

Cornea

Pupil

Lens

Aqueous humor

Anterior chamber

Anterior cavity

Posterior chamber

Ciliary body

Optic disk

Optic nerve

Fovea centralis

Retina

Choroid

FIGURE 25-9 An illustration of the components of the optical system

prevent blindness or any vision loss from resulting. When eye drops, oral medication, or laser treatments have failed to control the patient's glaucoma condition, a trabeculectomy may be performed. This procedure treats glaucoma with an incision into the trabecular tissue of the eye to drain the excess fluid that has accumulated. In some cases, a drainage tube is inserted.

EXAMPLES

65850	Trabeculectomy ab externo
66170	Fistulization of sclera for glaucoma; trabeculectomy ab externo in absence of previous surgery

Vitrectomy

Patients diagnosed with diabetes mellitus are at risk for ophthalmic manifestations of their abnormal glucose levels. Diabetic retinopathy is the most common; it is a condition that causes damage to the tiny blood vessels inside the retina. In cases where the bleeding in the eye is severe, a vitrectomy, the surgical removal of vitreous gel from the center of the eye, may be necessary.

EXAMPLES

65810	Paracentesis of anterior chamber of eye (separate procedure); with removal of vitreous and/or discission of anterior hyaloid membrane, with or without air injection
67005	Removal of vitreous, anterior approach (open sky technique or limbal incision); partial removal

Foreign Object in Eye

We all know . . . things happen. Tiny specks of dirt, gravel, debris, etc. can fly into one's eyes and may need to be surgically removed. In those cases where the foreign body is difficult to remove, the patient may be admitted to the hospital to have a surgical extirpation. Read the documentation carefully to identify the specific part of the eye from which the object is removed, as well as the direction of the approach.

EXAMPLES

65205	Removal of foreign body, external eye; conjunctival superficial
67413	Orbitotomy without bone flap (frontal or transconjunctival approach); with removal of foreign body
67430	Orbitotomy with bone flap or window, lateral approach (e.g., Kroenlein); with removal of foreign body
68530	Removal of foreign body or dacryolith, lacrimal passages

Dacryocystorhinostomy

Nasolacrimal duct (NLD) stenosis is a condition that may be congenital or acquired. A patient may acquire an NLD stenosis as a result of a granulomatous disease, such as sarcoidosis; a sinus condition; or the formation of dacryoliths (calculus in the lacrimal duct or sac). A dacryocystorhinostomy (DCR) is the standard of care for an NLD obstruction. DCR can be performed using a percutaneous approach by way of a facial incision, or the approach may be via the natural opening of the nose endoscopically. The procedure is designed to bypass the obstructed nasolacrimal duct and enable tear drainage directly into the nose from the lacrimal sac.

Fornix
The conjunctival fornix is the area between the eyelid and the eyeball. The superior fornix is between the upper lid and eyeball; the inferior fornix is between the lower lid and the eyeball [plural: fornices].

EXAMPLES

68801	Dilation of lacrimal punctum, with or without irrigation
68815	Probing of nasolacimal duct, with or without irrigation; with insertion of tube or stent

 LET'S CODE IT! SCENARIO

Delores Leon was diagnosed with a herniated orbital mass, OD (right inferior orbit). Dr. Marconi performed an excision of the mass and repair. From his notes, "The lower lid was everted and the inferior **fornix** *examined. The herniating mass was viewed and measured at 0.81 cm in diameter. Westcott scissors were used to incise the conjunctival fornices. The herniating mass was then clamped, excised, and cauterized. It appeared to contain mostly fat tissue, which was sent to pathology. The inferior fornix was repaired using running suture of 6-0 plain gut. Bacitracin ointment was applied to the eye followed by an eye pad."*

Let's Code It!

The procedure performed was "*excision of the mass and repair, right inferior orbit.*"

In the CPT Alphabetic Index, turn to *excision* and review the long list of anatomical sites below. What did Dr. Marconi excise? Not the eye (that would be removal of the eyeball). He removed a "*mass* from the eye orbit" and then "*repaired* the orbit."

(continued)

There is no listing for *mass,* but you should remember from medical terminology class (or look it up in a medical dictionary) that another term for *mass* is *lesion.* In the Alphabetic Index, find:

Excision . . . Lesion . . . another long list. On your scratch pad, write down the codes suggested next to the word *Orbit*—61333, 67412, 67420—so that you can check them out. However, while you are here, also write down the codes suggested for *Conjunctiva*—68110–68130. Why? Because in the body of the notes, it states "*incise the conjunctival fornices.*" This is why it is so important to read the complete notes and not just code from the procedure statement at the top.

Now, let's turn to the main portion of the CPT and find the complete code descriptions:

61333	**Exploration of orbit (transcranial approach); with removal of lesion**
67412	**Orbitotomy without bone flap (frontal or transconjunctival approach); with removal of lesion**
67420	**Orbitotomy with bone flap or window, lateral approach (eg, Kroenlein); with removal of lesion**
68110	**Excision of lesion, conjunctiva; up to 1 cm**
68115	**Excision of lesion, conjunctiva; over 1 cm**
68130	**Excision of lesion, conjunctiva; with adjacent sclera**

Which code description matches the physician's notes accurately? **68110.** Good work!

 YOU CODE IT! CASE STUDY

Ronald Jackson, a 49-year-old male, was working in a metal shop. As he was trimming a steel bar, some metal splinters got into his eye. Fortunately, Dr. Draman found that the metal pieces presented superficial damage and had not embedded themselves in Ronald's conjunctiva. Dr. Draman removed all the metal pieces and placed a patch over Ronald's eye.

You Code It!

Go through the steps and determine the procedure code(s) that should be reported for this encounter between Dr. Draman and Ronald Jackson.

Step #1: Read the case carefully and completely.

Step #2: Abstract the scenario. Which key words or terms describe what service the physician provided to the patient during this encounter?

Step #3: Are there any details missing or incomplete for which you would need to query the physician? [If so, ask your instructor.]

Step #4: Determine the correct CPT procedure code or codes to explain the details about what was provided to the patient during this encounter.

Step #5: Check for any relevant guidance, including reading all of the symbols and notations.

Step #6: Do you need to append any modifiers to ensure complete and accurate information is provided?

Step #7: Double-check your work.

Answer:

Did you determine this to be the correct code?

    65205   **Removal of foreign body, external eye; conjunctival superficial**

Good for you!

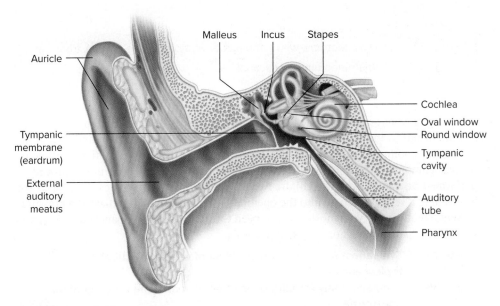

FIGURE 25-10 The auditory system

The Auditory System

The auditory system of the human body is referenced in three sections (Figure 25-10).

The Outer Ear

- Auricle (pinna).
- External acoustic meatus (also known as the external auditory canal).
- Eardrum (the tympanic membrane).

EXAMPLES

69100	Biopsy external ear
69209	Removal of impacted cerumen using irrigation/lavage, unilateral
69310	Recontruction of external auditory canal (meatoplasty) (e.g., for stenosis due to injury, infection) (separate procedure)

The Middle Ear

- Auditory ossicles: malleus, incus, and stapes.
- Oval window.
- Eustachian tube (auditory tube), which connects the middle ear to the nasopharynx (throat).

EXAMPLES

69421	Myringotomy, including aspiration and/or eustachian tube inflation requiring general anesthesia
69535	Resection temporal bone, external approach

The Inner Ear

- Semicircular canals.
- Cochlea.

Tympanostomy

When a patient has a middle ear infection (otitis media), pressure caused by the buildup of fluid or pus in the middle ear compresses the eardrum, causing pain and decreasing the patient's ability to hear. A lack of treatment can result in a perforation of the tympanic membrane. Tympanostomy (ear tube surgery) is a relatively common procedure performed on about 2 million children each year in the United States. It involves the insertion of a ventilating tube into the opening of the tympanum to relieve the pressure.

When reporting a tympanostomy, you need to know what type of anesthesia was provided to the patient: local or general anesthesia.

69433 Tympanostomy (requiring insertion of ventilating tube), local or topical anesthesia

69436 Tympanostomy (requiring insertion of ventilating tube), general anesthesia

These codes report the insertion of the tube into one ear only. When the physician performs this for both ears at the same encounter, you will need to append modifier 50 Bilateral procedure to the correct procedure code.

Sometimes, over a period of time, the tubes naturally fall out. However, when the physician must go in and surgically remove the tubes under general anesthesia, this procedure will be reported separately:

69424 Ventilating tube removal requiring general anesthesia

YOU CODE IT! CASE STUDY

Anna Mendoza, a 33-year-old female, has been deaf since she was 11. She is admitted today for Dr. Eberhardt to put a cochlear implant in her left ear. It is expected that Anna will gain back much of her hearing.

You Code It!

Go through the steps, and determine the procedure code(s) that should be reported for this encounter between Dr. Eberhardt and Anna Mendoza.

Step #1: Read the case carefully and completely.

Step #2: Abstract the scenario. Which key words or terms describe what service the physician provided to the patient during this encounter?

Step #3: Are there any details missing or incomplete for which you would need to query the physician? [If so, ask your instructor.]

Step #4: Determine the correct CPT procedure code or codes to explain the details about what was provided to the patient during this encounter.

Step #5: Check for any relevant guidance, including reading all of the symbols and notations.

Step #6: Do you need to append any modifiers to ensure complete and accurate information is provided?

Step #7: Double-check your work.

Answer:

Did you determine this to be the correct code?

69930 Cochlear device implantation, with or without mastoidectomy

25.14 Organ Transplantation

Lung Transplantation

Special guidelines help you report any lung transplant. However, as soon as you begin to read the notation shown before codes 32850–32856, you will see that the editors of the CPT book use the term lung **allotransplantation** in addition to **transplantation**. These words have a very similar meaning.

A lung transplant requires three steps, which can be performed by a single physician or a team of physicians, with each physician submitting his or her own claim. Each step has its own code.

Cadaver Donor Pneumonectomy

Because a human cannot live without lungs, the donor has to be deceased (a cadaver) prior to the harvesting of the organ. This portion of the transplant, or allotransplantation, procedure should be identified with the code

> **32850** Donor pneumonectomy(s) (including cold preservation), from cadaver donor

Backbench Work

The actual preparation of the cadaver lung allograft prior to the transplant procedure is known as *backbench work*. The actual preparation of the cadaver donor lung allograft prior to the transplant procedure is coded by using either of the following:

> **32855** Backbench standard preparation of cadaver donor lung allograft prior to transplantation . . . ; unilateral

or

> **32856** Backbench standard preparation of cadaver donor lung allograft prior to transplantation . . . ; bilateral

Recipient Lung Allotransplantation

The final code for the entire operation identifies the placement of the allograft in the patient (the recipient). The selection of a code from the range 32851–32854 is determined by whether the procedure is performed unilaterally or bilaterally and with or without a cardiopulmonary bypass.

> **32851** Lung transplant, single; without cardiopulmonary bypass
> **32852**   with cardiopulmonary bypass
> **32853** Lung transplant, double (bilateral sequential or en bloc); without cardiopulmonary bypass
> **32854**   with cardiopulmonary bypass

Allotransplantation
The relocation of tissue from one individual to another (both of the same species) without an identical genetic match.

Transplantation
The transfer of tissue from one site to another.

 GUIDANCE CONNECTION

Read the additional explanations in the in-section guidelines within the **Surgery** section, subhead **Respiratory System,** subsection **Lung Transplantation,** directly above code 32850 in your CPT book.

CPT **LET'S CODE IT! SCENARIO**

Abbey Reason, a 15-year-old female, was diagnosed 3 years ago with idiopathic pulmonary fibrosis, a chronic interstitial pulmonary disease. Corticosteroid therapy has not improved her condition, so Dr. Flemming admitted her today for a double-lung transplantation. The harvesting of the allograft and the preparation of the cadaver donor double-lung allograft were done by Dr. Orenge. Dr. Flemming only performed the actual lung transplant, en bloc, along with a cardiopulmonary bypass. Abbey tolerated the procedure well and has an excellent prognosis.

Let's Code It!

The notes indicate that Dr. Flemming performed only one of the three steps. Therefore, you will have only one code on his claim form for Abbey's surgery.

(continued)

Let's go to the Alphabetic Index and look for *transplant*. Read down until you find *lung*. You know that Abbey received a *double-lung* transplant, *en bloc, with a bypass*. That information leads to the suggested code 32854. Now go to the numeric listing to check the complete code description.

32854   **Lung transplant, double (bilateral sequential or en bloc); with cardiopulmonary bypass**

Terrific! This code matches the notes.

Heart/Lung Transplantation

Similar to the components of the lung transplantation that we reviewed earlier, a heart transplant, with or without a lung allotransplantation, requires three steps to be performed by a single physician or a team of physicians. Each step has its own codes.

Cadaver Donor Cardiectomy with or without a Pneumonectomy

A human cannot live without a heart or lungs, so the donor has to be deceased (a cadaver) prior to any organ harvesting. This portion of the transplant or allotransplantation procedure is identified with the code 33930 (heart and lungs) or 33940 (heart alone):

33930   **Donor cardiectomy-pneumonectomy (including cold preservation)**

or

33940   **Donor cardiectomy (including cold preservation)**

Backbench Work

The actual preparation of the cadaver donor heart, or heart and lung, allograft prior to the transplant procedure is known as *backbench work*. The second portion of the transplant is coded by using either of the following:

33933   **Backbench standard preparation of cadaver donor heart/lung allograft to transplantation, including dissection of allograft from surrounding soft tissues to prepare aorta, superior vena cava, inferior vena cava, and trachea for implantation**

or

33944   **Backbench standard preparation of cadaver donor heart allograft to transplantation, including dissection from surrounding soft tissues to prepare aorta, superior vena cava, inferior vena cava, pulmonary artery, and left atrium for implantation**

Recipient Heart with or without Lung Allotransplantation

The third code for the entire operation identifies the placement of the allograft into the patient (the recipient). Select the code from either of the following:

33935   **Heart-lung transplant with recipient cardiectomy-pneumonectomy**

or

33945   **Heart transplant with or without recipient cardiectomy**

The codes for the insertion of the transplanted organs include the removal of the damaged or diseased organs.

Liver Transplantation

Again, the components that we have reviewed for the other organ transplants are involved with a liver allotransplantation.

Donor Hepatectomy

A human can live without a portion of the liver, so the donor can be either deceased (a cadaver) or living. The best code for this portion of the transplant process is determined by whether or not the donor is living, and if living, what percentage or portion of the liver is donated.

47133   **Donor hepatectomy (including cold preservation), from cadaver donor**

or

47140   **Donor hepatectomy (including cold preservation), from living donor; left lateral segment only (segments II and III)**

or

47141   **Donor hepatectomy (including cold preservation), from living donor; total left lobectomy (segments II, III, and IV)**

or

47142   **Donor hepatectomy (including cold preservation), from living donor; total right lobectomy (segments V, VI, VII, and VIII)**

Backbench Work

The actual preparation of the whole liver graft prior to the transplant procedure is coded with

47143   **Backbench standard preparation of cadaver donor whole liver graft prior to allotransplantation, including cholecystectomy, if necessary, and dissection and removal of surrounding soft tissues to prepare the vena cava, portal vein, hepatic artery, and common bile duct for implantation; without trisegment or lobe split**

47144   **with trisegment split of whole liver graft into 2 partial liver grafts (i.e., left lateral segment [segments II and III] and right trisegment [segments I and IV through VIII])**

47145   **with lobe split of whole liver graft into 2 partial liver grafts (i.e., left lobe [segments II, III, and IV] and right lobe [segments I and V through VIII])**

In certain cases, and almost always if the donor is living, some reconstruction of the liver will be required prior to the transplantation. If the notes indicate that a venous and/or arterial anastomosis was also performed, then you will need to use

47146   **Backbench reconstruction of cadaver or living donor liver graft prior to allotransplantation; venous anastomosis, each**

Recipient Liver Allotransplantation

The third code for the entire operation identifies the placement of the allograft in the patient (the recipient): orthotopic (normal position) or heterotopic (other than normal position).

47135   **Liver allotransplantation; orthotopic, partial or whole, from cadaver or living donor, any age**

Pancreas Transplantation

Again, the components that we have reviewed for the other organ transplants are involved with a pancreatic allotransplantation.

Cadaver Donor Pancreatectomy

A pancreas graft has to come from a deceased (a cadaver) donor.

GUIDANCE CONNECTION

Read the additional explanations in the in-section guidelines within the **Surgery** section, subhead **Digestive System,** subsection **Pancreas Transplantation,** directly above code 48550 in your CPT book.

48550	Donor pancreatectomy (including cold preservation), with or without duodenal segment for transplantation

Backbench Work

When the preparation of the pancreas graft prior to the transplant procedure is routine, you use the following code:

48551	Backbench standard preparation of cadaver donor pancreas allograft prior to transplantation, including dissection of allograft from surrounding soft tissues, splenectomy, duodenotomy, ligation of bile duct, ligation of mesenteric vessels, and Y-graft arterial anastomoses from iliac artery to superior mesenteric artery and to splenic artery

However, in certain cases, some reconstruction of the pancreas will be required prior to the transplantation. If the notes indicate that a venous and/or arterial anastomosis was performed, then you have to use

48552	Backbench reconstruction of cadaver donor pancreas allograft prior to allotransplantation; venous anastomosis, each

Recipient Pancreatic Allotransplantation

The final code for the entire operation identifies the placement of the allograft in the patient (the recipient). For this, use the following code:

48554	Transplantation of pancreatic allograft

Renal (Kidney) Transplantation

The same three components exist for renal transplantation as for the other organ transplants.

Donor Nephrectomy

A human can live without one kidney, so the donor can be either deceased (a cadaver) or living.

50300	Donor nephrectomy (including cold preservation); from cadaver donor, unilateral or bilateral

or

50320	Donor nephrectomy (including cold preservation); open, from living donor

or

50547	Laparoscopy, surgical; donor nephrectomy (including cold preservation), from living donor

Backbench Work

Performing the routine preparation of the allograft is coded differently, depending upon whether the donor is living or a cadaver.

50323	Backbench standard preparation of cadaver donor renal allograft prior to transplantation, including dissection and removal of perinephric fat, diaphragmatic and retroperitoneal attachments, excision of adrenal gland, and preparation of ureter(s), renal vein(s), and renal artery(s), ligating branches, as necessary

or

50325	Backbench standard preparation of living donor renal allograft prior to transplantation, including dissection and removal of perinephric fat,

diaphragmatic and retroperitoneal attachments, excision of adrenal gland, and preparation of ureter(s), renal vein(s), and renal artery(s), ligating branches, as necessary

In certain cases, some reconstruction of the kidney will be required prior to the transplantation. If the notes indicate that a venous, arterial, and/or ureteral anastomosis was performed, then you have to use one of the following codes:

50327   **Backbench reconstruction of cadaver or living donor renal allograft prior to allotransplantation; venous anastomosis, each**

or

50328   **Backbench reconstruction of cadaver or living donor renal allograft prior to allotransplantation; arterial anastomosis, each**

or

50329   **Backbench reconstruction of cadaver or living donor renal allograft prior to allotransplantation; ureteral anastomosis, each**

Recipient Renal Allotransplantation

The final code for the entire operation identifies the placement of the allograft in the patient (the recipient). Choose the code by whether or not a recipient nephrectomy (the removal of the organ being replaced) is performed at the same time by the same physician:

50360   **Renal allotransplantation; implantation of graft; without recipient nephrectomy**

or

50365   **Renal allotransplantation; implantation of graft; with recipient nephrectomy**

GUIDANCE CONNECTION

Read the additional explanations in the in-section guidelines located within the **Surgery** section, subhead **Urinary System,** subsection **Renal Transplantation,** directly above code 50300 in your CPT book.

YOU CODE IT! CASE STUDY

PATIENT: Ethan Norwood IV

PROCEDURE PERFORMED: Percutaneous kidney transplant biopsy.

DESCRIPTION OF PROCEDURE: After informed written consent was obtained from the patient, he was taken to the ultrasound suite and placed in the supine position on the stretcher with the left side propped up slightly with towels for optimal exposure of the transplant. The kidney transplant was localized in the left iliac fossa with ultrasound and a point overlying the lower pole was marked on the skin. The area was then prepped with Betadine and covered with a sterile fenestrated drape. Lidocaine 1% was infiltrated at the mark superficially and then to less than 1 cm, as indicated by ultrasound, to the surface of the kidney. A small incision was made at the anesthetized site with a #11 blade. A 16-gauge Monopty biopsy gun was then introduced through the incision to a depth of less than 1 cm and fired. A core tissue was obtained and placed in 10% formalin. The procedure was repeated once more, again yielding a core tissue. It was divided between formalin and Michel's solution. The procedure was then terminated. Firm pressure was applied to the biopsy site after each pass including 5 minutes after the last pass. A Band-Aid was then placed over the incision. A final ultrasound scan showed no obvious evidence of hematoma. A pressure dressing was applied. The patient tolerated the procedure well. There were no apparent complications. He has been returned to the floor in satisfactory condition and orders have been written for frequent vital signs, hematocrit, exam parameters.

Ava Ferrer, MD

(continued)

Read the details about the biopsy that Dr. Ferrer performed and determine the most accurate way to report it.

Step #1: Read the case carefully and completely.

Step #2: Abstract the scenario. Which key words or terms describe what service the physician provided to the patient during this encounter?

Step #3: Are there any details missing or incomplete for which you would need to query the physician? [If so, ask your instructor.]

Step #4: Determine the correct CPT procedure code or codes to explain the details about what was provided to the patient during this encounter.

Step #5: Check for any relevant guidance, including reading all of the symbols and notations.

Step #6: Do you need to append any modifiers to ensure complete and accurate information is provided?

Step #7: Double-check your work.

Answer:

Did you determine these to be the codes?

50200	**Renal biopsy; percutaneous, by trocar or needle**
76942	**Ultrasonic guidance for needle placement (e.g., biopsy, aspiration, injection, localization device), imaging supervision and interpretation**

Did you find the radiology code for the ultrasound, too? You will learn more about coding for radiology services in our next chapter of this textbook. However, to get to this code, all you had to do is read the guideline notation beneath code 50200.

(For radiological supervision and interpretation, see 76942, 77002, 77012, 77021)

This notation not only told you how to report the ultrasound service for this biopsy; it also informed you that it was not already included in the 50200 code.

25.15 Operating Microscope

When a surgeon performs microsurgery, he or she has to use an operating microscope. In such cases, you must code the use of the microscope (69990) in addition to the procedure in which the microscope is used.

+69990 **Microsurgical techniques, requiring use of operating microscope (List separately in addition to code for primary procedure.)**

There are two guidelines with regard to this add-on code:

1. Do not append modifier 51 Multiple Procedures to the code for the microscope. It is not an additional procedure. Code 69990 indicates the use of a special technique or tool, making modifier 51 incorrect.

2. There are some codes that already include the use of the operating microscope. Therefore, adding code 69990 is redundant. The tough part here is that none of the codes that already include use of the operating microscope include this information in their description. Following, and in many CPT books above the code description, is the list of codes to which you are *not* permitted to add code 69990 because it is already included:

15756–15758	31531	49906
15842	31536	61548
19364	31541	63075–63078
19368	31545	64727
20955–20962	31546	64820–64823
20969–20973	31571	64912–64913
22551–22552	43116	65091–68850
22856–22861	43180	0184T
26551–26554	43496	0308T
26556	46601	0402T
31526	46607	0583T

> **GUIDANCE CONNECTION**
>
> Read the additional explanations in the in-section guidelines within the **Surgery** section, subhead **Operating Microscope,** directly above code 69990 in your CPT book.

EXAMPLE

19364   Breast reconstruction with free flap

(Do not report code 69990 in addition to code 19364.)

As you can see, the codes involved are throughout the *Surgery* section of the CPT. You might want to go through and mark or highlight the codes, should you be coding for a physician who works with an operating microscope.

 ## LET'S CODE IT! SCENARIO

PATIENT: Olivia Prima

DATE OF PROCEDURE: 07/22/2019

PREOPERATIVE DIAGNOSIS: Right vocal cord lesion

POSTOPERATIVE DIAGNOSIS: Respiratory papilloma

PROCEDURE: Microscopic laryngoscopy with biopsy and papilloma shave

SURGEON: Serita Frapenstein, MD

ASSISTANT: Morris Bershic, MD

ANESTHESIA: General endotracheal

COMPLICATIONS: None

SPECIMENS REMOVED: Biopsy samples sent from the anterior commissure of the vocal cord

INDICATION FOR PROCEDURE: The patient is a 37-year-old female with a 6-month history of isolated hoarseness with a vocal cord lesion on direct laryngoscopy, who presents for biopsy of the vocal cord lesion.

DESCRIPTION OF PROCEDURE: The patient was brought to the operating room, and an appropriate plane of anesthesia was obtained via endotracheal intubation.

The head of the bed was turned 90 degrees. The Dedo laryngoscope was used to visualize the base of tongue, the bilateral vallecula, both surfaces of the epiglottis, the aryepiglottic folds, the bilateral pyriform sinuses, and hypopharynx. All of these areas were clear of any lesions or mucosal abnormalities. The true vocal cords were noted to have papillomatous lesions on the right inferior aspect of the cord and the anterior commissure. The false cords and ventricles were clear.

The patient's larynx was suspended via the laryngoscope. Biopsy samples were taken for frozen and permanent specimens from the anterior commissure lesion. This came back to confirm papilloma. Next, the operating microscope was brought into the field to obtain a detailed visualization of the vocal cord lesion. A straight shaver was then utilized to remove the papillomatous tissue on the right vocal cord. Care was taken to preserve the mucosa on that side and not injure the vocal cord. This was done unilaterally again on the right. Appropriate hemostasis was obtained.

The patient tolerated the procedure well. The operating microscope was removed from the field. The patient was extubated and taken to recovery in stable condition with no immediate complications.

(continued)

As you read in the operative reports, Dr. Frapenstein performed a *laryngoscopy* using an operating microscope. First, you must determine the code for the laryngoscopy. Find this in the CPT Alphabetic Index.

Laryngoscopy

with Operating Microscope or Telescope 31526, 31531, 31536, 31541, 31545, 31546, 31561, 31571

Turn to the main section and find the codes suggested. Remember, you are obligated to read ALL of these code descriptions to determine which one is most accurate.

31526	Laryngoscopy direct, with or without tracheoscopy; diagnostic, with operating microscope or telescope
31531	Laryngoscopy direct, operative, with foreign body removal; with operating microscope or telescope
31536	Laryngoscopy direct, operative, with biopsy; with operating microscope or telescope
31541	Laryngoscopy direct, operative, with excision of tumor and/or stripping of vocal cords or epiglottis; with operating microscope or telescope
31545	Laryngoscopy direct, operative, with operating microscope or telescope, with submucosal removal of non-neoplastic lesion(s) of vocal cord; reconstruction with local tissue flap(s)
31546	Laryngoscopy direct, operative, with operating microscope or telescope, with submucosal removal of non-neoplastic lesion(s) of vocal cord; reconstruction with graft(s) (includes obtaining autograft)
31561	Laryngoscopy direct, operative, with arytenoidectomy; with operating microscope or telescope
31571	Laryngoscopy direct, operative, with injection into vocal cord(s), therapeutic; with operating microscope or telescope

Now that you know, specifically, what these codes report, go back to the operative notes and abstract the details, beyond laryngoscopy + operating microscope.

The documentation reads, *"Biopsy samples were taken."* . . . This leads you to code 31536. However, the documentation also states,

"A straight shaver was then utilized to remove the papillomatous tissue on the right vocal cord."

[*NOTE:* Use your medical dictionary if you don't already know that papillomatous tissue is benign.]

. . . This might lead to code 31545 or 31546, except there is documentation that *"Care was taken to preserve the mucosa,"* so you know that submucosal tissue was not removed. And there is no mention of a reconstruction being performed.

So, you can confidently report code 31536. One more thing to check . . . do you need to report a second code for the use of the operating microscope? Turn to code 69990 and read the guideline carefully. Code 31536 is included in the "*Do not report 69990*" notation.

You also know that code 31536 includes the specific detail that an operating microscope was used, therefore meaning that this tells the whole story and reporting 69990 would just be repetitive. Now, you know the accurate way to report this procedure:

31536   Laryngoscopy direct, operative, with biopsy; with operating microscope or telescope

Good job!

Chapter Summary

When coding surgical procedures, you have the challenge of determining which services are included in the procedure code, which services are part of the global package, and which services must be coded separately.

In addition, it is important to remember that the *Surgery* section of the CPT book not only includes codes for reporting services provided in an operating room under general anesthesia but also includes codes for reporting simple and small procedures such as removing a splinter.

When reporting surgical procedures, it is important to (1) identify the components of the operation and (2) determine which services are included in the code's description and which services require a separate code. The *Surgery* section of the CPT book is divided into subsections identified by the body system upon which the technique was performed.

CODING BITES

CPT Surgical Package

- Subsequent to the decision for surgery, one related E/M encounter on the date immediately prior to or on the date of the procedure (including history and physical).
- Local infiltration, metacarpal/metatarsal/digital block, or topical anesthesia.
- The procedure itself.
- Immediate postoperative care, including dictating operative notes and talking with the family and other physicians/health care professionals.
- Writing orders.
- Evaluation of the patient in the postanesthesia recovery area.
- Typical postoperative follow-up care.

You Interpret It! Answers

1. Diagnostic, **2.** Therapeutic, **3.** Therapeutic, **4.** Prophylactic, **5.** Open, **6.** Percutaneous, **7.** Endoscopic, **8.** Included, **9.** Not included; report separately, **10.** Not included; report separately, **11.** 90 days, **12.** Zero days, **13.** 90 days, **14.** Zero days, **15.** Zero days

CHAPTER 25 REVIEW
CPT Surgery Section

Enhance your learning by completing these exercises and more at mcgrawhillconnect.com!

Let's Check It! Terminology

Match each key term to the appropriate definition.

Part I

1. **LO 25.2** The length of time allotted for postoperative care included in the surgical package, which is generally accepted to be 90 days for major surgical procedures and up to 10 days for minor procedures.

2. **LO 25.5** The process of taking skin or tissue (on the same body or another).

3. **LO 25.5** The area or part of the body from which skin or tissue is removed with the intention of placing that skin or tissue in another area or body.

4. **LO 25.1** The methodology or technique used by the physician to perform the procedure, service, or treatment.

5. **LO 25.2** The accepted principles of conduct, services, or treatments that are established as the expected behavior.

6. **LO 25.5** A method of sealing an opening in the skin involving a multilayered closure and a reconstructive procedure such as scar revision, debridement, or retention sutures.

7. **LO 25.5** The full-thickness removal of a lesion, including margins; includes (for coding purposes) a simple closure.

A. Complex Closure

B. Donor Area

C. Excision

D. Full-Thickness

E. Global Period

F. Harvesting

G. Intermediate Closure

8. LO 25.5 The area, or site, of the body receiving a graft of skin or tissue.

9. LO 25.5 A multilevel method of sealing an opening in the skin involving one or more of the deeper layers of the skin.

10. LO 25.5 A method of sealing an opening in the skin (epidermis or dermis), involving only one layer. It includes the administration of a local anesthesia and/or chemical or electrocauterization of a wound not closed.

11. LO 25.5 A measure that extends from the epidermis to the connective tissue layer of the skin.

H. Recipient Area

I. Simple Closure

J. Standard of Care

K. Surgical Approach

Part II

1. LO 25.6 Surgically opening the fracture site, or another site in the body nearby, in order to treat the fractured bone.

2. LO 25.6 The treatment of a fracture without surgically opening the affected area.

3. LO 25.6 The insertion of fixation instruments (such as pins) placed across the fracture site. It may be done under x-ray imaging for guidance purposes.

4. LO 25.6 The surgical removal of a vertebral posterior arch.

5. LO 25.8 Either of the two major veins in the leg that run from the foot to the thigh near the surface of the skin.

6. LO 25.14 The relocation of tissue from one individual to another (both of the same species) without an identical genetic match.

7. LO 25.14 The transfer of tissue from one site to another.

8. LO 25.6 The immobilization of a joint using a surgical technique.

9. LO 25.6 The attempted return of the fracture or dislocation to its normal alignment manually by the physician.

10. LO 25.13 The area between the eyelid and the eyeball.

A. Allotransplantation

B. Arthrodesis

C. Closed Treatment

D. Fornix

E. Laminectomy

F. Manipulation

G. Open Treatment

H. Percutaneous Skeletal Fixation

I. Saphenous Vein

J. Transplantation

Let's Check It! Concepts

Choose the most appropriate answer for each of the following questions.

Part I

1. LO 25.2 The global surgical package includes all *except*

   a. preprocedure evaluation and management.

   b. general anesthesia.

   c. the procedure.

   d. follow-up care.

2. LO 25.3 The global period is determined by

   a. the type of anesthesia provided.

   b. the size of the excision.

   c. the location of the donor site.

   d. the standard of care.

3. LO 25.1 Which of the following is an example of a diagnostic test not included in the global package?

   a. Closure

   b. Local infiltration

   c. Biopsy

   d. Metacarpal block

4. LO 25.2 When a procedure is planned as a series of procedures, each service after the first should be appended with the modifier

   a. 76   b. 79   c. 58   d. 59

5. LO 25.4 When a surgeon does not provide preoperative or postoperative care to the patient upon whom he or she operates, the procedure code should be appended with modifier

    a. 54   **b.** 55   **c.** 56   **d.** 77

6. LO 25.5 Excision of lesions is reported

    a. with total measurement of all lesions removed in one code.

    b. with only the largest lesion coded.

    c. with each lesion coded separately.

    d. as a part of the total surgical procedure.

7. LO 25.5 The code for excision of a lesion includes this type of repair.

    a. Intermediate   **b.** Complex

    c. None   **d.** Simple

8. LO 25.5 If the surgeon performs a reexcision of a lesion during a later encounter with the patient, append the procedure code with modifier

    a. 58   **b.** 59   **c.** 51   **d.** 77

9. LO 25.5 If multiple wounds located on the same anatomical site are repaired with the same complexity, report this procedure by

    a. coding each wound separately.

    b. coding only the largest wound.

    c. adding all the lengths together and coding the total.

    d. coding the average of all the wounds repaired.

10. LO 25.5 The elements of determining the most accurate code for a skin graft include all *except*

    a. the size of the recipient area.

    b. the type of donor.

    c. the location of the recipient area.

    d. the type of graft.

Part II

1. LO 25.6 Codes within the musculoskeletal subsection include

    a. x-rays.   **b.** casts.

    c. medications.   **d.** shoes.

2. LO 25.13 Which of the following is/are part of the inner ear?

    a. Auditory ossicles   **b.** Oval window

    c. Eustachian tube   **d.** Semicircular canals

3. LO 25.7 Thoracotomy, with biopsy of pleura, would be coded

    a. 32096   **b.** 32097   **c.** 32098   **d.** 32400

4. LO 25.14 Backbench work during a transplant process is

    a. the harvesting of an organ from a donor.

    b. the implantation of the new organ.

    c. the documentation of the surgery.

    d. the preparation of the organ.

5. LO 25.8 When an arterial graft is performed, which of the following codes, in addition to the code for the bypass procedure, would be assigned if the graft is harvested from the femoropopliteal vein?

    a. 35600   **b.** 35500   **c.** 35572   **d.** 35601

6. LO 25.11 Vulvectomy, radical, partial; with unilateral inguinofemoral lymphadenectomy would be coded

    a. 56620   **b.** 56630   **c.** 56631   **d.** 56632

7. LO 25.8 The code for an endovascular repair of an iliac aneurysm includes all *except*

    a. introduction of graft.

    b. stent deployment.

    c. balloon angioplasty.

    d. pacemaker.

8. LO 25.9 A laparoscopy, surgical, gastric restrictive procedure; with gastric bypass and Roux-en-Y gastroenterostomy of 145 cm would be coded

    a. 43846   **b.** 43847   **c.** 43644   **d.** 43645

9. LO 25.12 Code 62263 includes all of the following *except*

    a. percutaneous insertion of an epidural catheter.

    b. extensive dural grafting.

    c. procedure injections.

    d. multiple adhesiolysis sessions over the course of 2 or more days.

10. LO 25.10 A physician who only interprets the results of a urodynamic procedure must append the code with

    a. modifier 32   **b.** modifier 26

    c. modifier 53   **d.** modifier 51

Let's Check It! Guidelines

Refer to the Surgery Guidelines and fill in the blanks accordingly.

concomitant	supervision	session	independently	Follow-up
component	Introduction	technique	therapeutic	integral
usually	guidelines	"separate procedure"	management	guidance
59	date	modifiers	itself	diagnostic
addition	one	Radiology	Evaluation and Management	surgical
designated	only	destruction	separately	post-operative

1. Guidelines to direct general reporting for services are presented in the _____.

2. Services rendered in the office, home, or hospital, consultations, and other medical services are listed in the _____ Services section.

3. _____ care for diagnostic procedures includes _____ that care related to recovery from the diagnostic procedure itself.

4. Care of the condition for which the _____ procedure was performed or of other _____ conditions is not included and may be listed _____.

5. Follow-up care for _____ surgical procedure includes only that care which is _____ a part of the _____ service.

6. When more than _____ procedure/service is performed on the same _____, same _____ or during a _____ period, several CPT _____ may apply.

7. The codes designated as _____ should not be reported in _____ to the code for the total procedure or service of which it is considered an _____ component.

8. However, when a procedure or service that is _____ as a "separate procedure" is carried out _____ or considered to be unrelated or distinct from other procedures/services provided at that time, it may be reported by _____, or in addition to other procedures/services by appending modifier _____ to the specific "separate procedure" code to indicate that the procedure is not considered to be a _____ of another procedure, but is a distinct, independent procedure.

9. When imaging _____ or imaging _____ and interpretation is included in a surgical procedure, _____ for image documentation and report, included in the guidelines for _____, will apply.

10. Surgical _____ is a part of a surgical procedure and different methods of destruction are not ordinarily listed separately unless the _____ substantially alters the standard _____ of a problem or condition.

Let's Check It! Rules and Regulations

Please answer the following questions from the knowledge you have gained after reading this chapter.

1. LO 25.1   Explain the difference between prophylactic, diagnostic, and therapeutic treatments.
2. LO 25.4   What does the notation "Separate Procedure" tell a professional coder?
3. LO 25.5   What is the formula to find the correct coded size of an excised lesion?
4. LO 25.5   Differentiate between intermediate closure repair and complex closure repair.
5. LO 25.15   When a surgeon performs microsurgery, he or she has to use an operating microscope. What code identifies the use of the microscope?

YOU CODE IT! Basics

First, identify the procedural main term in the following statements; then code the procedure or service.

Example: Dr. Slaughter drains an ovarian cyst, vaginal approach:

a. main term: *Drainage*   b. procedure: *58800*

1. Dr. Ladd performs a fine-needle aspiration using ultrasound-guidance imaging; first lesion:

   a. main term: _____   b. procedure: _____

2. Dr. Dingle performs paring of six soft corn lesions:

   a. main term: _____   b. procedure: _____

3. Dr. Gunter removes 10 skin tags:

   a. main term: _____   b. procedure: _____

4. Dr. Strobel performs an insertion of a nonbiodegradable drug delivery contraception implant:

   a. main term: _____   b. procedure: _____

5. Dr. Amerson performs cryotherapy for acne:

   a. main term: _____   b. procedure: _____

6. Mark Latham was accidentally shot in the arm; Dr. Quattlebaum explores and enlarges the wound to remove the bullet. Code the exploration of the wound:

   a. main term: _____   b. procedure: _____

7. Dr. Hunter applies a uniplane external fixation device for temporary stabilization of a radial fracture:

   a. main term: _____   b. procedure: _____

8. Dr. Preston performs an arthroscopic repair of a rotator cuff tear:

   a. main term: _____   b. procedure: _____

9. Roy has an implanted single-chamber pacemaker; Dr. Terrence removes the existing pulse generator, tests the existing lead, and inserts a new dual-chamber system for an upgrade:

   a. main term: _____   b. procedure: _____

10. Dr. Shumpert performs a infratentorial craniotomy to remove a hematoma; intracerebellar:

    a. main term: _____   b. procedure: _____

11. Dr. Wattel performs an epidermal facial chemical peel:

    a. main term: _____   b. procedure: _____

12. Dr. Rudner performs a breast reconstruction with free flap:

    a. main term: _____   b. procedure: _____

13. Dr. Payton excises a malignant lesion from the neck that measured 2.9 cm with margins:

    a. main term: _____   b. procedure: _____

14. Dr. Charne excises an ischial pressure ulcer with a primary suture:

    a. main term: _____   b. procedure: _____

15. Dorothy Loman had a small partial-thickness burn on her hand. Dr. Beariman performed a debridement and dressing of the injury:

    a. main term: _____   b. procedure: _____

YOU CODE IT! Practice

Using the techniques described in this chapter, carefully read through the case studies and determine the most accurate surgery CPT code(s) and modifier(s), if appropriate, for each case study.

1. Jack Friedman, a 41-year-old male, was in a fight at a soccer game and was hit in the head with a bottle, which caused some deep lacerations in his scalp. Dr. Girald performed a layered closure of the wounds: one 2.0 cm, one 4.5 cm, and two lacerations that were 1.0 cm each in length.

2. Bobby Sherman, a 36-year-old male, cut his left thumb at work on a construction site 2 weeks ago. He did not get any treatment for the wound, which became infected. Today, Dr. Ravenell admitted Bobby to Westward Hospital and amputated the thumb. The procedure is made more complicated by the spread of the infection to the surrounding tissues, as Dr. Ravenell fights to save as much of the hand as possible.

3. Patricia Atkins, a 31-year-old female, has been diagnosed with pleural effusion. Patricia is having difficulty breathing and is admitted to the hospital, where Dr. Jamison performs a percutaneous pleural drainage and inserts an indwelling catheter. Dr. Jamison is aided by image guidance. Patricia tolerates the procedure well and is breathing easier.

4. Kevin Benchley, a 52-year-old male, has been diagnosed with benign prostatic hyperplasia (BPH). Kevin and Dr. Derek, his urologist, have discussed the options, and Kevin has elected to proceed with a TURP. Kevin is taken to the OR, where he is placed under general anesthesia and the transurethral electrosurgical resection of prostate, complete, is performed without complication. Code the TURP procedure.

5. Dr. Albertson performed a lumbar laminectomy, 2 vertebral segments, for decompression on Grace James on September 15. One month later, as originally planned, Dr. Albertson brought Grace back into the OR to implant an epidural drug infuser with a subcutaneous reservoir. Code both procedures.

6. Bridgette Smith found a sore on her neck. The lab test identified it as a malignant lesion, and Dr. Payas excised the lesion, which measured 2.9 cm with margins.

7. Alice Milton, a 39-year-old female, was diagnosed with an abdominal wall incisional hernia, which was repaired using prosthetic mesh. Alice has had recurrent infections. Alice is taken to the OR, where Dr. Gilroy debrides the infected subcutaneous tissue and removes the prosthetic mesh.

8. Samantha DaVita, a 74-year-old female, has a permanent subcutaneous implanted defibrillator system, which is not functioning properly. Samantha is taken to the OR, where Dr. Meetze removes and replaces the implanted defibrillator pulse generator and subcutaneous electrode; 25 minutes of moderate sedation was achieved. The new defibrillator system is tested and is working within normal limits. The nurse monitored Samantha's vital signs during the procedure. Samantha tolerated the procedure well.

9. Having trouble hearing, Ruth Ann Marcelle, a 73-year-old female, came to see Dr. Assiss, an otolaryngologist. After examination, Dr. Assiss uses a curette to remove the impacted earwax from both ears. Ruth Ann was amazed at the improvement in her hearing and left the office feeling much better.

10. One week ago, Dr. Alden performed a ureteroneocystostomy with cystoscopy and ureteral stent placement laparoscopically on Brad Vitalli. Brad is admitted to the hospital today because Dr. Alden must perform an open procedure to drain a renal abscess that was discovered. Dr. Alden drained the abscess. Brad tolerated the procedure well. Code the drainage of Brad's renal abscess.

11. Frank Chestnut, a 17-year-old male, came to see Dr. Quartermain for the first time. He was in a fight at school and got punched in the jaw, dislocating his temporomandibular joint. Dr. Quartermain performed a closed treatment of the temporomandibular dislocation. The dislocation did not require any wiring or fixation.

12. Dr. Quinn ordered a catheter aspiration with fiberscope of Stephan's tracheobronchial tree. The procedure was performed at Stephan's bedside in his hospital room. The patient received 15 minutes of conscious sedation. Stephan is a 34-year-old male.

13. Colleen Sizmauski, a morbidly obese 27-year-old female, was admitted for a gastric restrictive procedure. In addition to the gastric bypass performed by Dr. Lafferty, Colleen's small intestine was reconstructed to limit absorption.

14. Dr. Macintosh performed the backbench preparation of a cadaver donor heart allograft prior to Dr. Gantt's performing the transplantation. Code for Dr. Mackintosh's work.

15. Hannah Lopez, a 53-year-old female, hurt her eye in an accident. Dr. Dawson examined her and noticed that her cornea was scratched. It was not a perforating laceration. Dr. Dawson repaired the laceration of the cornea in the office.

  YOU CODE IT! Application

The following exercises provide practice in the application of abstracting the physicians' notes and learning to work with documentation from our health care facility, Prader, Bracker, & Associates. These case studies are modeled on real patient encounters. Using the techniques described in this chapter, carefully read through the case studies and determine the most accurate surgery CPT code(s) and modifier(s), if appropriate, for each case study.

PRADER, BRACKER, & ASSOCIATES

A Complete Health Care Facility

159 Healthcare Way • SOMEWHERE, FL 32811 • 407-555-6789

PATIENT: PENNETTA, OSCAR

ACCOUNT/EHR #: PENNOS001

Admission Date: 10/09/19

Discharge Date: 10/09/19

DATE: 10/09/19

Preoperative DX: Lacerations of arm, hand, and leg

Postoperative DX: Same

Procedure: Layered closure of leg laceration; simple closure of arm and hand lacerations

Surgeon: Gregg Wilson, MD

Assistant: None

Anesthesia: General

INDICATIONS: The patient is a 4-year-old male brought to the emergency room by his mother. He was helping his father install a new window when the window fell and shattered. Oscar suffered lacerations on his left hand, left arm, and left leg.

PROCEDURE: The patient was placed on the table in supine position. Satisfactory anesthesia was obtained. The area was prepped, and attention to the deeper laceration of the left thigh, right above the patella, was first. A layered closure was performed, and the 5.1-cm laceration was closed successfully with sutures. The lacerations on the upper extremity, a 2-cm laceration on the left hand at the base of the fifth metacarpal and the 3-cm laceration on the left arm, just below the joint capsule in the posterior position, were successfully closed with 4-0 Vicryl, as well. The patient tolerated the procedures well and was transported to the recovery room.

GW/mg   D: 10/09/19 09:50:16   T: 10/09/19 12:55:01

(continued)

Determine the most accurate surgery CPT code(s) and modifier(s), if appropriate.

WESTON HOSPITAL

629 Healthcare Way • SOMEWHERE, FL 32811 • 407-555-6541

PATIENT: DRESDEN, NELDA

ACCOUNT/EHR #: DRESNE001

Admission Date: 11/01/19

Discharge Date: 11/01/19

DATE: 11/01/19

Preoperative DX: Toxic epidermal necrolysis

Postoperative DX: Same

Procedure: Xenogaft

Surgeon: William Dresser, MD

Assistant: None

Anesthesia: Local

INDICATIONS: The patient is a 29-year-old female with a diagnosis of toxic epidermal necrolysis as a result of a reaction to procainamide, previously prescribed by a physician no longer in attendance.

PROCEDURE: The patient was placed on the table in supine position. Local anesthesia was administered. As soon as patient stated a complete loss of feeling in the left forearm, the dermal xenograft proceeded. Procedure was repeated for right forearm.

A total of 150 sq. cm of grafting was successfully completed.

Bandages were applied. A prescription for Darvocet N100 po q4–6h prn was given to the patient before discharge.

Follow-up appointment in office scheduled for 10 days.

WD/mg   D: 11/01/19 09:50:16   T: 11/01/19 12:55:01

Determine the most accurate surgery CPT code(s) and modifier(s), if appropriate.

WESTON HOSPITAL

629 Healthcare Way • SOMEWHERE, FL 32811 • 407-555-6541

PATIENT: APPON, CYNTHIA

ACCOUNT/EHR #: APPOCY001

DATE: 09/23/19

Attending Physician: Regina Glasser, MD

Preoperative DX: C5 compression fracture

Postoperative DX: Same

Procedure: C5 corpectomy and fusion fixation with fibular strut graft and Atlantis plate

---

(continued)

Anesthesia: General endotracheal

This is a 31-year-old female status post assault. The patient sustained a C5 compression fracture. MRI scan showed compression with evidence of posterior ligamentous injury. The patient was subsequently set up for the surgical procedure. The procedure was described in detail, including the risks. The risks included but were not limited to bleeding, infection, stroke, paralysis, death, CSF leak, loss of bladder and bowel control, hoarse voice, paralyzed vocal cord, death, and damage to adjacent nerves and tissues. The patient understood the risks. The patient also understood that bank bone instrumentation would be used and that the bank bone could collapse and the instrumentation could fail or break, or the screws could pull out. The patient provided consent.

The patient was taken to the OR. The patient was induced. An endotracheal tube was placed. A Foley was placed. The patient was given preoperative antibiotics. The patient was placed in slight extension. The right neck was prepped and draped in the usual manner. A linear incision was made over the C5 vertebral body. The platysma was divided. Dissection was continued medial to the sternocleidomastoid to the prevertebral fascia. This was cauterized and divided. The longus colli was cauterized and elevated. The fracture was visualized. A spinal needle was used to verify the location using fluoroscopy. The C5 vertebral body was drilled out. The bone was saved. The disks above and below were removed. The posterior longitudinal ligament was removed. The bone was quite collapsed and fragmented. Distraction pins were then packed with bone removed from the C5 vertebral body prior to implantation. A plate was then placed with screws in the C4 and C6 vertebral bodies. The locking screws were tightened. The wound was irrigated. Bleeding was helped with the bipolar. The retractors were removed. The incision was approximated with simple interrupted Vicryl. The subcutaneous tissue was approximated, and skin edges were approximated subcuticularly. Steri-Strips were applied. A dressing was applied. The patient was placed back in an Aspen collar. The patient was extubated and transferred to recovery.

RG/mgr   D: 09/23/19 12:33:08 PM   T: 09/25/19 3:22:54 PM

Determine the accurate surgery CPT code(s) and modifier(s), if appropriate.

WESTON HOSPITAL

629 Healthcare Way • SOMEWHERE, FL 32811 • 407-555-6541

PATIENT: WHEATON, MARLA

ACCOUNT/EHR #: WHEAMA001

Admission Date: 09/18/19

Discharge Date: 09/18/19

DATE: 09/18/19

Preoperative DX: High-grade squamous intraepithelial lesion of the cervix

Postoperative DX: Same

Operation: Loop electrosurgical excision procedure (LEEP) and endocervical curettage (ECC)

Surgeon: Ralph L. Goff, MD

Assistant: None

Anesthesia: General by LMA

Findings: Large ectropion, large nonstaining active cervix essentially encompassing the entire active cervix

(continued)

Specimens: To pathology

Disposition: Stable to recovery room

PROCEDURE: The patient was taken to the OR, where she was placed in the supine position and administered general anesthesia. She was then placed in candy cane stirrups and prepped and draped in the usual fashion. Her vaginal vault was not prepped. The coated speculum was then placed and the cervix exposed. It was then painted with Lugol and the entire active cervix was nonstaining with the clearly defined margins where the stain began to be picked up. The cervix was injected with approximately 7 cc of lidocaine with 1% epinephrine. Using a large loop, the anterior cervix was excised, and then the posterior loop was excised in separate specimens. Because of the size of the lesion, one piece in total was not accomplished. Prior to the excision, the endocervical curettage was performed, and specimens were collected. All specimens were sent to pathology. The remaining cervical bed was cauterized and then painted with Monsel for hemostasis. The case was concluded with this. Instruments were removed. The patient was taken down from candy cane stirrups, awakened from the anesthesia, and taken to the recovery room in stable condition.

RLG/mgr   D: 09/23/19 12:33:08 PM   T: 09/25/19 3:22:54 PM

Determine the accurate surgery CPT code(s) and modifier(s), if appropriate.

WESTON HOSPITAL

629 Healthcare Way • SOMEWHERE, FL 32811 • 407-555-6541

PATIENT: UPTON, MAXINE

ACCOUNT/EHR #: UPTOMA001

DATE: 09/25/19

Diagnosis: Medulloblastoma

Procedure: Central Venous Access Device (CVAD) insertion

Physician: Vincent Hoyt, MD

Anesthesia: Conscious sedation

PROCEDURE: Patient is a 4-year-old female, with a recent diagnosis of malignancy. Due to an upcoming course of chemotherapy, the CVAD is being inserted to ease administration of the drugs. The patient was placed on the table in supine position and 1 mg of Versed was administered IM; moderate sedation was achieved, 13 minutes. Maxine's vital signs were monitored by the nurse. The incision was made to insert a central venous catheter, centrally. During the placement of the catheter, a short tract (nontunneled) was made as the catheter was advanced from the skin entry site to the point of venous cannulation. The catheter tip was set to reside in the subclavian vein. The patient was gently aroused from the sedation and was awake when transported to the recovery room.

VH/mg   D: 09/25/19 09:50:16   T: 09/25/19 12:55:01

Determine the accurate surgery CPT code(s) and modifier(s), if appropriate.

CPT Radiology Section

Learning Outcomes

After completing this chapter, the student should be able to:

LO 26.1   Distinguish the different types of imaging.

LO 26.2   Abstract the different reasons for imaging services.

LO 26.3   Identify the technical components from professional components.

LO 26.4   Apply the guidelines accurately regarding the number of views.

LO 26.5   Apply the guidelines to determine how to code the administration of contrast materials.

LO 26.6   Recognize diagnostic radiologic services.

LO 26.7   Interpret accurately into CPT codes to report mammography services.

LO 26.8   Discern how to report bone and joint studies.

LO 26.9   Decide when to code radiation treatments.

LO 26.10 Determine how to accurately report nuclear medicine services.

Key Terms

Angiography
Arthrography
Computed Tomography (CT)
Computed Tomography Angiography (CTA)
Fluoroscope
Magnetic Resonance Arthrography (MRA)
Magnetic Resonance Imaging (MRI)
Nuclear Medicine
Radiation
Sonogram
Venography

 STOP!   Remember, you need to follow along in your CPT code book for an optimal learning experience.

26.1 Types of Imaging

Health care professionals use medical imaging technologies to see inside the body to support medical decision making and accurate diagnostics. Radiologic services, also known as *interventional radiology,* can be used to investigate a potential condition (diagnostically), measure the progress of a disease or condition, or aid in the actual reduction or prevention of disease or other condition (therapeutically).

Many, many years ago, radiology was simply known as x-ray because this was the extent of the equipment. Now, technology has made tremendous advancements in the science of imaging, and health care professionals can screen, diagnose, monitor, and treat patients much more effectively and efficiently.

X-Rays (Radiography)

Radiography is the term that describes the use of x-rays to visualize the visceral aspects (internal structures) of the human body. An x-ray tube emits a type of electromagnetic radiation that is passed through and recorded on the opposite side of the anatomical site being investigated by a digital detector (the digital version of film). Radiologists can identify bone, muscle, and soft tissue on the image because each absorbs the radiation at differing levels. The resulting contrast records a two-dimensional image for evaluation and analysis.

Clinical Applications

- Chest x-rays are most commonly used to analyze aspects of the lungs.
- Skeletal x-rays are frequently used to identify and diagnose fractures, dislocations, and other abnormalities of the bones.
- Abdominal x-rays are used to determine obstructions in any organs within the cavity, or to illuminate the presence of air or fluid.
- Dental x-rays are employed to detect abnormalities such as dental caries or abscesses.

Computed Tomography (CT) Scans

A computed tomography (CT) scanner is similar to radiography in that it is constructed of an x-ray tube and detectors. During a CT scan, an x-ray beam is emitted, aimed through the anatomical site being studied, and recorded by the detectors, which reconstruct the emissions in order to create a two- or three-dimensional image that results in a cross-sectional slice through the patient at that point. Each consecutive image is acquired at a slightly different angle, providing a more complete picture of the internal aspects.

Contrast media may be used to enable differentiation of the various structures of similar density throughout the body. The contrast materials enable the identification of various abnormalities, including hemorrhaging and malignant tissue.

Clinical Applications

- Brain function
- Neck/head
- Vascular system

Magnetic Resonance Imaging (MRI)

Magnetic resonance imaging (MRI) provides three-dimensional views of internal body organs, in real time, with greater visibility of variations within soft tissues, making visualization of brain, spine, muscles, joints, and other structures more informative. The images are captured utilizing a multiplanar modality (various body planes without changing the position of the patient). Similarly to CT scans, contrast materials may be used to illuminate specific visceral aspects.

Clinical Applications

- Measuring volumes of brain structures.
- Measurement of brain tissue.
- Soft tissue damage.

Positron Emission Tomography (PET)

Unlike CT or MRI, PET studies metabolic activity and/or body function. A radioactive medication is administered via IV enabling the areas of abnormal metabolism as well as the detection of tumors and other dysfunctions, not typically detectable by other means, to be captured.

Clinical Applications

- Detection and staging of cancer.
- Diagnosis of certain dementias such as Alzheimer's disease.
- Evaluation of coronary artery disease.

Nuclear Medicine

Nuclear medicine employs the administration of radioactive tracers to enable images of internal organs. The radioactive tracer produces gamma radiation, enabling a gamma camera to capture two-dimensional or three-dimensional images.

Nuclear medicine might also be used for therapeutic purposes. For instance, a larger dose of therapeutic radiation (a radiopharmaceutical specific to the particular diagnosis) may be used to eradicate malignant cells.

Clinical Applications

- Assessing the metabolic activity of a skeletal structure.
- Comparing blood flow to the myocardium at exercise and rest.
- Determining renal perfusion and drainage.
- Comparing pulmonary ventilation and perfusion.
- Assessing the thyroid gland's appearance and function.

Fluoroscopy

Fluoroscopy also utilizes x-rays to visualize internal organ structure and function. The emission of the x-ray beams is continuous, producing a real-time, dynamic image. High-density contrast agents, such as barium, might be administered to enable comparative data.

Clinical Applications

- Hysterosalphingography (HSG).
- Retrograde urethrogram.
- Micturating cysto-urethrogram.
- Fistulography.
- Guidance for procedures, such as the reduction of a fracture.

Ultrasound (Sonography)

Ultrasound, also known as sonography, uses high-frequency sound waves to capture cross-sectional images of visceral organs, including the arteries, veins, and lymph nodes. There are several different types of ultrasound:

- *A-mode* indicates a one-dimensional ultrasonic measurement procedure.
- *M-mode* is also a one-dimensional ultrasonic measurement procedure; however, it includes the movement of the trace so that there can be a recording of both amplitude and velocity of the moving echo-producing structures.
- *B-scan* indicates a two-dimensional ultrasonic scanning procedure with a two-dimensional display.
- *Real-time scan* indicates that a two-dimensional ultrasonic scanning procedure with a display was performed, and included both the two-dimensional structure and motion with time.

Ultrasound also may be used as a visual guide for percutaneous surgical procedures.

Clinical Applications

- Abdominal cavity.
- Pelvic area [*NOTE:* Codes are different for an obstetrical ultrasound vs. nonpregnant pelvic area].
- Cardiovascular structures, i.e., echocardiography.

Angiography

During an angiography, x-rays are used to identify obstruction or stenosis of an artery or vein, as well as other problems with the cardiovascular system. Contrast dyes may be administered to illuminate a specific vessel to enable visualization of blood flow and blockages.

Clinical Applications

- Tracking blood flow through arteries.
- Identifying blood vessel malformations (thrombi, aneurysms).
- Discovering arteriosclerosis.

 LET'S CODE IT! SCENARIO

PATIENT: Bonnie Suzett-Ellenton

DATE OF STUDY: 06/08/2019

REFERRING PHYSICIAN: Lawrence Chorino, MD

RE: MRI OF THE LUMBAR SPINE

Comparison is made to an earlier exam.

TECHNIQUE: Multiplanar images were obtained using multiple pulse sequences to the lumbar spine. Because of the postoperative nature of the lumbar spine, additional axial and sagittal postgadolinium T1-weighted images were obtained.

Plain films are not available for comparison; therefore, it will be assumed there is a normal complement of lumbar vertebrae. Scanning was performed on 0.3-Tesla open bore scanner.

FINDINGS: The examination shows lumbar vertebrae to be in normal overall alignment with preservation in vertebral body heights and normal signal within the marrow. For descriptive purposes of this study, a fairly small disc is noted at the S1–S2 interspace. The tip of the conus lies near the lower body of L1; we believe this nomenclature is the same as that used on the prior exam.

Transaxial images show postsurgical changes from prior right semi-hemilaminectomy at the S1 vertebra. Examination does show the presence of a small annular disc bulge and perhaps some early annular spurring; however, the traversing S1 nerve roots are unimpeded, and there is no evidence of recurrent focal disc herniation. There is some normal enhancement seen involving the soft tissues, presumably of a postoperative nature.

At the L4–L5 level, there is likewise no evidence of focal disc herniation or significant central spinal stenosis.

The L3–L4 interspace shows trace annular bulging without focal disc herniation or stenosis. L1–L2 and L2–L3 interspaces show a normal appearance on sagittal imaging.

IMPRESSION: MR examination of the lumbar spine with postsurgical changes from previous right semi-hemilaminectomy at L5-S1 level on the right.

While there may be some minimal annular bulging and annular spurring at this level, there is no discrete focal disc herniation, and traversing S1 nerve roots are not compromised.

The remainder of the lumbar interspaces may show some very minimal disc bulging; however, there is no focal disc herniation or central spinal stenosis. The cause of the patient's right lower extremity radicular symptoms cannot easily be explained on the basis of findings.

Jason Kunerreth, MD

Chief of Radiology

Let's Code It!

Dr. Kunerreth supervised and analyzed the MRI of Bonnie's lumbar spine. Turn to the Alphabetic Index of CPT and look for the term that MRI stands for . . .

(continued)

Magnetic Resonance Imaging (MRI)

Go back and read the documentation to determine if the MRI was done for diagnostic purposes or as guidance for another procedure. This was to determine the patient's current condition; therefore, it is a diagnostic procedure.

Magnetic Resonance Imaging (MRI)
Diagnostic
    Spine
        Cervical 72141, 72142, 72156
        Lumbar. 72148, 72149, 72158
        Thoracic 72146, 72147, 72157

What part of Bonnie's spine was examined? Her *lumbar* spine. Now, you need to turn to the *Main Section* and check out all three of the suggested codes.

72148   **Magnetic resonance (e.g., proton) imaging, spinal canal and contents, lumbar; without contrast material**

72149   **Magnetic resonance (e.g., proton) imaging, spinal canal and contents, lumbar; with contrast material**

72158   **Magnetic resonance (e.g., proton) imaging, spinal canal and contents, without contrast material, followed by contrast material(s) and further sequences; lumbar**

Does the documentation mention the use of contrast materials? Yes, it does. See the sentence in the section titled **TECHNIQUE:**

> *"Because of the postoperative nature of the lumbar spine, additional axial and sagittal postgadolinium T1-weighted images were obtained."*

Gadolinium is a contrast material. *Postgadolinium* means after the contrast material was introduced. *"Additional . . . images"* tells you that both without contrast and with contrast images were captured.

Now you know how to report Dr. Kunerreth's services . . .

72158   **Magnetic resonance (e.g., proton) imaging, spinal canal and contents, without contrast material, followed by contrast material(s) and further sequences; lumbar**

26.2 Purposes for Imaging

Screening or Diagnostic

Identifying whether an imaging service is performed as a screening or a diagnostic tool can be important in determining the correct code for the procedure. This designation refers to the reason the physician ordered the test.

A screening image is typically performed as part of a regular preventive checkup. This is ordered because the standard of care and the calendar have matched up. For example, a screening mammogram will be ordered the same time every year for a woman over the age of 50. There are no signs or symptoms that would prompt the test. It is just the wise thing to do to make certain all is fine.

A diagnostic image is taken to assist in the identification and/or confirmation of a suspected condition or diagnosis. In these cases, the physician would identify specific signs or symptoms that led him or her to decide this test was needed.

There are times when an imaging session for a patient begins as a screening test and becomes a diagnostic test while the patient is still there. With technology providing instant imaging, the radiologist can review the images almost immediately after they have been taken, while the patient is still on the premises. This eliminates a patient's needing to come back at another time to retake an image that was not clear or the technician's having to take additional views because the radiologist identified a suspicious element. When a screening test turns into a diagnostic test, report only the diagnostic imaging service because that will include the screening aspect of the procedure.

> **EXAMPLES**
>
> 74261   Computed tomography (CT) colonography, diagnostic, including image postprocessing; without contrast material
>
> 74263   Computed tomography (CT) colonography, screening, including image postprocessing

Image Guidance

When a procedure is conducted percutaneously, the physician cannot see into the body. Therefore, in order to ensure that the needle or scalpel finds the correct spot on an internal organ, image guidance will be used. This may be as simple as a fine needle aspiration to a biopsy to a more complex surgical procedure.

In some cases, the CPT book will provide you with a code that includes the imaging guidance; for example:

10007   **Fine needle aspiration biopsy, including fluoroscopic guidance; first lesion**

10009   **Fine needle aspiration biopsy, including CT guidance; first lesion**

10021   **Fine needle aspiration biopsy, without imaging guidance; first lesion**

33289   **Transcatheter implantation of wireless pulmonary artery pressure sensor for long-term hemodynamic monitoring, including . . . radiological supervision and interpretation, and pulmonary artery angiography, when performed**

Often, the CPT book will alert you to the need for a second code to report this additional service with a notation below the code, such as

(For radiological supervision and interpretation, see 76942, 77002, 77012, 77021)

And more code options can be found in the *Radiology* section of CPT:

- Ultrasonic Guidance Procedures: 76930–76965
- Other Procedures: 76970–76999
- Fluoroscopic Guidance: 77001–77003
- Computed Tomography Guidance: 77011–77014
- Magnetic Resonance Imaging Guidance: 77021–77022

 YOU CODE IT! CASE STUDY

Every year, Margarette Sanchez gets a mammogram the week before her birthday. She feels fine and no lumps were noted during her gynecologist's manual exam. Margarette arrives at the Women's Imaging Center for her annual exam.

You Code It!

Determine the correct code or codes to report the provision of Margarette's annual mammogram.

Step #1: Read the case carefully and completely.

Step #2: Abstract the scenario. Which key words or terms describe what service the physician provided to the patient during this encounter?

(continued)

Step #3: Are there any details missing or incomplete for which you would need to query the physician? [If so, ask your instructor.]

Step #4: Determine the correct CPT procedure code or codes to explain the details about what was provided to the patient during this encounter.

Step #5: Check for any relevant guidance, including reading all of the symbols and notations.

Step #6: Do you need to append any modifiers to ensure complete and accurate information is provided?

Step #7: Double-check your work.

Answer:

Did you determine this to be the correct code?

77067   **Screening mammography, bilateral (2-view study of each breast), including computer-aided detection (CAD) when performed**

Good job!

26.3 Technical vs. Professional

Essentially, there are two primary components of any radiologic procedure: the technical and the professional (referred to as supervision and interpretation in the CPT). This is not to say that radiologic technicians are not professionals. The designation is merely to divide the services provided so that it can be determined which facility or practitioner should be paid for what.

> ### EXAMPLE
>
> Jerod Paley, a 41-year-old male, was sent to the Kinsey Imaging Center to get an x-ray, three views, of his skull after he was hit in the head by a bat at a softball game.
>
> The x-ray equipment is owned by the facility. Kris Chappel, the x-ray technician who will operate the equipment, is a member of the facility's staff, and Dr. Briscoe, a board-certified radiologist who will interpret the films and send a report of this evaluation to Jerod's physician, is also a staff member of the center. Therefore, Kinsey Imaging's coding specialist will ask the insurance company for reimbursement for both the technical procedure (the use of the equipment, materials, and the staff to work and maintain that equipment) and the professional aspect (the cost and work to supervise and interpret the films). For Jerod's case, the code to be reported is **70250 Radiologic examination, skull; less than 4 views.**

Purchasing (or leasing) and maintaining imaging equipment is very expensive and cannot be supported by every health care facility. In addition, physicians who are specially trained radiologists are not necessarily staff members of all health care facilities with the equipment. Therefore, circumstances may arise when the technical procedure and the professional service must be billed separately. In those cases, the coder who is responsible for charging for the professional services must use modifier 26 to identify the separation of the components.

26   **Professional Component:** *Certain procedures are a combination of a physician component and a technical component. When the physician component is reported separately, the service may be identified by adding modifier 26 to the usual procedure number.*

CODING BITES

You learned in medical terminology class that the suffix *-graphy* means the recording of an image and the suffix *-scopy* means to look or view. We tend to think of all these procedures and services as radiology. However, not all of them are coded from the *Radiology* section of the CPT book.

For example, cardiography is listed in the *Medicine* section. Therefore, always use the Alphabetic Index to help point you toward the correct area of the book. It will save you time in the long run.

EXAMPLE

Walter Wasser, a 31-year-old male, was brought into the emergency department of a small hospital near his farm after he fell off a ladder onto his back while working in the barn. The physician sent Walter to radiology for x-rays of his entire thoracic, lumbar, and sacral spine (two views). The hospital does not have a staff radiologist, so Dr. Chen is brought over to evaluate the x-rays and write the report for the physician.

The hospital, which owns the equipment and pays the salary of the technician, will bill the insurance carrier for the technical portion of the examination, using code 72082-TC.

Dr. Chen's coding specialist will send in a claim for Dr. Chen's interpretation only, the professional services he provided. In order to make this clear on the claim form, the modifier **26 Professional Component** will be appended to the code for the radiologic examination; the code that will be reported on his claim form will be 72082-26.

As you have already learned, sometimes the CPT book will save you work. Certain radiologic examination codes distinguish the technical component and professional component of services for you. One of the easiest ways to identify such cases is by the notation within the code's description that specifies the code is for radiologic supervision and interpretation only.

EXAMPLE

70015   Cisternography, positive contrast, radiological supervision and interpretation

From the example, you can see that code 70015 excludes the technical component. If you are coding for the physician's services only, that makes it easy. If you are coding for the facility for the technical aspect, you need to add modifier TC Technical Component. After a while, you will learn the details about the procedures performed by all of the professionals in your health care facility, and you will be able to identify the components easily. It just takes some practice.

  LET'S CODE IT! SCENARIO

Roland Dellman, an 8-year-old male, is brought into the emergency department by ambulance. He was skateboarding off a homemade ramp and fell on his neck and shoulder. Dr. Tyner suspects a broken clavicle and orders a complete radiologic exam of the area. This facility does not have a radiologist on staff at this time, so the facility took the x-ray and the digital images were electronically sent to Radiology Associates in another state. Dr. Neuman reads the films and sends a report to Dr. Tyner confirming the fracture. Code for Dr. Neuman.

Let's Code It!

The physician's notes state that a *radiologic exam* of Roland's *clavicle* was performed. Let's turn to the Alphabetic Index under *radiology*. Note that the choices are not going to satisfy our needs. Therefore, let's try an alternate term for radiology: x-ray. Turn to *x-ray,* and you find a long list of anatomical sites. Next to the word *clavicle* you see only one suggested code. Let's go to the numeric listing and read the complete description:

(continued)

73000   Radiologic examination; clavicle, complete

This is exactly what Dr. Tyner ordered for Roland. And the facility only provided the technical component, so the coder would report:

73000-TC   Radiologic examination; clavicle, complete, technical component

The coder for Radiology Associates would report **73000-26** to be reimbursed for Dr. Neuman's work. Good job!

 LET'S CODE IT! SCENARIO

*Jalyssa Miland, a 35-year-old female, is 10-weeks pregnant. This is her first pregnancy, and twins run in her family. In order to determine how many fetuses there are, Dr. Ruber orders a **sonogram**. Iona Appell is the technician at the imaging center next door to Dr. Ruber's office. The Kinsey Imaging Center performs Jalyssa's real-time transabdominal exam and sends the documentation to Dr. Ruber so that he can read and interpret the results. A single fetus was observed.*

Let's Code It!

You are Dr. Ruber's coder, and his notes state that a sonogram of Jalyssa was performed at the imaging center. We know that she is pregnant, and this is why she is having the test done, so the anatomical site of the examination is her *pregnant uterus*.

Turn to the Alphabetic Index under *sonography,* and the CPT book tells you to *see echography,* which is the type of technology that sonograms use. Turn to *echography* (caution—not echo*cardio*graphy; this is not of Jalyssa's heart), and find a list of anatomical sites. Looking for *pregnant uterus,* you see a range of suggested codes. Let's go to the numeric listing and read the complete description of the first one.

76801   Ultrasound, pregnant uterus, real time with image documentation, fetal and maternal evaluation, first trimester (<14 weeks 0 days), transabdominal approach; single or first gestation

Great! The very first code seems to match the notes perfectly. However, to make certain you are using the best, most appropriate code, you will want to read through all the suggested codes.

Remember, you are coding for Dr. Ruber. With regard to Jalyssa's radiologic exam, he provided the interpretation—the professional component only. Therefore, the claim form you prepare should show this code as **76801-26.**

26.4 Number of Views

Throughout the *Radiology* section of the CPT book, radiologic examinations are often described by the number of views taken by the technician.

Sonogram
The use of sound waves to record images of internal organs and tissues; also called an *ultrasound.*

EXAMPLE

73060   Radiologic examination, humerus, minimum of 2 views

The "two views" refers to the number of angles, or perceptions, from which the images were taken, such as anterior and posterior. Such codes represent the norm, or standard, in imaging when it comes to these certain anatomical sites.

The most common angles, or pathways, of imaging include:

AP   *Anteroposterior:* Front to back.
PA   *Posteroanterior:* Back to front.
O   *Oblique:* At an angle.
RAO   *Right anterior oblique:* At an angle from the right front.
LAO   *Left anterior oblique:* At an angle from the left front.
LPO   *Left posterior oblique:* At an angle from the left back.
Lat   *Lateral (lat):* From one side to the other side.

In those cases when the radiologist takes fewer than the minimum number of views included in the description, you have to append the radiologic code with modifier 52 Reduced Services.

52   **Reduced Services:** Under certain circumstances a service or procedure is partially reduced or eliminated at the physician's discretion. Under these circumstances, the service provided can be identified by its usual procedure number and the addition of modifier 52, signifying that the service is reduced. This provides a means of reporting reduced services without disturbing the identification of the basic service.

 YOU CODE IT! CASE STUDY

Carly-Ann Price, an 18-month-old female, is brought into the office of her pediatrician, Dr. Lattel. She fell off the couch onto a hard tile floor and it appears that her hip is painful to her. Dr. Lattel has his staff take an x-ray of the pelvis and hip to determine if there is a fracture. He orders only the anteroposterior view to be taken. He does not subject his patients to radiology exposure unnecessarily, and he believes that the one view will tell him what he needs to know. The x-ray confirms a hairline fracture, and he applies a cast.

You Code It!

Go through the steps, and determine the code(s) that should be reported for the radiologic service Dr. Lattel provided to Carly-Ann.

Step #1: Read the case carefully and completely.

Step #2: Abstract the scenario. Which key words or terms describe what service the physician provided to the patient during this encounter?

Step #3: Are there any details missing or incomplete for which you would need to query the physician? [If so, ask your instructor.]

Step #4: Determine the correct CPT procedure code or codes to explain the details about what was provided to the patient during this encounter.

Step #5: Check for any relevant guidance, including reading all of the symbols and notations.

Step #6: Do you need to append any modifiers to ensure complete and accurate information is provided?

Step #7: Double-check your work.

Answer:

Did you determine this to be the correct code?

    73501   **Radiologic examination, hip, unilateral, with pelvis when performed; 1 view**

Good job!

26.5 Procedures With or Without Contrast

Some imaging examinations use contrast materials to gain a clearer picture of an organ or anatomical site. The phrase "with contrast" means that the technician or physician gave the patient a substance to enhance the image. For example, arthrography is used to identify abnormalities that may be present within a joint (wrist, hip, shoulder, knee). Gadolinium is injected into the joint that is to be visualized to provide better-quality images of the patient's condition. In other procedures, different substances are injected. For example, when myelography is done to examine a patient's spinal cord and nerves, an injection of x-ray dye may be used to more clearly visualize a patient's disc herniation, bone spurs, or vertebral stenosis.

1. When radiographic **arthrography** is performed, use an additional code for the supervision and interpretation of the appropriate joint. This includes the use of a **fluoroscope**.

> **EXAMPLE**
>
> Dr. Horace, a radiologist, supervised a radiographic arthrography of Porter Maison's ankle; later the interpreted results were reported with this code:
>
> 73615   Radiologic examination, ankle, arthrography, radiological supervision and interpretation

2. Imaging "with contrast" has some guidelines that you have to know in order to code accurately.

   a. If the code description includes the term "with contrast," such as **computed tomography (CT)** with contrast, **computed tomography angiography (CTA)** with contrast, **magnetic resonance arthrography (MRA)** with contrast, or **magnetic resonance imaging (MRI)** with contrast, the injection of the contrast materials, when administered intravenously, is already included in the code and should *not* be reported separately.

   b. If the contrast material is injected intra-articularly (into a joint) or intrathecally (into a tendon or sheath), an additional code is reported for the appropriate injection.

   c. Providing contrast materials orally and/or rectally alone does not constitute an exam "with contrast."

> **EXAMPLE**
>
> Dr. Groder injected Vincent Speck's elbow intrathecally with contrast materials to do a radiographic arthrography for his tennis elbow. This is reported with these codes:
>
> 73085   Radiologic examination, elbow, arthrography, radiological supervision and interpretation
> 20550   Injection(s); single tendon sheath, or ligament, aponeurosis (e.g., plantar "fascia")

3. When a CT or MR arthrography is performed without radiographic arthrography, you will need three different codes:

   a. A code for the injection of the contrast material into the specific joint.

   b. A code for the appropriate CT or MR.

   c. A code for the imaging guidance (fluoroscopy) of the placement of the needle to inject the contrast material.

GUIDANCE CONNECTION

Read the additional explanations in the **Radiology Guidelines (Including Nuclear Medicine and Diagnostic Ultrasound)**, subhead **Administration of Contrast Material(s)**, in your CPT book directly in front of the Radiology section that lists all the codes.

Arthrography
The recording of a picture of an anatomical joint after the administration of contrast material into the joint capsule.

Fluoroscope
A piece of equipment that emits x-rays through a part of the patient's body onto a fluorescent screen, causing the image to identify various aspects of the anatomy by density.

Computed Tomography (CT)
A specialized computer scanner with very fine detail that records imaging of internal anatomical sites; also known as computerized axial tomography (CAT).

Computed Tomography Angiography (CTA)
A CT scan using contrast materials to visualize arteries and veins all over the body.

Magnetic Resonance Arthrography (MRA)
MR imaging of an anatomical joint after the administration of contrast material into the joint capsule.

Magnetic Resonance Imaging (MRI)
A three-dimensional radiologic technique that uses nuclear technology to record pictures of internal anatomical sites.

Other types of radiologic procedures include

- *Positron emission tomography (PET):* Uses a variety of radiopharmaceuticals that mimic natural sugars, water, proteins, and oxygen and collect in various tissues and organs. It is a time-exposure picture of cellular biologic activities.
- *Bone density scan (DEXA):* Used most often for osteoporosis screenings; enables assessment of bone minerals in spine, hip, and other skeletal sites.
- *Nuclear medicine scan:* Used to assess organ system function.

 LET'S CODE IT! SCENARIO

Mark Silver, an 81-year-old male, has been having problems with his memory and his walking. After an extensive examination, his neurologist, Dr. Chernuchin, orders an MRI, brain, with and without contrast, to determine if Mark is suffering from hydrocephalus.

Let's Code It!

This is very straightforward. Mark had an *MRI* of his *brain* taken. Let's go to the Alphabetic Index and look this up. Under *magnetic resonance imaging (MRI)*, you see the list of anatomical sites, including *brain*, which suggests code range 70551–70553. (*NOTE: Intraoperative*, indented below *brain*, means that the MRI was performed during surgery. This was not the case for Mark, according to the physician's notes.) Let's go to the numeric listing and read the descriptions.

70551   Magnetic resonance (e.g., proton) imaging, brain (including brain stem); without contrast material
70552   with contrast material(s)
70553   without contrast material, followed by contrast material(s) and further sequences

Dr. Chernuchin's notes state that the MRI is *with and without contrast*. That means both types of imaging were done. Code 70551 describes without contrast, and code 70552 includes the contrast. When you keep reading, you see that code 70553 is the correct code because, as the notes state, it includes both sequences: without the contrast followed by with contrast materials. Of course, you also will add the appropriate HCPCS Level II codes to report the contrast materials used.

CODING BITES

Appropriate HCPCS Level II codes from the range Q9951–Q9969, based on the number of units, should be assigned to report the contrast materials supplied.

26.6 Diagnostic Radiology

Diagnostic Angiography

The coding of the process of imaging the body's blood vessels, diagnostic **angiography**, carries certain guidelines affecting the use of the codes.

1. In some cases, interventional coding guidelines don't permit you to report a diagnostic angiography when it is performed at the same time as a therapeutic interventional procedure. This rule applies when the patient has already been diagnosed and has scheduled a therapeutic intervention to correct the problem. As you have already learned, you must read the guidelines and the code descriptions carefully.

> **Angiography**
> The imaging of blood vessels after the injection of contrast material.

EXAMPLE

Dr. Victoria performed a left internal and external carotid arterial angiography to check for blockage and immediately performed an intervention procedure. You would report this by using codes

36224	Selective catheter placement, internal carotid artery, unilateral, with angiography of the ipsilateral intracranial carotid circulation and all associated radiological supervision and interpretation, includes angiography of the extracranial carotid and cervicocerebral arch, when performed
+36227	Selective catheter placement, external carotid artery, unilateral, with angiography of the ipsilateral external carotid circulation and all associated radiological supervision and interpretation (List separately in addition to code for primary procedure.)

2. In other cases, the diagnostic angiography *should be coded separately* even though it is done at the same session as an interventional procedure. This is true if one of the following conditions has been met:

   a. A full diagnostic study is done, no prior catheter-based angiographic study is available, and the decision to intervene is determined by the diagnostic study.

   b. The patient's condition has changed since a previously done study.

   c. The patient's condition changes during the interventional procedure that requires a diagnostic procedure to look at vessels outside of the area.

   d. The prior diagnostic angiography did not show the applicable anatomy and/or pathology being treated at the session.

EXAMPLE

Thelma Hadid had a diagnostic angiography of her adrenal gland 1 year ago. Since then, her condition has deteriorated. Therefore, Dr. Carnicki first performs a diagnostic procedure. Because this shows changes, at the same session, he performs an interventional procedure.

> **GUIDANCE CONNECTION**
>
> Read the additional explanations in the in-section guidelines within the **Radiology** section, subhead **Vascular Procedures,** subsection **Aorta and Arteries,** directly above code 75600 in your CPT book.

3. Diagnostic angiography is included with the code for an interventional procedure and should *not* be coded separately when that diagnostic angiography is performed for any of the following:

   a. Vessel measurement.

   b. Postangioplasty or stent angiography.

   c. Contrast injections, angiography, road mapping, and/or fluoroscopic guidance for the interventional procedure.

LET'S CODE IT! SCENARIO

Alene Ransom, a 61-year-old female, has had two mild heart attacks in the past 2 years. Today, Alene is at the Beyers Ambulatory Surgical Center for a diagnostic angiography to quantify the degree of blockage suspected in her left renal artery. Dr. Black performs the procedure, which includes placing the catheter directly in the renal artery. Later that day, Dr. Black dictates a report indicating that Alene's left renal artery is 50% blocked.

Let's Code It!

The notes indicate that a *left renal angiography* was performed on Alene. Let's go to the Alphabetic Index and look up *angiography*. You know that Alene's renal artery was examined, and the Alphabetic Index suggests codes 36251–36254. Let's check the complete descriptions in the numeric listings:

36251 **Selective catheter placement (first-order), main renal artery and any accessory renal artery(s) for renal angiography, including arterial puncture and catheter placement(s), fluoroscopy, contrast injection(s), image postprocessing, permanent recording of images, and radiological supervision and interpretation, including pressure gradient measurements when performed, and flush aortogram when performed; unilateral**

36252 **bilateral**

The difference between these two code descriptions is that 36251 is for a unilateral procedure and 36252 is for a bilateral procedure. Alene had only her left renal artery examined. One side is unilateral, leading us to the correct code of **36251.**

Diagnostic Venography

Venography
The imaging of a vein after the injection of contrast material.

The codes for reporting diagnostic **venography** have guidelines similar to those for diagnostic angiography.

1. Some interventional procedure codes include the diagnostic venography when done at the same time as the procedure. You must read the descriptions carefully to determine if this is the case.

2. Diagnostic venography done at the same time as an interventional procedure *should be coded separately* if one of the following conditions has been met:

    a. A full diagnostic study is done, no prior catheter-based venographic study is available, and the decision to intervene is determined by this diagnostic study.

    b. The patient's condition has changed since a previously done study.

    c. The patient's condition changes during the interventional procedure and requires a diagnostic procedure to look at vessels outside of the area.

    d. The prior diagnostic venography did not show the applicable anatomy and/or pathology being treated at the session.

3. Diagnostic venography is included with the code for an interventional procedure and should *not* be coded separately when that diagnostic venography is performed for any of the following:

    a. Vessel measurement.

    b. Postangioplasty or stent venography.

    c. Contrast injections, venography, road mapping, and/or fluoroscopic guidance for the interventional procedure.

GUIDANCE CONNECTION

Read the additional explanations in the in-section guidelines within the **Radiology** section, subhead **Vascular Procedures,** subsection **Veins and Lymphatics,** directly above code 75801 in your CPT book.

LET'S CODE IT! SCENARIO

Charles Baseman, a 55-year-old male, flew in yesterday from Australia, a 26-hour airplane ride. Since getting off the plane, he has been having pain in his right calf. Dr. Vernon performed a diagnostic venography to determine if Charles has deep vein thrombosis (DVT). After completing the procedure, he wrote a report with his interpretation, which was sent to Charles's internist.

Let's Code It!

Dr. Vernon performed a *diagnostic venography* of Charles's *right leg*. Let's go to the Alphabetic Index and find *venography*. Beneath *venography,* you see the anatomical site *leg* with the suggested code range 75820–75822. Let's look at the code descriptions in the numeric listings:

75820   **Venography, extremity, unilateral, radiological supervision and interpretation**
75822   **Venography, extremity, bilateral, radiological supervision and interpretation**

The difference between these two codes is that 75820 is a unilateral procedure and 75822 is a bilateral procedure. Charles had only his right leg examined, making it a unilateral procedure and making **75820** the correct code.

Transcatheter Procedures

Therapeutic transcatheter radiologic supervision and interpretation codes, when associated with intervention, already include

1. Vessel measurement.
2. Postangioplasty or stent venography.
3. Contrast injections, angiography/venography, road mapping, and/or fluoroscopic guidance for the interventional procedure.

Transcatheter therapeutic radiologic and interpretation services *are* separately reportable from diagnostic angiography/venography done at the same time *unless* they are specifically included in the code descriptor.

 GUIDANCE CONNECTION

Read the additional explanations in the in-section guidelines within the **Radiology** section, subhead **Vascular Procedures,** subsection **Transcatheter Procedures,** directly above code 75894 in your CPT book.

 LET'S CODE IT! SCENARIO

Dr. Grubman is in the OR today to perform a transcatheter placement of an intravascular stent, percutaneously, in Olivia Samuel's common iliac.

Let's Code It!

You are Dr. Grubman's coding specialist, so you are going to code only the radiologic supervision and interpretation of the *transcatheter* procedure, as well as the placement of the stent itself. Let's go to *transcatheter* in the Alphabetic Index. You will notice that, if you go to *placement* under *transcatheter,* you see *intravascular stents* indented below. Here, the Alphabetic Index suggests some Category III codes (0075T, 0076T) along with code ranges 37215–37218, 37236–37239, and 92928–92929.

When you turn to the codes, you realize that they are in the **Surgery** section, not **Radiology**. However, they are the only codes offered by the Alphabetic Index, so let's take a look at them all. Notice

37236   **Transcatheter placement of an intravascular stent(s) (except lower extremity artery(s) for occlusive disease, cervical carotid, extracranial vertebral or intrathoracic carotid, intracranial or coronary), open or percutaneous, including radiological supervision and interpretation and including all angioplasty within the same vessel, when performed; initial artery**

(continued)

But we are coding for Dr. Grubman's radiologic supervision and interpretation for the procedure as well as the stent placement. Notice that the description for code 37236 includes "radiological supervision and interpretation."

Perfect!

Diagnostic Ultrasound

CODING BITES

If the reason that an organ was not visible is documented in the patient's record, you are permitted to code this as "complete."

When reporting diagnostic ultrasound services, you need to abstract specific details about the anatomical sites viewed. As the coding specialist, you must read the report and pay attention to whether the exam was "complete" or "limited" and choose the correct code. The description of an ultrasound exam as being "complete" is determined by the specific number of elements, such as organs or areas, that are surveyed during the test. However, sometimes the full list is not visualized. For example, an organ may have been previously removed surgically, or another organ may be blocking the view. The report that is submitted for the patient's record, after the exam, should note everything that was studied—as well as those elements that should have been but were not, along with why they were not.

You will find information regarding what is included in a complete exam in the guidelines shown below each of the ultrasound subheadings: **Abdomen and Retroperitoneum, Pelvis—Obstetrical, Pelvis—Nonobstetrical.**

Should an ultrasound exam be performed *without* a thorough evaluation of an organ or anatomical region *and* recording of the image *and* a final, written report, you are not permitted to code the procedure separately.

GUIDANCE CONNECTION

Read the additional explanation in the in-section guidelines within the **Radiology** section, subhead **Diagnostic Ultrasound,** directly above code 76506 in your CPT book.

> **EXAMPLE**
>
> **Abdomen and Retroperitoneum**
>
> A complete ultrasound examination of the abdomen (76700) consists of real-time scans of the liver, gallbladder, common bile duct, pancreas, spleen, kidney, and the upper abdominal aorta and inferior vena cava including any demonstrated abdominal abnormality.

Let's say an ultrasound examination is done on Herman Smith's abdomen. The documentation includes the physician's (radiologist's) interpretation of all organs except the gallbladder. The patient had his gallbladder removed 1 year prior to this ultrasound exam. As long as this fact is also documented, code 76700 for a complete ultrasound examination of the abdomen is accurate.

You already know that an ultrasound may be called a *sonogram.* However, other definitions are important for you to know so that you can determine the best, most appropriate code. The following terms identify the type of scan:

- *A-mode* indicates a one-dimensional ultrasonic measurement procedure.
- *M-mode* is also a one-dimensional ultrasonic measurement procedure; however, it includes the movement of the trace so that there can be a recording of both amplitude and velocity of the moving echo-producing structures.
- *B-scan* indicates a two-dimensional ultrasonic scanning procedure with a two-dimensional display.
- *Real-time scan* indicates that a two-dimensional ultrasonic scanning procedure with a display was performed and included both the two-dimensional structure and motion with time.

CODING BITES

Ultrasound services are especially dangerous to code from superbills instead of notes. Make certain you get the complete documentation before choosing a code.

If the report indicates that a Doppler evaluation of vascular structures, or another diagnostic vascular ultrasound study, was performed, it should be coded separately with the codes from the **Noninvasive Vascular Diagnostic Studies** subsection, codes 93880–93998.

 YOU CODE IT! CASE STUDY

Eriq Taleni, a 57-year-old male, was sent to the Kinsey Imaging Center by Dr. Rayman to have an ophthalmic biometry by ultrasound echography, A-scan. After performing the exam, Dr. Turner, the radiologist, wrote in his report that a second test using intraocular lens power calculation might be necessary to further clarify the condition of the eye. Dr. Rayman determined that Eriq should wait before having the second test.

You Code It!

Go through the steps, and determine the codes that should be reported for the service provided to Eriq Taleni by Dr. Turner.

Step #1: Read the case carefully and completely.

Step #2: Abstract the scenario. Which key words or terms describe what service the physician provided to the patient during this encounter?

Step #3: Are there any details missing or incomplete for which you would need to query the physician? [If so, ask your instructor.]

Step #4: Determine the correct CPT procedure code or codes to explain the details about what was provided to the patient during this encounter.

Step #5: Check for any relevant guidance, including reading all of the symbols and notations.

Step #6: Do you need to append any modifiers to ensure complete and accurate information is provided?

Step #7: Double-check your work.

Answer:

Did you determine this to be the correct code?

> **76516** **Ophthalmic biometry by ultrasound echography, A-scan**

Good job!

26.7 Mammography

Until researchers can find a way to prevent breast cancer, the best weapon in the health care arsenal is early detection—finding the malignancy when it is tiny and easier to eradicate. Mammography, low-dose radiology, is considered the best method for identifying a small, otherwise undetectable lump or microcalcification. Mammography employs low-energy x-rays specifically designed to take and record images of breast tissue for the discovery of breast lesions.

> **77065** **Diagnostic mammography, including computer-aided detection (CAD) when performed; unilateral**
>
> **77066** **Diagnostic mammography, including computer-aided detection (CAD) when performed; bilateral**
>
> **77067** **Screening mammography, bilateral (2-view film study of each breast), including computer-aided detection (CAD) when performed**

At times, computer-aided detection (CAD) is used in conjunction with the x-ray imaging. CAD transitions the x-ray image into a digital image, which is then scanned by a computer, searching for anything that might be abnormal.

 YOU CODE IT! CASE STUDY

Every year, Donna Simmons, a 47-year-old female, came in for her annual well-woman exam, and then would go over to the Imaging Center for her screening mammogram. This year, Dr. Douglas felt a lump during Donna's manual exam, so he ordered a diagnostic mammogram for the left breast and a screening mammogram for the right. These mammograms were provided the next day at the Imaging Center.

You Code It!

Read the case study of Donna's encounter at the Imaging Center, and determine the correct code or codes.

Step #1: Read the case carefully and completely.

Step #2: Abstract the scenario. Which key words or terms describe what service the physician provided to the patient during this encounter?

Step #3: Are there any details missing or incomplete for which you would need to query the physician? [If so, ask your instructor.]

Step #4: Determine the correct CPT procedure code or codes to explain the details about what was provided to the patient during this encounter.

Step #5: Check for any relevant guidance, including reading all of the symbols and notations.

Step #6: Do you need to append any modifiers to ensure complete and accurate information is provided?

Step #7: Double-check your work.

Answer:

Did you determine these to be the correct codes?

77065	Diagnostic mammography, including computer-aided detection (CAD) when performed; unilateral
77067-52	Screening mammography, bilateral (2-view film study of each breast), including computer-aided detection (CAD) when performed, reduced services

Good job!

26.8 Bone and Joint Studies

There are many reasons a physician may need information about a patient's bone structure and strength, and several imaging techniques that could be used to provide the most accurate data.

- Bone age studies enable the physician to identify the degree of maturation of a child's bones.
- CT scanography has surpassed orthoroentgenogram in the last decade to determine leg length discrepancies.
- Osseous survey is a radiologic procedure used to identify fractures, tumors, and degenerative conditions of the bone.
- Bone mineral density (BMD) scanning, also called dual-energy x-ray absorptiometry (DXA or DEXA) or bone densitometry, is an enhanced form of x-ray technology that is used to measure bone loss.

YOU CODE IT! CASE STUDY

Rachel VanHeusen, a 65-year-old female, arrived at the Kinsey Imaging Center to have a DEXA bone density study, both axial and appendicular skeleton. Dr. Underwood, the staff radiologist, analyzed the images and wrote a report.

You Code It!

The Kinsey Imaging Center performed a DEXA bone density study for both the axial and appendicular skeleton of Rachel VanHeusen. Review the details, and determine the code or codes for this service.

Step #1: Read the case carefully and completely.

Step #2: Abstract the scenario. Which key words or terms describe what service the physician provided to the patient during this encounter?

Step #3: Are there any details missing or incomplete for which you would need to query the physician? [If so, ask your instructor.]

Step #4: Determine the correct CPT procedure code or codes to explain the details about what was provided to the patient during this encounter.

Step #5: Check for any relevant guidance, including reading all of the symbols and notations.

Step #6: Do you need to append any modifiers to ensure complete and accurate information is provided?

Step #7: Double-check your work.

Answer:

Did you accurately determine these to be the codes?

77080	Dual-energy X-ray absorptiometry (DXA), bone density study, 1 or more sites; axial skeleton (e.g., hips, pelvis, spine)
77081-59	Dual-energy X-ray absorptiometry (DXA), bone density study, 1 or more sites; appendicular skeleton (peripheral) (e.g., radius, wrist, heel), Distinct procedural service

26.9 Radiation Oncology

Radiation oncology is performed to treat malignant neoplasms and other carcinomas, commonly known as cancer.

The codes in this subsection already include certain services:

- Initial consultation.
- Clinical treatment planning.
- Simulation.
- Medical radiation physics.
- Dosimetry (the determination of the correct dosage).

Radiation
The high-speed discharge and projection of energy waves or particles.

- Treatment devices.
- Special services.
- Clinical treatment management procedures.
- Normal follow-up care during treatment and for 3 months following the completion of the treatment.

Radiation oncology services may be provided in varying degrees of intensity and are usually determined in the planning process. Therefore, the preparation for the sequence of treatments must be coded accurately. Some professionals may describe the planning as simple, intermediate, or complex. However, others may provide the detail, leaving you to match the components performed with the level of service.

Here are the specifics involved in each level:

- *Simple planning* involves one treatment area with one port, or parallel opposed ports, with simple or no blocking.
- *Intermediate planning* involves two separate treatment areas, three or more converging ports, multiple blocks, or special time–dose constraints.
- *Complex planning* involves three or more separate treatment areas, highly complex blocking, custom shielding blocks, tangential ports, special wedges or compensators, rotational or special beam consideration, or a combination of therapeutic methods.

Just to keep you on your toes, you will find the same terms *(simple, intermediate, complex)* also used to describe the simulation applied, with different definitions. The good news is that the same terms relate to the same elements involved in the process.

With simulation, there is one additional descriptor:

- *Simple simulation:* a single treatment area with either a single port or parallel opposed ports, simple or no blocking.
- *Intermediate simulation:* three or more converging ports, two separate treatment areas, multiple blocks.
- *Complex simulation:* tangential portals, three or more treatment areas, rotation or arc therapy, complex blocking, custom shielding blocks, brachytherapy source verification, hyperthermia probe verification, any use of contrast materials.
- *Three-dimensional computer-generated:* reconstruction of the size and mass of the tumor and the normal tissues that surround the tumor site.

If you work in a facility that provides proton beam treatments and/or clinical brachytherapy for patients, you will note that the CPT book has different definitions for the same three terms: simple, intermediate, and complex.

 LET'S CODE IT! SCENARIO

PATIENT: Craig Bennington

DATE OF PROCEDURE: 09/25/2019

PREOPERATIVE DIAGNOSIS: Adenocarcinoma of the prostate

POSTOPERATIVE DIAGNOSIS: Adenocarcinoma of the prostate

PROCEDURE PERFORMED: Prostate brachytherapy

SURGEON: Carlos Arias, MD

(continued)

ANESTHESIA: General anesthesia via LMA

COMPLICATIONS: None

DRAINS: One 18-French Foley catheter per urethra

INDICATIONS FOR PROCEDURE: This patient has a new diagnosis of adenocarcinoma of the prostate diagnosed due to a very slowly rising PSA. His current PSA level is only 2.0, but prostate ultrasound biopsies were performed showing adenocarcinoma of the prostate at the left base of the prostate, and two biopsies were positive out of eight with a Gleason score of 6. Treatment options have been discussed, and he wishes to proceed with prostate brachytherapy. Informed consent has been obtained.

DESCRIPTION OF PROCEDURE: The patient was placed on the operating table in the supine position. General anesthesia was administered via LMA. He was then placed in the dorsal lithotomy position and sterilely prepped and draped in the usual fashion. The prostate ultrasound was inserted. The prostate was visualized using the preplanned study as a guide. Intracavitary application of prostate brachytherapy was performed. The patient tolerated the procedure well and had no immediate intraoperative or postoperative complications.

We implanted a total of 54 iodine-125 radioactive seeds through 12 needles with each seed containing 0.373 millicurie per seed. During the procedure, the patient received 4 mg of Decadron IV and 400 mg of Cipro IV. Subsequent fluoroscopy showed good distribution of the seeds throughout the prostate. The patient will have a CAT scan of the pelvis and simulation for his seed localization. Total target dose is 14,500 cGy.

The patient will be discharged with prescriptions for Cardura 1 mg a day for a month with two refills; Tylenol No. 3 one t.i.d. p.r.n. for pain, a total of 20; Pyridium Plus one b.i.d. for 10 days; Cipro 500 mg b.i.d. for 5 days; and prednisone 10 mg t.i.d. for a week.

Discharge instructions were explained to the patient and his wife. He will return to see Dr. Ferguson, his oncologist, in 2 weeks and Dr. Victors, his urologist, in 4 weeks for a follow-up.

Let's Code It!

Dr. Arias performed brachytherapy, so turn to this term in the CPT Alphabetic Index.

Brachytherapy

Read down the listing of the types of brachytherapic methods. Notice the documentation states, *"Intracavitary application of prostate brachytherapy was performed,"* which leads you to

Intracavitary Application 0395T, 77761-77763

Now, look up each of these codes and read each complete description to find the one that matches:

0394T **High dose rate electronic brachytherapy, skin surface application, per fraction, includes basic dosimetry, when performed**

0395T **High dose rate electronic brachytherapy, interstitial or intracavitary treatment, per fraction, includes basic dosimetry, when performed**

77761 **Intracavitary radiation source application; simple**

77762 **Intracavitary radiation source application; intermediate**

77763 **Intracavitary radiation source application; complex**

Analyze each of these codes' descriptions. Code 0394T or 0395T cannot be accurate for this encounter because there is no mention of electronic brachytherapy being used. Codes 77761, 77762, and 77763 are essentially the same except for the level of intensity: simple, intermediate, or complex.

Do you know which level is described in the documentation? No, so you need to query the physician. The physician responds by adding a notation in the patient's chart that this was a low-dose (simple) application. Now you have what you need to report:

77761 **Intracavitary radiation source application; simple**

Good work!

26.10 Nuclear Medicine

Nuclear Medicine
Treatment that includes the injection or digestion of isotopes.

Nuclear medicine uses tiny quantities of radioactive material, also known as tracers, in conjunction with a scintillation or gamma camera to record the emissions from the tracers to create an image of the anatomical site. Several types of nuclear medicine tests are used to identify a health concern:

- Bone scans are used to investigate injuries (fractures, sprains, and strains) as well as tumors.
- Thyroid uptake scans are used to assess thyroid function and record the structure of the gland.
- Lung scans are used to determine the presence of blood clots. In addition, scans can be valuable to calculate the flow of air into and out of the lungs.
- Hepatobiliary scans can provide information to evaluate the function of the liver and the gallbladder.
- Gallium scans can be used to identify the presence of infection and some types of tumors.

In addition to the diagnostic benefits of nuclear medicine, this methodology also can be used therapeutically to treat hyperthyroidism and thyroid cancer and to help to correct blood imbalances.

One important point that you have to know as a coding specialist working with nuclear medicine procedures is that the codes presented in the CPT book do not include diagnostic or therapeutic radiopharmaceuticals (the drugs or isotopes used in the treatments). Therefore, you have to code them separately. If the insurance carrier accepts HCPCS Level II codes, you will use them. You will learn all about HCPCS Level II codes in Part IV of this textbook.

Radiopharmaceutical therapy, the administration of nuclear drugs, whether given to the patient orally, intravenously, intracavitarily, interstitially, or intra-arterially, are reported with codes 79005–79999.

Also note that any chemical pathology or chemical analysis done in connection with the provision of nuclear medicine treatments should be coded separately from the *Pathology and Laboratory* section of the CPT book.

 YOU CODE IT! CASE STUDY

Nadya Bartlett, a 43-year-old female, had gained a great deal of weight recently, with no change in her diet or exercise regimen. After a thorough examination, Dr. Posner ordered nuclear imaging of her thyroid, with uptake. Radiopharmaceuticals were administered intravenously. The report came back to Dr. Posner with the multiple determinations of Nadya's exam.

You Code It!

Go through the steps of coding, and determine the radiology code or codes that should be reported for this encounter between Dr. Posner and Nadya Bartlett.

Step #1: Read the case carefully and completely.

Step #2: Abstract the scenario. Which key words or terms describe what service the physician provided to the patient during this encounter?

(continued)

Step #3: Are there any details missing or incomplete for which you would need to query the physician? [If so, ask your instructor.]

Step #4: Determine the correct CPT procedure code or codes to explain the details about what was provided to the patient during this encounter.

Step #5: Check for any relevant guidance, including reading all of the symbols and notations.

Step #6: Do you need to append any modifiers to ensure complete and accurate information is provided?

Step #7: Double-check your work.

Answer:

Did you determine this to be the correct code?

> **78014** **Thyroid imaging (including vascular flow, when performed); with single or multiple uptake(s) quantitative measurement(s) (including stimulation, suppression, or discharge, when performed)**

Great job!

Chapter Summary

Health care technology has advanced tremendously in the area of radiology and imaging. It is important that, as a coding specialist, you understand the differences among the types of radiologic methods, as well as the components of each. Procedures with contrast and without contrast, CT scans, MRIs, sonograms, and so many more enable professionals to look inside the patient in a noninvasive manner, and it is your job to obtain the correct reimbursement for every procedure.

CODING BITES

Isotopes Used in Nuclear Medicine

Lutetium-177	A therapeutic radioisotope with just enough gamma to enable imaging.
Yttrium-90	Treatment of cancer, particularly non-Hodgkin's lymphoma and liver cancer, and it is being used more widely, including for arthritis treatment.
Iodine-131	Treats thyroid for malignancy and other abnormal conditions such as hyperthyroidism (overactive thyroid).
Phosphorus-32	Controls an excess of red blood cells (RBCs).
Caesium-131, Palladium-103, Iodine-125, and Radium-223	Used for brachytherapy.

CHAPTER 26 REVIEW
CPT Radiology Section

Let's Check It! Terminology

Match each key term to the appropriate definition.

1. LO 26.6   The imaging of a vein after the injection of contrast material.

2. LO 26.3   The use of sound waves to record images of internal organs and tissues; also called an *ultrasound*.

3. LO 26.6   The imaging of blood vessels after the injection of contrast material.

4. LO 26.5   A piece of equipment that emits x-rays through a part of the patient's body onto a fluorescent screen, causing the image to identify various aspects of the anatomy by density.

5. LO 26.5   A three-dimensional radiologic technique that uses nuclear technology to record pictures of internal anatomical sites.

6. LO 26.5   A specialized computer scanner with very fine detail that records imaging of internal anatomical sites.

7. LO 26.9   The high-speed discharge and projection of energy waves or particles.

8. LO 26.5   The recording of a picture of an anatomical joint after the administration of contrast material into the joint capsule.

9. LO 26.10 Treatment that includes the injection or digestion of isotopes.

10. LO 26.5 MR imaging of an anatomical joint after the administration of contrast material into the joint capsule.

11. LO 26.5 A CT scan using contrast materials to visualize arteries and veins all over the body.

A. Angiography

B. Arthrography

C. Computed Tomography (CT)

D. Computed Tomography Angiography (CTA)

E. Fluoroscope

F. Magnetic Resonance Arthrography (MRA)

G. Magnetic Resonance Imaging (MRI)

H. Nuclear Medicine

I. Radiation

J. Sonogram

K. Venography

Let's Check It! Concepts

Choose the most appropriate answer for each of the following questions.

1. LO 26.3 The professional component of radiologic services includes

   a. repair of the equipment.
   b. interpretation of the imaging.
   c. supplies.
   d. training.

2. LO 26.1 Interventional radiologic services are provided with the intent of all *except*

   a. diagnosing a condition.

   b. preventing the spread of a disease.

   c. measuring the progress of a disease.

   d. testing the equipment.

3. LO 26.10 Dani Thompson presents for a thyroid carcinoma metastases imaging; limited area (neck and chest only). What radiology code would you assign?

   a. 78012   **b.** 78013   **c.** 78014   **d.** 78015

4. LO 26.5 The phrase "with contrast" means that the technician or radiologist

   a. administered a substance to enhance the image.

   b. used a black background behind the patient.

   c. took the image a second time, to compare to the first.

   d. used a blue background beneath the patient.

5. LO 26.4 If the code description includes the phrase "two views" and the radiology reports show that only one view was taken, you should code the service

   a. with that code alone.

   b. with that code plus the modifier 52.

   c. with that code plus the modifier 53.

   d. with that code plus the modifier 22.

6. LO 26.6 Therapeutic transcatheter radiologic supervision and interpretation codes, when associated with intervention, include all of the following *except*

   a. vessel measurement.

   b. postangioplasty or stent venography.

   c. catheter placement.

   d. contrast injections, angiography/venography, road mapping, and/or fluoroscopic guidance for the interventional procedure.

7. LO 26.4 RPO stands for

   a. right procedure operation.   b. regional protocol obstetric.

   c. right posterior oblique.   d. right preventive oblique.

8. LO 26.9 Radiation for the treatment of a malignant neoplasm is most often used for

   a. diagnostic purposes.

   b. therapeutic purposes.

   c. research purposes.

   d. prevention purposes.

9. LO 26.1 An x-ray is the same as

   a. a CTA.   b. a CT.   c. an MRI.   d. a radiologic exam.

10. LO 26.10 Nuclear medicine uses tiny quantities of radioactive material, also known as _____, in conjunction with a scintillation or gamma camera to record the emissions from the _____ to create an image of the anatomical site.

   a. isotopes, tracers   b. tracers, isotopes

   c. tracers, tracers   d. tracers, drugs

Let's Check It! Guidelines

Refer to the Radiology Guidelines and fill in the blanks accordingly.

Imaging	joint	arthrography	new
contrast	surgical	not	Medicine
injection	analog	MR	integral
access	"with contrast"	rarely	enhancement
descriptors	intravascular	signed	without
qualify	included	needle	service

1. A service that is _____ provided, unusual, variable, or _____ may require a special report.

2. _____ may be required during the performance of certain procedures or certain imaging procedures may require surgical procedures to _____ the imaged area.

3. Many services include image guidance, and imaging guidance is _____ separately reportable when it is included in the base service.

4. When imaging is not included in a _____ procedure or procedure from the _____ section, image guidance codes or codes labeled "radiological supervision and interpretation" may be reported for the portion of the _____ that requires imaging.

5. The phrase _____ used in the codes for procedures performed using contrast for imaging _____ represents contrast material administered intravascularly, intra-articularly, or intrathecally.

6. For intra-articular injection, use the appropriate _____ injection code.

7. If radiographic _____ is performed, also use the arthrography supervision and interpretation code for the appropriate joint.

8. If computed tomography or magnetic resonance arthrography are performed _____ radiographic arthrography, use the appropriate joint _____ code, the appropriate CT or _____ code, and the appropriate imaging guidance code for _____ placement for contrast injection.

9. Injection of _____ contrast material is part of the "with contrast" CT, computed tomographic angiography, magnetic resonance imaging and magnetic resonance angiography procedure.

10. Oral and/or rectal _____ administration alone does not _____ as a study "with contrast."

11. A written report _____ by the interpreting individual should be considered an _____ part of a radiologic procedure or interpretation.

12. With regard to CPT _____ for imaging services, "images" must contain anatomic information unique to the patient for which the imaging service is provided. "Images" refer to those acquired in either an _____ or digital manner.

Let's Check It! Rules and Regulations

Please answer the following questions from the knowledge you have gained after reading this chapter.

1. **LO 26.3** Differentiate between the technical component and professional component and identify the modifiers that represent each component.

2. **LO 26.2** What is the difference between a screening image and a diagnostic image? Why is it important for the professional coder to know the difference?

3. **LO 26.2** When a screening test turns into a diagnostic test, what service(s) should be reported?

4. **LO 26.9** What is radiation oncology? What do the codes in this subsection already include?

5. **LO 26.10** What are the types of nuclear medicine tests that are used to identify a health concern?

YOU CODE IT! Basics

First, identify the procedural main term in the following statements; then code the procedure or service.

Example: Dr. Bradford performs a CT scan of the brain without contrast material:

a. main term: *CT*   **b.** procedure: *70450*

1. Dr. Gray takes an eye x-ray for detection of foreign body:

   a. main term: _____   **b.** procedure: _____

2. Dr. Robertson takes a CT scan of the pelvis with contrast:

   a. main term: _____   **b.** procedure: _____

3. Dr. Banks performs a renal ultrasound, complete, real-time with image documentation:

   a. main term: _____   **b.** procedure: _____

4. Dr. Hicks takes a panoramic x-ray:

   a. main term: _____   **b.** procedure: _____

5. Dr. Louche administers brachytherapy, intracavitary radiation, 8 sources:

   a. main term: _____   **b.** procedure: _____

6. Dr. Pullets performs a liver SPECT (single photon emission computed tomography) with vascular flow tomography:

   a. main term: _____   **b.** procedure: _____

7. Dr. Roof completes PET imaging of a heart:

   a. main term: _____   **b.** procedure: _____

8. Dr. Darby performs a ureteral reflux study:

   a. main term: _____   **b.** procedure: _____

9. Dr. Allister takes a unilateral x-ray of ribs, 2 views:

   a. main term: _____   **b.** procedure: _____

10. Dr. Alexander completes kidney imaging morphology:

    a. main term: _____   **b.** procedure: _____

11. Dr. Steiner performs a DXA scan, hips:

    a. main term: _____   **b.** procedure: _____

12. Dr. Smyth completes a radiopharmaceutical localization of inflammatory process; whole body:

    a. main term: _____   **b.** procedure: _____

13. Dr. Benton performs radiopharmaceutical therapy by intra-articular administration:

    a. main term: _____   **b.** procedure: _____

14. Dr. Gilbert completes an angiography, extremity (arm), bilateral, radiological supervision and interpretation:

    a. main term: _____   **b.** procedure: _____

15. Dr. Johannson performs an MRI, spinal canal and contents, lumbar; without contrast material:

    a. main term: _____   **b.** procedure: _____

YOU CODE IT! Practice

Using the techniques described in this chapter, carefully read through the case studies and determine the most accurate radiology CPT code(s) and modifier(s), if appropriate, for each case study.

1. Edith Shapin, a 24-year-old female, is pregnant for the first time and is at approximately 11-weeks gestation. She is brought into the diagnostic center for a fetal biophysical profile with nonstress testing.

2. William Browne, a 15-year-old male, is brought into Dr. Jenkins's office with severe right leg pain. Dr. Jenkins takes x-rays of his right femur, AP and PA, to determine whether or not Bill's leg is fractured.

3. Martha Lightfood, an 82-year-old female, was brought into Dr. Morrison's office by her daughter because Martha was complaining of a sharp pain in her chest. After a negative EKG, Dr. Morrison had a quantitative differential pulmonary perfusion and ventilation study performed, which confirmed a pulmonary embolism. Martha was taken immediately by ambulance to the hospital. Code the quantitative differential pulmonary perfusion and ventilation study only.

4. Dr. Logan saw Jason Miolo, a 38-year-old male, with a swollen right eye and loss of vision. Dr. Logan ordered a CT with contrast of the right eye and area, which revealed marked proptosis of the right orbit, thrombosis, and enlargement of the right superior ophthalmic vein.

5. Carl Gadsden, a 66-year-old male, was diagnosed with intrinsic laryngeal cancer, supraglottic T1 tumor. With the tumor confined to one subsite in the supraglottis, Dr. Yoshihashi provided radiation treatment delivery, with a single port, simple block, of 4.5 MeV.

6. Olivia Kane, a 33-year-old female, came into Kinsey Imaging Center for her annual screening mammogram. Due to her family history of malignant neoplasms of the breast (both her mother and sister have been diagnosed), the mammogram was ordered with computer-aided detection (CAD).

7. Brianna Haralson, a 24-year-old female, is brought into Dr. Duncan's office with sharp pains in her lower right abdomen, shooting across to the left side. Dr. Duncan ordered some blood work and an MRA to confirm the suspected diagnosis of acute appendicitis. Code the MRA.

8. Charles Gresham, a 40-year-old male, was in training at Cape Canaveral when he hit his head in a weightlessness simulator, causing him to lose consciousness for 3 minutes. Charles was transported to the nearest hospital, where Dr. Neumours, the ED on-call physician, took a skull x-ray, three views, and did an MRI without contrast of Charles's brain.

9. Jonelle Graybar, a 73-year-old female, was experiencing pain in her back that radiated around her trunk. She was also suffering with spastic muscle weakness. Dr. Maxwell ordered a radioisotope bone scan of Jonelle's lumbar spinal area. The scan identified a metastatic invasion of L1–L3.

10. Maxine Zeigleman, newly diagnosed with metastatic lumbar spinal tumors, has been referred to Dr. Appleton for the creation of a simple radiation therapy plan.

11. Vernon Unger had been diagnosed with a malignancy and came today for intravenous radiopharmaceutical therapy.

12. Before beginning a series of treatments, Anna Hogan came to the Diagnostic Imaging Center for a metabolic evaluation PET scan of her brain.

13. Ira Morgan, a 16-month-old male, was brought to radiology for a real-time, limited, static ultrasound of his hips.

14. Xavier Pollack, a 62-year-old male, arrived at the Kinsey Imaging Center to have a SPECT (single photon emission computed tomography) performed on his left kidney.

15. Dr. Astrone performed a complete ultrasound evaluation of Alden Roberts's pelvis. The procedure included evaluation and measurement of Alden's urinary bladder, evaluation of his prostate and seminal vesicles, and pathology of his enlarged prostate.

 YOU CODE IT! Application

The following exercises provide practice in the application of abstracting the physicians' notes and learning to work with documentation from our Kinsey Imaging Center. These case studies are modeled on real patient encounters. Using the techniques described in this chapter, carefully read through the case studies and determine the most accurate radiology CPT code(s) and modifier(s), if appropriate, for each case study. You are coding for the radiologist.

KINSEY IMAGING CENTER

951 SYDNEY STREET • SOMEWHERE, FL 32811 • 407-555-3573

PATIENT: SAVOY, MARCELLA

ACCOUNT/EHR#: SAVOMA001

DATE: 09/17/19

Procedure Performed: MRI, Spinal canal, thoracic, 3 views

                       CT, abdomen/pelvis

(continued)

Radiologist: Keith Robbins, MD

Referring Physician: Oscar R. Prader, MD

INDICATIONS: Probable metastatic disease, T1–T3, asymptomatic; metastatic mucinous adenocarcinoma of unknown primary

IMPRESSIONS: MRI scans also showed edema at T1, T2, and T3, but no obvious metastatic disease. In the course of her evaluation, a CT of the abdomen and pelvis showed some mild common bile duct dilation, but no obvious primary malignancy.

Keith Robbins, MD

KR/mg   D: 09/17/19 09:50:16   T: 09/20/19 12:55:01

Determine the most accurate radiology CPT code(s) and modifier(s), if appropriate.

KINSEY IMAGING CENTER

951 SYDNEY STREET • SOMEWHERE, FL 32811 • 407-555-3573

PATIENT: JAQUARD, JOEL

ACCOUNT/EHR#: JAQUJO001

DATE: 10/01/19

Procedure Performed: X-rays, skull, two views

CT, soft tissue of neck, with contrast

MRI, brain stem

Radiologist: Robyn Campbell, MD

Referring Physician: Renee O. Bracker, MD

INDICATIONS: Concussion, after fall from ladder

IMPRESSIONS: 1. Full muscle and tendon retraction of the supraspinatus and infraspinatus structures.

2. Bruising and possible microfractures to the skull at occipital base.

3. Other partial tearing of the superior aspect of the semispinalis capitis

RC/mg   D: 10/01/19 09:50:16   T: 10/02/19 12:55:01

Determine the most accurate radiology CPT code(s) and modifier(s), if appropriate.

KINSEY IMAGING CENTER

951 SYDNEY STREET • SOMEWHERE, FL 32811 • 407-555-3573

PATIENT: BURMAN, CECILIA

ACCOUNT/EHR#: BURMCE001

DATE: 10/17/19

Procedure Performed: MRI, brain, no contrast

MRA, brain, no contrast

MRA, neck, no contrast

(continued)

Radiologist: Eryn Alberts, MD

Clinical Information: Evaluate for VP shunt

No prior studies available for a comparison

TECHNICAL INFORMATION: The examination was performed without the use of intravenous contrast material.

INTERPRETATION: Evaluation of the posterior fossa demonstrates hydrocephalus versus low pressure communicating hydrocephalus.

Eryn Alberts, MD

EA/mg   D: 10/17/19 09:50:16   T: 10/20/19 12:55:01

Determine the most accurate radiology CPT code(s) and modifier(s), if appropriate.

KINSEY IMAGING CENTER

951 SYDNEY STREET • SOMEWHERE, FL 32811 • 407-555-3573

PATIENT: TREMONT, GARETT

ACCOUNT/EHR#: TREMGA001

DATE: 11/05/19

EXAMINATION: Chest and abdomen

CLINICAL HISTORY: Fever

CHEST: AP supine and lateral films demonstrate no evidence of alveolar infiltrate or consolidation or pleural effusion. The mediastinal structures are not enlarged. There is very mild increase in central bronchovascular markings. There is no evidence of focal destructive bone lesion.

IMPRESSION: No infiltrate.

ABDOMEN: Supine and erect films demonstrate mild to moderate dilatation of loops of small bowel with short air/fluid levels on the erect film. The large bowel is within normal limits in size but is visualized to the level of the splenic flexure. There is no air visualized in the remainder of the colon. The findings are not specific but consistent with ileus. Further clinical correlation is advised. There is no evidence of focal destructive bone lesion. There is no suspicious calcification in the upper abdomen.

IMPRESSIONS: Abdominal bowel pattern, not specific, consistent with ileus.

Milton Harrison, MD

MH/mg   D: 11/05/19 09:50:16   T: 11/07/19 12:55:01

Determine the most accurate radiology CPT code(s) and modifier(s), if appropriate.

KINSEY IMAGING CENTER

951 SYDNEY STREET • SOMEWHERE, FL 32811 • 407-555-3573

PATIENT: WILLARD, NADINE

ACCOUNT/EHR#: WILLNA001

DATE: 09/29/19

(continued)

Procedure Performed: CT angiography of the head, without contrast and with contrast

Radiologist: Kevin Linnard, MD

Referring Physician: Renee O. Bracker, MD

INDICATIONS: Left CVA

IMPRESSIONS: The current study is compared with the previous one of 05-25-14.

Compared with the previous study, there is a focal area of hypodensity present in the right posterior cerebral arterial distribution adjacent to the falx, a finding suspicious for a small acute infarction, non-hemorrhagic, most likely the parieto-occipital branch.

No other abnormality detected. There are no intra- or extra-axial hemorrhages. There is no significant midline shift or hydrocephalus.

Small new area as described above is suspicious for an area of acute infarction in the right posterior cerebral arterial distribution, likely the occipital branch. Please clinically correlate.

Kevin Linnard, MD

KL/mg   D: 09/29/19 09:50:16   T: 09/30/19 12:55:01

Determine the most accurate radiology CPT code(s) and modifier(s), if appropriate.

27 CPT Pathology & Lab Section

Key Terms

Cytology
Etiology
Gross Examination
Laboratory
Microscopic
 Examination
Pathology
Qualitative
Quantitative
Specimen
Surgical Pathology

Learning Outcomes

After completing this chapter, the student should be able to:

LO 27.1 Recognize key factors involved in pathology testing.
LO 27.2 Identify testing methodologies and sources.
LO 27.3 Report panel codes when qualified.
LO 27.4 Analyze blood test reports to ensure accurate reporting.
LO 27.5 Discern clinical chemistry studies.
LO 27.6 Interpret details about molecular diagnostic testing.
LO 27.7 Distinguish immunologic, microbiologic, and cytopathologic testing.
LO 27.8 Abstract the correct details to report surgical pathology testing.
LO 27.9 Append the correct modifier, when required.
LO 27.10 Accurately interpret the abbreviations used most often in pathology and laboratory reports.

 STOP! Remember, you need to follow along in your <u>CPT</u> code book for an optimal learning experience.

27.1 Specimen Collection and Testing

As physicians and health care professionals work to help their patients, very often they need medical science to guide them. The guidance frequently comes from tests performed by professionals working in a **laboratory**, studying the evolution of a patient's disease. This type of study is called **pathology**, which includes **etiology**.

Pathology and lab testing help detect the early presence of disease, ruling out or confirming conditions that might have similar symptoms yet need to be treated differently. The results of these tests also may predict the occurrence of disease in the future. You probably already know from your own experiences the importance of such work. Your annual physical has possibly included blood tests to measure your cholesterol. Physicians order blood work to confirm pregnancy or a urinalysis to determine if a symptom could be the result of an infection. Testing takes time and the expertise of professionals educated in interpreting the results. It also takes materials and resources.

A specimen sent to the lab for testing may be from any number of different sources:

- Blood
- Urine

Laboratory
A location with scientific equipment designed to perform experiments and tests.

Pathology
The study of the nature, etiology, development, and outcomes of disease.

Etiology
The original source or cause for the development of a disease; also, the study of the causes of disease.

- Other bodily fluids, such as
  - sputum
  - sperm
  - mucus
- Tissue
- An organ

CODING BITES

Every pathology or lab test requires specimens to examine. In some cases, you may need to report the collection of the specimen separately.

For example:

36415   Collection of venous blood by venipuncture
83930   Osmolality; blood

Be alert to the fact that the collection of the specimen may be provided at a separate facility from the lab, in which case, each facility would report the code for the part performed.

CODING BITES

When you code pathology and laboratory work, you may be reporting the work provided by the professional performing the test and interpreting the results (the pathologist), or you may be reporting for the facility that provided the testing.

As a coding specialist, you may work for a health care organization that has a laboratory within its facilities, a billing company that codes everything, or an independent facility that does nothing other than taking and analyzing **specimens**. In any case, you should understand the different aspects of pathology and lab testing and procedures, as well as the guidelines involved in coding the services.

Specimen
A small part or sample of any substance obtained for analysis and diagnosis.

 LET'S CODE IT! SCENARIO

Cynthia Cardamen, a 33-year-old female, was not feeling well, so she went to see her family physician, Dr. Slater. After talking with her and performing an exam, Dr. Slater began to suspect that Cynthia had diabetes mellitus, type 2. Reagan Dram, the nurse, obtained a specimen of capillary blood from Cynthia's left index finger and took it to Abbey Carmichael, who ran their in-house lab, for a glucose test to be performed. She used a reagent strip to perform the test and delivered the results to Dr. Slater.

Let's Code It!

There are two steps to this test: the collection of the specimen and the testing of that blood to determine Cynthia's glucose level.

Let's turn to the CPT Alphabetic Index, and find

Collection and Processing
Specimen
      Capillary Blood...............36416

Now, turn to the *Main Section* of CPT and find

36416   **Collection of capillary blood specimen (e.g., finger, heel, ear stick)**

Now, we must report the test that Abbey will perform on this blood specimen. Dr. Slater ordered a blood glucose test. Turn in the Alphabetic Index to

Glucose
Blood Test.................82947, 82948, 82950

(continued)

This time, we have three different codes to investigate.

82947   **Glucose; quantitative, blood (except reagent strip)**
82948   **Glucose; blood, reagent strip**
82950   **Glucose; post glucose dose (includes glucose)**

Compare the details in these code descriptions to the details you have in the documentation. Code 82948 matches.

36416   **Collection of capillary blood specimen (e.g., finger, heel, ear stick)**
82948   **Glucose; blood, reagent strip**

Good work!

27.2 Testing Methodology and Desired Results

Although no one expects you, as the coding specialist, to be completely knowledgeable about the details of laboratory and pathology testing, you will need certain information about how the tests are performed in order to code them correctly. This may begin with exactly what type of properties are needed, going beyond just the name of the test itself.

Types of Test Results

Quantitative
The counting or measurement of something.

Qualitative
The determination of character or essential element(s).

Two of the types of results that lab tests can evidence are **quantitative** and **qualitative**. These details can support a physician's medical decision making, especially when trying to determine an accurate diagnosis or identify the success of a treatment, or lack of success of a treatment.

For example, serum calcium tests are used to assess parathyroid function and calcium metabolism. The quantitative results (total amount of calcium in the blood) also can be used to check on patients with renal failure.

Other tests you may be familiar with are white blood cell (WBC) count (quantitative) and differential count (qualitative and quantitative) tests. These tests are part of routine blood testing. The quantitative totals can provide important diagnostic details—for example, an increased white blood cell count usually identifies the presence of an infection, inflammation, tissue necrosis, or leukemic neoplasia, while a decreased total white blood cell count can be present due to bone marrow failure, indicating a potential immunocompromised patient.

> ### EXAMPLES
> **Calcium**
>
> 82310   Calcium; total
> 82330   Calcium; ionized
> 82331   Calcium; after calcium infusion test
> 82340   Calcium; urine quantitative, timed specimen
>
> **White Blood Cell**
>
> 85004   Blood count; automated differential WBC count
> 85007   Blood count; blood smear, microscopic examination with manual differential WBC count
>
> *(continued)*

| 85008 | Blood count; blood smear, microscopic examination without manual differential WBC count |
| 85009 | Blood count; manual differential WBC count, buffy coat |

The guidelines tell you that, if the documentation does not specify, you may assume that the examination performed was quantitative. However, remember that documentation is absolute in the health care industry. Therefore, it is recommended that you query the lab technician or pathologist and request that the report include this important detail.

Testing Methodologies

For other testing, you might see the details about the methodology of the testing. Some of the terms you will notice in test descriptions and their codes include

- By dipstick.
- Automated or nonautomated.
- With or without microscopy.
- Visual or gross inspection.

These terms refer to the methods that the lab technicians use to test the specimen and obtain the results.

 LET'S CODE IT! SCENARIO

Margaret O'Hanahan came to see Dr. Marinson. She states that she has been feeling a stinging pain when she urinates. She confirms some lower back aches but denies hematuria. Dr. Marinson asks Margaret to go into the bathroom and provide a urine sample, which is then tested in the office by dipstick, automated without microscopy.

Let's Code It!

Dr. Marinson is performing a *urinalysis, by dipstick, automated.* Turn to *urinalysis* in your CPT Alphabetic Index.

Urinalysis
Automated.........81001, 81003

These two listings fit the details according to the documentation, so turn to the *Main Section* and read these code descriptions.

81000	Urinalysis, by dip stick or tablet reagent for bilirubin, glucose, hemoglobin, ketones, leukocytes, nitrite, pH, protein, specific gravity, urobilinogen, any number of these constituents; nonautomated, with microscopy
81001	Urinalysis, by dip stick or tablet reagent for bilirubin, glucose, hemoglobin, ketones, leukocytes, nitrite, pH, protein, specific gravity, urobilinogen, any number of these constituents; automated, with microscopy
81002	Urinalysis, by dip stick or tablet reagent for bilirubin, glucose, hemoglobin, ketones, leukocytes, nitrite, pH, protein, specific gravity, urobilinogen, any number of these constituents; nonautomated, without microscopy
81003	Urinalysis, by dip stick or tablet reagent for bilirubin, glucose, hemoglobin, ketones, leukocytes, nitrite, pH, protein, specific gravity, urobilinogen, any number of these constituents; automated, without microscopy

(continued)

Go back to the scenario and abstract the details about the test. The documentation states, "*dipstick, automated without microscopy.*" When you read all of these code descriptions, you can see that only one accurately reports this specific test:

81003   Urinalysis, by dip stick or tablet reagent for bilirubin, glucose, hemoglobin, ketones, leukocytes, nitrite, pH, protein, specific gravity, urobilinogen, any number of these constituents; automated, without microscopy

Good work!

In addition to how the test is performed, you must also know the type of specimen involved in the testing and, sometimes, how many specimens or sources are involved. The type of specimen being tested may change the code. Consider a physician ordering a potassium test. Let's go to the Alphabetic Index for *potassium.*

EXAMPLE

Potassium.................. 84132
Urine........................... 84133

The first code in the example, listed next to the word *potassium,* is code 84132, but it does not contain any additional descriptors. However, the second code, listed under *potassium,* indicates that it would be the code used if the potassium were tested from the patient's urine rather than blood (serum). When you look at the codes' complete descriptions in the numeric listing, you see the details shown.

EXAMPLE

84132   Potassium; serum, plasma, or whole blood
84133   urine

The listings clearly show that there is a difference as to which code is correct based on the source of the specimen.

In certain circumstances, an analysis may be performed on multiple specimens collected at different times or from different sources. In these cases, the guidelines tell you to code each source and each specimen separately. However, be certain to always read the code descriptions carefully. Some codes already include multiple tests and/or multiple sources.

 LET'S CODE IT! SCENARIO

Gilian Morrison, RN, performs a rapid influenza test using a commercial test kit in the office to determine if Hester Childs has the virus. This way the results can be provided while Hester is still in with Dr. Alberts. When complete, Nurse Morrison visually reads the result as positive.

Let's Code It!

For this scenario, you are going to focus only on reporting the provision of the rapid influenza test. The first place you look in the CPT Alphabetic Index is under the word *Test.* However, there is nothing there, so let's look up the term *Influenza.* There are several choices. Let's analyze them.

The first two choices are titled *Influenza A* and *Influenza B*. There is nothing in the notes about which this might be. Before querying the nurse or doctor, let's keep reading.

The next listing is *Influenza Vaccine*. There is nothing in the notes stating that Hester was given a vaccination, so this is not applicable to this encounter.

The last listing category is titled *Influenza Virus*. This could be possible because the notes state the test was given to "determine if Hester has the virus." Two codes are suggested here:

Antibody..86710
Detection
    by Immunoassay with Direct Optical Observation............................87804
    by Nucleic Acid...87501–87503

Let's turn to the *Main Section* of CPT, look for these two possible codes in the **Pathology and Laboratory** section, and read the complete code descriptions.

86710   **Antibody; influenza virus**

87804   **Infectious agent antigen detection by immunoassay with direct optical observation; influenza**

When you read the scenario and the complete code description, you can see how code **87804** matches accurately.

27.3 Panels

A pathology report, such as the one shown in Figure 27-1, will typically itemize the tests performed for the patient along with the results of each test.

When you turn to the **Pathology and Laboratory** section of the CPT book, you will notice that many codes include a long list of tests within one code's description. These groupings of tests commonly performed at the same time are called *panels*.

EXAMPLE

80051   Electrolyte panel

This panel must include the following:

Carbon dioxide (82374)
Chloride (82435)
Potassium (84132)
Sodium (84295)

```
                              LIPID PROFILE
-------------------------------------------------------------------------
Day                    2
Date              05/16/05
Time                0610                          Reference        U
-------------------------------------------------------------------------
CHOLESTEROL            166                        (140-200)        M
TRIGLYCERIDE           104                        (35-160)         M
HDL                     83                        (35-85)          M
LDL (CALC)             63(a)                       (60-129)         M
VLDL (CALC)             20                        (5-40)           M
CHOL/HDL RATIO         2.0(b)                                       R


NOTES:   (a)   LDL GOAL:
               <100 FOR PATIENTS WITH CHD, DM OR VASCULAR DISEASE.
         (b)   LOWEST CHD RISK
```

FIGURE 27-1 Sample lab report showing the tests run as part of a lipid profile

This example shows you that, in order for you to report code 80051 legally and accurately, the lab must have performed all four tests: carbon dioxide, chloride, potassium, and sodium.

If the lab performed fewer than *all* the tests listed in a panel, you must report the code for each test separately; you are *not* permitted to use the panel code.

Again, the CPT book will help you. Should you have to code any of the tests separately, each test code is given in parentheses right next to the name of the test listed there. From our example, next to carbon dioxide, you can see the number 82374. Turn to code 82374, and you will see that it is the code for testing carbon dioxide alone.

Let's say, instead of fewer tests than those listed in a panel, the lab performs more tests. The guidelines state that you are to report those additional tests, those not included in the panel code, separately and additionally.

 LET'S CODE IT! SCENARIO

Concerned that Keisha Evans, a 51-year-old female, might be suffering from hypercholesterolemia, Dr. Rawlins ordered blood work, including a total cholesterol serum test, lipoprotein (direct measurement of high-density lipoprotein), and triglycerides. He also added a potassium serum test to the order.

Let's Code It!

The lab performed four tests: *total cholesterol serum test, lipoprotein (direct measurement of high-density lipoprotein), triglycerides,* and *potassium serum.* When you look up the tests individually, you are directed to codes for each. However, when it comes to pathology and laboratory coding, you must take an extra step.

Turn to the numeric listings at the beginning of the **Pathology and Laboratory** section, where you find the standardized panels listed. Review the list of tests included in each of the panels and match it with the list of tests Dr. Rawlins ordered. You see that code **80061 Lipid Panel** includes three of the four tests performed.

80061   Lipid Panel

Since none of the panels includes all four tests, you use the lipid panel code and code the potassium test additionally, code 84132.

84132   Potassium; serum, plasma, or whole blood

Therefore, you have two codes for the lab work's claim: 80061 and 84132.
   Good job!

 GUIDANCE CONNECTION

Read the additional explanations in the in-section guidelines located within the **Pathology and Laboratory** section, subhead **Organ or Disease-Oriented Panels,** directly above code 80047 in your CPT book.

27.4 Blood Test Documentation

Determining the code for a blood test can be complex, as you are learning in this chapter. The lab report (see Figure 27-2) is an important part of the documentation you will have to report the performing of the tests.

- *Bicarbonate:* Kidneys and lungs keep bicarbonate balanced to maintain homeostatic pH levels (ensure a balance of acid and alkali levels). Abnormal levels can indicate dysfunction of these organs (kidneys and lungs).

- *Blood culture:* This test measures the presence of bacteria or yeast in the blood, which is used to confirm (or deny) a suspected infection or sepsis.

- *Blood differential (Diff):* This test measures numbers of WBCs, which are used to identify presence of infection. Normal is less than 20%.

- *Blood urea nitrogen (BUN):* This test measures kidney function. A low count might indicate malnutrition, while a high count may identify the presence of heart failure, kidney disease, or liver disease. Normal range: 7–20 milligrams per deciliter (mg/dL).

- *Creatinine:* This test measures levels of this chemical excreted by the kidneys. It is used to determine muscle damage, dehydration, and/or kidney dysfunction. Normal range: 0.8–1.4 mg/dL.

- *Erythrocyte sedimentation rate (ESR):* This test measures the speed with which red blood cells cling together, fall, and settle in the bottom of a glass tube within 60 minutes. It is used to detect inflammatory, neoplastic, infectious, and necrotic processes. When inflammation is present, the higher the rate, the greater the amount of inflammation. Normal range: male = up to 15 millimeters per hour (mm/h); female = up to 20 mm/h.

- *Glucose:* This test measures the level of sugar in the blood. Low levels may indicate hypoglycemia or liver disease, whereas high levels may indicate hyperglycemia (diabetes) or hyperthyroidism. Normal range: 70–99 mg/dL.

- *Hematocrit (HCT):* This test identifies the percentage of RBCs, which is used to identify anemia. Low counts may indicate bone marrow damage or vitamin deficiency, while high counts may indicate congenital heart disease, renal problems, or pulmonary disease. Normal range: 34%–45%.

- *Hemoglobin (Hgb):* This test measures oxygen being carried by the RBCs. Low counts may indicate bone marrow damage or vitamin deficiency, while high counts may indicate congenital heart disease, renal problems, or pulmonary disease. Normal range: 11.5–15.5 grams per deciliter (g/dL).

- *Mean corpuscular hemoglobin (MCH):* This test measures the amount of hemoglobin in RBCs. A low number may indicate an iron deficiency, whereas a high number may indicate a vitamin deficiency. Normal range: 27–34 picograms (pg).

- *Mean corpuscular volume (MCV):* This test identifies the average size of the RBCs. Small size may indicate an iron deficiency, whereas a large reading may indicate a vitamin deficiency. Normal range: 80–100 femtoliters (fL).

LABORATORIES

	Augusta, GA.	Orlando, FL	Tampa, FL
	Tel:	Tel:	Tel:
	Fax:	Fax:	Fax:

Patient:
DOB:　　　　　Age:　Yrs　Sex:
PID:
Phone:
Episode:
Notes:
Copy to:

Collecting Time:	03/26/20	08:27	PHYSICIAN
Log in DT/TM:	03/27/20	00:57	550
Report DT/TM:	03/27/20	05:02	
Reprint DT/TM:	03/31/20	10:07	
FASTING: Y	Priority: R		Physician:

P96

TEST NAME	RESULT	UNITS	REF RANGE	LAB
COMPREHENSIVE METABOLIC PANEL WITH eGFR				ORL
Sodium	139	mEq/L	(133–146)	
Potassium	3.9	mEq/L	(3.5–5.4)	
Chloride	101	mEq/L	(97–110)	
Carbon Dioxide	31	mEq/L	(21–33)	
Anion Gap	7.0	mEq/L	(5.0–15.0)	
Glucose	96	mg/dL	(65–100)	
BUN	11	mg/dL	(8–25)	
Creatinine	0.64	mg/dL	(0.6–1.4)	
eGFR African American	113	mL/min	(>60)	
eGFR Non-African Am.	98	mL/min	(>60)	
BUN/Creatinine Ratio	17		(6–28)	
Calcium	9.3	mg/dL	(8.2–10.6)	
Total Protein	7.2	g/dL	(6.0–8.3)	
Albumin	4.5	g/dL	(3.5–5.7)	
Globulin	2.7	g/dL	(1.6–4.2)	
A/G Ratio	1.7		(0.9–2.5)	
Bilirubin Total	0.5	mg/dL	(0.1–1.30	
Alkaline Phosphatase	87	U/L	(35–126)	
AST (SGOT)	17	U/L	(5–43)	
ALT (SGPT)	11	U/L	(7–56)	
TSH	4.199	uIU/mL	(0.550–4.780)	ORL
Free T4	1.16	ng/dL	(0.89–1.76)	ORL
LIPID PANEL				
Cholesterol	H　243	mg/dL	(80–199)	
Triglycerides	188	mg/dL	(30–150)	
HDL Cholesterol	55	mg/dL	(40–110)	
LDL Cholesterol Calc	141	mg/dL	(30–130)	
VLDL Cholesterol Calc	28	mg/dL	(10–60)	
Risk Ratio (CHOL/HDL)	3.6	Ratio	(0.0–5.0)	
Non-HDL Cholesterol	145	mg/dL		

Cholesterol/HDL	Ratio	Interpretation:	
Gender	CVD	Risk Category	
Female			
	Average Risk		4.4
	Twice Average Risk		71

Printed at: 03/31/20　10:07　　　　　　　"CONTINUED REPORT"

FIGURE 27-2 Pathology report showing a list of all of the individual blood tests run for the patient, including results and reference ranges

- *Partial thromboplastin time (PTT):* This test measures factors I (fibrinogen), II (prothrombin), V, VIII, IX, X, XI, and XII. Inadequate quantities of these factors cause the PTT to be prolonged, a delay in the clotting of the blood that increases the opportunity for the patient to hemorrhage. Normal PTT: 60–70 seconds.

- *Platelet count:* Low platelet counts can indicate a clotting disorder, putting the patient at risk for hemorrhage. Low levels may indicate pernicious anemia, lupus, or a viral infection, while high levels may identify leukemia. Normal range: 150–400 thousand per microliter (K/mcL).

- *Potassium:* This test measures levels of potassium in the blood. Low potassium levels can cause muscle cramps and/or weakness; abnormal levels (too high or low) can result in an abnormal heartbeat. Low levels can identify use of corticosteroids or diuretics, while high levels may signify kidney failure, diabetes, or Addison's disease. Normal range: 3.7–5.2 milliequivalents per liter (mEq/L).

- *Prothrombin time (PT):* This test evaluates the clotting ability of factors I (fibrinogen), II (prothrombin), V, VII, and X. Low quantities of these clotting factors result in a prolonged PT. PT results include the use of the international normalized ratio (INR) value as well as absolute numbers. Normal PT result: 85%–100% in 11–12.5 seconds and an INR of 0.8–1.1.

- *Sodium:* This test determines if the balance between sodium and liquid in the blood is at the correct proportion. Low levels of sodium can identify the use of diuretics or adrenal insufficiency, while high levels may indicate dehydration or kidney dysfunction. High levels of sodium can lead to hypertension. Normal range: 136–144 mEq/L.

 YOU CODE IT! CASE STUDY

Rosalyn Alvarez, an 84-year-old female, complained to Dr. Files that she was having severe cramps in her legs and hands. She said it has been getting worse the last few months. In Rosalyn's chart, it notes that she has been on diuretics, so Dr. Files orders blood work to quantify her creatinine levels to check on her kidney function. Thelma Brooks, RN, performed the venipuncture and sent the blood specimen to the lab.

You Code It!

Determine the code for the pathology lab testing Rosalyn's blood to quantify the potassium levels.

Step #1: Read the case carefully and completely.

Step #2: Abstract the scenario. Which key words or terms describe what service the physician provided to the patient during this encounter?

Step #3: Are there any details missing or incomplete for which you would need to query the physician? [If so, ask your instructor.]

Step #4: Determine the correct CPT procedure code or codes to explain the details about what was provided to the patient during this encounter.

Step #5: Check for any relevant guidance, including reading all of the symbols and notations.

Step #6: Do you need to append any modifiers to ensure complete and accurate information is provided?

Step #7: Double-check your work.

Answer:

Did you determine this to be the code?

82565   Creatinine; blood

Good job!

27.5 Clinical Chemistry

The lab tests that are most commonly performed use chemical processes to distinguish qualities and quantities of elements in the specimens provided. Typically, the specimens are samples of a patient's blood or urine. Tests with which you might be familiar include the following:

- *Blood glucose* (sugar) is used to diagnose conditions such as diabetes mellitus (hyperglycemia) or hypoglycemia.
- *Electrolytes* are used to diagnose metabolic or kidney disorders.
- *Enzymes* can be released into the bloodstream by a damaged or diseased organ. The presence of creatine kinase can indicate damage after a heart attack, or amylase and lipase elevations may be a sign of cancer of the pancreas and/or pancreatitis.
- *Hormones,* such as cortisol, in quantities too high or too low might indicate the malfunction of the patient's adrenal glands.
- *Lipids* (fatty substances) can signal coronary heart disease or liver disease.
- *Metabolic substances,* such as uric acid, at incorrect levels can identify the presence of gout.
- *Proteins* identified at the wrong levels on electrophoresis can point to malnutrition or certain infections.

Many tests can be easily performed in the physician's office with a small amount of blood or urine. Companies have created kits that make measuring such elements as simple as dipping a little slip of special paper into the patient's specimen. It means that you have a much greater opportunity to code any number of tests.

GUIDANCE CONNECTION

Read the additional explanations in the in-section guidelines located within the **Pathology and Laboratory** section, subhead **Chemistry,** directly above code 82009 in your CPT book.

YOU CODE IT! CASE STUDY

Charles Endicott, a 31-year-old male, is an up-and-coming stockbroker who does not pay much attention to a proper diet. He came to see his physician, Dr. Falacci, because he has been experiencing episodes of light-headedness. Dr. Falacci asks his assistant, Carla Falco, to do a quantitative blood glucose test. Carla takes a blood sample, goes to the back, and checks the specimen. The results indicate that Charles has hypoglycemia.

You Code It!

Go through the steps, and determine the pathology/lab code(s) that should be reported for this encounter.

Step #1: Read the case carefully and completely.

Step #2: Abstract the scenario. Which key words or terms describe what service the physician provided to the patient during this encounter?

Step #3: Are there any details missing or incomplete for which you would need to query the physician? [If so, ask your instructor.]

Step #4: Determine the correct CPT procedure code or codes to explain the details about what was provided to the patient during this encounter.

Step #5: Check for any relevant guidance, including reading all of the symbols and notations.

Step #6: Do you need to append any modifiers to ensure complete and accurate information is provided?

Step #7: Double-check your work.

Answer:

Did you determine this to be the correct code?

82947   **Glucose; quantitative, blood (except reagent strip)**

Good work!

27.6 Molecular Diagnostics

Molecular diagnostic tests investigate infectious disease, oncology concerns (malignant neoplasms), hematology (the study of blood and its disorders), neurology, and inherited disorders (genetics).

Specifically, genetic testing involves the analysis of specimens to identify any presence of a genetic disorder. Research and technology have developed testing methodologies for more than 2,000 diseases that can be performed to provide peace of mind, or early detection of diseases and conditions that are passed from parents to child via their genes.

The ability for parents-to-be to determine if they have any conditions that might be passed on to their future children has been found to be an important part of family planning. After conception, embryos and fetuses can be tested to reassure parents, to enable physicians to treat some conditions in utero, or to enable the family to be prepared with accommodations before the baby arrives.

Adults with a family or personal history of a genetic disorder may be tested to provide the option for preventive health care services or treatment as early as possible.

Pharmacogenomic Testing

Physicians are trained to determine the correct medication and dosage to prescribe for their patients based on several factors, including age, weight, personal history, general health, and allergies/sensitivities. In recent years, researchers have discovered that an individual's genes also may affect the efficacy of a specific drug, explaining why one version of a drug may really help one patient while having no or little benefit to another. Evolving from these discoveries has been the development of pharmacogenomic tests to provide specific information that will assist the physician with a more accurate and effective prescription.

GUIDANCE CONNECTION

Read the additional explanations in the in-section guidelines located within the **Pathology and Laboratory** section, subhead **Molecular Pathology,** on the pages directly before code 81170 in your CPT book.

 YOU CODE IT! CASE STUDY

Parker Thomasini, a 4-year-old male, has a cousin who was diagnosed with cystic fibrosis last year. Recently, he has been wheezing and has a dry, nonproductive cough. The fact that his cousin has cystic fibrosis means that Parker has a 25% chance of carrying the disease. Therefore, Dr. Preston ordered a molecular diagnostic test for the mutation of delta F 508 deletion in his DNA by sequencing, single segment.

You Code It!

Go through the steps, and determine the pathology/lab code(s) that should be reported for this encounter.

Step #1: Read the case carefully and completely.

Step #2: Abstract the scenario. Which key words or terms describe what service the physician provided to the patient during this encounter?

Step #3: Are there any details missing or incomplete for which you would need to query the physician? [If so, ask your instructor.]

Step #4: Determine the correct CPT procedure code or codes to explain the details about what was provided to the patient during this encounter.

Step #5: Check for any relevant guidance, including reading all of the symbols and notations.

Step #6: Do you need to append any modifiers to ensure complete and accurate information is provided?

Step #7: Double-check your work.

(continued)

Answer:

Did you determine this to be the correct code?

> **81220**   **CFTR (cystic fibrosis transmembrane conductance regulator) (e.g., cystic fibrosis) gene analysis; common variants (e.g., ACMG/ACOG guidelines)**

Good job!

GUIDANCE CONNECTION

Read the additional explanations in the in-section guidelines located within the **Pathology and Laboratory** section, subhead **Microbiology,** directly above code 87003 in your CPT book.

27.7 Immunology, Microbiology, and Cytopathology

Immunology

Immunology is the study of the body's immune system—how it works and what can go wrong. Immunologic tests identify problems that may occur when a disease causes the body's defense system to attack itself (called an *autoimmune disease*) or when a disease causes a malfunction of the body's immune system (called an *immunodeficiency disorder*). The tests also can evaluate the compatibility of tissues and organs for transplantation.

Conditions and diseases that you may be familiar with, which fall into this category, include rheumatoid arthritis, allergies, and, of course, human immunodeficiency virus (HIV).

LET'S CODE IT! SCENARIO

Nigel Winthrope, a 19-year-old male, was diagnosed with hemophilia many years ago. As a result of a blood transfusion, he contracted HIV. He has come today for lab work to check on his T-cell count, an indicator of whether the HIV is progressing.

Let's Code It!

Nigel is having a test to determine the *count* of *T cells* in his blood. Let's turn to the Alphabetic Index to the letter *T.*

Are you surprised at the many listings with *T cell* in the heading? Read through them all carefully. Remember that Nigel does not have leukemia; he has HIV. Keep going down the list to *T Cells,* under which you see *Count,* with the suggested code 86359.

The complete code description in the numeric listing shows us

> **86359**   **T cells; total count**

Good job!

Microbiology

Microbiologic tests use many different methods to study bacteria, fungi, parasites, and viruses. The specimens used in the tests might be blood, urine, sputum (mucus, also called *phlegm*), feces (stool), cerebrospinal fluid (CSF), and other bodily fluids. Blood cultures are used to diagnose bacterial infections of the blood, sputum cultures can identify respiratory infections like pneumonia, and stool cultures can confirm the presence of pinworms and other parasites.

Code descriptions in this subsection may include some specific terms, such as

- *Presumptive identification.* This is the pathologic identification of colony morphology; growth on selective media (such as a culture or slide); gram stains; or other tests such as catalase, oxidase, indole, or urease. For example: 87081 Culture, presumptive, pathogenic organisms, screening only.

- *Definitive identification.* This is the pathologic identification of the genus or species that requires additional testing, such as biochemical panels or slide cultures. For example: 87106 Culture, fungi, definitive identification, each organism, yeast.

 LET'S CODE IT! SCENARIO

Sally Tong, a 5-year-old female, went to a picnic at the park with her playgroup and had a hamburger, cooked very rare. Later that evening, her parents rushed her to the hospital because she was vomiting and had severe diarrhea. Dr. Warner ordered an infectious agent antigen enzyme immunoassay for E. coli O157. Fortunately, the test was negative, and it turned out that she just had eaten too much ice cream and milk.

Let's Code It!

Dr. Warner ordered "*an infectious agent antigen enzyme immunoassay*" for Sally to determine if she was suffering from *Escherichia coli (E. coli).* Let's go to the Alphabetic Index to *immunoassay* and find *infectious agent* below it, with the suggested codes 86317–86318, 87449–87451. Let's go to the numeric listings and read the complete code descriptions.

86317   Immunoassay for infectious agent antibody, quantitative, not otherwise specified (For immunoassay techniques for antigens, see 83516, 83518, 83519, 83520, 87301–87450, 87810–87899)

The code description states *antibody,* but the notes say *antigen.* Luckily, the CPT book is guiding you via the parenthetical notation below the code description, which directs you to a long list of codes. The descriptions for 83516, 83518, 83519, and 83520 do not come any closer to Dr. Warner's notes. Let's turn to the next set of suggested codes:

87301   Infectious agent antigen detection by immunoassay technique (e.g., enzyme immunoassay [EIA], enzyme-linked immunosorbent assay [ELISA], immunochemiluminometric assay [IMCA]), qualitative or semiquantitative, multiple-step method; adenovirus enteric types 40/41

Read down the list a little farther:

87335   Escherichia coli O157

When you read the complete description, you get the following:

87335   Infectious agent antigen detection by immunoassay technique (e.g., enzyme immunoassay [EIA], enzyme-linked immunosorbent assay [ELISA], immunochemiluminometric assay [IMCA]), qualitative or semiquantitative, multiple-step method; Escherichia coli O157

Sometimes, even with the CPT book pointing at codes, it may take a lot of reading to be certain you have the best, most appropriate code.

Cytopathology and Cytogenetic Studies

Cytology is the study of one cell at a time to discover abnormal cells present in tissue or bodily fluids. Cytologic testing is used to detect cancer cells and infectious organisms and to screen for fetal abnormalities.

    Specimens used in cytopathologic testing are obtained by fine-needle aspirations (as in amniocentesis), scraping of tissue surfaces (as in Pap smears), and collection of bodily fluids (as with sputum or seminal fluid, or sperm).

Cytology
The investigation and identification of cells.

LET'S CODE IT! SCENARIO

Rosalie Panesca, a 47-year-old female, came to see Dr. Sizemore for her annual well-woman checkup. In addition to the examination, Dr. Sizemore took a Pap smear, to be examined using cytopathological testing, specifically, the Bethesda reporting system with manual screening. Rosalie's examination showed she was completely healthy.

Let's Code It!

Dr. Sizemore took a *smear* of tissue for a cytopathologic examination of Rosalie's cervical cells using *the Bethesda reporting system.*

Let's go to the Alphabetic Index to *cytopathology, smears, cervical or vaginal,* with five more choices as to the type: Automated Screen, Hormone Evaluation, Manual Screen, Partially Automated Screen, and Physician Interpretation—each with its own suggested codes. Go back to the documentation and see if you can find any terms that will help you narrow this down. The notes state, "*Bethesda reporting system with manual screening.*" In the Alphabetic Index, you can see that cytopathology, smears, cervical or vaginal, manual screen suggests 88150, 88153, 88164, 88165. Let's go to the *Main Section* and read the complete code descriptions.

Before you begin reading all the code descriptions, read the paragraph of instructions directly before code 88141. You will note that these instructions tell you to "Use codes 88164–88167 to report Pap smears that are examined using the Bethesda System of reporting." That saves you quite a lot of time. Reading that one small paragraph directs you to the four best codes:

88164   **Cytopathology, slides, cervical or vaginal (the Bethesda System); manual screening under physician supervision**

88165   **Cytopathology, slides, cervical or vaginal (the Bethesda System); with manual screening and rescreening and under physician supervision**

88166   **Cytopathology, slides, cervical or vaginal (the Bethesda System); with manual screening and computer-assisted rescreening under physician supervision**

88167   **Cytopathology, slides, cervical or vaginal (the Bethesda System);with manual screening and computer-assisted rescreening using cell selection and review under physician supervision**

Which of these four codes most accurately describes the pathology test done for Rosalie? No rescreening or computer-assisted rescreening is documented. This means the most accurate code for this test is

88164   **Cytopathology, slides, cervical or vaginal (the Bethesda System); manual screening under physician supervision**

Great job!

27.8 Surgical Pathology

Surgical Pathology
The study of tissues removed from a living patient during a surgical procedure.

Gross Examination
The visual study of a specimen (with the naked eye).

Microscopic Examination
The study of a specimen using a microscope (under magnification).

When a biopsy is taken during a surgical procedure (or is the surgical procedure itself), the specimen is sent to the lab for testing. The testing, typically performed immediately upon receipt from the OR, is called **surgical pathology**. Its purpose, much like that of other testing and studies, is to provide the information necessary to diagnose a disease or condition and to set forth a treatment plan. In such cases, all the steps (taking the specimen, testing, diagnosis, and treatment) may occur during one surgical session. The benefit of this quick and immediate process is that there is less trauma for the patient, who has to undergo anesthesia and an invasive procedure only once. In addition, it saves money for the patient, the facility, and the third-party payer.

Codes 88300–88309 represent six levels of surgical pathologic testing. The codes include accession, the testing itself, and the written report from the pathologist. The codes (with the exception of 88300) also include both **gross examination** (also known as macroscopic examination) of the specimen and **microscopic examination**.

The first level, code 88300, is applicable for any and all specimens that are examined only by visual, or gross, examination. It means that the sample has not been looked at under a microscope.

88300   Level I – Surgical pathology, gross examination only

Codes 88302–88309 recognize the various amounts of work required by the pathologist or physician doing the examination to determine the accurate condition of the specimen. Don't worry—you don't have to study pathology to decide which level to use properly to represent the work done. Each code level is determined by the anatomical site from where the specimen was taken. Under each, the sites are listed in alphabetic order. However, you have to know what happened in the OR to find the correct code because that will change the level involved.

Reading the Lab Report

You may find a report, such as the one shown in Figure 27-3, that shows the results of the surgical pathology along with the pathologist's interpretation.

The physician's operative report may state a tissue biopsy was taken; however, you may need more details from the pathologist's report so you can code this accurately. Remember, when you are reporting a code or codes from the *Pathology and Laboratory* section of CPT, you are reporting *for the pathologist,* not the surgeon. The code from the *Surgery* section of CPT will report the *collection* of the specimen, while the code from the *Pathology and Laboratory* section will report the *testing* of the specimen.

GUIDANCE CONNECTION

Read the additional explanations in the in-section guidelines located within the **Pathology and Laboratory** section, subhead **Surgical Pathology,** directly above code 88300 in your CPT book.

 YOU CODE IT! CASE STUDY

Hildy French, an 11-year-old female, was taken to the OR to have her tonsils removed. However, due to additional symptoms, Dr. Anachino did a biopsy and sent a specimen of Hildy's tonsils to the lab for surgical pathologic examination. The report came back from the lab that Hildy had a malignant neoplasm of her tonsils. Dr. Anachino surgically removed additional sections to be certain that the entire tumor had been removed. Hildy tolerated the procedure well and was taken to the recovery room.

You Code It!

Go through the steps, and determine the pathology/lab code(s) that should be reported for this encounter.

Step #1: Read the case carefully and completely.

Step #2: Abstract the scenario. Which key words or terms describe what service the physician provided to the patient during this encounter?

Step #3: Are there any details missing or incomplete for which you would need to query the physician? [If so, ask your instructor.]

Step #4: Determine the correct CPT procedure code or codes to explain the details about what was provided to the patient during this encounter.

Step #5: Check for any relevant guidance, including reading all of the symbols and notations.

Step #6: Do you need to append any modifiers to ensure complete and accurate information is provided?

Step #7: Double-check your work.

Answer:

Did you determine this to be the correct code?

88305   Level IV – Surgical pathology, gross and microscopic examination; Tonsil, biopsy

Good work!

HILL MCGRAW PATHOLOGY LABORATORIES INC.
Warren R. Mulford, MD,. Director
123 Learning Way • Academia, FL 12345

PATIENT INFORMATION	PHYSICIAN INFORMATION

Name: NICOLE GABRINI
Sex: Female
D.O.B: 09/07/01
Patient ID: 55899
Patient Phone: 555-456-5555

JOSE MARKETTEN, MD
456 Healing Lane
Suite 505
Academia, FL 12345
555-399-5555

SPECIMEN INFORMATION

COLLECTED: 04/29/20
Reported: 05/01/20
Received: 04/30/20

Accession # IF_16_6971
Other Accession (IC):

PATHOLOGY REPORT

CLINICAL INFORMATION

A. Right upper extremity—Scabies vs Eczema
B. Left lower extremity—Scabies vs Eczema
C. Right lower extremity—Scabies vs Eczema

Terrell Rodriguez, PA-C

SPECIMEN DATA

GROSS DESCRIPTION:

A. The specimen is a punch biopsy received in immunofluorescence transport medium that measures 0.1 × 0.4 × 0.1 cm. The specimen is flash frozen and multiple 4 micron sections are cut for manual immunofluorescence staining. The sections are probed with fluorescein labeled antihuman antibodies against IgG, IgA, IgM, C3, C5b-9, and fibrinogen.

B. Received is a 0.2 cm punch biopsy of skin, submitted complete. The specimen is received in formalin.

C. Received is a 0.2 cm punch biopsy of skin, submitted complete. The specimen is received in formalin.

MICROSCOPIC DESCRIPTION:
All positive and negative controls stained appropriately as required.

RESULTS

DIAGNOSIS:

A. DIRECT IMMUNOFLUORESCENCE, RIGHT UPPER EXTREMITY—NEGATIVE (See Note)
Note: There is no IgG, IgA, IgM, C3, C5b-9, and fibrinogen deposition seen in this specimen. There is no immunofluorescence evidence of connective tissue, vasculitis, dermatitis herpetiformis, porphyria cutanea tarda, pseudoporphyria, or autoimmune blistering disease; however, clinical histologic and, if pertinent, serologic correlation is recommended. Multiple immunoreactant dilutions and sections were performed.

B. PUNCH BIOPSY, LEFT LOWER EXTREMITY—STASIS ECZEMA, TRAUMATIZED AND IMPETIGINIZED
Note: PAS is negative for fungus. Multiple deeper sections have been reviewed and no mite or mite elements identified. There is an impetiginized ulcer with bacterial colonization of the stratum corneum containing neutrophils and serum exudate. The papillary dermis contains a capillary proliferation, a few neutrophils, rare eosinophils and dermal cicatrix. These histopathologic features are consistent with traumatized and impetiginized stasis eczema. There is no evidence of scabies.

C. PUNCH BIOPSY, RIGHT LOWER EXTREMITY—STASIS ECZEMA, TRAUMATIZED AND IMPETIGINIZED
Note: PAS is negative for fungus. Multiple deeper sections have been reviewed and no mite or mite elements identified. There is an impetiginized ulcer with bacterial colonization of the stratum corneum containing neutrophils and serum exudate. The papillary dermis contains a capillary proliferation, a few neutrophils, rare eosinophils and dermal cicatrix. These histopathologic features are consistent with traumatized and impetiginized stasis eczema. There is no evidence of scabies.

Noah W. Wegner, MD Dermatopathologist (electronic signature)

FINAL REPORT

FIGURE 27-3 Sample pathology report showing details and analysis of a surgical specimen

Pathologic Testing on Bone Marrow

Medical Necessity for Bone Marrow Testing

Although not performed as commonly as blood tests or urinalysis (because obtaining the specimen is complex), pathologic examination of a patient's bone marrow has many possible uses, including:

- To serve as a diagnostic tool for suspected myeloma, leukemia, myelodysplastic syndromes, and myeloproliferative disorders.
- To assess a current diagnosis of thrombocytopenia, anemia, or leukopenia.
- To measure quantities of stored iron and marrow cellularity.
- To determine neoplasm, infection, fibrosis, or other infiltrative bone disease.
- To enable staging of lymphoma and/or other malignant neoplasms.

A patient may have abnormal blood counts for which an explanation has yet to be identified, or the patient may have other abnormal cells evidenced in circulating blood. These, as well as a current diagnosis of a bone marrow–related disease (such as lymphoma) or indications that a malignancy has metastasized into the marrow, are standard-of-care justifications to obtain and study a bone marrow specimen.

Collection of the Specimen

Typically, the specimen is taken from the posterior superior iliac spine of the pelvis to acquire a sampling of the blood-forming cells in the marrow space. Evaluation of a specimen taken by biopsy is considered to be more accurate than one obtained by aspiration because the quantity of material gathered is greater and therefore more likely to provide a representative sampling of a wider scope.

When coding for bone marrow biopsy, the first procedure to be reported is for obtaining the specimen, using either 38220 Bone marrow; aspiration only or 38221 Bone marrow, biopsy, needle or trocar.

Note that the abstraction of bone marrow from a patient is not performed solely for the lab. Therefore, it is very important to identify, from the documentation, not only how the bone marrow was taken but also for what purpose. For example, bone marrow aspiration for platelet-rich stem cell injections are not reported with 38220 but with code 0232T Injection(s), platelet-rich plasma, any site, including image guidance, harvesting and preparation when performed. Harvesting bone marrow for transplantation is reported with either 38230 Bone marrow harvesting for transplantation; allogeneic or 38232 Bone marrow harvesting for transplantation; autologous.

When both a bone marrow biopsy and a bone marrow aspiration are performed on a Medicare beneficiary during the same encounter, do not report code 38220. Instead, use code G0364 Bone marrow aspiration performed with bone marrow biopsy through the same incision on the same date of service.

Pathologic Testing

Next, the specimen will be sent to the laboratory for analysis. A bone marrow specimen, obtained by either biopsy or aspiration, can enable a hematologist/pathologist to investigate the patient's hematopoiesis (the process of forming blood cells), as well as the shape, size, and quantity of red and white blood cells and megakaryocytes (very large bone marrow cells that produce blood platelets). Blood cell formation is primarily the responsibility of the red bone marrow, specifically in the sternum, ribs, and iliac bones (pelvis).

Code 88305 Level IV – Surgical pathology, gross and microscopic examination reports both evaluation of the bone marrow biopsy specimen by the naked eye (gross examination) and visualization of the specimen using a microscope. When the documentation states that the specimen was obtained by aspiration, instead of 88305, the analysis is reported with 85097 Bone marrow; smear interpretation.

It is not uncommon for a decalcification procedure and/or iron staining to be performed at the same time as the surgical pathologic examination. When documentation confirms this, report these procedures separately using +88311 Decalcification procedure (list separately in addition to code for surgical pathology examination) and/or 88313 Special stain including interpretation and report; Group II, all other (e.g., iron, trichrome) except stain for microorganisms, stains for enzyme constituents, or immunocytochemistry and immunohistochemistry.

Per CPT parenthetical instruction, you should report one unit of 88313 for each special stain on each surgical pathologic block, cytologic specimen, or hematologic smear. Check documentation or query the pathologist performing the testing to ensure that the notes are clear as to how many blocks, specimens, or smears are tested so that you can report the accurate number of codes.

Immunophenotyping by flow cytometry provides the identification of cell-specific antibodies, enabling a more accurate determination of cell percentages as well as identification of abnormal cell patterns. Report this test using 88184 Flow cytometry, cell surface, cytoplasmic, or nuclear marker, technical component only; first marker and +88185 each additional marker, as appropriate.

Because 88184 and 88185 are specifically limited to the technical component only, you will need a code to report the interpretation service separately. Note that no modifiers (neither TC nor 26) are necessary because these details are already included in the code descriptors, as follows:

88187	Flow cytometry, interpretation; 2 to 8 markers
88188	Flow cytometry, interpretation; 9 to 15 markers
88189	Flow cytometry, interpretation; 16 or more markers

Fluorescent in situ hybridization (FISH) analysis (88365 In situ hybridization [e.g., FISH], per specimen; initial single probe stain procedure) is usually performed after the analysis of the bone marrow, the results of which will direct the specific DNA probes to be conducted. FISH analysis is better than an overall karyotype test because it can find smaller pieces of chromosomes that may be missing or may have extra copies.

 YOU CODE IT! CASE STUDY

Danielle Lee, a 37-year-old female, has a history of chronic myeloid leukemia (CML) and came to our facility today for a bone marrow aspiration, right side posterior iliac crest. Dr. Hansen used a 15-gauge needle to obtain the aspirate including an aspirate clot. The patient tolerated the procedure well.

You Code It!

Part 1: *Go through the steps of coding, and determine the code or codes that should be reported for this encounter between Dr. Hansen and Danielle Lee.*

Step #1: Read the case carefully and completely.

Step #2: Abstract the scenario. Which key words or terms describe what service the physician provided to the patient during this encounter?

Step #3: Are there any details missing or incomplete for which you would need to query the physician? [If so, ask your instructor.]

Step #4: Determine the correct CPT procedure code or codes to explain the details about what was provided to the patient during this encounter.

Step #5: Check for any relevant guidance, including reading all of the symbols and notations.

Step #6: Do you need to append any modifiers to ensure complete and accurate information is provided?

Step #7: Double-check your work.

(continued)

Answer:

Did you determine this to be the correct code for obtaining the bone marrow specimen?

    38220   **Diagnostic bone marrow; aspiration(s)**

Part 2: *Dr. Uker, a certified pathologist, wrote this report after testing the bone marrow.*

PATHOLOGY REPORT:

The following specimens were reviewed:

- peripheral smear of bone marrow aspirate and clot section
- iron stain

Determine the code or codes that should be reported for Dr. Uker.

Answer:

Did you determine these to be the correct codes for the pathology testing?

    85097   **Bone marrow; smear interpretation**
    88313   **Special stain including interpretation and report; Group II, all other (e.g., iron, trichrome) except stain for microorganisms, stains for enzyme constituents, or immunocytochemistry and immunohistochemistry**

27.9 Modifiers for Laboratory Coding

If your health care facility uses an outside laboratory that bills your office, you include the charges for the lab work on the claim form that you file. In such instances, you must append the CPT code for the lab test with modifier 90. If the outside lab bills the patient's insurance directly, you will not include the test code or modifier on the claim form you submit.

    90   **Reference (Outside) Laboratory:** When laboratory procedures are performed by a party other than the treating or reporting physician, the procedure may be identified by adding modifier 90 to the usual procedure number.

Also on occasion, you may find that a lab test has to be repeated, on the same day for the same patient, in order to get several readings of a level or measurement. When this is documented, append modifier 91:

    91   **Repeat Clinical Diagnostic Laboratory Test:** In the course of treatment of the patient, it may be necessary to repeat the same laboratory test on the same day to obtain subsequent (multiple) test results. Under these circumstances, the laboratory test performed can be identified by its usual procedure number and the addition of modifier 91. (**Note:** This modifier may not be used when tests are rerun to confirm initial results; due to testing problems with specimens or equipment; or for any other reason when a normal, one-time, reportable result is all that is required. This modifier may not be used when other code[s] describe a series of test results [e.g., glucose tolerance tests, evocative/suppression testing]. This modifier may only be used for laboratory test[s] performed more than once on the same day on the same patient.)

The use of testing kits is increasing in health care facilities because they make it easier to obtain fast, accurate results. When a testing kit is being used, append modifier 92.

    92   **Alternative Laboratory Platform Testing:** When laboratory testing is being performed using a kit or transportable instrument that wholly or in part consists of a single use, disposable analytical chamber, the service may be identified by adding modifier 92 to the usual laboratory procedure code (HIV testing 86701–86703, and 87389). The test does not require permanent dedicated space, hence by its design may be hand carried or transported to the vicinity of the patient for immediate testing at that site, although location of the testing is not in itself determinative of the use of this modifier.

YOU CODE IT! CASE STUDY

Dr. Georges is implementing a new treatment protocol for Priscilla Roper. He ordered that qualitative urinalysis be performed first thing in the morning, again at noon, and again at 5:00 p.m. Erline Cutter, RN, collected the specimens from Priscilla's catheter and sent them to the lab for each of the tests.

You Code It!

Review the scenario, and report the appropriate code or codes for the pathology lab's work.

Step #1: Read the case carefully and completely.

Step #2: Abstract the scenario. Which key words or terms describe what service the physician provided to the patient during this encounter?

Step #3: Are there any details missing or incomplete for which you would need to query the physician? [If so, ask your instructor.]

Step #4: Determine the correct CPT procedure code or codes to explain the details about what was provided to the patient during this encounter.

Step #5: Check for any relevant guidance, including reading all of the symbols and notations.

Step #6: Do you need to append any modifiers to ensure complete and accurate information is provided?

Step #7: Double-check your work.

Answer:

Did you determine this to be the code?

> **81005-91x3**   **Urinalysis; qualitative or semiquantitative, except immunoassays, repeat clinical diagnostic laboratory test, three tests**

Proprietary Laboratory Analyses

New diagnostic laboratory tests have been adopted to investigate the presence of very specific elements, such as colorectal adenomatous polyps or Helicobacter pylori detection and antibiotic resistance. These codes are unusual for the CPT code set, in that they are all alphanumeric and end with the letter "U".

For example:

> **0005U**   **Oncology (prostate) gene expression profile by real-time RT-PCR of 3 genes (ERG, PCA3, and SPDEF), urine, algorithm reported as risk score**

27.10 Pathology and Lab Abbreviations

Abbreviations for pathology and laboratory tests are used in reports from labs all over the country. Some of the most common are shown in Table 27-1.

TABLE 27-1 Abbreviations and Acronyms for Most Common Diagnostic and Laboratory Tests

ABG	Arterial blood gases
ACE	Angiotensin-converting enzyme
ACT	Activated clotting time
AFP	Alpha-fetoprotein
A/G	Albumin/globulin ratio
AIT	Agglutination inhibition test
ALP	Alkaline phosphatase
ALT	Alanine aminotransferase
AMA	Antimitochondrial antibody
ANA	Antinuclear antibody
APTT	Activated partial thromboplastin time
AST	Aspartate aminotransferase
BASO	Basophiles
BMC	Bone mineral content
BMD	Bone marrow density
BST	Blood serologic test
BUN	Blood urea nitrogen
CBC	Complete blood count
CEA	Carcinoembryonic antigen
CK	Creatine kinase
CMV	Cytomegalovirus
CO_2	Carbon dioxide
CPK	Creatine phosphokinase
DIC	Disseminated intravascular coagulation
DIFF	Differential
EIA	Enzyme immunoassay
EOS	Eosinophil count
ESR	Erythrocyte sedimentation rate
FBS	Fasting blood sugar
GTT	Glucose tolerance test
HCT	Hematocrit
HDL	High-density lipoprotein
HGB	Hemoglobin
HPF	High-power field
INR	International normalization ratio
LD	Lactic dehydrogenase
LDL	Low-density lipoprotein
LFT	Liver function tests
LPF	Low-power field
LYMPHS	Lymphocytes
MCH	Mean corpuscular hemoglobin

(continued)

MCHC	Mean corpuscular hemoglobin concentration
MCV	Mean corpuscular volume
MONO	Monocyte count
MPV	Mean platelet volume
NEUT	Neutrophils
PAP	Prostatic acid phosphatase
PH	Hydrogen ion concentration
PLT	Platelet
PSA	Prostate-specific antigen
PT	Prothrombin time
PTT	Partial thromboplastin time
RBC	Red blood cells
RDW	Red cell distribution width
RF	Rheumatoid factor
RPR	Rapid plasma reagin test
SEGS	Segmented neutrophils
SGOT	Serum glutamicoxaloacetic transaminase
SGPT	Serum glutamicpyruvic transaminase
SMA	Sequential multiple analyzer
SP GRAV	Specific gravity
STS	Serologic test for syphilis
T&C	Type and crossmatch
TSH	Thyroid-stimulating hormone
UA	Urinalysis
WBC	White blood cell

Chapter Summary

Pathology and laboratory tests provide health care professionals with definitive evidence as to the condition that may be interfering with a patient's good health. That proof will help direct the physician toward a more accurate diagnosis and a beneficial treatment plan. Lab tests are an invaluable part of the health care toolbox and must be coded accurately.

CODING BITES

Common Abbreviations Used in Pathology Testing

PT = Prothrombin time, which is used to evaluate bleeding and clotting disorders
CBC = Complete blood count, which includes the following tests:
WBC = White blood cell count
RBC = Red blood cell count
PLT = Platelet count, which is used to diagnose or monitor bleeding and clotting disorders
HCT = Hematocrit
HGB = Hemoglobin concentration, which is the concentration of the oxygen-carrying pigment in red blood cells
DIFF = Differential blood count

Remember that the CBC includes the WBC, RBC, HCT, HGB, platelet count, and differential count. Therefore, you are not to code those tests separately.

CHAPTER 27 REVIEW
CPT Pathology & Lab Section

Let's Check It! Terminology

Match each key term to the appropriate definition.

1. LO 27.7 The investigation and identification of cells.

2. LO 27.2 The counting or measurement of something.

3. LO 27.8 The study of tissues removed from a living patient during a surgical procedure.

4. LO 27.8 The study of a specimen using a microscope (under magnification).

5. LO 27.1 A location with scientific equipment designed to perform experiments and tests.

6. LO 27.1 The study of the nature, etiology, development, and outcomes of disease.

7. LO 27.8 The visual study of a specimen (with the naked eye).

8. LO 27.1 The study of the causes of disease.

9. LO 27.1 A small part or sample of any substance obtained for analysis and diagnosis.

10. LO 27.2 The determination of character or essential element(s).

A. Cytology

B. Etiology

C. Gross Examination

D. Laboratory

E. Microscopic Examination

F. Pathology

G. Qualitative

H. Quantitative

I. Specimen

J. Surgical Pathology

Let's Check It! Concepts

Choose the most appropriate answer for each of the following questions.

1. LO 27.10 What is the correct abbreviation for a liver function test?

   a. INR   **b.** LDL   **c.** LPF   **d.** LFT

2. LO 27.7 What code(s) would you assign for a blood compatibility test by incubation technique, 2 units?

   a. 86920

   c. 86921

   b. 86921, 86921

   d. 86922, 86921

3. LO 27.1 A specimen can be

   a. blood.

   c. sputum.

   b. urine.

   d. all of these.

4. LO 27.3 When not all of the tests listed in a panel are performed, you should

   a. code the panel with modifier 52.

   b. code the panel alone.

   c. code the tests individually.

   d. code the panel with modifier 53.

5. LO 27.2 The guidelines tell you that, if the documentation does not specify, you may assume that the examination performed was _____.

   a. qualitative

   c. quantitative

   b. measured

   d. none of these

6. LO 27.5 The lab test most commonly performed using a chemical process to identify hyperglycemia uses
   a. hormones.
   b. blood glucose.
   c. electrolytes.
   d. lipids.

7. LO 27.9 What modifier would you append to a CPT code for a lab test that has to be repeated, on the same day for the same patient, in order to get several readings of a level or measurement?
   a. 99
   b. 90
   c. 92
   d. 91

8. LO 27.4 This test identifies the percentage of RBCs, which is used to identify anemia.
   a. BUN
   b. ESR
   c. Hgb
   d. HCT

9. LO 27.8 Surgical pathology may include
   a. gross examination.
   b. microbiology.
   c. genetic testing.
   d. nuclear medicine.

10. LO 27.6 _____ testing involves the analysis of specimens to identify any presence of a genetic disorder.
    a. Infectious
    b. Oncology
    c. Genetic
    d. Hematology

Let's Check It! Guidelines

Refer to the Pathology and Laboratory Guidelines and fill in the blanks accordingly.

multiple	rarely	same
definition	technologists	special
separate	effort	85999
extent	may	physician

1. Services in Pathology and Laboratory are provided by a physician or by _____ under responsible supervision of a _____.

2. It is appropriate to designate _____ procedures that are rendered on the _____ date by _____ entries.

3. Unlisted hematology and coagulation procedure is represented by code _____.

4. A service that is _____ provided, unusual, variable, or new _____ require a _____ report.

5. Pertinent information should include an adequate _____ or description of the nature, _____, and need for the procedure; and the time, _____, and equipment necessary to provide the service.

Let's Check It! Rules and Regulations

Please answer the following questions from the knowledge you have gained after reading this chapter.

1. LO 27.1 Differentiate between pathology and etiology.
2. LO 27.2 What is the difference between *quantitative* and *qualitative*?
3. LO 27.7 What is cytopathology? What is cytologic testing used for, and how are specimens obtained?
4. LO 27.8 What are the purpose and benefit of surgical pathology?
5. LO 27.9 If your health care facility uses an outside laboratory that bills your office, and you include the charges for the lab work on the claim form, what modifier must you append?

YOU CODE IT! Basics

First, identify the procedural main term in the following statements; then code the procedure or service.

Example: Dr. Gleason performs a definitive drug test for barbiturates:

a. main term: *Drug Assay* **b.** procedure: *80345*

1. Dr. McElory completes a drug monitoring of total digoxin:

    a. main term: _____   **b.** procedure: _____

2. Dr. Gavin performs a bleeding time test:

    a. main term: _____   **b.** procedure: _____

3. Dr. Kaufmann completes a tuberculosis skin test:

    a. main term: _____   **b.** procedure: _____

4. Dr. Lovece performs an HLA crossmatch test, first dilution:

    a. main term: _____   **b.** procedure: _____

5. Dr. Sox completes a blood typing compatibility test by spin technique:

    a. main term: _____   **b.** procedure: _____

6. Dr. Dickenson performs a urine bacterial culture quantitative colony count:

    a. main term: _____   **b.** procedure: _____

7. Dr. Campos performs an HBsAg (hepatitis B surface antigen) immunoassay test:

    a. main term: _____   **b.** procedure: _____

8. Dr. Hearon performs a forensic necropsy:

    a. main term: _____   **b.** procedure: _____

9. Dr. Busby completes a mature oocytes cryopreservation:

    a. main term: _____   **b.** procedure: _____

10. Dr. Klausing performs a blood cell count with automated differential WBC count:

    a. main term: _____   **b.** procedure: _____

11. Dr. Reilly completed a creatine kinase, total:

    a. main term: _____   **b.** procedure: _____

12. Dr. Flemington performs an RPR syphilis test:

    a. main term: _____   **b.** procedure: _____

13. Dr. Jensen completes a CMV (cytomegalovirus) antibody IgM:

    a. main term: _____   **b.** procedure: _____

14. Dr. Vance performs a bilirubin, total; direct test:

    a. main term: _____   **b.** procedure: _____

15. Dr. Humphrey completes a direct Coombs test:

    a. main term: _____   **b.** procedure: _____

 YOU CODE IT! Practice

Using the techniques described in this chapter, carefully read through the case studies and determine the most accurate pathology and laboratory CPT code(s) and modifier(s), if appropriate, for each case study.

1. Walter Winegarten, a 42-year-old male, was feeling rundown and tired all the time. So, Dr. Stevenson, thinking that Walter might have anemia, ordered a complete CBC, automated with an automated differential WBC count.

2. Deidra Lowe, a 23-year-old female, has been living on the street and in shelters and comes to the free clinic for a checkup because she is 5-months pregnant. Dr. Ashton orders a complete CBC, automated and appropriate manual differential WBC count, hepatitis B surface antigen, rubella antibody, qualitative syphilis test, RBC antibody screening, blood typing ABO, and Rh factor.

3. Vivian Praxis, a 3-year-old female, is at the office of her pediatrician, Dr. Ashley, for her regular checkup. Dr. Ashley notices that Vivian is very small for her age and orders a growth hormone stimulation panel to be done.

4. Jay Zeeman, a 36-year-old male, went to the shore with his friends and feasted on raw oysters and beer. About 7 hours later, after getting home, he began to cough and vomit, and he found blood in his stool. He went to the walk-in clinic, where Dr. Lanahan ran a smear test for ova and parasites, particularly *Anisakis*.

5. Gregg Abernathy, a 41-year-old male, was diagnosed with prostate cancer last week. Before beginning radiation treatments, which will make him unable to have children, he comes today to submit his sperm for cryopreservation.

6. Rudy Porter, a 71-year-old male, has a history of gastrointestinal problems, including intestinal polyps. After taking a special kit home, he submits fecal specimens for an occult blood test by immunoassay.

7. Tiffany Matheson, a 28-year-old female, just got a new job with the space industry. As a condition of her employment, she came to the lab today for a presumptive drug test for alcohol, amphetamines, and barbiturates. The test was performed and the results were read by direct optical observation; they confirmed negative outcomes for all drugs.

8. Caitlyn Deloach, a 21-year-old female, was found unconscious by her roommate and brought into the emergency department by ambulance. The roommate stated that Caitlyn was very depressed, and she feared that Caitlyn might have taken an overdose of her medication. Dr. Leroy ordered a therapeutic drug assay for phenobarbital.

9. Rulon Cutler, a 25-year-old male, is overweight, bordering on obese, and Dr. Jacobs is concerned that he may be developing diabetes, so he orders an insulin tolerance panel for adrenocorticotropic hormone (ACTH) insufficiency.

10. Shawn McCully, a 51-year-old female, goes to her physician, Dr. Kahlil, for her annual checkup, which includes a nonautomated urinalysis with microscopy for glucose, ketones, and leukocytes. Dr. Kahlil's assistant, Donna, performs the test, by dipstick, in the office. The results are normal.

11. Margaret Calhoun, a 23-year-old female, got drunk at a party and had unprotected sex. She came into the clinic today for an HIV-1 and HIV-2 single assay test.

12. At the doctor's suggestion, Margaret Calhoun (previous scenario) also was tested for syphilis, qualitative (VDRL).

13. Georgia Stuart, a 37-year-old female, is pregnant for the first time. Dr. Ferguson performed an amniocentesis to do a chromosome analysis, count 15 cells, 1 karyotype, with banding. The results showed that the baby is fine.

14. Sean Olin, a 61-year-old male, was in the operating room for Dr. Tanger to perform a subtotal resection of his pancreas. Surgical pathology showed no malignancy.

15. Chad Snell, a 22-day-old male, was born at 33-weeks gestation, and there is concern that he may have hyperbilirubinemia. Therefore, Dr. Bateman performed a total transcutaneous bilirubin.

 YOU CODE IT! Application

The following exercises provide practice in the application of abstracting the physicians' notes and learning to work with documentation from our health care facility, Millard Pathology & Diagnostic Labs. These case studies are modeled on real patient encounters. Using the techniques described in this chapter, carefully read through the case studies and determine the most accurate pathology and laboratory CPT code(s) and modifier(s), if appropriate, for each case study. You are coding for the pathologist.

MILLARD PATHOLOGY & DIAGNOSTIC LABS

753 LITTLE WEST RD • SOMEWHERE, FL 32811 • 407-555-9371

PATIENT: MEDFORD, ROBERT

ACCOUNT/EHR #: MEDFRO001

DATE: 10/17/20

(continued)

Procedure Performed: Comprehensive metabolic panel

Pathologist: Derrick Castel, MD

Referring Physician: Oscar R. Prader, MD

INDICATIONS: Routine physical exam

IMPRESSIONS:

Albumin 3.9

Bilirubin Small*

Calcium 8.9

Carbon dioxide (CO_2) 28

Chloride 96 L C

Creatinine 1.2

Glucose 102

Phosphatase, alkaline 90

Potassium 3.9

Protein, total 30*

Sodium 138

Transferase, alanine amino (ALT) (SGPT) 30

Transferase, aspartate amino (AST) (SGOT) 29

Urea nitrogen (BUN) 18

* = Abnormal, L = Low, H = High

Derrick Castel, MD

DC/mg   D: 10/17/20 09:50:16   T: 10/20/20 12:55:01

Determine the most accurate pathology and laboratory CPT code(s) and modifier(s), if appropriate.

MILLARD PATHOLOGY & DIAGNOSTIC LABS

753 LITTLE WEST RD • SOMEWHERE, FL 32811 • 407-555-9371

PATIENT: INGER, TERRENCE

ACCOUNT/EHR #: INGETE001

DATE: 09/29/20

Procedure Performed: Tissue, skin, head, mutation identification

Pathologist: Peter Havner, MD

Referring Physician: Oscar R. Prader, MD

INDICATIONS: Suspected melanoma

(continued)

IMPRESSIONS: Abnormal cells present, by surgical pathology, gross and microscopic examination

Peter Havner, MD

PH/mg   D: 09/29/20 09:50:16   T: 09/30/20 12:55:01

Determine the most accurate pathology and laboratory CPT code(s) and modifier(s), if appropriate.

MILLARD PATHOLOGY & DIAGNOSTIC LABS
753 LITTLE WEST RD • SOMEWHERE, FL 32811 • 407-555-9371

PATIENT: WALLER, FELIX

ACCOUNT/EHR #: WALLFE001

DATE: 11/15/20

Procedure Performed: Surgical pathology, gallbladder, gross and microscopic examination

Pathologist: Peter Havner, MD

Referring Physician: Renee O. Bracker, MD

INDICATIONS: R/O malignancy

IMPRESSIONS: All tissues unremarkable

Surgical pathology, gross and microscopic examination of gallbladder

Peter Havner, MD

PH/mg   D: 11/15/20 09:50:16   T: 11/20/20 12:55:01

Determine the most accurate pathology and laboratory CPT code(s) and modifier(s), if appropriate.

MILLARD PATHOLOGY & DIAGNOSTIC LABS
753 LITTLE WEST RD • SOMEWHERE, FL 32811 • 407-555-9371

PATIENT: DALTON, ANGELA

ACCOUNT/EHR #: DALTAN001

DATE: 09/23/20

Procedure Performed: Rectal biopsies, gross and microscopic examination

Pathologist: Walter Alchemy, MD

Referring Physician: Matthew Appellet, MD

INDICATIONS: Inflammatory bowel disease

IMPRESSIONS: All tissues normal

Surgical pathology, gross and microscopic examination, colon biopsy

Walter Alchemy, MD

WA/mg   D: 09/23/20 09:50:16   T: 09/25/20 12:55:01

Determine the most accurate pathology and laboratory CPT code(s) and modifier(s), if appropriate.

MILLARD PATHOLOGY & DIAGNOSTIC LABS

753 LITTLE WEST RD • SOMEWHERE, FL 32811 • 407-555-9371

PATIENT: PRIMERO, GINO

ACCOUNT/EHR #: PRIMGI001

DATE: 06/17/20

Procedure Performed: Mass (fat tissue), upper eyelid gross and microscopic examination

Pathologist: Derrick Castel, MD

Referring Physician: Renee O. Bracker, MD

INDICATIONS: Herniated orbital fat pad, OD

IMPRESSIONS: Carcinoma in situ

Surgical pathology, gross and microscopic examination, soft tissue tumor, extensive resection

---

Derrick Castel, MD

DC/mg   D: 06/17/20 09:50:16   T: 06/20/20 12:55:01

Determine the most accurate pathology and laboratory CPT code(s) and modifier(s), if appropriate.

Design elements: ©McGraw-Hill

28

CPT Medicine Section

Learning Outcomes

After completing this chapter, the student should be able to:

LO 28.1 Interpret the guidelines for coding the administration of immunizations.

LO 28.2 Apply the guidelines to accurately report injections and infusions.

LO 28.3 Determine the correct coding parameters for reporting psychiatric services.

LO 28.4 Abstract physicians' notes to accurately report dialysis and gastroenterology services.

LO 28.5 Identify specifics to correctly report ophthalmology and otorhinolaryngologic services.

LO 28.6 Determine how to accurately report cardiovascular services.

LO 28.7 Recognize the details required for accurately reporting pulmonary function testing.

LO 28.8 Report accurately the provision of immunology services.

LO 28.9 Interpret the specifics for accurately reporting neurologic services.

LO 28.10 Abstract the required details for reporting physical medical and rehabilitation services.

LO 28.11 Employ the guidelines to accurately report alternative medicine services: acupuncture, osteopathic, and chiropractic treatments.

LO 28.12 Abstract documentation for reporting special and other services.

 STOP! Remember, you need to follow along in your <u>CPT</u> code book for an optimal learning experience.

GUIDANCE CONNECTION

Read the additional explanations in the in-section guidelines located within the **Medicine** section, subheads **Immune Globulins, Serum or Recombinant Products,** directly above code 90281; **Immunization Administration for Vaccines/Toxoids,** directly above code 90460; and **Vaccines, Toxoids,** directly above code 90476, all in your CPT book.

Immunization
To make someone resistant to a particular disease by vaccination.

28.1 Immunizations

Immunizations, also known as vaccinations, are developed to train a patient's immune system against a specific pathogen. Immunization sera work to build immune memory by creating antibodies, similar to special forces, that are ready to battle should a specific bacterium or virus invade. This system is designed to prevent, or at least limit, the damage done by invading pathogens. Immunization of a patient includes two parts: the medication itself and the administration of the medication. Each part is coded separately.

The medication may be an immune globulin, an antitoxin, a vaccine, or a toxoid. Codes 90281–90399 and 90476–90756 are available for you to identify specific drugs. You must be diligent and read all of the options for the specific vaccines because there may be several choices with small differences that are still important to accuracy. For example, there are actually 24 different codes (90653–90689) to report an influenza virus vaccine, each identifying a different version. The physician's documentation should provide you with the specifics you need to identify the version that was used. If not, you must query so you can report the correct code.

 LET'S CODE IT! SCENARIO

Phillip Landstone, a 21-year-old male, came in so Dr. Micah can administer a flu vaccine before he starts volunteering at Community Hospital. Dr. Micah documents that the vaccine was trivalent, split virus, 0.5 mL dosage, administered IM.

Let's Code It!

The documentation states that Dr. Micah administered a *trivalent, split virus* influenza vaccination to Phillip. Turn to the CPT Alphabetic Index and find

Vaccination
Vaccine Administration
   See Immunization Administration
Vaccines and Toxoids
   See Vaccines and Toxoids

This is great! The Alphabetic Index is reminding you that, when reporting the administration of a vaccination (or other injection), you will need two codes: one for the administration + one for the serum (what is inside that syringe).
    As long as you are here, let's find the suggestion(s) for the serum—the influenza vaccine itself.

Vaccines and Toxoids

Read down the list until you find something that matches what you abstracted from the documentation. Do you see . . .

Influenza

Read down the indented list below *Influenza* to find

Influenza
  Trivalent, Split Virus (IIV3)...........................90654–90658, 90660, 90673
    for Intradermal Use..90654
    for Intramuscular Use...90655–90658
    Increased Antigen Content 90662

The documentation states, "*trivalent, split virus, administered IM.*" This matches, so turn to the suggested codes to read the entire code descriptions.

90655	**Influenza virus vaccine, trivalent (IIV3), split virus, preservative free, 0.25 mL dosage, for intramuscular use**
90656	**Influenza virus vaccine, trivalent (IIV3), split virus, preservative free, 0.5 mL dosage, for intramuscular use**
90657	**Influenza virus vaccine, trivalent (IIV3), split virus, 0.25 mL dosage, for intramuscular use**
90658	**Influenza virus vaccine, trivalent (IIV3), split virus, 0.5 mL dosage, for intramuscular use**

As you read these four code descriptions, you can see that there are two differences: preservative free or not + the dosage. There is no mention that the vaccine was preservative free, so this narrows down the options to 90657 and 90658. What was the dosage? The documentation states, "*0.5 mL dosage.*" Now, you can determine the accurate code for this vaccine is

90658	**Influenza virus vaccine, trivalent (IIV3), split virus, 0.5 mL dosage, for intramuscular use**

(continued)

Now, you need to go back to the Alphabetic Index, this time to the main term "Immunization Administration."

Immunization Administration

Each Additional Vaccine/Toxoid...........................90472, 90474
    with Counseling...90461
One Vaccine/Toxoid 90471, 90473
    with Counseling...90460

Dr. Micah documented only one vaccine was administered; there is no documentation of any counseling. Turn to the *Main Section* to code 90471 so you can read the entire code description:

90471 **Immunization administration (includes percutaneous, intradermal, subcutaneous, or intramuscular injections); 1 vaccine (single or combination vaccine/toxoid)**

90473 **Immunization administration by intranasal or oral route; 1 vaccine (single or combination vaccine/toxoid)**

Go back to the documentation to check what route of administration was used. The documentation states, "*administered IM.*" IM is the abbreviation for *intramuscular.* This fact eliminates 90473 as an option, and you know what code to report.

Good job! You now can report codes **90471** and **90658** for Dr. Micah's service to Phillip with confidence!

If more than one vaccine was administered during the same encounter, there may be a combination code available for those vaccinations that are typically provided together, such as the MMR (Measles, Mumps, Rubella) or the DTaP (Diphtheria, Tetanus toxoids, and Acellular Pertussis vaccines). It is illegal to report these vaccines individually if they are administered in a combination.

Medications can be given, or administered, to the patient in several different ways: percutaneous, intradermal, subcutaneous (SC), or intramuscular (IM) injections; intranasal (INH) or oral (ORAL); intra-arterial (IA) or intravenous (IV). The method of administration will help you find the correct administration codes 90460–90461 and 90471–90474.

When more than one vaccine is provided on the same date, use the add-on codes for the administration of the additional injections. You will find that most of the codes are offered in sets: the first injection, administration, or hour and then the add-on code for each additional injection, administration, or hour.

 LET'S CODE IT! SCENARIO

Isaac Nelson, a 5-year-old male, came to Dr. Rubino for his MMR vaccine so that he can start kindergarten next month. Dr. Rubino administered an injection subcutaneously. Dr. Rubino met face-to-face with Isaac's mother and discussed the importance of the vaccine, as well as indications of a reaction that she should watch for. Isaac chose a red balloon as his prize for being a good patient.

Let's Code It!

Dr. Rubino gave Isaac *one subcutaneous injection* of the *MMR vaccine.* Do you know what *MMR* stands for? Even if you don't know that it is an acronym for *measles, mumps, and rubella,* you can look it up in the Alphabetic Index under *MMR shots.* The suggested code is 90707. The numeric listing confirms

90707 **Measles, mumps, and rubella virus vaccine (MMR), live, for subcutaneous use**

The description matches Dr. Rubino's notes exactly. However, the code will reimburse Dr. Rubino's office only for the drug itself, not Dr. Rubino's time and expertise in administering the injection and counseling the family. You could go back to the Alphabetic Index, or you could read the instructional paragraph at the beginning of the

(continued)

Vaccines, Toxoids subsection (where you found the code 90707). You will see that this paragraph tells you that you must use these codes "in addition to an immunization administration code(s) 90460–90474." Let's turn to the first code, 90460, and read the description:

90460   **Immunization administration through 18 years of age via any route of administration, with counseling by physician or other qualified health care professional; first or only component of each vaccine or toxoid administered**

+90461   **each additional vaccine or toxoid component administered (list separately in addition to code for primary procedure)**

Now, you have the codes to reimburse Dr. Rubino for the MMR vaccine, as well as his time and expertise in administering the injection and talking with Isaac's mother. Remember, the MMR vaccine is a combination vaccine with three components. So, you will need to report four codes:

90707, 90460, 90461, 90461

Good job!!

NOTE: If Dr. Rubino had not spent time face-to-face with Isaac and his mother, 90460 and 90461 would not be used. Instead you would use codes 90471, +90472, +90472, which do not include the phrase "when the physician counsels the patient/family" in the code description.

28.2 Injections and Infusions

The administration of fluids (such as saline solution to hydrate a patient suffering from dehydration), pharmaceuticals (such as medications for treatment or preventive purposes), or dyes (such as those used for diagnostic testing) is coded from the **Injections and Infusions** subsection, which includes codes 96360–96379.

Some of these terms may sound familiar to you because we discussed them earlier when reviewing the various ways drugs can be administered into the body. In Figure 28-1, do you see how the needle illustrating an *intradermal* injection has its tip pointing into the dermis (*intra* = within + *dermal* = dermis)? The injection that is

> **CODING BITES**
>
> When a drug is provided to a patient, two types of codes are reported: one for the administration—being discussed here—plus one for the drug itself—discussed in the chapter *HCPCS Level II.*

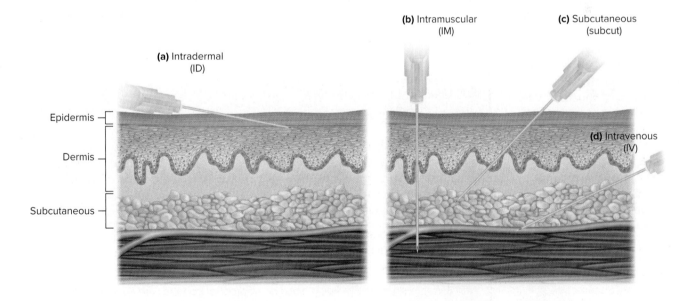

(a) Intradermal (ID)
(b) Intramuscular (IM)
(c) Subcutaneous (subcut)
(d) Intravenous (IV)

Epidermis
Dermis
Subcutaneous

FIGURE 28-1 An illustration showing various injection routes

Infusion
The introduction of a fluid into a blood vessel.

Injection
Compelling a fluid into tissue or cavity.

CODING BITES

The administration of chemotherapy drugs is *not* coded from the **Injections and Infusions** subsection, but from the **Chemotherapy Administration** subsection, codes 96401–96549.

Push
The delivery of an additional drug via an intravenous line over a short period of time.

GUIDANCE CONNECTION

Read the additional explanations in the in-section guidelines located within the **Medicine** section, subheads **Hydration,** directly above code 96360, and **Therapeutic, Prophylactic, Diagnostic Injections and Infusions (Excludes Chemotherapy and Other Highly Complex Drug or Highly Complex Biologic Agent Administration),** directly above code 96365, both in your CPT book.

---

delivered *subcutaneously* has the tip of the needle all the way down into the fatty tissue layer. And the *intramuscular* (*intra* = within + *muscular* = muscle) injection leads down to the layer of muscle that lies below the fatty tissue layer.

The **infusion** and **injection** codes include certain standard parts involved in administering liquids. Services included and therefore not reported separately are

- The administration of a local anesthetic.
- The initiation of the IV.
- Accessing an indwelling IV, subcutaneous catheter, or port.
- Flushing the line at the completion of the infusion.
- The appropriate supplies: tubing, syringes, and so on.

The guidelines for coding injections and infusions provide further direction when coding these services:

- When more than one infusion is provided into one IV site, report only the first service.
- Should more than one IV site be used, report the appropriate services for each site.
- Report different drugs or materials and that service separately.
- Report infusion time as the actual time the fluid is provided.

An IV or intra-arterial **push** is described by the CPT guidelines as

- An injection administered to the patient and then observed continuously by the health care professional who administered the drug.

or

- An infusion that lasts 15 minutes or less.

Multiple Administrations

When more than one injection or infusion is provided to a patient at the same encounter, there is a specific order in which you need to report the codes. The sequencing guidelines are different for those reporting physician services than for those reporting for the facility.

When you are reporting for the physician's, or other health care professional's, services, you must read the notes carefully to determine the main diagnosis or reason for the treatment. The primary reason for the injection or infusion should be reported first, as the "initial" service, no matter in what order the injections were administered.

EXAMPLE

Wendy comes to see her physician because she has been vomiting a lot over the last several days. Dr. Kilmer identifies that she has become dehydrated due to this excessive vomiting. Dr. Kilmer gives Wendy an intramuscular (IM) injection of an antiemetic (a drug to stop vomiting) and then gives her an IV infusion, 45 minutes, of normal saline for hydration. The primary reason for the encounter is Wendy's excessive vomiting; therefore, the injection of the antiemetic is the "initial" service, followed by the hydration infusion service.

96372	Therapeutic, prophylactic, or diagnostic injection; subcutaneous or intramuscular
96360	Intravenous infusion, hydration; initial, 31 minutes to 1 hour

NOTE: Remember, you will also need an additional code for the specific antiemetic medication that was inside that injection, as well as an additional code for the saline.

When you are reporting services on behalf of a facility rather than the providing professional, the order is determined by the type of service provided as well as the reason for that service:

1. Chemotherapy service.
2. Therapeutic, prophylactic, and diagnostic services.
3. Hydration services.

Then, the specific service hierarchy is

1. Infusions.
2. Pushes.
3. Injections.

 LET'S CODE IT! SCENARIO

Melissa Fusion, a 51-year-old female, postmastectomy for malignant neoplasm of the breast, has been having chemotherapy treatments. She was seen today for nausea and vomiting as a result of this therapy. Dr. Saludo ordered an antiemetic 10 mg IV push and another antiemetic IV infusion over 30 minutes.

Let's Code It!

Melissa received two medications via two different routes of administration: *IV push* and *IV infusion*. Therefore, you need two codes.

The notes report that an intravenous push, which is an injection given intravenously, was given. Let's turn to the Alphabetic Index and look up *injection, intravenous*.

> **Injection**
> Intravenous...96379

Keep reading below that and you will see

> **Injection**
> Intravenous push 96374–96376

That looks perfect. Turn to the numeric listing and read the complete descriptions. You see that 96374 matches the notes:

96374 **Therapeutic, prophylactic or diagnostic injection (specify substance or drug); intravenous push, single or initial substance/drug**

You also know that Melissa was given an *infusion, intravenously,* and that it was for *therapeutic* reasons—to eliminate her nausea and vomiting. Let's go to the Alphabetic Index and look up *infusion, intravenous, therapeutic*.

> **Infusion**
> Intravenous
>   Diagnostic/Prophylactic/Therapeutic...........................96365–96368, 96379
>   Hydration...96360, 96361

When you turn to the numeric listing to check the code descriptions, you see that codes 96360–96361 are for hydration only. Look through the complete descriptions for the next grouping, 96365–96368, and you see that the best, most accurate code is

96367 **Intravenous infusion, for therapy, prophylaxis, or diagnosis (specify substance or drug); additional sequential infusion of a new drug/substance, up to 1 hour**

The notes indicate that Melissa was given the infusion after the first (sequentially) for 30 minutes. Excellent!
Therefore, the claim form for this encounter with Melissa will show **96374** and **96367.**
Great job!

GUIDANCE CONNECTION

Read the additional explanations in the in-section guidelines located within the **Medicine** section, subhead **Chemotherapy and Other Highly Complex Drug or Highly Complex Biologic Agent Administration,** directly above code 96401 in your CPT book.

Chemotherapy Administration

Codes 96401–96549 cover the different methods of chemotherapy dispensation that may be used with one patient. Each method (such as steroidal agents and biologic agents) and/or each technique (such as infusion or IV push) should be coded separately. The codes include the following services:

- The administration of a local anesthetic.
- The initiation of the IV.
- Accessing an indwelling IV, subcutaneous catheter, or port.
- Flushing the line at the completion of the infusion.
- The appropriate supplies: tubing, syringes, and so on.
- The preparation of the chemotherapy agent(s).

YOU CODE IT! CASE STUDY

Andrew Gitner is admitted today for his chemotherapy, which consists of an antineoplastic drug, 500 mg IV infusion over 3 hours. Dr. Munch is in attendance during Andrew's treatment.

You Code It!

Go through the steps, and determine the code(s) that should be reported for this encounter between Dr. Munch and Andrew Gitner.

Step #1: Read the case carefully and completely.

Step #2: Abstract the scenario. Which key words or terms describe what service the physician provided to the patient during this encounter?

Step #3: Are there any details missing or incomplete for which you would need to query the physician? [If so, ask your instructor.]

Step #4: Determine the correct CPT procedure code or codes to explain the details about what was provided to the patient during this encounter.

Step #5: Check for any relevant guidance, including reading all of the symbols and notations.

Step #6: Do you need to append any modifiers to ensure complete and accurate information is provided?

Step #7: Double-check your work.

Answer:

Did you determine these to be the correct codes?

96413	Chemotherapy administration, intravenous infusion technique; up to 1 hour, single or initial substance/drug
+96415	each additional hour (List separately in addition to code for primary procedure) [for second hour]
+96415	each additional hour (List separately in addition to code for primary procedure) [for third hour]

28.3 Psychiatry, Psychotherapy, and Biofeedback

Sometimes we become so focused on physical health care issues that we forget the health care professionals who treat mental health concerns. This area is a great opportunity for coding specialists because more and more health care plans cover psychotherapy and psychiatric services. Codes 90785–90911 provide details on such services.

Psychiatry services are categorized as:

- Interactive Complexity
- Psychiatric Diagnostic Procedures
    - Psychotherapy
    - Psychotherapy for Crisis
    - Other Psychotherapy
    - Other Psychiatric Services or Procedures

Once the type of therapy is determined, the next factor to consider is how much time the provider spent face-to-face with the patient.

There is a difference between *psychiatric* E/M and *medical* E/M, so, lastly, you must abstract from the documentation whether the physician or therapist provided *medical* E/M services in addition to the therapy session at the same time or on the same day.

When medical E/M services are provided at the same time or on the same date, and are documented as separately identified—specifically different from those issues covered by the therapy—then a code from the *Evaluation and Management (E/M)* section of the CPT book may be appropriate.

GUIDANCE CONNECTION

Read the additional explanations in the in-section guidelines located within the **Medicine** section, subhead **Psychiatry,** directly above code 90785 in your CPT book

---

 LET'S CODE IT! SCENARIO

Taylor Loeb, a 32-year-old male, was sent to Dr. Panjab for psychotherapy to deal with anger management issues. Dr. Panjab spent 45 minutes with Taylor in her office.

Let's Code It!

Taylor saw Dr. Panjab in *her office* for psychotherapy for *45 minutes.* Let's look in the Alphabetic Index under *psychotherapy,* beneath which you see *family* of patient, for crisis, group other than multifamily, individual patient, and several more, as choices. The notes indicate that Taylor had an individual psychotherapy session. The Alphabetic Index suggests codes 90832–90834 and 90836–90838. Let's look at the numeric listing and see which of these matches Dr. Panjab's notes.

90834 **Psychotherapy, 45 minutes with patient**

+90836 **Psychotherapy, 45 minutes with patient when performed with an evaluation and management service (List separately in addition to the code for primary procedure.)**

The next issue to consider is whether Dr. Panjab provided medical E/M services at the same time. According to her notes, she did not. This means that code 90834 is the code to report.

Great job!

Telemedicine Synchronous Services

Several codes within the **Psychiatry** subsection qualify to be provided using telemedicine synchronous services, as noted by the star (★) symbol to the left of the code: 90791, 90792, 90832, 90833, 90834, 90836, 90837, 90838, 90845, 90846, 90847, and 90863.

As you learned in the chapter *CPT and HCPCS Level II Modifiers* in the section *Service-Related Modifiers*, the documentation for these encounters must confirm that the content of the physician/patient meeting is sufficient to meet the requirements for the code to be reported whether the service was provided face-to-face or with the use of synchronous telemedicine services (as indicated by appending modifier 95).

YOU CODE IT! CASE STUDY

Adam has been acting out, often losing his temper and getting violent, since his parents divorced. After individual sessions, Dr. Eisenberg holds a family psychotherapy session with Adam and his parents. As Adam's mother had moved about 1 hour away, and Adam's father was at work, Dr. Eisenberg used Skype to connect the whole family for the 50-minute session. Dr. Eisenberg's notes indicate good progress was made.

You Code It!

Dr. Eisenberg used technology to have one session with an entire family. Determine the appropriate code to report this service.

Step #1: Read the case carefully and completely.

Step #2: Abstract the scenario. Which key words or terms describe what service the physician provided to the patient during this encounter?

Step #3: Are there any details missing or incomplete for which you would need to query the physician? [If so, ask your instructor.]

Step #4: Determine the correct CPT procedure code or codes to explain the details about what was provided to the patient during this encounter.

Step #5: Check for any relevant guidance, including reading all of the symbols and notations.

Step #6: Do you need to append any modifiers to ensure complete and accurate information is provided?

Step #7: Double-check your work.

Answer:

Did you determine this to be the correct code?

90847-95 **Family psychotherapy (conjoint psychotherapy) (with patient present), 50 minutes, synchronous telemedicine service rendered via a real-time interactive audio and video telecommunications system**

28.4 Dialysis and Gastroenterology Services

Dialysis

Dialysis is an artificial process used to clean the blood by removing excess water and waste products when the individual's body cannot do this. In addition to hospitals providing this service, independent centers and home health agencies help patients receive treatment. The correct code for reporting dialysis service is determined by the patient's age, where the services are provided, and the level of physician services during the encounters.

Physician services provided during a dialysis month included in these codes are

- Determination of the dialysis cycle.
- Outpatient E/M of the dialysis visits.
- Telephone calls.
- Patient management.
- Face-to-face visit with the patient.

Hemodialysis

Hemodialysis is a process that uses a mechanical dialyzer to extract blood via an intravenous catheter to filter out waste products and excess fluids, and returns the "cleaned" blood back into the patient via an intra-arterial catheter. Typically, three sessions a week are provided.

Prior to beginning ongoing hemodialysis treatments, the nephrologist will order the insertion of either an arteriovenous fistula (AVF) or an arteriovenous graft (AVG). For more information on these procedures, see the additional explanations in the in-section guidelines located within the *Surgery* section, subhead **Dialysis Circuit,** directly above code 36901 in your CPT book.

Hemodialysis procedures are reported with one of two codes determined by the number of evaluations provided by the physician during the encounter:

GUIDANCE CONNECTION

Read the additional explanations in the in-section guidelines located within the **Medicine** section, subhead **Dialysis,** subsections **Hemodialysis,** directly above code 90935; **Miscellaneous Dialysis Procedures,** directly above code 90945; and **End-Stage Renal Disease Services,** directly above code 90951, all in your CPT book.

90935   Hemodialysis procedure with single evaluation by a physician or other qualified physician or other health care professional

90937   Hemodialysis procedure requiring repeated evaluation(s) with or without substantial revision of dialysis prescription

When the hemodialysis services are performed by a nonphysician health care professional in the patient's residence, including a private home, assisted living center, group home, nontraditional provider home, custodial care facility, or a school, use this code:

99512   Home visit for hemodialysis

When hemodialysis is provided via an AV fistula, graft, or catheter, there are Category II codes to report this service:

4052F   Hemodialysis via functioning arteriovenous (AV) fistula [ESRD]
4053F   Hemodialysis via functioning arteriovenous (AV) graft [ESRD]
4054F   Hemodialysis via catheter [ESRD]

Access flow studies may be provided to determine the effectiveness of the dialysis process.

90940   Hemodialysis access flow study to determine blood flow in grafts and arteriovenous fistulae by an indicator method

93990   Duplex scan of hemodialysis access (including arterial inflow, body of access and venous outflow)

Other Renal Therapies

There are other types of dialysis provided to patients with renal failure, including

- *Peritoneal dialysis,* which uses a catheter connected to the abdominal cavity, using the peritoneal membrane to filter the blood.

- *Hemofiltration,* which is a process that uses mechanical filtration circuit to clean the blood of waste products and excess fluid using a convection process.

These types of renal therapies are reported with one of two codes:

90945   Dialysis procedure other than hemodialysis, with single evaluation by a physician or other qualified physician or other health care professional

90947   Dialysis procedure other than hemodialysis, requiring repeated evaluation(s) by a physician or other qualified health care professional, with or without substantial revision of dialysis prescription

When these services are provided at the patient's home by a nonphysician professional, use these:

99601   **Home infusion/specialty drug administration, per visit (up to 2 hours)**

+99602   **each additional hour (List separately in addition to code for primary procedure.)**

End-Stage Renal Disease (ESRD)

When a patient is diagnosed with end-stage renal disease (ESRD), dialysis services are reported on a monthly basis, rather than for each individual encounter, with a code from the range 90951–90966. The correct code for reporting dialysis service is determined by

- *Patient's age:* Grouped into ranges: younger than 2 years of age, 2–11 years of age, 12–19 years of age, and 20 years of age and older.
- *Where the services are provided:* Outpatient facility or home dialysis.
- *Level of physician services:* Number of face-to-face visits by a physician.

If a facility does not provide a full month of services to a patient, for whatever reason, then you should use one code from the range 90967–90970, determined by the age of the patient, multiplied by each day of service.

 LET'S CODE IT! SCENARIO

Glory Anders, a 61-year-old female, was diagnosed with ESRD 6 months ago. She has just moved to Springfield to be closer to her daughter and began her daily dialysis on June 20 at the Southside Dialysis Center. Prepare the claim for dialysis services for June.

Let's Code It!

Glory has *ESRD* and has received *dialysis* as an *outpatient* from Southside Dialysis Center. Let's look up *dialysis* in the Alphabetic Index. You can see in the listing for *end-stage renal disease,* there is a reference: "*See* End-Stage Renal Disease Services, Dialysis." Let's turn, in the Alphabetic Index, to this listing. Under this header, you will see Dialysis with the suggested code range of 90951–90970, with further clarification by the location at which the dialysis service was provided. What does the documentation state? ". . . *at the Southside Dialysis Center.*" This helps narrow down the suggested codes to Outpatient . . . 90951–90962.

When you turn to the numeric listing, you read that codes 90951–90962 are only for a full month of treatment. Glory received *11 days* of treatment from the facility (June 20 through June 30 is 11 days), so you have to find the code to report each day of service to Glory. Codes 90967–90970 report dialysis "less than a full month of service, per day" and are broken down by the patient's age. Glory is *61 years old,* bringing us to the following code:

90970   **End-stage renal disease (ESRD) related services for dialysis less than a full month of service, per day; for patients 20 years of age and over**

Great! So the code will read **90970 × 11.**

Gastroenterology Services

A limited number of tests and services for the gastroenterological system—from the patient's mouth down the esophagus to the stomach through the intestinal tract to the rectum—are included in the *Medicine* section of the CPT book. The Alphabetic Index will guide you to the best, most appropriate code in the best section, depending upon the service provided.

Paulina Porter, a 39-year-old female, has been battling with indigestion for over a year. After trying virtually every over-the-counter medication possible, she came to see Dr. Dahl, who decided to administer an esophageal acid reflux test. The test was administered in the office using a nasal catheter intraluminal impedance electrode. The 45-minute test was recorded and analyzed and interpreted by Dr. Dahl.

You Code It!

Go through the steps, and determine the procedure code(s) that should be reported for the test provided by Dr. Dahl to Paulina Porter.

Step #1: Read the case carefully and completely.

Step #2: Abstract the scenario. Which key words or terms describe what service the physician provided to the patient during this encounter?

Step #3: Are there any details missing or incomplete for which you would need to query the physician? [If so, ask your instructor.]

Step #4: Determine the correct CPT procedure code or codes to explain the details about what was provided to the patient during this encounter.

Step #5: Check for any relevant guidance, including reading all of the symbols and notations.

Step #6: Do you need to append any modifiers to ensure complete and accurate information is provided?

Step #7: Double-check your work.

Answer:

Did you determine this to be the correct code?

91037 **Esophageal function test, gastroesophageal reflux test with nasal catheter intraluminal impedance electrode(s) placement, recording, analysis and interpretation**

28.5 Ophthalmology and Otorhinolaryngologic Services

Ophthalmology

Ophthalmologists are commonly called *eye doctors* or *vision specialists.* However, be careful not to confuse them with **optometrists**, who are eyeglass specialists.

The **Ophthalmology** subsection of the CPT book reports services provided by an ophthalmologist. General services, codes 92002–92014, are divided in two ways:

1. *The relationship between the patient and the physician: new patient or established patient.* Remember this from E/M coding? As a reminder, a new patient is one who has not received any services or treatments from the ophthalmologist (or any other physician with the same specialty in the same group practice) within the last 3 years.

2. *The level of service: intermediate or comprehensive.* An intermediate service is similar to a problem-focused evaluation. That is, the patient has a new or existing specific condition to be addressed by the physician. The comprehensive service is more of a general evaluation of the patient's entire visual system.

Ophthalmologist
A physician qualified to diagnose and treat eye disease and conditions with drugs, surgery, and corrective measures.

Optometrist
A professional qualified to carry out eye examinations and to prescribe and supply eyeglasses and contact lenses.

It is important to remember that these general services include both technical examinations and medical decision-making services. Therefore, it is not appropriate to code any of those services separately.

However, special services may be coded separately if provided at the same time as general services or E/M services. The documentation must be specific in its identification of the additional services. (Of course, special services can be provided alone and coded as such.) Codes 92015–92499 are used to report other ophthalmologic services.

LET'S CODE IT! SCENARIO

Warren Preston, a 61-year-old male, has been having a problem with blurred vision and pain in his eyes. His father has glaucoma, which makes Warren at high risk for the disease. Therefore, Dr. Coreley is going to perform a bilateral visual field examination and a serial tonometry with multiple measurements. None of these services is done as a part of a general ophthalmologic service provided to Warren.

Let's Code It!

Dr. Coreley is giving Warren a "*bilateral visual field examination and a serial tonometry*" today. Let's go to the Alphabetic Index and look at *visual field, exam.* The Alphabetic Index suggests codes 92081–92083. Let's take a look at the numeric listing's code description:

92081 **Visual field examination, unilateral or bilateral, with interpretation and report; limited examination (e.g., tangent screen, Autoplot, arc perimeter, or single stimulus level automated test, such as Octopus 3 or 7 equivalent)**

It matches the notes. Now, you need to code the second test, the tonometry. You see that the Alphabetic Index shows *tonometry, serial* and suggests code 92100. Let's take a look at the complete code description:

92100 **Serial tonometry (separate procedure) with multiple measurements of intraocular pressure over an extended time period with interpretation and report, same day (e.g., diurnal curve or medical treatment of acute elevation of intraocular pressure)**

That's great! You are ready to create the claim form for Warren's tests: codes **92081** and **92100.** Good job!

 GUIDANCE CONNECTION

Read the additional explanations in the in-section guidelines located within the **Medicine** section, subhead **Ophthalmology,** directly above code 92002 in your CPT book.

Otorhinolaryngologic Services

Otorhinolaryngology
The study of the human ears, nose, and throat (ENT) systems.

In the **Special Otorhinolaryngologic Services** portion of the *Medicine* section are codes for special services that are not usually included in an office visit or evaluation encounter in the field of **otorhinolaryngology**.

Throughout the listings for codes 92502–92700, you will see all types of tests and services that can help health care professionals diagnose and treat conditions relating to a patient's ears, nose, and throat and their functions.

 YOU CODE IT! CASE STUDY

Darlene Watson came with her husband, Albert, to see Dr. Hudman because of the problems Albert has been having sleeping. Darlene noticed that Albert snores terribly during the night and has, at times, abruptly stopped making noise. She is concerned that he may have actually stopped breathing during one of his episodes. Dr. Hudman performed a nasopharyngoscopy with an endoscope to check Albert's adenoids and lingual tonsils. The results of the exam indicated that Albert is suffering from sleep apnea.

You Code It!

Go through the steps, and determine the code(s) that should be reported for this test provided by Dr. Hudman to Albert Watson.

Step #1: Read the case carefully and completely.

Step #2: Abstract the scenario. Which key words or terms describe what service the physician provided to the patient during this encounter?

Step #3: Are there any details missing or incomplete for which you would need to query the physician? [If so, ask your instructor.]

Step #4: Determine the correct CPT procedure code or codes to explain the details about what was provided to the patient during this encounter.

Step #5: Check for any relevant guidance, including reading all of the symbols and notations.

Step #6: Do you need to append any modifiers to ensure complete and accurate information is provided?

Step #7: Double-check your work.

Answer:

Did you determine this to be the correct code?

92511   Nasopharyngoscopy with endoscope (separate procedure)

That is exactly what Dr. Hudman did. In addition, he did not perform it as a part of any other service, so it was a separate procedure. Excellent!

 GUIDANCE CONNECTION

Read the additional explanations in the in-section guidelines located within the **Medicine** section, subhead **Special Otorhinolaryngologic Services,** directly above code 92502 in your CPT book.

28.6 Cardiovascular Services

When reporting cardiovascular services from the *Medicine* section of CPT, you will find both diagnostic and therapeutic services for conditions of the heart and its vessels. As you look through the descriptions of the codes in this section, you might think that some appear to be surgical in nature (an atherectomy), while others appear to be imaging (radiologic), such as an echocardiogram. Regardless of what you think, the CPT book is structured the way it is, and it is your job as a coding specialist to find the best, most appropriate code to represent the service or treatment provided by the physician or other health care professional for whom you are reporting. Again, this is why it is so important that you take nothing for granted, read all notations and instructions carefully, and use the Alphabetic Index to guide you through the numeric listings.

Cardiovascular Therapeutic Services

A variety of procedures relating to the heart are included in the **Cardiovascular** subsection *Therapeutic Services and Procedures* that might seem more appropriate for other places in the CPT book. For example, the inclusion of intravascular ultrasound and percutaneous transluminal coronary balloon angioplasty illustrates the importance of using the Alphabetic Index to locate the correct range of codes for the procedures performed.

 YOU CODE IT! CASE STUDY

Ransom Sweeney was in Dr. Plenmen's office when Ransom went into cardiac arrest. Dr. Plenmen immediately performed cardiopulmonary resuscitation (CPR). The nurse called 911, and Ransom was taken to the hospital after regaining consciousness and being stabilized.

You Code It!

Go through the steps, and determine the code(s) that should be reported for the service provided by Dr. Plenmen for Ransom Sweeney.

Step #1: Read the case carefully and completely.

Step #2: Abstract the scenario. Which key words or terms describe what service the physician provided to the patient during this encounter?

Step #3: Are there any details missing or incomplete for which you would need to query the physician? [If so, ask your instructor.]

Step #4: Determine the correct CPT procedure code or codes to explain the details about what was provided to the patient during this encounter.

Step #5: Check for any relevant guidance, including reading all of the symbols and notations.

Step #6: Do you need to append any modifiers to ensure complete and accurate information is provided?

Step #7: Double-check your work.

Answer:

Did you determine this to be the correct code?

92950 **Cardiopulmonary resuscitation (e.g., in cardiac arrest)**

It matches the notes perfectly. Good work!

Cardiography

The electronic measurement of heart rhythms very often uses an electrocardiograph (ECG, also called an EKG, machine). Services involving an electrocardiogram are coded from the **Cardiography** subsection.

Implantable and Wearable Cardiac Device Evaluations

Technology has provided physicians with the ability to monitor a person's heart function under various circumstances. You learned how to code the implantation of these devices in the *CPT Surgery Section* chapter of this book, subsection *Cardiovascular System.*

These incredible measuring devices must be programmed, and then data must be gathered by using in-person and/or remote transmission and interpreted by the physician. The codes in this subsection report these services.

Echocardiography

Echocardiography is different from electrocardiography. As the name indicates, an echocardiogram uses ultrasound (sound waves to produce an echo), rather than a measurement by electronic impulses, as with the ECG.

When coding echocardiography, the codes already include

- The exam (the recording of the images of the organ or anatomical areas being studied).
- The interpretation and report of the findings.

You are not permitted to use these codes for echocardiograms that have been taken when no interpretation or report has been done.

Cardiac Catheterization

The codes available for reporting cardiac catheterization include the following:

- The introduction of the **catheter(s)**.
- The positioning and repositioning of the catheter(s).
- Recording of the intracardiac and intravascular pressure.
- Obtaining blood samples for the measurement of blood gases, dilution curves, and/or cardiac output with or without electrode catheter placement.
- Final evaluation and report of the procedure.

Catheter
A thin, flexible tube, inserted into a body part, used to inject fluid, to extract fluid, or to keep a passage open.

CODING BITES

The provision of a cardiac catheterization may require as many as five codes. The determination of how many of these codes you are responsible for reporting will depend upon for whom you are coding (which professional or facility):

1. The professional service for the catheterization . . . procedure code + modifier 26.
2. The administration of the dye . . . procedure code + modifier 51.
3. The radiologist's supervision and interpretation for the guidance for the injection of the dye . . . procedure code + modifier 26.
4. The procedure itself, such as coronary artery angiography.
5. The radiologist's supervision and interpretation of the images.

 LET'S CODE IT! SCENARIO

Mason Franks, a 4-month-old male, was experiencing cyanotic episodes, known as "blue" spells. Dr. Zahn, his pediatrician, performed a transthoracic echocardiogram, which identified a ventricular septal defect and hypertrophied walls of the right ventricle. He then performed a right cardiac catheterization that confirmed a diagnosis of a tetralogy of Fallot.

Let's Code It!

Dr. Zahn performed two tests on little Mason: first, a *transthoracic echocardiogram* and, second, a *right cardiac catheterization.* Let's go to the Alphabetic Index and look for the echocardiogram or echocardiography. Beneath *echocardiography,* you see *transthoracic* with a series of suggested codes. But before you go on, take a look at the indented listing below *transthoracic* for *congenital cardiac anomalies.* Mason is only 4 months old, and his heart problems are congenital; therefore, those are likely the more accurate codes. Let's take a look at the complete descriptions in the numeric listing for the suggested codes 93303 and 93304.

93303 **Transthoracic echocardiography for congenital cardiac anomalies; complete**

This matches the notes. Now, we must code the catheterization. In the Alphabetic Index, under *catheterization,* you find *cardiac,* and indented below that you find a notation, "*See* Cardiac Catheterization." Therefore, look back and find this header in the Alphabetic Index.

Under the *Cardiac Catheterization* header, read down to find *congenital cardiac anomalies* . . . 93530–93533. Let's take a look at the complete description:

93530 **Right heart catheterization, for congenital cardiac anomalies**
93531 **Combined right heart catheterization and retrograde left heart catheterization, for congenital cardiac anomalies**
93532 **Combined right heart catheterization and transseptal left heart catheterization through intact septum with or without retrograde left heart catheterization, for congenital cardiac anomalies**
93533 **Combined right heart catheterization and transseptal left heart catheterization through existing septum opening, with or without retrograde left heart catheterization, for congenital cardiac anomalies**

Excellent. Now, you can see how terms you learned from coding the first procedure—congenital cardiac anomalies—make coding the second procedure easier. From all of those code choices, there is only one that matches the documentation:

93530 **Right heart catheterization, for congenital cardiac anomalies**

It is a small example of how practice and experience will make the entire coding process go more smoothly for you.

Electrophysiologic Procedures

Intracardiac electrophysiologic studies (EPS) codes include

- The insertion of the electrode catheters (usually performed with two or more catheters).
- The repositioning of the catheters.
- Recording of electrograms both before and during the pacing or programmed stimulation of multiple locations of the heart.
- Analysis of the recorded electrograms.
- Report of the procedure and the findings.

There are cases when a diagnostic EPS is followed by treatment (**ablation**) of the problem at the same encounter. When ablation is done at the same time as an EPS, you must code it separately.

Ablation
The destruction or eradication of tissue.

GUIDANCE CONNECTION

Read the additional explanations in the in-section guidelines located within the **Medicine** section, subhead **Cardiovascular,** subsections **Cardiography,** directly above code 93000; **Cardiovascular Monitoring Services,** directly above code 93224; **Implantable, Insertable, and Wearable Cardiac Device Evaluations,** directly above code 93264; **Echocardiography,** directly above code 93303; **Cardiac Catheterization,** directly above code 93451; and **Intracardiac Electrophysiological Procedures/Studies,** directly above code 93600, all in your CPT book.

Noninvasive Vascular Studies

Codes 93880–93998 are provided for reporting noninvasive vascular studies of the arteries and veins of a patient and include the following:

- Preparation of the patient for the testing.
- Supervision of the performance of the tests.
- Recording of the study.
- Interpretation and report of the findings.

Codes are chosen by the type of study done: noninvasive physiologic, transcranial Doppler (TCD), or **duplex scan**.

CODING BITES

If the device used does *not* record the test, then you may not use a separate code for the service.

Duplex Scan
An ultrasonic scanning procedure to determine blood flow and pattern.

 YOU CODE IT! CASE STUDY

Dr. Robbins was giving Teena Salazar her annual physical examination. She had a low-grade fever, and swelling and cyanosis were evident on her lower right leg. Concerned that she might have deep-vein thrombophlebitis, he performed a duplex Doppler ultrasonogram to study the arteries in her leg.

You Code It!

Go through the steps, and determine the code(s) that should be reported for this test performed on Teena Salazar.

Step #1: Read the case carefully and completely.

(continued)

Step #2: Abstract the scenario. Which key words or terms describe what service the physician provided to the patient during this encounter?

Step #3: Are there any details missing or incomplete for which you would need to query the physician? [If so, ask your instructor.]

Step #4: Determine the correct CPT procedure code or codes to explain the details about what was provided to the patient during this encounter.

Step #5: Check for any relevant guidance, including reading all of the symbols and notations.

Step #6: Do you need to append any modifiers to ensure complete and accurate information is provided?

Step #7: Double-check your work.

Answer:

Did you determine this to be the correct code?

93926   Duplex scan of lower extremity arteries or arterial bypass grafts; unilateral or limited study

Good job!

28.7 Pulmonary

Codes 94002–94799 in the Pulmonary subsection identify procedures and tests on the pulmonary system and include

- The exam and/or laboratory procedure.
- Interpretation of the findings.

Pulmonary Function Testing

Pulmonary function testing is performed to measure the ability of the patient's lungs to inspire (bring air into the lungs) and expire (expel gases from the body) as well as measure the efficacy of the lungs to transfer oxygen into the circulatory system of the body.

Spirometry

Spirometry, the basis of pulmonary function testing, measures the quantity of airflow during expiration (exhaling), as well as the speed of this action. The results of this assessment can provide indications of a wide range of lung diseases.

94010   Spirometry, including graphic record, total and timed vital capacity, expiratory flow rate measurement(s), with or without maximal voluntary ventilation

94060   Bronchodilation responsiveness, spirometry as in 94010, pre- and post-bronchodilator administration

Lung Volume Measurement

Measurement of lung volumes can be done in several ways:

- Plethysmography is used to determine total lung capacity, residual volume, functional residual capacity, and airway resistance.
- Helium dilution and/or nitrogen washout are used to measure lung volumes, distribution of ventilation, and closing volume.

Diffusing Capacity

A test for diffusing capacity uses an inhaled tracer gas and is measured during expiration. The comparison between the amount of gas acquired during inspiration and the amount exhaled evidences the effectiveness of air and gases moving from the lungs into the blood.

+94729   **Diffusing capacity (e.g., carbon monoxide, membrane)**

 GUIDANCE CONNECTION

Read the additional explanations in the in-section guidelines located within the **Medicine** section, subhead **Pulmonary,** subsection **Pulmonary Diagnostic Testing and Therapies,** directly above code 94010 in your CPT book.

 YOU CODE IT! CASE STUDY

Carmine Allen, a 2-day-old male, was born at 35-weeks gestation, with a birth weight of 1,450 g. After exhibiting hypotension, peripheral edema, and oliguria, Carmine was diagnosed by Dr. Yanger with respiratory distress syndrome. Dr. Yanger performed the initiation of continuous positive airway pressure ventilation (CPAP).

You Code It!

Go through the steps, and determine the code(s) that should be reported for this treatment provided to Carmine.

Step #1: Read the case carefully and completely.

Step #2: Abstract the scenario. Which key words or terms describe what service the physician provided to the patient during this encounter?

Step #3: Are there any details missing or incomplete for which you would need to query the physician? [If so, ask your instructor.]

Step #4: Determine the correct CPT procedure code or codes to explain the details about what was provided to the patient during this encounter.

Step #5: Check for any relevant guidance, including reading all of the symbols and notations.

Step #6: Do you need to append any modifiers to ensure complete and accurate information is provided?

Step #7: Double-check your work.

Answer:

Did you determine this to be the correct code?

    94660   **Continuous positive airway pressure ventilation (CPAP) initiation and management**

Excellent!

28.8 Allergy and Clinical Immunology

Codes 95004–95199 cover allergy and clinical immunology procedures. Allergies can be responsible for many different reactions in the human body. Beyond the typical sneezing and watery eyes, outcomes can cause anything from hives and rashes to behavioral problems, sleeplessness, and even death.

Often, when there is concern or suspicion that a patient may be suffering from an allergic reaction, the physician will begin with allergy sensitivity tests. In these cases,

CODING BITES

The process of desensitizing can take weeks, months, or years, so pay close attention to the dates of service.

small yet potent samples of the suspected allergen are given to the patient in one of a number of methods: percutaneously (scratch, puncture, or prick), intracutaneously (intradermal), inhalation, or ingestion. Then the patient is watched, and the body's reaction to the allergen is documented. The results of the tests tell the physician to which elements the patient is considered allergic.

Once an allergy is identified, immunotherapy may be provided. The therapy is a way of retraining the patient's immune system, or desensitizing it, so that the body no longer views the particles as a threat.

EXAMPLE

Dr. Bagg conducted percutaneous scratch testing with immediate reactions on Shelley to identify the cause of her asthma. He tested her for a dozen common allergens. Report this with **95004 Percutaneous tests × 12** tests.

 ## LET'S CODE IT! SCENARIO

PATIENT: Marina Louongo

REASON FOR VISIT: Skin testing to environmental allergens.

HISTORY OF PRESENT ILLNESS: The patient was a long-standing patient of Dr. Yeager in Masonville, her previous hometown in the north side of the state, and had received immunotherapy for the past several years. She was referred to us by her new neighbor.

She had been getting injections for grass/ragweed/plantain, cat/dog/mold, dust mite, and trees. She states she has been having some difficulty with local reactions and swelling to the tree injection. She is using Tylenol before and after injections along with ice, which has helped somewhat. She gets injections every 3 weeks. Patient states she had an episode one time where her arms swelled significantly and she required oral prednisone. She typically has allergy symptoms in February, March, November, and December with rhinitis, congestion, and itchy eyes. She was going to get dust covers for her pillow and mattress but hasn't gotten around to it. Her bedroom is carpeted. She denies smoking.

CURRENT MEDICATIONS: Flonase and Clarinex prior to injections.

PHYSICAL EXAMINATION: She is a healthy-appearing, well-nourished, well-developed 27-year-old female in no acute distress.

Skin testing via prick was positive to birch 2+, beech 2+, ash 0/1+, hickory 1+, mite DF 2+, mite DP 2+, histamine 3+, grass 3+, mugwort 1+, oak 4+, and maple 3+.

IMPRESSION: Seasonal and perennial allergic rhinitis.

RECOMMENDATIONS:
1. Continue immunotherapy here with birch/oak/maple, mite DF/DP, grass/mugwort.
2. Continue Flonase two sprays per nostril daily during the spring and fall.
3. Environmental control measures regarding dust and pollen.
4. Report was sent to Dr. Yeager, along with patient's signed Release of Information form so we can get copies of her previous medical records.

Alvin Birchwood, MD

Let's Code It!

Dr. Birchwood did percutaneous skin prick testing on Marina. Turn in the CPT Alphabetic Index and find

> **Allergy Tests**
> Skin Tests
> Allergen Extract...................... 95004, 95024, 95027

(continued)

Turn to the *Main Section* of CPT and read carefully the complete code descriptions for all three of these suggestions.

95004   **Percutaneous tests (scratch, puncture, prick) with allergenic extracts, immediate type reaction, including test interpretation and report, specify number of tests**

95024   **Intracutaneous (intradermal) tests with allergenic extracts, immediate type reaction, including test interpretation and report, specify number of tests**

95027   **Intracutaneous (intradermal) tests, sequential and incremental, with allergenic extracts for airborne allergens, immediate type reaction, including test interpretation and report, specify number of tests**

Which of these is supported by Dr. Birchwood's documentation? Did you determine . . .

95004   **Percutaneous tests (scratch, puncture, prick) with allergenic extracts, immediate type reaction, including test interpretation and report, specify number of tests**

Correct! Now, how many tests were performed? The documentation states: "birch, beech, ash, hickory, mite DF, mite DP, histamine, grass, mugwort, oak, maple."

A total of 11 tests were performed, so you can report **95004 × 11** with confidence. Good work!

28.9 Neurology and Neuromuscular Procedures

GUIDANCE CONNECTION

As with so many other headings in this section, the neurology and neuromuscular procedure codes (95782–96020) include the recording of the test as well as the physician's interpretation and report of the findings.

Acronyms often seen in this arena of health care services include:

EEG	Electroencephalogram
EMG	Electromyogram
EOG	Electrooculogram
MEG	Magnetoencephalography

Read the additional explanations in the in-section guidelines located within the **Medicine** section, subhead **Neurology and Neuromuscular Procedures,** directly following code 95251 in your CPT book.

 LET'S CODE IT! SCENARIO

Ian Ellington, a 47-year-old male, was having a hard time staying awake during the day and asleep during the night. Dr. Bruse sent him down the hall to have a polysomnography, with three additional parameters, to rule out sleep apnea.

Let's Code It!

Dr. Bruse ordered a *polysomnography* on Ian to see if he has *sleep apnea*. Let's turn to the Alphabetic Index and find

    Polysomnography......................95782, 95783, 95808–95811

As you read through the complete code descriptions in the numeric listing, you will see that, because Dr. Bruse ordered *three additional parameters,* the best code is

95808   **Polysomnography; any age, sleep staging with 1–3 additional parameters of sleep, attended by a technologist**

Excellent!

Central Nervous System Assessments

When a patient exhibits problems with cognitive processes, testing may evaluate the extent of the condition so that a treatment plan can be established. It is expected that the results of the tests in the **Central Nervous System** subsection (codes 96105–96146) will be formulated into a report to be used in the creation of a treatment plan.

 GUIDANCE CONNECTION

Read the additional explanations in the in-section guidelines located within the **Medicine** section, subhead **Central Nervous System Assessments/Tests (eg, Neuro-Cognitive, Mental Status, Speech Testing),** directly above code 96105 in your CPT book.

 YOU CODE IT! CASE STUDY

Oliver Gates, a 3-year-old male, does not appear to be meeting certain milestones. Dr. Saunders performed a developmental test known as an Early Language Milestone Screening and spent 85 minutes assessing his motor skills, social, and language functions. Once the test was interpreted, he sent his report and contacted a speech therapist to consult on a treatment plan.

You Code It!

Go through the steps, and determine the code(s) that should be reported for this screening test performed on Oliver.

Step #1: Read the case carefully and completely.

Step #2: Abstract the scenario. Which key words or terms describe what service the physician provided to the patient during this encounter?

Step #3: Are there any details missing or incomplete for which you would need to query the physician? [If so, ask your instructor.]

Step #4: Determine the correct CPT procedure code or codes to explain the details about what was provided to the patient during this encounter.

Step #5: Check for any relevant guidance, including reading all of the symbols and notations.

Step #6: Do you need to append any modifiers to ensure complete and accurate information is provided?

Step #7: Double-check your work.

Answer:

Did you determine this to be the correct code?

96112	Developmental testing administration (including assessment of fine and/or gross motor, language, cognitive level, social, memory and/or executive functions by standardized developmental instruments when performed) by physician or other qualified health care professional, with interpretation and report, first hour
+96113	each additional 30 minutes

Good work!

28.10 Physical Medicine and Rehabilitation

Physiatrists are health care professionals who specialize in physical medicine and rehabilitation, focusing their skills and knowledge to evaluate and treat traumatic injuries, illnesses, and resulting disabilities affecting components of the nervous system and musculoskeletal systems. The goals of these health care encounters are most often centered around maximizing the patient's physical function and improving quality of life.

Physical therapy focuses on working with patients who have been injured or disabled by an illness, with the goal of helping them restore their mobility. These sessions educate patients with methodologies to manage their physical situations, promote healing, and prevent further deterioration of physical abilities.

Occupational therapy connects patients with activities they can participate in to improve their quality of life, and sometimes independence. The positive outcomes of these therapies include disabled students gaining inclusion in school and social events, as well as working with patients to function despite cognitive or physical changes.

Throughout the **Physical Medicine and Rehabilitation** subsection and its components, note that some groups of codes require the provider to have direct (face-to-face) contact with the patient during the course of the treatment and others do not.

> **CODING BITES**
>
> Codes 97010–97799 are used to report each distinct procedure provided to the patient. Modifier 51 cannot be used with any of these codes.

 YOU CODE IT! CASE STUDY

DATE OF PHYSICAL THERAPY EVALUATION: 05/31/2019

DATE OF INJURY: 03/18/2019

HISTORY OF PRESENT ILLNESS: The patient is a 19-year-old male who was the driver in an MVA. He was struck from behind by a tractor trailer, causing his car to fishtail, landing beneath the truck's trailer. He is single and lives with his parents while he finishes college. His injuries have halted his education for now, but he is determined to reenroll at a future date. He depends, right now, on someone to transport him to our facility.

ASSESSMENT AND PLAN: The patient is a 19-year-old male, status post multiple trauma.
  For full assessment notes, including exam and clinical presentation of characteristics, see attached notes.

1. Rehabilitation: Toe-touch weightbearing, left lower extremity. Weightbearing as tolerated, left upper extremity. PT, OT, speech language pathology, therapeutic recreation, and psychology to see and treat.
2. Deep venous thrombosis prophylaxis: The patient is on Fragmin. The patient is to have his Dopplers repeated.
3. Gastrointestinal prophylaxis: The patient is not on anything but complains of systemic nausea. We will start Pepcid 20 mg b.i.d.
4. Bowel and bladder: Overflow urinary incontinence. We will place Foley and start Urecholine 12.5 mg p.o. t.i.d.
5. Pain: Not well controlled. Start Oramorph 15 mg with Percocet for breakthrough and schedule before therapies.

DISPOSITION: The patient will likely be discharged to home with any equipment and modifications PRN.

You Code It!

Dr. Gerald Foxglove was called in to perform a predischarge physical therapy evaluation.

Step #1: Read the case carefully and completely.

Step #2: Abstract the scenario. Which key words or terms describe what service the physician provided to the patient during this encounter?

Step #3: Are there any details missing or incomplete for which you would need to query the physician? [If so, ask your instructor.]

Step #4: Determine the correct CPT procedure code or codes to explain the details about what was provided to the patient during this encounter.

Step #5: Check for any relevant guidance, including reading all of the symbols and notations.

Step #6: Do you need to append any modifiers to ensure complete and accurate information is provided?

Step #7: Double-check your work.

(continued)

Answer:

Did you determine this to be the correct code?

> **97163**   **Physical therapy evaluation; high complexity, requiring these components: a history of present problem with 3 or more personal factors and/or comorbidities that impact the plan of care; an examination of body systems using standardized tests and measures addressing a total of 4 or more elements from any of the following: body structures and functions, activity limitations, and/or participation restrictions; a clinical presentation with unstable and unpredictable characteristics; and clinical decision-making of high complexity using standardized patient assessment instrument and/or measurable assessment of functional outcome.**

GUIDANCE CONNECTION

Read the additional explanations in the in-section guidelines located within the **Medicine** section, subhead **Acupuncture,** directly above code 97810 in your CPT book.

28.11 Acupuncture, Osteopathic, and Chiropractic Treatments

Acupuncture

The health care industry is always evolving and incorporating new techniques into its accepted methods for helping patients. The techniques of acupuncture (codes 97810–97814) are thousands of years old but are newly accepted by Western medicine and health insurance payers.

Acupuncture services are measured in 15-minute increments of direct provider-patient contact. While the needles may be in place for a longer period of time, you are permitted to report only the time actually spent with the patient.

 LET'S CODE IT! SCENARIO

Josie Rossini, a 57-year-old female, was having a problem with menopause. Because of the reported concerns about hormone replacement therapy (HRT), she decided to try acupuncture. After discussing her symptoms and a treatment plan, Dr. Kini inserted several needles. The needles were removed 20 minutes later. Dr. Kini reviewed the follow-up plan and made an appointment for Josie's next visit. Dr. Kini spent 30 minutes in total face-to-face with Josie, who reported marked improvement.

Let's Code It!

Dr. Kini's treatment of Josie included *30 minutes face-to-face time* and *several needles* during the *acupuncture* treatment. Let's turn to the Alphabetic Index and look up *acupuncture.*

> **Acupuncture**
> With Electrical Stimulation 97813–97814
> Without Electrical Stimulation 97810–97811

There is no mention of electrical stimulation being used in Josie's treatment, so turn to the codes recommended for *without electrical stimulation.*

> **97810**   **Acupuncture, 1 or more needles; without electrical stimulation, initial 15 minutes of personal one-on-one contact with the patient**
> **+97811**   **without electrical stimulation, each additional 15 minutes of personal one-on-one contact with the patient, with reinsertion of needles(s) (List separately in addition to code for primary procedure.)**

The first code, 97810, reports Dr. Kini's services, but only for the first 15 minutes. You have to add the second code, 97811, to report the remainder of the time so that the doctor can be reimbursed for the total 30 minutes for the session.

Osteopathic Manipulative Treatments

Codes 98925–98929, to report osteopathic manipulative treatments (OMT), are defined by the number of body regions involved in the encounter. Ten regions are identified with the codes:

- Head
- Cervical
- Thoracic
- Rib cage
- Upper extremities
- Lumbar
- Sacral
- Abdominal/visceral
- Pelvic
- Lower extremities

Chiropractic Manipulative Treatment

Similar to the osteopathic treatment codes, chiropractic manipulative treatment (CMT) codes 98940–98943 are determined by the number of regions treated during an encounter. The codes use spinal or extraspinal descriptions and are identified as follows:

Spinal Regions

- Cervical, including atlanto-occipital joint.
- Thoracic, including costovertebral and costotransverse joints.
- Lumbar.
- Sacral.
- Pelvic, including the sacroiliac joint.

Extraspinal Regions

- Head, including temporomandibular joint (but not the atlanto-occipital).
- Upper extremities.
- Rib cage, excluding costotransverse and costovertebral joints.
- Abdomen.
- Lower extremities.

GUIDANCE CONNECTION

Read the additional explanations in the in-section guidelines located within the **Medicine** section, subhead **Osteopathic Manipulative Treatment,** directly above code 98925 in your CPT book.

GUIDANCE CONNECTION

Read the additional explanations in the in-section guidelines located within the **Medicine** section, subhead **Chiropractic Manipulative Treatment,** directly above code 98940 in your CPT book.

 YOU CODE IT! CASE STUDY

Evan LaVelle, a 37-year-old male who is 6 ft 6 in. tall, has pain in his neck and spine. Dr. Eisenberg, a chiropractor, provides CMT to his cervical, thoracic, lumbar, sacral, and pelvic regions to alleviate Evan's pain.

You Code It!

Go through the steps, and determine the code(s) that should be reported for this CMT encounter.

Step #1: Read the case carefully and completely.

(continued)

Step #2: Abstract the scenario. Which key words or terms describe what service the physician provided to the patient during this encounter?

Step #3: Are there any details missing or incomplete for which you would need to query the physician? [If so, ask your instructor.]

Step #4: Determine the correct CPT procedure code or codes to explain the details about what was provided to the patient during this encounter.

Step #5: Check for any relevant guidance, including reading all of the symbols and notations.

Step #6: Do you need to append any modifiers to ensure complete and accurate information is provided?

Step #7: Double-check your work.

Answer:

Did you determine this to be the correct code?

98942   **Chiropractic manipulative treatment (CMT); spinal, five regions**

Good job!

28.12 Other Services Provided

Education and Training for Patient Self-Management

Technological and other health care treatment and pharmaceutical advancements have made it easier for the average patient to care for him- or herself or for a caregiver to administer treatments formerly provided exclusively by a physician. Of course, this is not something that should be done without guidance, so it is important that the patient or caregiver is taught how to administer treatment properly. Education and training for patient self-management are reported by using codes 98960–98962.

> **EXAMPLE**
> - Teaching a diabetic patient how to self-administer insulin injections.
> - Teaching a caregiver how to change a dressing.

GUIDANCE CONNECTION

Read the additional explanations in the in-section guidelines located within the **Medicine** section, subhead **Non-Face-to-Face Nonphysician Services,** directly above code 98966 in your CPT book.

Non-Face-to-Face Nonphysician Services

Nurses and allied health care professionals extend the ability of a physician to communicate with patients. When a qualified nonphysician member of the health care team provides an assessment and management service to an established patient via telephone or online electronic contact, this service is reported with a code from 98966–98969.

Special Services, Procedures, and Reports

There are times when a health care professional is required to provide a service or write a report that is outside the normal realm of his or her responsibilities or outside of the scope of other codes in the CPT book. In those cases, match the circumstance to one of the descriptions in the **Special Services, Procedures, and Reports** subsection (codes 99000–99091). Each code identifies a different special situation.

GUIDANCE CONNECTION

Read the additional explanations in the in-section guidelines located within the **Medicine** section, subhead **Special Services, Procedures and Reports,** directly above code 99000 in your CPT book.

Medication Therapy Management Services

When a patient is prescribed multiple medications, especially when ordered by multiple providers, a pharmacist may step in to assess the list and intervene as necessary. The pharmacist can provide insights into potential drug interactions and duplications caused by secondary ingredients.

Medication Therapy Management Services (MTMS) codes can be reported when the following has been documented:

- Review of the pertinent patient history.
- Review of the medication profile for prescription and nonprescription drugs and herbal supplements.
- Specific recommendations for improving patient health outcomes.
- Recommendations to support the patient's treatment compliance.

The codes available to report these services are

99605   **Medication therapy management service(s) provided by a pharmacist, individual, face-to-face with patient, with assessment and intervention, if provided; initial 15 minutes, new patient**

99606   **Medication therapy management service(s) provided by a pharmacist, individual, face-to-face with patient, with assessment and intervention, if provided; initial 15 minutes, established patient**

+99607   **each additional 15 minutes (List separately in addition to code for primary service.)**

As stated in the CPT guidelines, these codes should not be used to report the provision of product-specific information at the time the product is provided to the patient or any other routine dispensing-related activities.

Home Health Procedures/Services

In the chapter *CPT Evaluation and Management Coding,* you learned about codes 99341–99350 for services provided by a physician at the patient's home. However, occasionally a health care professional in your facility *other than the physician* provides services to a patient at his or her home. The person may be a nurse or therapist, for example. For nonphysician clinical professionals, you must use the codes 99500–99602 from the **Home Health Procedures/Services** subsection in the *Medicine* section.

GUIDANCE CONNECTION

Read the additional explanations in the in-section guidelines located within the **Medicine** section, subhead **Home Health Procedures/Services,** directly above code 99500 in your CPT book.

YOU CODE IT! CASE STUDY

Eliot Sharpton is a Certified Diabetes Educator (CDE) and is meeting today with Robyn Wu. She was just diagnosed with type 2 diabetes mellitus. Eliot spends 30 minutes with her, using the standardized curriculum, to help Robyn adjust her diet, get some exercise in her routine, and answer questions about her medication.

You Code It!

Determine the correct code or codes to report Eliot Sharpton, CDE's training of Robyn Wu.

Step #1: Read the case carefully and completely.

Step #2: Abstract the scenario. Which key words or terms describe what service the physician provided to the patient during this encounter?

Step #3: Are there any details missing or incomplete for which you would need to query the physician? [If so, ask your instructor.]

Step #4: Determine the correct CPT procedure code or codes to explain the details about what was provided to the patient during this encounter.

Step #5: Check for any relevant guidance, including reading all of the symbols and notations.

Step #6: Do you need to append any modifiers to ensure complete and accurate information is provided?

Step #7: Double-check your work.

Answer:

Did you determine this to be the code?

98960 **Education and training for patient self-management by a qualified, nonphysician health care professional using a standardized curriculum, face-to-face with the patient (could include caregiver/family) each 30 minutes; individual patient**

Fantastic!

Chapter Summary

Many services provided by physicians, therapists, chiropractors, and other trained health care professionals deserve to receive reimbursement. The *Medicine* section contains information about these services. The variety of services included in the *Medicine* section emphasizes the fact that finding the correct code begins in the Alphabetic Index and culminates in the numeric listings.

CODING BITES

The *Medicine* section of the CPT book has codes for services that are supplied by health care professionals but not represented in any other sections. Services reported using codes from the *Medicine* section include these:

- Flu shots
- Vaccinations for the kids to go back to school
- Allergy shots
- Chiropractic services
- Psychotherapy
- Dialysis

- Hearing evaluations
- Vision checks
- Chemotherapy
- Acupuncture

Wherever you work as a coding specialist, there is an excellent chance you will be using this section. Let's go through it together.

CHAPTER 28 REVIEW
CPT Medicine Section

Mc Graw Hill **connect**

Enhance your learning by completing these exercises and more at mcgrawhillconnect.com!

Let's Check It! Terminology

Match each key term to the appropriate definition.

1. LO 28.2 The introduction of a fluid into a blood vessel.

2. LO 28.6 The destruction or eradication of tissue.

3. LO 28.2 The delivery of an additional drug via an intravenous line over a short period of time.

4. LO 28.6 A thin, flexible tube, inserted into a body part, used to inject fluid, to extract fluid, or to keep a passage open.

5. LO 28.5 A professional qualified to carry out eye examinations and to prescribe and supply eyeglasses and contact lenses.

6. LO 28.2 Compelling a fluid into tissue or cavity.

7. LO 28.5 A physician qualified to diagnose and treat eye disease and conditions with drugs, surgery, and corrective measures.

8. LO 28.6 An ultrasonic scanning procedure to determine blood flow and pattern.

9. LO 28.5 The study of the human ears, nose, and throat (ENT) systems.

10. LO 28.1 To make someone resistant to a particular disease by vaccination.

A. Ablation

B. Catheter

C. Duplex scan

D. Immunization

E. Infusion

F. Injection

G. Ophthalmologist

H. Optometrist

I. Otorhinolaryngology

J. Push

Let's Check It! Concepts

Choose the most appropriate answer for each of the following questions.

1. LO 28.1 When an immunization is given, you will need

   a. one code for administering the immunization.

   b. two codes: one for the administration and one for the drug.

   c. one code for the medication or drug.

   d. one HCPCS Level II code.

2. LO 28.2 When a patient receives infusion therapy via more than one IV site, code

   a. only the first site.

   b. all appropriate services for each site.

   c. infusion time instead of number of sites.

   d. only when chemotherapy is infused.

3. **LO 28.3** Which of the following codes identifies an encounter for psychotherapy, 60 minutes with patient?

   a. 90832

   b. 90834

   c. 90836

   d. 90837

4. **LO 28.4** Dialysis codes are reported by

   a. the patient's age.

   b. the number of days treated.

   c. the location of treatment (inpatient or outpatient).

   d. all of these.

5. **LO 28.5** An optometrist is qualified to

   a. diagnose and treat serious eye diseases.

   b. supply glasses and contact lenses.

   c. write prescriptions for the treatment of serious eye diseases.

   d. perform surgery.

6. **LO 28.6** What code would you assign for a duplex scan of the left radial artery?

   a. 93925   b. 93926

   c. 93930   d. 93931

7. **LO 28.12** Medication Therapy Management Services (MTMS) codes can be reported when all of the following have been documented *except*

   a. review of the pertinent patient examination.

   b. review of medication profile for prescription and nonprescription drugs and herbal supplements.

   c. specific recommendations for improving patient health outcomes.

   d. recommendations to support the patient's treatment compliance.

8. **LO 28.11** Chiropractic treatment codes are chosen by

   a. the time spent face-to-face with the patient.

   b. the total number of treatments in a month.

   c. the number of regions treated.

   d. the age of the patient.

9. **LO 28.9** Kinney Harris, a 41-year-old male, was in an automobile accident and was transported to the nearest hospital, unconscious. The ED physician, Dr. Alexander, attempted to awaken Kinney with stimulants without success. Dr. Alexander performs an EEG due to Kinney's comatose condition. What is the correct code for the EEG?

   a. 95812

   b. 95816

   c. 95822

   d. 95824

10. **LO 28.10** Betty Cannon receives an acupuncture treatment, two needles, for a total of 45 minutes of face-to-face time with Dr. Hamilton. What is/are the correct code(s) for this procedure?

   a. 97810

   b. 97810, 97811

   c. 97813, 97814

   d. 97810, 97811, 97811

Let's Check It! Guidelines

Refer to the Medicine Guidelines and fill in the blanks accordingly.

99070	not	Medicine	assessment
add-on	identified	itself	16 minutes
"Special Report"	"separate procedure"	independent	
independently	59	integral	
99600	Introduction	supply	
nomenclature	"Unlisted Procedure"	exempt	

1. In addition to the definitions and commonly used terms present in the _____, several other items unique to this section on _____ are defined or identified here.

2. All _____ codes found in the CPT codebook are _____ from the multiple procedure concept.

3. Add-on codes in the CPT codebook can be readily _____ by specific descriptor _____ which includes phrases such as "each additional" or "(List separately in addition to primary procedure.)"

4. The codes designated as _____ should not be reported in addition to the code for the total procedure or service of which it is considered an _____ component.

5. However, when a procedure or service that is designated as a "separate procedure" is carried out _____ or considered to be unrelated or distinct from other procedures/services provided at the time, it may be reported by _____, or in addition to other procedures/services by appending modifier _____ to the specific "separate procedure" code to indicate that the procedure is not considered to be a component of another procedure, but is a distinct, _____ procedure.

6. Supplies and materials over and above those usually included with the procedure(s) rendered are reported separately using code _____ or a specific _____ code.

7. A service or procedure may be provided that is _____ listed in this edition of the CPT code book. When reporting such a service, the appropriate _____ code may be used to indicate the service, identifying it by _____.

8. Unlisted home visit service or procedure is reported with code _____.

9. The psychotherapy services codes 90832–90838 include ongoing _____ and adjustment of psychotherapeutic interventions, and may include involvement of informants in the treatment process.

10. Do not report psychotherapy of less than _____ duration.

Let's Check It! Rules and Regulations

Please answer the following questions from the knowledge you have gained after reading this chapter.

1. LO 28.1 List five ways medication can be administered to a patient.

2. LO 28.2 Explain the *standard parts* included in infusion and injection codes.

3. LO 28.3 What are the categories of psychotherapy?

4. LO 28.4 What physician services are included in the codes during a dialysis month?

5. LO 28.6 What do the available codes for reporting a cardiac catheterization include?

(CPT) YOU CODE IT! BASICS

First, identify the procedural main term(s) in the following statements; then code the procedure or service.

Example: Alan Capshaw, PA, completes a home visit for mechanical ventilation care.

　　a. main term: *Ventilation Assist*　b. procedure: *99504*

1. Dr. Jameson performs a psychotherapy session with the patient, 45 minutes:

　　a. main term: _____　　b. procedure: _____

2. Dr. Graban completes a therapeutic repetitive transcranial magnetic stimulation (TMS), initial treatment:

　　a. main term: _____　　b. procedure: _____

3. Dr. Kantsiper performs biofeedback training, anorectal:

   a. main term: _____   **b.** procedure: _____

4. Dr. Abernethy completes a diagnostic transcutaneous electrogastrography:

   a. main term: _____   **b.** procedure: _____

5. Dr. Shutter fits a contact lens for management of keratoconus, initial fitting:

   a. main term: _____   **b.** procedure: _____

6. Dr. Sanning completes a positional nystagmus test:

   a. main term: _____   **b.** procedure: _____

7. Dr. Foldings performs a tympanometry and reflex threshold measurements:

   a. main term: _____   **b.** procedure: _____

8. Dr. Edge completes a right heart catheterization including measurement of oxygen saturation and cardiac output:

   a. main term: _____   **b.** procedure: _____

9. Dr. Pugh performs a duplex scan of lower extremity arteries; complete bilateral study:

   a. main term: _____   **b.** procedure: _____

10. Dr. McKee completes nitric oxide expired gas determination:

    a. main term: _____   **b.** procedure: _____

11. Dr. Middleton performs an unattended sleep study with simultaneous recording of heart rate, oxygen saturation, respiratory analysis, and sleep time:

    a. main term: _____   **b.** procedure: _____

12. Dr. Trezevant completes a manual muscle testing with report of extremity:

    a. main term: _____   **b.** procedure: _____

13. Dr. Reese performs a chemotherapy administration, intra-arterial; infusion technique, 45 minutes:

    a. main term: _____   **b.** procedure: _____

14. Dr. Kemper performs an anogenital (perineum) examination, magnified in childhood for suspected trauma:

    a. main term: _____   **b.** procedure: _____

15. Dr. Guinyard completes a home visit for prenatal monitoring and assessment including fetal heart rate and nonstress test:

    a. main term: _____   **b.** procedure: _____

 YOU CODE IT! Practice

Using the techniques described in this chapter, carefully read through the case studies and determine the most accurate Medicine section CPT code(s) and modifier(s), if appropriate, for each case study.

1. Marlene Overton, a 59-year-old female, has been suffering from bronchitis off and on for 2 years. Dr. Turner has ordered a pulmonary stress test for her. Dr. Turner notes that he wants her CO_2 and O_2 uptake measured during the test as well as an electrocardiogram to be recorded.

2. Grant Hughes, a 74-year-old male, has uncontrolled diabetes and comes into the emergency department complaining of signs of hyperglycemia. Dr. Hawkins gives him insulin subcutaneous and IV push to bring his blood sugar down. Code injection administration only.

3. After finding relief nowhere else, Rasheem Conner, a 42-year-old female, goes to Dr. Johnston, an acupuncturist, for treatment of her osteoarthritic knee. Dr. Johnston spends 15 minutes with the patient reviewing history and symptoms, palpating, and locating the points to treat, and inserts the needles and applies electrical stimulation. Rasheem is asked to rest. Dr. Johnston comes back in about 10 minutes later and spends 5 minutes monitoring the patient and restimulating the needles. Ten minutes later, Dr. Johnston sees that the pain and swelling in Rasheem's knee have reduced, removes the needles, and instructs Rasheem on home care measures. Dr. Johnston spent a total of 30 minutes in direct contact with Rasheem.

4. Darlene Overton, an 8-year-old female, is brought to Dr. Mackinaw by her mother after a referral from the school counselor and her pediatrician. Darlene is having difficulties with classwork. Mrs. Overton also tells Dr. Mackinaw that Darlene has a problem understanding speech in noisy environments. Darlene may have a

hearing deficiency that has not shown up in hearing tests before, and it may account for her declining work in class. Dr. Mackinaw performs a central auditory function evaluation, which takes 1 hour, with report.

5. Kent Egerton, a 13-year-old male, suffered from a severe asthma attack while at the playground. He was rushed to the clinic, where he was given a nebulizer treatment (nonpressurized inhalation).

6. Kenya Cantrell, a 41-year-old female, broke out in a rash, which would not go away. After trying multiple over-the-counter treatments, she went to Dr. Beech, who did a series of 11 allergenic extract scratch tests to see if he could identify an allergen. The tests pointed to an allergy to her new kitten.

7. Kenya (previous scenario) didn't want to give away her new kitten, so Dr. Beech prepared the allergenic extract and began immunotherapy injections. She received the first injection today.

8. Paul Kensington, a 51-year-old male, is beginning chemotherapy today with the administration of methotrexate, via IV push.

9. Darren Pinchot, a 24-year-old male, is a lifeguard at the beach and came into the emergency clinic with uncontrolled nausea and vomiting. Darren told Dr. Valentine that he was on the beach for 12 hours straight with no breaks because his replacement didn't show up. Dr. Valentine diagnosed him with severe dehydration and ordered 20 minutes of Zofran, IV infusion, and then saline for 4 hours.

10. Robin Gerstein, a 32-year-old female, comes to Duane Nettles, a licensed massage therapist, as prescribed by Dr. Luellen. Robin is pregnant and has been suffering from acute lower back pain for over a month. Duane performs therapeutic massage with effleurage on the left side and kneading on the iliac band, nerve stroking, and light compression on the gluteus for a total of 15 minutes.

11. Robert Kini, a 9-day-old male, was born prematurely, and Dr. Martin is concerned about Robert's heart. He performs a combined right heart catheterization and transseptal left heart catheterization through the intact septum, in order to measure the blood gases and record Robert's intracardiac pressure. Dr. Martin provides conscious sedation, 15 minutes, while the nurse monitors Robert's status during the procedure.

12. Felicia Gardener, a 6-year-old female, comes to see Dr. Kaplan for an evaluation of her cochlear implant. Dr. Kaplan reprograms the implant to improve Felicia's reception.

13. Alice Heath, a 73-year-old female, came to see Dr. Browne, her ophthalmologist, for an annual checkup of her eyes. Dr. Browne does a comprehensive evaluation of Alice's complete visual system.

14. Jalal Kalisz, a 68-year-old male, came to see Dr. McDaniel because he was having chest pain. Dr. McDaniel performed a routine ECG with 15 leads. After talking with Jalal and reviewing the ECG results, Dr. McDaniel determined that Jalal was having a bout of indigestion.

15. Cecil Rossini, an 18-year-old female, is a professional gymnast who pulled a muscle in her shoulder. Today, Dr. Salton measured her range of motion in the shoulder to confirm that the area has healed completely. Dr. Salton then wrote and signed the report.

 # YOU CODE IT! Application

The following exercises provide practice in the application of abstracting the physicians' notes and learning to work with documentation from our health care facilities. These case studies are modeled on real patient encounters. Using the techniques described in this chapter, carefully read through the case studies and determine the most accurate Medicine section CPT code(s) and modifier(s), if appropriate, for each case study.

WESTON HOSPITAL

629 Healthcare Way • SOMEWHERE, FL 32811 • 407-555-6541

PATIENT: HAUPTON, NICHOLAS

ACCOUNT/EHR #: HAUPNI001

DATE: 10/13/20

(continued)

Attending Physician: Jessica P. Turner, MD

PATIENT SERVICES:

IV fluid replacement for dehydration, intravenous, 58 minutes

Continuous pulse oximetry

Therapeutic warm water enema for intussusception

Robin P. Moss, RN

RPM/mg   D: 10/13/20 09:50:16   T: 10/15/20 12:55:01

Determine the most accurate Medicine section CPT code(s) and modifier(s), if appropriate.

SPELLING CHIROPRACTIC CENTER

A Complete Health Care Facility

159 Healthcare Way • SOMEWHERE, FL 32811 • 407-555-6789

PATIENT: CARMICHAEL, ABIGAIL

ACCOUNT/EHR #: CARMAB001

DATE: 10/21/20

Attending Physician: Philip M. Osburn, DC

Diagnosis: Lumbar stenosis, sciatica

Procedure: CMT; traction, manual

PROCEDURE: The patient was placed on the table.

Chiropractic manipulative treatment: spinal, thoracic

Chiropractic manipulative treatment: lower extremity, left

Manual traction: cervical & lumbar regions × 30 minutes

PMO/mg   D: 10/21/20 09:50:16   T: 10/25/20 12:55:01

Determine the most accurate Medicine section CPT code(s) and modifier(s), if appropriate.

NORTHSIDE PHYSICAL THERAPY CENTER

955 East Main Ave. • SOMEWHERE, FL 32811 • 407-555-1191

PATIENT: TRAULER, CASIE

ACCOUNT/EHR #: TRAUCA001

DATE: 09/30/20

Attending Physician: Laverne Aspiras, MD

Physical Therapist: Harvey Shaw

DX: Postsurgical carpal tunnel (CT) release LT

(continued)

TYPE OF THERAPY: Occupational therapy (hand) BIW × 3 weeks

VISIT # 1/6:

Reported Pain Level: 6/10

Patient reports: "I am still having pain in my hand and fingers."

1. Ultrasound for 10 minutes, 3 mgHz, 0.4 u/cm2 100% to scar at LT CT area

2. Massage: Retrograde, 4 minutes to LT hand

3. Manual therapy: Soft tissue mobilization, 7 minutes to scar at LT wrist

4. AROM and stretching, 4 minutes

5. Therapeutic exercise: 12 minutes, tendon glides, joint blocking, digit extension, median nerve glides, and desensitization with cold towels (tolerated up until #5)

Pain level: 4–5/10. Pt still with heavy scar tissue adhesions in CT area. Pt still having pain in fingertips and numbness, reportedly up arm and into his neck.

Harvey Shaw

HS/mg   D: 09/30/20 09:50:16   T: 09/30/20 12:55:01

Determine the most accurate Medicine section CPT code(s) and modifier(s), if appropriate.

PRADER, BRACKER, & ASSOCIATES

A Complete Health Care Facility

159 Healthcare Way • SOMEWHERE, FL 32811 • 407-555-6789

PATIENT: PASTNERNAC, ELSA

ACCOUNT/EHR #: PASTEL001

DATE: 10/07/20

Attending Physician: Walter P. Henricks, MD

Referring Physician: Renee O. Bracker, MD

Pt is a 69-year-old female who recently had a stroke. She is here on referral from Dr. Bracker for an assessment of her aphasia.

Assessment of expressive and receptive speech and language function; language comprehension, speech production ability, reading, spelling, writing, using Boston Diagnostic Aphasia Examination.

Interpretation and report to follow.

Total time: 60 minutes

Walter P. Henricks, DC

WPH/mg   D: 10/07/20 09:50:16   T: 10/09/20 12:55:01

Determine the most accurate Medicine section CPT code(s) and modifier(s), if appropriate.

RAILS RADIOLOGY

A Complete Health Care Facility

159 Healthcare Way • SOMEWHERE, FL 32811 • 407-555-6789

PATIENT: CRESSENA, FRANCIE

ACCOUNT/EHR #: CRESFR001

DATE: 10/15/20

Attending Physician: James I. Cipher, MD

Radiologist: Rhonda E. Beardall, MD

Reason for Exam: MD order—pre-op clearance

EXAMINATION:

1. Chest two views

    Chest—AP and lateral views.

    Clinical history states evaluation: kidney stone with obstruction.

    Slightly elongated thoracic aorta. Prominent left ventricle. No pulmonary vascular congestion. No acute inflammatory infiltrates in the lungs.

2. ECG, 12 leads

    Unremarkable.

Rhonda E. Beardall, MD

REB/mg   D: 10/15/20 09:50:16   T: 10/17/20 12:55:01

Determine the most accurate Medicine section CPT code(s) and modifier(s), if appropriate.

Design elements: ©McGraw-Hill

Physicians' Services Capstone

29

Patients come to a physician for help to feel better, or to maintain good health. You have learned that CPT codes are one of three code sets used to report WHAT the physician did for the patient during a specific encounter. Now, this chapter provides you with case studies so you can get some hands-on practice using CPT to report physician services.

For each of the following case studies, read through the documentation, and determine:

- Which code or codes report WHAT the physician did for this patient.

- If any modifiers are necessary, and if so, which modifiers, and in what order.

- If more than one code is required, the sequence in which to report the codes.

Remember, the notations, symbols, and Official Guidelines—both before each section as well as those in some subsections—are there to help you get it correct.

CASE STUDY #1: PAUL HENDRICKS

Marlena Hendricks brought her 13-year-old son, Paul, into my office as a walk-in. Paul stated that he fell through a sliding glass door, while chasing his brother, and sustained three lacerations: left knee, right knee, and left hand.

After physical examination, Dr. Smyth determined that the wounds of both knees and left hand required debridement and suture repair using 1% lidocaine for topical anesthetic.

Left knee: 5.5 cm laceration involving deep subcutaneous tissue and fascia, repaired with layered closure. Some debridement was performed.

Right knee: 7.2 cm laceration repaired with a single-layer closure.

Left hand: 2.5 cm laceration of the dermis, repaired with simple closure.

Plan: Instructions for keeping bandages and area clean, and change of bandages provided to Mrs. Hendricks. Follow-up in 10 days for suture removal. Call office PRN any problems or complications.

CASE STUDY #2: MARIA CURRY

Maria Curry, a 39-year-old female, status post right knee arthroplasty, was referred to our rehabilitation clinic for a physical therapy evaluation by Dr. Hanson, her orthopedic surgeon. Patient was diagnosed with degenerative osteoarthritis approximately 2 years ago. As part of my evaluation, I completed a range of motion measurement on both legs. The physician was provided with a copy of my evaluation and a written report was developed.

CASE STUDY #3: SABRINA BARBARA

Sabrina Barbara, a 23-year-old gravida 1 para 1 by cesarean delivery, presented to the emergency department in active labor. She is at 38-weeks gestation and was visiting her parents here in town. She lives 250 miles away in another state. Patient delivered vaginally in the elevator on the way up to obstetrics. The emergency services physician, Dr. Zebbria, delivered the baby. The patient will follow up with her obstetrician for postpartum care.

CASE STUDY #4: ROGER FORCHETTA

Roger Forchetta, a 33-year-old male, came in to our ophthalmology office today. I last saw him 6 years ago when he had a corneal ulcer on his right eye. This is now cleared. He states that over the last few weeks, his vision is "a bit off."

I began with a complete, interval history. He denied any specific trauma or problems with his eyes prior to this latest concern. Overall, this patient is a healthy male with an admitted diet filled with a great deal of fast food and restaurant food.

His external ocular and adnexal areas were unremarkable, free from injury or infection. The patient has a normal corneal anterior chamber and iris but with very slow dilating pupils. Ophthalmoscopy shows there is no pseudoexfoliation, but there are dense juvenile nuclear cataracts on both eyes, the right greater than the left.

I counseled him regarding cataract surgery of this right eye first, and then the left eye; the need for postop correction; a 4- to 6-week recovery time; and the type of procedure. He agreed to schedule the procedure for next Friday. Kathy, my assistant, obtained the appropriate consent form signatures.

CASE STUDY #5: CAMILLE FIELDS

Camille Fields, a 67-year-old female, came into our Allergy & Immunology Clinic with urticarial rash over a large portion of her body.

Patient has a history of hysterectomy at age 35. She has current diagnoses of generalized osteoporosis, severe bone pain, and risk of bone fractures. After failure of prior treatments for osteoporosis (bisphosphonates, alendronate, and risedronic acid) and experiencing major side effects—gastrointestinal erosion with biphosphonates and alendronate, and severe gastrointestinal bleeding, severe muscle and joint pain, fever, flu symptoms, conjunctivitis, episcleritis, and uveitis with risedronic acid—she was referred to Dr. Lantana for alternate therapies of her condition. All symptoms were intense and persistent. Dr. Lantana prescribed denosumab. He administered Prolia, 60 mg subq into abdomen and told her to come back in 6 months.

On the day after the first administration of denosumab, the patient developed a generalized urticarial rash (thighs, abdomen, bilateral breast area, back) accompanied by bilateral facial angioedema and pruriginous injuries in the area of drug administration (the abdomen). The symptoms started 2 h after the first administration and resolved completely after 15 days with the administration of antihistamines and oral corticoids and the application of local corticoids.

She came here, to our office, to determine if the denosumab was the instigator of the allergic reaction, or if other sources were to blame. She agreed to a skin prick test (SPT) with denosumab, along with house dust mites, cat and dog dander, olive, grass pollen, and latex, which we performed today.

A positive reaction was defined as a wheal with a diameter at least 3 mm larger than that obtained by a negative control, shown at the test spot of denosumab.

We discussed a rapid desensitization protocol and she agreed. We began with an initial subcutaneous dose of 0.005 mg, which will gradually be increased in an 8-hour cycle until a cumulative dose of 60 mg.

CASE STUDY #6: BELINDA PETTAWAY

Oscar Pettaway brought his unconscious 3-year-old daughter, Belinda, into the emergency department after finding her on the floor of the bathroom. An empty bottle of his wife's thyroid medication, Synthroid, was lying by her side. Oscar told the physician on call, Dr. Rubinstein, that his wife had just refilled the prescription.

Dr. Rubinstein immediately evaluated Belinda's condition and, after obtaining permission from Oscar, ordered a gastric aspiration and lavage be done immediately, due to the poisoning.

CASE STUDY #7: JOSEPH GREESON

PATIENT: Joseph Greeson

S: The last time I saw this 29-year-old male was 6 months ago for his annual checkup. He came in today stating that he has been feeling feverish × 3 days and noticed increased redness on his arm last night and this morning. He denies joint pain. He explained that yesterday he was playing with his girlfriend's new dog and it bit him on the right forearm. The dog is a stray and has had no shots, and the patient states that he believes he accidentally provoked the dog by getting too rough with it.

O: Temp 99.2 degrees, pulse 68, resp 20, weight 142. Right arm reveals four puncture wounds with secondary cellulitis around the area. The area is warm to the touch and is erythematous.

A: Infected dog bite.

P: Patient is given 1 gram of Rocephin IM today. Follow up in 24 hours. A bandage was applied. He was given a rabies immune globulin (RIg), human, IM. Tylenol is recommended PRN for pain. The patient is given a prescription for Erythromycin 333 mg t.i.d. for 10 days.

CASE STUDY #8: MONIQUE KENNARD

Monique Kennard, a 17-year-old female, came into our office today. She is accompanied by her mother, who is very worried about her daughter. Patient states she has been experiencing wheezing × 10 days. She states the symptoms are worse at night. She was seen a week ago at this clinic and started on a 5-day course of azithromycin without improvement. Yesterday she was seen at an urgent care clinic and prescribed an albuterol inhaler, amoxicillin/clavulonic acid, and methylprednisolone. Symptoms continued to worsen throughout the day. Patient reports chest pain attempting to swallow the amoxicillin/clavulonic acid tablets. Chest pain involves her left upper chest; it does not radiate. The quality is "heavy."

VS: 97.9°F, HR 85, RR 25, BP 144/101, SaO$_2$ 97%

HEAD/NECK: She is awake and alert, NAD (no apparent distress), HEENT (head, eyes, ears, nose, throat), NC/AT (normocephalic and atraumatic), EOMI (extraocular movements intact). Left EAC (external auditory canal) is swollen shut; right is occluded with cerumen. Oropharynx is pink and moist.

HEART: RRR (regular rate and rhythm)

LUNGS: No wheezing, but patient is stridorous

ABDOMEN: Benign/unremarkable

EXTREMITIES: Normal pulses × 4, CN II–XII grossly intact

INTEGUMENTARY: Dermatologic exam reveals no rash

ALLERGIES: NKDA (no known drug allergies)

PMHx (Past Medical History): Unremarkable

SocHx (Social History): Patient denies EtOH (ethanol, alcohol). Denies smoking but states positive for secondhand tobacco exposure.

PLAN: Orders written for CXR (chest x-ray) to be done at imaging center across the road. Nurse to perform venipuncture for specimens for comprehensive metabolic panel; CBC complete, automated; and automated differential WBC count.

Patient to return once results are in.

CASE STUDY #9: HARRISON PARKER

Harrison Parker, a 69-year-old right-handed male, was referred to me for a neurologic evaluation by his internist, Dr. Brady, for a tremor that has been present for approximately 20 years.

Patient states that the tremor began insidiously and has progressed gradually. It now involves both hands and affects his handwriting, drinking coffee and other liquids with a cup, and general work that requires manual dexterity. Other people occasionally notice a tremor in his head.

He is otherwise healthy, although he feels his balance is not quite as good as it used to be. A glass of beer or wine markedly decreases the tremor severity. His mother and daughter also have tremor. Patient denies smoking.

On examination, he has a rather regular tremor of approximately 8 cycles per second (Hz) with his hands extended and also on finger-nose-finger maneuver. Mild regular "waviness" is seen when writing or drawing spirals. His tone is normal, although when performing voluntary movements with one hand there is a "ratchety" quality felt in the tone of the contralateral arm. Occasional tremor is also noted in the head and voice.

Diagnosis: Probable essential tremor (ET)

Next diagnostic step: MRI of brain and cervical spine + Labs (CBC + TSH) done in our facility today.

Nurse Montana drew blood specimens.

Next step in therapy: Primidone or propranolol

CASE STUDY #10: TORI BENSIO

PATIENT: Tori Bensio

Preop Diagnosis: Acute cholecystitis, cholelithiasis

Postop Diagnosis: Acute cholecystitis, cholelithiasis

Procedure: Laparoscopic cholecystectomy

Surgeon: Anthony DeTaglia, MD

Assistant: Robyn Acculo, MD

Anesthesiologist: Benjamin Sullivan, MD

Anesthesia: General endotracheal

Findings at Surgery: Pericholecystic adhesions, large gallstones

DESCRIPTION OF OPERATION: This otherwise healthy patient was brought to the OR and after the induction of general endotracheal anesthesia, the patient's abdomen was prepped and draped in the usual sterile manner and a small infraumbilical incision was made in the skin and carried down to the linea alba, which was grasped with a clamp and incised in a vertical manner. The peritoneum was entered under direct vision. Stay sutures were placed in the fascia. The Hasson introducer was placed. Pneumoperito-neum was established, and following this, three additional trocars were placed in the abdomen: one in the left epigastrium and two in the right upper quadrant, all 5 mm. Following this, the gallbladder was grasped with cephalad retraction of the gallbladder fundus and lateralward retraction of the gallbladder infundibulum. The dissector was employed to take down the peritoneum overlying the gallbladder infundibulum and cystic duct junction. When this was well delineated on both the anterior and posterior surfaces of the cystic duct, the 5-mm endoscopic clip applier was inserted and two clips were placed on the patient's side, on the gallbladder side of the cystic duct, which was transected. Further dissection in the triangle of Calot revealed the cystic artery, which was handled in an identical manner. The remainder of the dissection was performed by using the Bovie spatula cautery, and the liver bed was dry. A 10- to 15-mm camera change-out was performed, and the camera was inserted into the left epigastric port. A toothed clamp was passed through the umbilicus to grasp the gallbladder, which was then removed through the umbilicus in a standard manner. Following this, the operative field was copiously irrigated with saline and the return was clear. All three upper abdominal ports were seen to exit the abdomen under direct vision, and with the Has-son introducer removed, the fascial incision was closed with a 2-0 Vicryl figure-of-eight suture. The skin at the umbilicus was closed with a 4-0 Maxon subcuticular suture. Steri-strips were applied at all sites. The patient tolerated the procedure well.

ADDENDUM: There were three cystic artery branches; each was doubly clipped and transected.

Code for both Dr. DeTaglia and Dr. Sullivan.

CASE STUDY #11: ENID REYNOLDS

EMERGENCY DEPARTMENT

HISTORY OF PRESENT ILLNESS: The patient came in today for possible reaction to immunotherapy. She has been seeing Dr. Oligby for allergic rhinitis and asthma. She states that she is currently building on immunotherapy and yesterday received injections with oak/birch/maple 100 PNU 0.3 mL, grass and ragweed 100 BAU 0.3 mL, cat/dog 50 BAU 0.3 mL, and mite and mold mix 100 units 0.3 mL. The patient tells me after the immunotherapy, she went home and within hours felt some chest tightness. The patient used her albuterol inhaler, but the chest tightness got worse and she ended up taking her Symbicort 160/4.5 two puffs as well as some Claritin. She continued to feel lethargic and out of breath. She also had an itchy area on her left arm where she received the cat/dog injection. She was able to go to sleep that night but woke twice due to wheezing and used her albuterol inhaler and went back to sleep. When she woke up this morning, she was very tired and dizzy and could not catch her breath. She used her albuterol inhaler once or twice this morning as well as the Symbicort and took a tablet of Zyrtec. Then, around 9 or 9:30, when she was at work, she felt her tongue swelling. During this time, she felt she couldn't breathe normally. The albuterol inhaler did not have any benefit; neither did the other medications she tried. She tells me she had no rash, hives, or vomiting and is not coughing. She tells me she has not been sick this week. No fever. She has been off of her Symbicort since November because she felt her asthma is fine. She has had no recent trouble with asthma. No recent exposure to animals, dust, or other allergens. She is on no new medications. She has no pets at home and continues to avoid turkey and chicken and has no new foods during this time. She has a history of anxiety and panic attacks and does feel she is having one now.

MEDICATIONS: Topamax for migraine headaches, Lexapro

ALLERGIES: NKDA

PHYSICAL EXAMINATION:

GENERAL: The patient is a healthy-appearing, well-nourished, well-developed 45-year-old female in no acute distress but does appear to be breathing heavy and very shaky and panicky.

VITAL SIGNS: Height is 63 inches. Weight is 132 pounds. Blood pressure is 106/70.

HEENT: Tympanic membranes are normal. Throat is clear. I did not appreciate any swelling of the tongue or angioedema.

NECK: Supple without adenopathy

LUNGS: Completely clear

HEART: Regular rate and rhythm without murmur

STUDIES: I administered spirometry when she was a little bit more relaxed and achieved an FEV1 of 3.1 liters or 88% of predicted, FEF25–75 is 118% of predicted. Graphic record was placed in patient's chart.

IMPRESSION:

1. The patient appears to be having some anxiety and panic now. It is hard to say whether this started with some mild asthma symptoms as a result of her immunotherapy or if this is purely an anxiety issue.
2. Allergic asthma
3. Allergic rhinitis

RECOMMENDATIONS:

1. We recommend a cutback of the dose of immunotherapy at the next visit to oak/birch/maple 100 PNU at 0.2 mL, grass and ragweed 100 BAU at 0.2 mL, cat/dog 50 BAU at 0.2 mL, and mite and mold mix 100 units at 0.2 mL
2. Restart Symbicort 160/4.5 two puffs twice daily
3. Zyrtec 10 mg daily for the next week and prior to immunotherapy

4. Albuterol two puffs every 4 hours as needed

5. The patient should follow up if symptoms do not clear in the next day or two

6. Report to be sent to Dr. Oligby

7. Patient discharged at 16:55

CASE STUDY #12: ARNOLD TITLEMAN

OPERATION: Colonoscopy to the cecum

DESCRIPTION OF PROCEDURE: The patient was taken to the outpatient endoscopy suite where he was monitored for pulse oximetry and blood pressure monitoring. He was turned to the left side and given 50 mg of Demerol with 2 mg of Versed, IV, titrated during the procedure; the nurse monitored Arnold's vital signs for a total of 28 minutes.

An Olympus video colonoscope was inserted in the patient's anus and directed up to the rectum, sigmoid colon, descending colon, around the splenic flexure, through the transverse colon, around the hepatic flexure, ascending colon, and cecum. The ileocecal area was inspected and appeared grossly normal.

Terminal ileum was cannulated, appeared grossly normal. The scope was then slowly withdrawn back through the entire colon, rectum, and anus and no gross abnormality or lesion was identified. Mucosa pattern appeared normal. The patient tolerated the procedure well. He will be discharged home with instructions to follow up for a surveillance colonoscopy.

CASE STUDY #13: DARLIN EVERSTANG

OPERATIONS:

1. Flexible bronchoscopy
2. Cervical mediastinoscopy with biopsy and thyroid isthmusectomy

PROCEDURE: This otherwise normally healthy patient was brought to the operative suite and placed in supine position. After satisfactory induction of general endotracheal anesthesia, a flexible Olympus bronchoscope was passed through the endotracheal tube visualizing the distal trachea, carina, and right and left main stem bronchi of the primary and secondary divisions. No evidence of any endobronchial tumor was noted. The scope was then withdrawn.

The patient was then prepped and draped in the usual sterile fashion. A shoulder roll was placed. A curvilinear incision was made above the suprasternal notch in the line of a skin crease. Dissection was carried down through the subcutaneous tissue down through the platysma muscle. The strap muscles were next identified and laterally retracted. We continued our dissection down to the pretracheal space. A thyroid isthmusectomy was done without any problems; this gave me clear access to the pretracheal space. A pretracheal plane was next developed. A mediastinoscope was placed. I saw multiple, firm right paratracheal lymph nodes. After first aspirating these structures to make sure they are not vascular in nature, generous biopsies were taken and sent to pathology for examination. Frozen section analysis revealed these to be consistent with lymphoma. Excellent hemostasis was obtained. The wound was irrigated using warm antibiotic saline solution. The wound was then closed in layers using Vicryl sutures. Dressings were applied. Marcaine 0.25% was used as a regional block. The patient tolerated the procedure and was sent to the recovery room in stable condition.

CASE STUDY #14: DAVIDA PRAGER

PROCEDURE: Needle-localized biopsy, right breast

DESCRIPTION OF PROCEDURE: After proper consent was obtained, the patient (48-year-old female) was brought to the operating room and placed on the table in a supine position. Patient was given 2 mg of midazolam HCL, IV, titrated during the procedure; the nurse monitored Davida's vital signs for a total of 15 minutes.

The right breast area was prepped and draped in a sterile manner. Plain Marcaine 0.5% solution was injected for local anesthesia in the perioperative region. A curvilinear incision was made medial to the insertion site of the wire, as the wire was noted to pass medially in the breast. The preoperative localization films were reviewed, noting that the clip was posterior to the wire. The dissection was carried out with cautery to remove a core of tissue around the wire, being more generous on the posterior aspect around the wire and especially near the end of the wire, taking a very generous area of tissue posteriorly; in fact, it was all the way down to the pectoralis fascia at that site. The specimen was removed, noting that the wire was within the mid portion of removed tissue with a large amount of surrounding tissue. This was submitted for radiographic analysis and the wire was noted to be within the large specimen. However, the clip could not be visualized. For this reason, the operative area was inspected with fluoroscopy with diligence and there was no evidence of any residual clip within the right breast tissue or within the drapes around the right breast. The Ray-Tec sponge was also evaluated with fluoroscopy and direct inspection and no clip was noted. The suction canister and tubing were also evaluated with fluoroscopy and no clip was noted. At this point, due to the generous size of the biopsy specimen, decision was made to not blindly remove any further breast tissue. I suspect that the clip may have become stuck to a Ray-Tec sponge or other instrument during this procedure and came out of the wound and fell out of the field of dissection. The operative area was irrigated, noted to hemostatic, and closed in layers using interrupted #3-0 Vicryl suture to close deep dermis and running #4-0 subcuticular Vicryl suture to close the skin. Benzoin, Steri-Strips, and sterile gauze dressings were placed. The patient had her sedation stopped and she was taken to the recovery area.

CASE STUDY #15: HENRY SYSTONA

OPERATION: Orbitotomy on the right with biopsy of right lacrimal gland

DESCRIPTION OF OPERATION: The patient was brought to the major operating room where general endotracheal anesthesia was induced. Lateral lid crease of the right eye was marked, and I marked the incision to extend lateral to the lateral canthus in case a lateral orbitotomy became necessary, pending the biopsy. The area of the lateral upper lid, beyond the lateral canthus, was injected with approximately 5 cc of 50:50 mix of 2%

Xylocaine with 1:100,000 epinephrine, 0.75% Marcaine with 1:100,000 epinephrine. He was prepped and draped in the usual manner for sterile oculoplastic surgery.

Attention was turned to the right upper lid. A lateral lid crease incision was made with a 15 blade. Dissection was carried down through the orbicularis to the superior orbital rim using the Colorado needle. The periosteum of the superior and lateral orbital rim was incised with the Colorado needle. Freer elevator was then used to reflect the periorbital off the lateral orbital wall and lateral orbital roof. Prior to proceeding with the orbital dissection, a 4-0 silk suture was placed on the insertion of the lateral rectus muscle for traction to better identify lateral rectus if an orbitotomy became necessary.

It was obvious, as the periorbital and lacrimal gland were lifted off the superotemporal orbit, that the lacrimal gland was enlarged with an infiltrative mass. Periosteum was opened near the posterior third of the mass and a modest biopsy was taken. It was then opened at the anterior edge and a biopsy was taken from this portion. Clinically, the biopsies looked like a lymphomatous infiltrate. These were sent for frozen section, and frozen section did reveal lymphomatous infiltrate consistent with non-Hodgkin lymphoma. Because of the need for special studies, more tissue was excised and as much of the infiltrative mass that was safely excisable was excised.

Bleeders were cauterized with the Colorado needle and the use of cottonoids saturated with 1:100,000 epinephrine. After adequate hemostasis was obtained, the 4-0 silk was removed from the lateral rectus muscle. The periosteum was closed with 2 interrupted 5-0 Vicryl, and the skin was closed with a running 5-0 fast-absorbing gut. Polysporin ointment was placed in the right eye and along the wound. The patient was awakened and taken to the recovery room in good condition. Estimated blood loss less than 10 cc. He tolerated the procedure well without complications.

Design elements: ©McGraw-Hill

PART IV

DMEPOS & TRANSPORTATION

There is another portion to the procedure coding system that professional coding specialists use to report services and treatments. HCPCS (pronounced "hick-picks") is the acronym for Healthcare Common Procedure Coding System. You have learned about the CPT codes used to report physician services and outpatient facility services. This part of this textbook will give you the opportunity to learn about HCPCS Level II codes (referred to as HCPCS codes).

DMEPOS is a combination abbreviation that stands for

- *DME = Durable Medical Equipment*
- *P = Prosthetics*
- *O = Orthotics*
- *S = Supplies*

Transportation refers to moving a patient from one point to another, such as ambulance services.

30 HCPCS Level II

Key Terms

Advanced Life Support (ALS)
Basic Life Support (BLS)
Chelation Therapy
DMEPOS
Durable Medical Equipment (DME)
Durable Medical Equipment Regional Carrier (DMERC)
Enteral
Not Otherwise Specified (NOS)
Orthotic
Parenteral
Prosthetic
Self-Administer
Specialty Care Transport (SCT)

Learning Outcomes

After completing this chapter, the student should be able to:

LO 30.1 Abstract physician's notes to identify the category of HCPCS Level II codes needed.

LO 30.2 Employ the Alphabetic Index to find suggested HCPCS Level II codes.

LO 30.3 Distinguish the types of services, products, and supplies reported with HCPCS Level II codes.

LO 30.4 Follow the directions supplied by the notations and symbols.

LO 30.5 Utilize the additional information provided by Appendices.

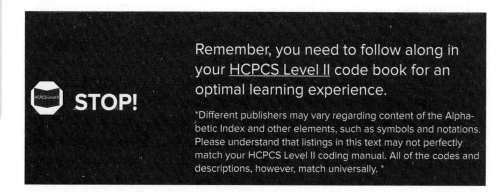

STOP!

Remember, you need to follow along in your <u>HCPCS Level II</u> code book for an optimal learning experience.

Different publishers may vary regarding content of the Alphabetic Index and other elements, such as symbols and notations. Please understand that listings in this text may not perfectly match your HCPCS Level II coding manual. All of the codes and descriptions, however, match universally.

30.1 HCPCS Level II Categories

HCPCS Level II codes and modifiers are listed in their own book and are used to report services, procedures, and supplies that are not properly described in the CPT book. There are almost 5,000 HCPCS codes, each represented by five characters: one letter followed by four numbers.

EXAMPLES

C9460	Injection, cangrelor, 1 mg
R0076	Transportation of portable EKG to facility or location, per patient

HCPCS Level II codes cover specific aspects of health care services, including

- Durable medical equipment
  - e.g., a wheelchair or a humidifier
- Pharmaceuticals administered by a health care provider
  - e.g., a saline solution or a chemotherapy drug

- Medical supplies provided for the patient's own use
  - e.g., an eye patch or gradient compression stockings
- Dental services
  - e.g., all services provided by a dental professional
- Transportation services
  - e.g., ambulance services
- Vision and hearing services
  - e.g., trifocal spectacles or a hearing screening
- **Orthotic** and **prosthetic** procedures
  - e.g., scoliosis braces or postsurgical fitting

Not all insurance carriers accept HCPCS Level II codes, but Medicare and Medicaid want you to use them. It is your responsibility as a coding specialist to find out whether each third-party payer with which your facility works accepts HCPCS Level II codes. If not, you have to ask for the payer's policies on reporting the services and supplies covered by HCPCS Level II.

Orthotic
A device used to correct or improve an orthopedic concern.

Prosthetic
Fabricated artificial replacement for a damaged or missing part of the body.

EXAMPLES

Medicare accepts HCPCS Level II codes and therefore requires you to code an injection of tetracycline, 200 mg, with two codes (for administration of the shot and the drug inside the syringe).

96372	Therapeutic, prophylactic or diagnostic injection (specify substance or drug injected); subcutaneous or intramuscular
J0120	Injection, tetracycline, up to 250 mg

Yankee Health Insurance does not accept HCPCS Level II codes. This payor includes reimbursement for the drug in the CPT code for the actual injection. Therefore, you would only report the one code to get paid for both the service (the giving of the shot) and the material (the drug inside the syringe).

96372	Therapeutic, prophylactic or diagnostic injection (specify substance or drug injected); subcutaneous or intramuscular

---

The process for using HCPCS Level II codes is the same as coding from the CPT book. You abstract the key words from the physician's notes regarding the services and procedures, look those key words up in the Alphabetic Index of the appropriate book (CPT or HCPCS), confirm the code in the numeric listing, and report the service using that code. You know how to do this already! However, there are specific elements unique to HCPCS Level II coding that you need to know.

Understanding how to use HCPCS codes accurately will open new employment opportunities for you. In addition to hospitals, physician's offices, and outpatient clinics, nursing homes, home health care agencies, health care equipment and supply companies, and other facilities use these codes quite extensively.

CODING BITES

A physiatrist is a health care professional who uses physical methodologies to treat illness or injury.

These methodologies include electrical stimulation, heat/cold, light, water, exercise, manipulation, and mechanical devices.

 LET'S CODE IT! SCENARIO

Carole Shelton, a 47-year-old female, came to see Dr. Giardino, a podiatrist recommended by her primary care physician, complaining of acute pain in the ball of her left foot. She states that the pain has been ongoing for about

(continued)

2 months. After examination, and an x-ray of the foot, two views, Dr. Giardino took a walking boot, non-pneumatic, from the storage room and placed it on her foot. He instructed Carole to wear the boot at all times, except while in bed, for 6 weeks, and return for a follow-up evaluation.

Let's Code It!

Review the information in the scenario and abstract the services that Dr. Giardino provided: he evaluated her condition, took x-rays, and provided her with the boot (durable medical equipment).

You have learned about CPT coding, so you can determine that these two codes will be reported for this encounter:

99202	**Office visit, new patient, problem-focused**
73620	**Radiologic examination, foot; 2 views**

Now, you need to report the provision of the boot. It is only right that Dr. Giardino be reimbursed for providing this to the patient for her use at home. Turn in your HCPCS Level II code book to the Alphabetic Index, and find:

Walking splint, L4386

Go back to the documentation, which states, "*walking boot.*" Is a splint the same as a boot? I don't know, so turn in the Main Section of HCPCS Level II so you can read the complete code description.

L4386 **Walking boot, non-pneumatic, with or without joints, with or without interface material, prefabricated item that has been trimmed, bent, molded, assembled, or otherwise customized to fit a specific patient by an individual with expertise.**

Go back to the documentation. Is there any mention of customization, as mentioned in the description for code L4386? No, there is not. And the documentation does state that the boot came right out of Dr. Giardino's storage room. There are three other codes that describe a walking boot in this subsection of *Ancillary Orthotic Services*. Take a look at the full descriptions for L4360, L4361, and L4387 to see if any of these match the documentation. Aha! L4387 matches!

Now, you can report the three codes for this encounter with confidence: the two CPT codes + this one HCPCS Level II code.

L4387-LT **Walking boot, non-pneumatic, with or without joints, with or without interface material, prefabricated, off-the-shelf, left foot**

Good work!

CODING BITES

Never, never, never, never, never code from the Alphabetic Index. Always confirm the code in the Alphanumeric Listing before deciding which code to report.

30.2 The Alphabetic Index

Like the other coding books, the HCPCS Level II book has an Alphabetic Index as well as an Alphanumeric Listing.

The Alphabetic Index lists the Level II code descriptions in alphabetic order from A to Z. After abstracting the key terms from the provider's notes, you can look up key words in the Alphabetic Index by using the following:

- Brand name of the drug
- Generic name of the drug
- Medical supply item
- Orthotic
- Prosthetic
- Service
- Surgical supply

The Alphabetic Index will suggest a code or a range of codes, similarly to CPT's Alphabetic Index. Then, as you have done before, you look the suggestions up in the Alphanumeric Listing, read the complete description(s) and all of the symbols and notations, and determine the best, most accurate code. (*NOTE:* The Alphabetic Index in the HCPCS Level II book does not list *all* the codes included in the Alphanumeric Listing. So if you can't find what you are looking for in the Alphabetic Index, you might want to find something closely related to get you to the appropriate section of the book and then look around.)

This index includes many alternate terms identified by notations in the Alphanumeric Listings:

EXAMPLE

In the Alphabetic Index, you will see

    Abciximab, J0130

In the Table of Drugs, you will see

    ReoPro, J0130

In the Alphanumeric Listing, you will see:

    J0130   Injection, abciximab, 10 mg
                 Other: ReoPro

Deleted code descriptions are not included in the Alphabetic Index. However, the new code(s) that is to be used instead of the deleted code is listed:

EXAMPLE

In the Alphabetic Index, you will see

    Ventilator
        Home ventilator, any type, E0465, E0466
            used with invasive interface, E0465

In the Alphanumeric Listing, you will see:

    E0465   Home ventilator, any type, used with invasive interface,
                 (e.g., tracheostomy tube)

The Alphanumeric Listing shows a notation to use one code with another code.

EXAMPLE

In the Alphanumeric Listing, you will see

    D2953   Each additional indirectly fabricated post–same tooth
                 To be used with D2952

HCPCS Level II codes are listed in sections, grouped by the type of service, the type of supply item, or the type of equipment they represent. However, you should not assume that a particular item or service is located only in that specific section. Use the

Alphabetic Index to direct you to the correct category in the Alphanumeric Listing of the book. One type of service or procedure might be located under several different categories depending upon the details.

EXAMPLE

Transportation services may be identified by A, Q, R, or V codes.

Transportation
Ambulance, A0021–A0999, Q3019, Q3020
Corneal tissue, V2785
EKG equipment, portable, R0076

30.3 The Alphanumeric Listing Overview

The Alphanumeric Listing presents the codes in alphabetic order by the first letter and then numeric order beginning with the first number of that code. Let's go through all the sections together so you can get a general idea of the procedures, services, and supplies that are reported using these codes.

A0000–A0999 Transportation Services Including Ambulance

If a severely ill or injured individual must be moved, whether from home or an accident scene, to a health care facility or from one health care facility to another, transportation arrangements are made. The patient may need to be lying down or receiving continuous IV therapy. The health care professional may have to monitor the patient's vital signs and other issues constantly. The room for additional personnel, the ability to keep special equipment secure and functional, and the configuration of the seating so that everyone involved can be kept safe during the ride are all concerns that demand more than the average vehicle.

HCPCS Level II codes A0021–A0999 report the following transportation services:

- Ground ambulances
- Air ambulances (often a helicopter but not exclusively)
- Nonemergency transportation, such as a special van, a taxi cab, a car, or even a bus
- Additional or secondary related costs and fees

Advanced Life Support (ALS)
Life-sustaining, emergency care provided, such as airway management, defibrillation, and/or the administration of drugs.

Basic Life Support (BLS)
The provision of emergency CPR, stabilization of the patient, first aid, control of bleeding, and/or treatment of shock.

Specialty Care Transport (SCT)
Continuous care provided by one or more health professionals in an appropriate specialty area, such as respiratory care or cardiovascular care, or by a paramedic with additional training.

Coding Components

The transportation section codes are determined by the answers to these questions:

1. What type of vehicle was used to transport the patient?
   - Ground (ambulance, taxi, bus, minibus, van, etc.)
   - Air–fixed wing (such as an airplane)
   - Air–rotary wing (such as a helicopter)
2. What type of services did the patient need?
   - Emergency
   - Nonemergency
   - **Advanced life support (ALS)**
   - **Basic life support (BLS)**
   - **Specialty care transport (SCT)**

3. Did the ambulance have to wait?

4. How many miles did the ambulance have to travel from origin to destination?

5. Were extra personnel required?

Determining the answers to these five questions from the documentation will direct you to the best, most appropriate code or codes needed to properly report transportation services for a patient.

GUIDANCE CONNECTION

Read the guidelines within section **A,** sub-head **Transportation Services Including Ambulance A0000–A0999** in your HCPCS Level II book.

EXAMPLE

EMTs Garret Tyson and Peter Gromine were asked by Jason Aeronson to travel over the state line to the Morrison Nursing Center and transport his mother, Melinda Donner, a 93-year-old female, to the Bramington Nursing Center back near their home base and Jason's home. Ms. Donner requires ALS services during the ambulance transport. Upon arrival at Morrison Nursing Center, they had to wait 30 minutes for the staff to process Melinda out and release her to their care. The round trip was 52 miles. Pre-approval from Medicaid was documented.

A0021x52	Ambulance service, outside state per mile, transport, 52 miles round trip
A0420	Ambulance waiting time (ALS or BLS), one-half (1/2) hour increments

---

 ### LET'S CODE IT! SCENARIO

Priscilla DeLucca, an emergency medical technician (EMT), was called in as an extra ambulance attendant for the ALS ground transportation of Willow Lawarence, a 12-year-old autistic female.

Let's Code It!

Priscilla was called in as an *extra ambulance attendant*. When you look in the Alphabetic Index of the HCPCS Level II book, notice that this does not match any of the listings under *Ambulance* or *Attendant*. So let's turn to the range shown next to the term *Ambulance* in the index: A0021–A0999.

Although reading down the listing will take time, sometimes it is the best way to find the code you need. Fortunately, you won't have to read too far to reach:

A0424   Extra ambulance attendant, ground (ALS or BLS) or air (fixed or rotary winged); (requires medical review)

Transportation Codes in Other Sections

A few transportation codes in the HCPCS Level II book are in sections other than the A codes. This, of course, is an excellent example of why you should use the Alphabetic Index to find the best code in the Alphanumeric Listing—because there may be a better, more appropriate code in a section you might not otherwise examine. In all cases of temporary codes, you must confirm the acceptance of the temporary code by the third-party payer to whom you are billing.

The S series (S0000–S9999) consists of temporary codes and is not accepted by Medicare, according to the HCPCS Level II book. Medicaid programs and some private insurers, such as Blue Cross and Blue Shield Association, do accept S codes.

You must check with the organization or association in your state to confirm the acceptance of S codes. Here are two of the S codes that relate to transportation:

S0215   Non-emergency transportation; mileage, per mile

S9992   Transportation costs to and from trial location and local transportation costs (e.g., fares for taxicab or bus) for clinical trial participant and one caregiver/companion

The T codes (T1000–T9999) are used by Medicaid state agencies to report services, procedures, and other items for which there are no permanent national codes. You must communicate with the third-party payer to whom you are sending the claim to ensure that it accepts T codes. Here are some transportation services that may be reported using T codes:

T2001   Non-emergency transportation; patient attendant/escort

T2002   Non-emergency transportation; per diem

T2003   Non-emergency transportation; encounter/trip

T2004   Non-emergency transport; commercial carrier, multi-pass

T2005   Non-emergency transportation; stretcher van

T2007   Transportation waiting time, air ambulance and non-emergency vehicle, one-half (1/2) hour increments

T2049   Non-emergency transportation; stretcher van, mileage; per mile

 LET'S CODE IT! SCENARIO

Barry Camacho, a 79-year-old male, had a stroke 3 weeks ago. He has now improved sufficiently to be discharged from the hospital. However, he is not completely well. Barry is being transferred to a short-term rehabilitation facility to help him regain use of his legs and right arm. Ira Waxen, from Flomenhoff Ambulance Services, drove the wheelchair van to take Barry from McGraw Hospital to Flowers Nursing and Rehabilitation Center, a 12-mile ride.

Let's Code It!

Ira, the driver, will submit the documentation to you. He noted that he drove a *wheelchair van* to transport Barry from the hospital to the nursing facility. The notes also indicate that Barry is being discharged from the hospital and there is no indication that this is an emergency. In addition, the wheelchair van does not contain emergency equipment, so we know that this is a *non-emergency* trip.

Let's go to the Alphabetic Index and turn to *Wheelchair*. Go down the list to the indented term *Van, nonemergency*, A0130. Turn to the Alphanumeric Listing to check out the complete description of the code:

A0130   Non-emergency transportation: wheelchair van

This matches Ira's documentation, doesn't it? Yes. In addition, it is the only code shown for that portion of the service. However, you might also look in the Alphabetic Listing under *Transportation, nonemergency*, A0080–A0210, T2001–T2005. Once you review the complete descriptions of the suggested codes, you will see rather quickly that A0130 is the most specific and accurate.

Now, you must include a code for the mileage traveled by the van. Under *Transportation, non-emergency, wheelchair van*, you get the suggestion for codes A0130 and S0209. We already know that A0130 reports the use of the van itself. Let's find out what the description is for S0209:

S0209   Wheelchair van, mileage, per mile

also note just below this . . .

S0215   Non-emergency transportation; mileage per mile

(continued)

You also might notice:

A0380   **BLS mileage (per mile)**

A0390   **ALS mileage (per mile)**

A0425   **Ground mileage, per statute mile**

Five different codes appear applicable to reporting the mileage component of the service. Look at S0209 versus S0215 versus A0380, A0390, and A0425. You can see that the descriptions of A0380 and A0390 do not match your notes and would be considered upcoding! S0209 is more accurate and more specific in its description of the type of vehicle involved in the transportation. Therefore, as long as the insurance carrier accepts S codes, the claim form should show these codes:

A0130   **Non-emergency transportation: wheelchair van**

S0209   **Wheelchair van, mileage, per mile;**
                         Number of miles: twelve (12)

Great job!

Ambulance Origin/Destination

When reporting transportation services to insurance carriers, you have to identify the *origin of service* and the *destination of service*. The most common modifiers for the origin and the destination of service are one-letter codes that categorize locations.

D   **Diagnostic or therapeutic site other than P or H when these are used as origin codes**

E   **Residential, domiciliary, custodial facility (other than 1819 facility)**

G   **Hospital-based ESRD facility**

H   **Hospital**

I   **Site of transfer (e.g., airport or helicopter pad) between modes of ambulance transport**

J   **Free-standing ESRD facility**

N   **Skilled nursing facility (SNF) (1819 facility)**

P   **Physician's office**

R   **Residence**

S   **Scene of accident or acute event**

X   **Intermediate stop at physician's office on way to hospital (destination code only)**

A4000–A8004 Medical and Surgical Supplies and A9000–A9999 Administrative, Miscellaneous and Investigational

These codes cover medical supplies, surgical supplies, and some services related to **durable medical equipment (DME)**.

In almost every health care encounter, materials and supplies are used. The paper used to cover the examination table and the disposable cover on the digital thermometer are good examples. Such medical supplies are used by the health care facility itself. However, they are *not* the types of medical and surgical supplies to which the HCPCS Level II book refers. The codes in the HCPCS Level II book are for reporting supplies given to a patient to **self-administer** health care at home.

Durable Medical Equipment (DME)
Apparatus and tools that help individuals accommodate physical frailties, deliver pharmaceuticals, and provide other assistance that will last for a long time and/or be used to assist multiple patients over time.

Self-Administer
To give medication to oneself, such as a diabetic giving herself an insulin injection.

A Codes and B Codes

Let's begin by reviewing the subheadings throughout the A code and B code sections to get a good idea of which items are covered.

- **Miscellaneous Supplies:** The supplies used by a physician in the course of treatment (syringes, alcohol wipes, urine test strips, and so on) are included in the amount reimbursed for the provision of that treatment or service. The codes in miscellaneous supplies (HCPCS Level II) are used to report, and be reimbursed for, supplies provided to patients for their own use at home. For example, if a diabetic patient requires a daily insulin shot at home, he or she would need to have syringes available.

- **Vascular Catheters:** These codes report the use of a disposable drug delivery system (DDS) as well as implantable access catheters. The codes are not for reporting the physician's work to implant the catheter but for the facility to be reimbursed for the cost of the catheter itself.

- **Incontinence Appliances and Care Supplies** and **External Urinary Supplies:** The sections **Incontinence Appliances and Care Supplies** and **External Urinary Supplies** cover urinary supplies that a patient uses when he or she has been diagnosed with permanent, or chronic, incontinence.

- **Ostomy Supplies:** Patients who have had surgery to create an ostomy need supplies every day to make their medical situation easier to deal with and to enable them to live their lives more normally.

EXAMPLES

A4245	Alcohol wipes, per box
A4452	Tape, waterproof, per 18 sq in.
A4490	Surgical stocking above knee length, each
A4637	Replacement, tip, cane, crutch, or walker, each

You will also find codes in this section for

- Nonprescription drugs (also known as over-the-counter drugs)
- Exercise equipment
- Radiopharmaceutical diagnostic imaging agents
- Noncovered items and services

(*NOTE:* An item or service may be noncovered with regard to national standards but covered by your state or other third-party carrier. Never take anything for granted. Always ask!)

EXAMPLES

A9280	Alert or alarm device, not otherwise classified
A9505	Thallium T1-201, thallous chloride, diagnostic, per millicurie

 LET'S CODE IT! SCENARIO

Teresa Baum, a 55-year-old female, has been diagnosed with malignant neoplasm of the liver. She has lost all her hair because of the chemotherapy and radiation treatments. Dr. Colter prescribed a wig to help lift her spirits and self-esteem.

(continued)

B4000–B9999 Enteral and Parenteral Therapy

The B codes cover supplies, formulas, nutritional solutions, and infusion pumps for **enteral** and **parenteral** therapy. These codes report the supply of items related to providing nutrition to a patient by alternate means—other than by mouth and/or the digestive tract.

Enteral
Within, or by way of, the gastrointestinal tract.

Parenteral
By way of anything other than the gastrointestinal tract, such as intravenous, intramuscular, intramedullary, or subcutaneous.

EXAMPLES

B4083	Stomach tube—Levine type
B9006	Parenteral nutrition, infusion pump, stationary

C1000–C9999 CMS Hospital Outpatient Payment System

Codes from the *Temporary Hospital Outpatient PPS* category are used to report drugs, biologicals, devices for transitional pass-through payments for hospitals, and items classified in new-technology ambulatory payment classifications.

GUIDANCE CONNECTION

Read the guidelines within section **C,** subhead **CMS Hospital Outpatient Payment System (C1000– C9999)** in your HCPCS Level II book.

EXAMPLES

C1724	Catheter, transluminal atherectomy, rotational
C2636	Brachytherapy linear source, non-stranded, Palladium-103, per 1 mm
C9364	Porcine implant, Permacol, per square centimeter

D0000–D9999 Dental Procedures

The *Dental Procedures* category is the **Dental Procedures and Nomenclature (CDT)** code set, copyrighted by the American Dental Association.

The codes are used to report dental services, such as x-rays (Figure 30-1).

EXAMPLES

D0240	Intraoral—occlusal radiographic image
D1110	Prophylaxis—adult
D3310	Endodontic therapy, anterior tooth (excluding final restoration)

NOTE: Prophylaxis is also known as a dental cleaning, and *anterior (excluding final restoration)* is one of the codes that can be used to report root canal therapy.

FIGURE 30-1 An x-ray of teeth (bitewing view) is one type of dental service ©Design Pics Inc./Alamy

LET'S CODE IT! SCENARIO

Alvin Tunney, an 81-year-old male, came to Dr. Kahn for a complete maxillary denture. His old one was broken beyond repair, so Alvin needed something immediately.

Let's Code It!

Dr. Kahn provided Alvin with a *complete maxillary denture.* Let's go to the HCPCS Level II Alphabetic Index:

Dentures D5110–D5899

As you read the full list, you see that the reference matches Dr. Kahn's notes. Next, turn to the Alphanumeric Listing to see which code is the most accurate.

D5110   **Complete denture—maxillary**
D5120   **Complete denture—mandibular**
D5130   **Immediate denture—maxillary**
D5140   **Immediate denture—mandibular**

Is there additional information in the notes that will help us determine the best code? They state that Alvin needed the denture *immediately.* It leads us directly to this code:

D5130   **Immediate denture—maxillary**

Excellent!

E0100–E8002 Durable Medical Equipment

The E codes are used to identify certain pieces of durable medical equipment (DME) provided to a patient.

Science and technology have provided our society with great innovations that make life easier and more functional. Canes, walkers, and wheelchairs, among other items, help individuals move from one place to another without further assistance. Portable oxygen, humidifiers, vaporizers, and other equipment assist breathing, and pacemakers and electrical nerve stimulators help keep a heart beating. Some items are so commonplace that we take them for granted, yet only 10 years ago, patients would be forced to stay home all day every day. Other products, such as wheelchairs, have evolved into more convenient and accommodating pieces of equipment. Each item and every accessory costs money to build. Therefore, the health care facility or company should be reimbursed for giving, renting/leasing, or selling equipment. HCPCS Level II codes for DME are used in the reimbursement process.

Durable Medical Equipment

Durable medical equipment (DME) includes such items as canes, wheelchairs, and ventilators. However, to be accurate, Medicare has four qualifiers to determine whether an item can be classified as DME. These qualifiers are

1. The item can withstand repeated use.

2. The item is primarily used for medical purposes.

3. The item is used in the patient's home (rather than only in a health care facility).

4. The item would not be used if the individual were not ill or injured.

Most often, **DMEPOS** dealers supply DME to the patient. Such companies submit their claims not to Medicare or the state's Medicare fiscal intermediary (FI) but to their assigned **durable medical equipment regional carrier (DMERC)**, which is contracted by Centers for Medicare and Medicaid Services (CMS).

HCPCS E Code Subheadings

The DME E code section, codes E0100–E8002, is divided into subheadings. It is not the only section in the HCPCS Level II book having codes related to DME services and supplies; however, it is the section dedicated to them. Take a minute to look through its subheadings, and you should gain a clearer understanding of the items and services included here.

EXAMPLES

Walking Aids and Attachments (E0100–E0159)
- Canes
- Crutches
- Walkers

CODING BITES

Be careful not to confuse the HCPCS Level II E codes with ICD-10-CM E codes, which report endocrinological illnesses.

E0980   Safety vest, wheelchair

Letter followed by four numbers (from HCPCS Level II)

E09.8   Drug or chemical induced diabetes mellitus with unspecified complications

Letter followed by two numbers, a period, and possibly additional numbers or letters (from ICD-10-CM)

CODING BITES

Remember that a coding specialist's job is to report with the greatest specificity. There will be times when you will need a code from this section because it provides more specificity than a code from the CPT.

EXAMPLES

E0105	Cane, quad or three prong, includes canes of all materials, adjustable or fixed, with tips
E0156	Seat attachment, walker
E0242	Bathtub rail, floor base

G0000–G9999 Temporary Procedures/Professional Services

Codes from this section are used to report services and procedures that do not have an accurate code description in the main portion of the CPT book.

EXAMPLES

G0102	Prostate cancer screening; digital rectal examination
G0151	Services performed by a qualified physical therapist in the home health or hospice setting, each 15 minutes
G0268	Removal of impacted cerumen (one or both ears) by physician on same date of service as audiologic function testing

---

CODING BITES

Throughout section **G** are codes grouped as *Quality Measures*. These codes are used to report services related to the **Physician Quality Reporting System (PQRS)** and are only used when an appropriate CPT Category II code is not available.

H0001–H9999 Alcohol and Drug Abuse Treatment Services

When alcohol and drug treatment, as well as some other mental health services, is provided, some state Medicaid agencies will have you use codes from the *Alcohol and Drug Abuse Treatment* category.

EXAMPLES

H0005	Alcohol and/or drug services; group counseling by a clinician
H0038	Self-help/peer services, per 15 minutes
H2020	Therapeutic behavioral services, per diem

J0100–J8999 Drugs Other Than Chemotherapy Drugs and J9000–J9999 Chemotherapy Drugs

This *Drugs Administered* section provides you with codes to identify the specific drugs that are given to the patient by a health care professional in any way. This includes immunosuppressive drugs, inhalation solutions, and other miscellaneous drugs and solutions. These codes have nothing to do with the writing of a prescription or when a patient self-administers medication.

EXAMPLES

J0207	Injection, amifostine, 500 mg
J7100	Infusion, dextran 40, 500 mL
J7610	Albuterol, inhalation solution, compounded product, administered through DME, concentrated form, 1 mg

You will find that drugs identified in the code descriptions are most often the chemical, or generic, name of the pharmaceutical. At times the brand, or trade, name is listed in the Alphabetic Index and/or in the Table of Drugs in an appendix of your HCPCS Level II book. If your provider notes refer to a name that you cannot find in this book, you might need to look in the *Physician's Desk Reference* (PDR) to find an alternate name for the drug.

CODING BITES

If you do not have access to a Drug Directory, such as *Physician's Desk Reference* (PDR), you can find all the necessary information on pharmaceuticals at https://www.pdr.net/browse-by-drug-name.

EXAMPLE

Dr. Valentine asked the nurse to administer a 250 mg tablet, CellCept, PO, to Benjamin Rudon.

CellCept, generic name mycophenolate mofetil, is classified as an immunosuppressant.

- Neither name is listed in the Alphabetic Index of HCPCS.
- CellCept is listed in the **Table of Drugs.**
- Mycophenolate mofetil is listed in the **Table of Drugs.**

J7517   Mycophenolate mofetil, oral, 250 mg

In the chapter *CPT Medicine Section*, you learned about coding for the administration of pharmaceuticals (drugs). Those codes are used for reporting the services—the labor—of the health care professional who gives the patient the drug. You may remember that the different methods of administering drugs include

IA	**Intra-arterial administration**
IV	**Intravenous administration (e.g., gravity infusion, injections, and timed pushes)**

IM	Intramuscular administration
IT	Intrathecal
SC	Subcutaneous administration
INH	Inhaled solutions
VAR	Various routes for drugs that are commonly administered into joints, cavities, tissues, or topical applications, as well as other parenteral administrations
ORAL	Administered orally
OTH	Other routes of administration, such as suppositories or catheter injections

The codes in HCPCS Level II enable you to report and gain reimbursement for the actual drug or medication, as well as the syringe or IV bag used. The codes cover the pharmaceutical materials only—*not* the administration of the drug.

In some cases, you may find DME has been supplied to the patient to provide medication, or drugs. When the equipment is made available to an individual, it may need to be reported separately from the drug itself.

 LET'S CODE IT! SCENARIO

Janine Howell, a 55-year-old female, came in for her chemotherapy treatment. She is given Adriamycin, 30 mg/m², IV daily, as treatment for malignant lymphoma. She tolerates the treatment well, and is discharged home.

Let's Code It!

You learned in the *CPT Medicine Section* chapter that you will need one code for the administration of this drug therapy and a second code from HCPCS Level II to identify the specific drug administered.

Let's begin determining the code for the Adriamycin. Open your HCPCS Level II code book to the *Table of Drugs*. Did you find it listed? It is there but listed as *Adriamycin, PFS, RDF*. Is this the same? Check the HCPCS Level II code book's *Alphabetic Index*. It is not there. You know there must be a code for this, so adriamycin may be an alternate name. You will need to check the PDR. [*NOTE:* If you do not have access to the PDR, you can use PDR.net or Drugs.com.]

You will see in the listing for Adriamycin that:

Therapeutic Classification: Antineoplastics
Common Name: Doxorubicin hydrocholoride

Go back to the HCPCS Level II code book's *Table of Drugs*. Can you find it using the common name?

Doxorubicin HCL   10 MG   IV   J9000

Now, let's go into the Alphanumeric Listing and find the specific code and its full description.

J9000   Injection, doxorubicin HCL, 10 mg

Perfect! However, this code only reports the provision of 10 mg. The documentation states, "*30 mg.*" Therefore, you will need a multiplier.

J9000x3   Injection, doxorubicin HCL, 10 mg × 3

If you have your CPT code book nearby, try to determine the code for the administration of this medication. Did you determine this to be the correct code?

96413   Chemotherapy administration, intravenous infusion technique; up to 1 hour, single or initial substance/drug

Good work!

K0000–K9999 Temporary Codes Assigned to DME Regional Carriers

The K codes were developed for **durable medical equipment regional carriers (DMERCs)** to report services that are not currently identified by other codes.

> **EXAMPLES**
>
> K0001   Standard wheelchair
> K0462   Temporary replacement for patient-owned equipment being repaired, any type

L0100–L4999 Orthotics and L5000–L9999 Prosthetics

The codes included in the *Orthotic Procedures and Devices* and *Prosthetic Procedures and Devices* categories identify orthotic devices, orthopedic shoes, prosthetic devices, prosthetic implants, and scoliosis equipment.

An *orthotic* is a device used to correct or improve the function of a musculoskeletal concern or abnormality, whereas a *prosthetic* is an artificial replacement for a damaged or missing part of the body (see Figure 30-2).

> **EXAMPLES**
>
> *ORTHOTICS*
>
> L0170   Cervical, collar, molded to patient model
> L0984   Protective body sock, prefabricated, off-the-shelf, each
> L3809   Wrist-hand-finger orthosis (WHFO), without joint(s), prefabricated, off-the-shelf, any type
>
> *PROSTHETICS*
>
> L5100   Below knee, molded socket, shin, SACH foot
> L6100   Below elbow, molded socket, flexible elbow hinge, triceps pad
> L8020   Breast prosthesis, mastectomy form
>
> SACH = Solid-Ankle Cushioned Heel

FIGURE 30-2 Man with prosthetic leg running in the desert ©MichaelSvoboda/Getty Images

M0000–M1071 Other Medical Services

The codes in the *Other Medical Services* category cover cellular therapy, prolotherapy, intragastric hypothermia, intravenous **chelation therapy**, and fabric wrapping of an abdominal aneurysm (MNP).

P0000–P9999 Laboratory Services

HCPCS Level II codes in the *Pathology and Laboratory Services* category include codes for services not listed in the CPT book, including chemistry, toxicology, microbiology, screening Papanicolaou (Pap) procedures, and numerous blood products.

EXAMPLES

P2031	Hair analysis (excluding arsenic)
P7001	Culture, bacterial, urine; quantitative, sensitivity study
P9051	Whole blood or red blood cells, leukocytes reduced, CMV-negative, each unit

Q0000–Q9999 Temporary Codes Assigned by CMS

The Q codes replace the less specific codes that you may find elsewhere in the coding process for casting and splinting supplies when a health care professional cares for a patient with a fracture. The section also includes codes for certain drugs and services having nothing to do with the management of a fracture.

EXAMPLES

Q0113	Pinworm examinations
Q2017	Injection, teniposide, 50 mg
Q4049	Finger splint, static

R0000–R9999 Diagnostic Radiology Services

The codes in the *Diagnostic Radiology Services* section are used to report the hauling of portable radiologic equipment.

EXAMPLES

R0070	Transportation of portable X-ray equipment and personnel to home or nursing home, per trip to facility or location, one patient seen
R0075	Transportation of portable X-ray equipment and personnel to home or nursing home, per trip to facility or location, more than one patient seen
R0076	Transportation of portable EKG to facility or location, per patient

Chelation Therapy
The use of a chemical compound that binds with metal in the body so that the metal will lose its toxic effect. It might be done when a metal disc or prosthetic is implanted in a patient, eliminating adverse reactions to the metal itself as a foreign body.

CODING BITES
Remember that you must always choose the code with the greatest specificity.

S0000–S9999 Temporary National Codes Established by Private Payers

The *Temporary National Codes* section was developed by the Health Insurance Association of America (HIAA) and the Blue Cross Blue Shield Association (BCBSA) for use by the Medicaid program and other third-party payers. The codes cover supplies, services, and drugs for which there are no other codes.

EXAMPLES

S0081	Injection, piperacillin sodium, 500 mg
S0317	Disease management program; per diem
S2060	Lobar lung transplantation
S9024	Paranasal sinus ultrasound

T1000–T9999 Temporary National Codes Established by Medicaid

Planned for use by state agencies that administer Medicaid programs, the T codes are used to report services not otherwise described by any other code. Services represented in this category include nursing facility and home health–related services, substance abuse treatment, and training-related procedures.

EXAMPLES

T1013	Sign language or oral interpretive services, per 15 minutes
T2022	Case management, per month
T2045	Hospice general inpatient care; per diem

V0000–V9999 Vision, Hearing, Speech-Language Pathology Services

V0000–V2999 Vision Services

If not represented by any other codes, ophthalmic and optometric services and supplies may be coded from this V code category, including contact lenses, intraocular lenses, miscellaneous lenses, prostheses, spectacles, and other vision-related supplies.

EXAMPLES

V2118	Aniseikonic lens, single vision
V2321	Lenticular lens, per lens, trifocal
V2530	Contact lens, scleral, gas impermeable, per lens

V5000–V9999 Hearing and Speech-Language Pathology Services

Services related to hearing and speech-language pathology are included in this V code category and cover hearing tests, repair of augmentative communicative system, speech-language pathology screenings, and other hearing test–related supplies and equipment.

EXAMPLES

V5008	Hearing screening
V5100	Hearing aid, bilateral, body worn
V5364	Dysphagia screening

 YOU CODE IT! CASE STUDY

Alfonzo Doyle, a 20-year-old male, lost his eye in a skiing accident and has come to see Dr. Durran to receive his prosthetic eye. It is a custom-made, plastic prosthesis. Code for the prosthesis only.

You Code It!

Go through the steps of coding, and determine the code(s) that should be reported for the prosthetic provided by Dr. Durran to Alfonzo Doyle.

Step #1: Read the case carefully and completely.

Step #2: Abstract the scenario. Which key words or terms describe what service the physician provided to the patient during this encounter?

Step #3: Are there any details missing or incomplete for which you would need to query the physician? [If so, ask your instructor.]

Step #4: Determine the correct HCPCS Level II code or codes to explain the details about what was provided to the patient during this encounter.

Step #5: Check for any relevant guidance, including reading all of the symbols and notations.

Step #6: Do you need to append any modifiers to ensure complete and accurate information is provided?

Step #7: Double-check your work.

Answer

Did you find this to be the correct code?

V2623   **Prosthetic eye, plastic, custom**

Good job!

30.4 Symbols and Notations

Throughout many versions of a HCPCS Level II code book, you may see notations that will help you use the codes correctly and determine the best, most appropriate code available. Check the front of your code book for meanings.

 GUIDANCE CONNECTION

Read the guidelines in the **Introduction** and **HCPCS Level II Use and Convention** sections in your HCPCS Level II book.

HCPCS quarterly updates are posted on the website when available: https://www.cms.gov/medicare/coding/hcpcsreleasecodesets/hcpcs-quarterly-update.html.

Symbols

● Bullet

A large bullet (●), or solid circle, shown next to a code indicates that it is the first year that the code is included in this code set. That is, it marks a new code.

▲ Solid Triangle

A solid triangle (▲) shown next to a code lets you know that the code's description has been changed or adjusted since last year or that a rule or guideline regarding the code has changed.

EXAMPLES

- ▲ G8648   Risk-adjusted functional status change residual score for the knee impairment successfully calculated and the score was less than zero (<0)
- ▲ K0037   High mount flip-up footrest, each

○ Open Circle

An open circle (○) next to a code identifies that the code had been deleted but now has been restored (reinstated).

EXAMPLES

- ○ J3090   Injection, tedizolid phosphate, 1 mg
- ○ J3380   Injection, vedolizumab, 1 mg

⊘ Circle with Slash

A circle with a slash through it (⊘), also known as the Forbidden Symbol in the HCPCS Level II book, identifies a code that is not covered under the skilled nursing facility (SNF) prospective payment system (PPS).

EXAMPLES

- ⊘ L5970   All lower extremity prostheses, foot, external keel, SACH foot
- ⊘ L7367   Lithium ion battery, rechargeable, replacement

☑ Box with Check Mark

A check mark inside a square box (☑) marks a code description that identifies a specific quantity of material or supply. It is a reminder for you to check the detail in the notes and report the code not only for the item it represents but for the amount as well.

EXAMPLES

- ☑ J0894   Injection, decitabine, 1 mg
- ☑ K0073   Caster pin lock, each

♂ Male Symbol

The male symbol (♂) is placed next to codes that identify procedures, services, and equipment that can *only* be performed or used on a male patient.

♀ Female Symbol

The female symbol (♀) identifies codes used to report procedures, services, and equipment that can *only* be performed or used on a female patient.

🅐 Capital Letter A

The 🅐 symbol highlights the fact that a code is used only for procedures, services, and equipment that are performed or used on a patient of a certain age group. Read the code description carefully to ensure the age limitation of the code matches the patient.

🅜 Capital Letter M

The 🅜 symbol is used to remind you that the code describes maternity procedures, services, and equipment that are performed or used on a pregnant female 12–55 years of age.

~~Z1111~~ Any Code with a Line Through It

A line through the center of a code and its description means that the code has been deleted and may no longer be used.

Notations

Just as in the CPT book, you will find notations (below code descriptions in the Alphanumeric Listing) that guide you on the proper use of HCPCS Level II codes.

Always Report Concurrent to the xxx Procedure

This notation directs you to always report this code with a code for another specific procedure. The notation is similar to the "code also" instruction found in CPT or ICD-10-CM.

EXAMPLE

A4262   Temporary, absorbable lacrimal duct implant, each
Always report concurrent to the implant procedure.

A4263   Permanent, long-term, non-dissolvable lacrimal duct implant, each
Always report concurrent to the implant procedure.

In the previous example, the "A" code is for the implant itself, and the note reminds you that you have to code the physician's services for putting the implant into the patient.

See Also Code Z1111

The *see also code* notation cross-references this code with another code that may be similar in description. The notation serves as a reminder for you to double-check that you are using the most accurate code.

EXAMPLES

A4450   Tape, non-waterproof, per 18 square inches
See also code A4452

A4452   Tape, waterproof, per 18 square inches
See also code A4450

Clarifications of Coverage

Clarifications of coverage notations are worded differently from code to code but indicate when to use or *not* use the code. However, always check with the specific payer to whom you will be sending the claim.

EXAMPLES

A4570   Splint
Dressings applied by a physician are included as part of the professional service.

A6260   Wound cleansers, any type, any size
Surgical dressings applied by a physician are included as part of the professional service. Surgical dressings obtained by the patient to perform homecare as prescribed by the physician are covered.

Report in Addition to Code Z1111

When one code is to be reported with other codes, a notation *Report in addition to* (a particular *code*) will identify those circumstances. It not only tells you the circumstances but also tells you which code to use. You may notice that it is similar to an add-on code in CPT.

To Report, See Code Z1111

When a code has been deleted, you may find a notation that directs you to another HCPCS Level II code that can be used instead.

See Code(s): 00000

The notation *See* (a particular *code*) refers you to a CPT code for a description that is *potentially* better and may be more specific for reporting what was actually done or given to the patient.

Determine If an Alternative HCPCS Level II or a CPT Code Better Describes . . .

You will see the notation *Determine if an alternative HCPCS Level II or a CPT code better describes* beneath each miscellaneous, unlisted, unclassified, not otherwise classified (NOC), not otherwise listed, or **not otherwise specified (NOS)** code. The notation serves as a warning to you to make certain that there is no better or more specific code in either the CPT or elsewhere in this HCPCS Level II book that correctly reports the services or procedures performed.

Not Otherwise Specified (NOS)
The absence of additional details documented in the notes.

Use This Code for . . .

The notation *Use this code for* provides you with alternative names, brand names, and other terms that are also represented by the code's description.

> **EXAMPLES**
>
> J0585   Injection, onabotulinumtoxinA, 1 unit
> *Use this code for Botox, Botox Cosmetic*
>
> J1160   Injection, digoxin, up to 0.5 mg
> *Use this code for Lanoxin*

Pertinent Documentation to Evaluate Medical Appropriateness Should Be . . .

Some procedures are not automatically accepted as being medically necessary. The notation *Pertinent documentation to evaluate medical appropriateness should be* warns you up-front that you should include the proper documentation along with the claim *the first time* you submit it, rather than wait to be asked by the third-party payer, which would delay payment.

> **EXAMPLES**
>
> D2980   Crown repair, by report
> *Pertinent documentation to evaluate medical appropriateness should be included when this code is reported.*
>
> V2399   Specialty trifocal (by report)
> *Pertinent documentation to evaluate medical appropriateness should be included when this code is reported.*

Do Not Use This Code to Report . . .

The notation *Do not use this code to report* warns you of circumstances when you are not permitted to use a code.

> **EXAMPLE**
>
> D3220   Therapeutic pulpotomy (excluding final restoration)—removal of pulp coronal to the dentinocemental junction and application of medicament
> *Do not use this code to report the first stage of root canal therapy.*

Medicare Covers . . .

Throughout the HCPCS Level II book, you will see notations giving you information about coverage, particularly Medicare and Medicaid coverage. You should note that the book covers the entire nation and that both programs are state-administered. This means that you should still confirm the terms and policies of what is covered with your own state's fiscal intermediary (FI)—the agency or organization that is in charge of reimbursement for your state's program. Also check with other third-party payers to see if they will cover this item or service.

EXAMPLES

E0607   Home blood glucose monitor
         Medicare covers home blood-testing devices for diabetic patients when the devices are prescribed by the patient's physicians. Many commercial payers provide this coverage to non–insulin dependent diabetics as well.

Q0174   Thiethylperazine maleate, 10 mg, oral, FDA approved prescription antiemetic, for use as a complete therapeutic substitute for an IV antiemetic at the time of chemotherapy treatment, not to exceed a 48-hour dosage regimen
         Medicare covers at the time of chemotherapy if regimen doesn't exceed 48 hours. Submit on the same claim as the chemotherapy.

Code with Caution

When you see the notation *Code with caution* beneath a code, you need to go back and double-check the provider's notes carefully. If this is what was actually done, then be certain to attach documentation explaining why that method was used instead of the newer technique because it is surely going to be questioned.

EXAMPLES

M0301   Fabric wrapping of abdominal aneurysm
         Code with caution: This procedure has largely been replaced with more effective treatment modalities. Submit documentation.

P2028   Cephalin flocculation, blood
         Code with caution: This test is considered obsolete. Submit documentation.

CODING BITES

When you determine from the documentation that a different code may be more accurate than one indicated by the physician, you should query the physician to have him or her document complete accurate details.

 YOU CODE IT! CASE STUDY

Dr. Principe modified Miriam Collins's left orthopedic shoe by inserting a between-sole metatarsal bar wedge to accommodate Miriam's shrinking Achilles tendon. Dr. Principe checked off the code L3649 on the superbill. As the professional coding specialist, is this the best code available?

You Code It!

Go through the steps of coding, and determine the code(s) that should be reported for this product between Dr. Principe and Miriam Collins.

Step #1: Read the case carefully and completely.

Step #2: Abstract the scenario. Which key words or terms describe what service the physician provided to the patient during this encounter?

Step #3: Are there any details missing or incomplete for which you would need to query the physician? [If so, ask your instructor.]

Step #4: Determine the correct HCPCS Level II code or codes to explain the details about what was provided to the patient during this encounter.

(continued)

Step #5: Check for any relevant guidance, including reading all of the symbols and notations.

Step #6: Do you need to append any modifiers to ensure complete and accurate information is provided?

Step #7: Double-check your work.

Answer

Did you find this to be the correct code?

L3410   **Metatarsal bar wedge, between sole**

Now that's a much more specific code. Good job!

 LET'S CODE IT! SCENARIO

Rita Warren came with her husband, Ryan, to see Dr. Capshaw because of the problems Ryan was having sleeping. Dr. Capshaw had performed a nasopharyngoscopy and diagnosed Ryan with sleep apnea. At this encounter, Dr. Capshaw provided Ryan with an apnea monitor, complete with a recording feature, so that more data could be collected and Dr. Capshaw could further evaluate his condition.

Let's Code It!

Dr. Capshaw has supplied Ryan with an *apnea monitor with a recording feature*. This machine is considered durable medical equipment (DME). Ryan's insurance carrier accepts HCPCS Level II codes. Therefore, we have determined the code so that Dr. Capshaw can be reimbursed for the machine. Let's go to the Alphabetic Index and look up the word *monitor* because that is the key word that best describes this item. Beneath the word *monitor,* indented slightly, you see the word *apnea,* and the suggestion for the codes E0618 and E0619. This seems to be exactly what Dr. Capshaw described in his notes, so let's turn to the Alphanumeric Listing to read the complete description of the codes.

E0618   **Apnea monitor, without recording feature**

This matches the notes with one big exception. The code description specifically states *without* recording feature. Dr. Capshaw documented giving Ryan a monitor *with* a recording feature. Let's look at the other suggested code:

E0619   **Apnea monitor, with recording feature**

Excellent! It matches perfectly.

 LET'S CODE IT! SCENARIO

Dr. Bettesh provided Lauren Martins, a 79-year-old female, with a quad cane, after putting on a new handgrip. Code for the supply only.

Let's Code It!

When you pull out the key words that describe the items for which Dr. Bettesh should be reimbursed, you see that Lauren was provided with a *quad cane* and *new handgrip*.

It wouldn't be out of line to think that the codes are automatically going to be listed in the **Durable Medical Equipment** section, codes E0100–E8002. If you turned to that section directly, you would find the code for the

(continued)

quad cane rather quickly. It's right in the front. However, you could examine and search through the entire listing of 7,902 possible codes in the section and never find the correct code for the replacement handgrip. When you look these key words up in the Alphabetic Index first, you see very quickly, and more efficiently, that the codes you need are these:

E0105   **Cane, quad or three prong, includes canes of all materials, adjustable or fixed, with tips**
A4636   **Replacement, handgrip, cane, crutch, or walker, each**

It's great when the process works, isn't it? You bet!

30.5 Appendices

The HCPCS Level II book provides you with additional information in the back of the book to help you code more accurately. See Table 30-1.

CODING BITES

NOTE: The content of appendices may vary depending upon the publisher of the HCPCS Level II book used.

You may find additional details at https://www.cms.gov/ Medicare/Coding/ HCPCSRelease CodeSets/Alpha-Numeric-HCPCS.html.

TABLE 30-1 List of most common Appendices found in HCPCS Level II code books.

Appendices	Description
Table of Drugs	This is an alphabetic listing of drug names, along with the standard unit of administration, a particular method of administration, and a reference to its HCPCS Level II code.
Modifiers	This is an alphabetic list of all HCPCS Level II modifiers. You will learn more about these modifiers in Appendix B of this text.
Abbreviations and Acronymns	Abbreviations and acronyms are used throughout the health care industry. This appendix lists those used in HCPCS Level II descriptions to help you better understand the meaning of the codes.
CMS References	Certain components of the coding system change from time to time. Up-to-date manuals and information can be found online in the Centers for Medicare and Medicaid Services (CMS) manual system found at www.cms.hhs.gov/manuals. Included in each annual edition of some printed HCPCS Level II books are references to national coverage determinations made just prior to publication. As a student, this may be outside the scope of your studies. As you mature in your career, this reference will be very handy.
New, Changed, Deleted, and Reinstated HCPCS Codes	This appendix lists all HCPCS Level II codes that have experienced a change since the previous year's printed book. As a student, this will have little relevance for you. But when the new book comes out, it serves as an excellent reference for someone who may use the same code or codes over and over again.
Place of Service and Type of Service Codes	This appendix offers you a thorough explanation of each place of service (POS) and type of service (TOS) code required for boxes 24B and 24C of the CMS 1500 claim form.
Deleted Code Crosswalk	This is a list of all deleted codes from last year to this, and includes the new codes to use to report the service, when available.
Glossary	Key terms used throughout this code set are listed here, along with their definitions.
Physician Quality Reporting System (PQRS)	This appendix provides up-to-date details about codes used in this program.

CODING BITES

The list in ***Abbreviations and Acronyms*** appendix is not inclusive of all abbreviations and acronyms used in the health care industry. It is a good idea to keep a medical dictionary close by to reference those abbreviations not included in this appendix.

Chapter Summary

HCPCS Level II codes are updated quarterly and are officially effective January 1 of each year, with no grace period. Most printed versions of the book are published with those codes posted by the Centers for Medicare and Medicaid Services (CMS) as of November 1. Read the following notation in the introduction of the HCPCS Level II book:

"Because of the unstable nature of HCPCS Level II codes, everything has been done to include the latest information available at print time. Unfortunately, HCPCS Level II codes, their descriptions, and other related information change throughout the year. Consult the patient's payer and the CMS website to confirm the status of any HCPCS Level II code. The existence of a code does not imply coverage under any given payment plan."

CHAPTER 30 REVIEW
HCPCS Level II

Enhance your learning by completing these exercises and more at mcgrawhillconnect.com!

Let's Check It! Terminology

Match each key term to the appropriate definition.

1. **LO 30.3** The provision of emergency CPR, stabilization of the patient, first aid, control of bleeding, and/or the treatment of shock.

2. **LO 30.3** A company designated by the state or region to act as the fiscal intermediary for all DME claims.

3. **LO 30.3** By way of anything other than the gastrointestinal tract, such as intravenous, intramuscular, intramedullary, or subcutaneous.

4. **LO 30.4** An indication that more detailed information is not available from the physician's notes.

5. **LO 30.1** A device used to correct or improve an orthopedic concern.

6. **LO 30.3** Life-sustaining, emergency care is provided, such as airway management, defibrillation, and/or the administration of drugs.

7. **LO 30.3** Apparatus and tools that help individuals accommodate physical frailties, provide pharmaceuticals, and provide other assistance that will last for a long time and/or be used to assist multiple patients over time.

8. **LO 30.3** Within, or by way of, the gastrointestinal tract.

9. **LO 30.1** Fabricated artificial replacement for a damaged or missing part of the body.

10. **LO 30.3** The use of a chemical compound that binds with metal in the body so that the metal will lose its toxic effect. It might be done when a metal disc or prosthetic is implanted in a patient, eliminating adverse reactions to the metal itself as a foreign body.

11. **LO 30.3** Continuous care provided by one or more health professionals in an appropriate specialty area, such as respiratory care or cardiovascular care, or by a paramedic with additional training.

A. Advanced Life Support (ALS)

B. Basic Life Support (BLS)

C. Chelation Therapy

D. Durable Medical Equipment (DME)

E. Durable Medical Equipment Regional Carrier (DMERC)

F. Enteral

G. Not Otherwise Specified (NOS)

H. Orthotic

I. Parenteral

J. Prosthetic

K. Specialty Care Transport

Let's Check It! Concepts

Choose the most appropriate answer for each of the following questions.

1. LO 30.4 The symbol of a circle with a line through it ⊘ means

    a. a new code.

    b. a revised code.

    c. a code exempt from a particular modifier.

    d. a service not covered under the skilled nursing facility payment system.

2. LO 30.4 The box with a check mark in it ☑ indicates a code description that

    a. includes a quantity measurement.

    b. is always covered by Medicare.

    c. is approved for reimbursement at a higher rate.

    d. includes refills.

3. LO 30.3 The J codes are used to bill insurance carriers for

    a. prescription drugs patients get at the drugstore.

    b. drugs administered by a health care professional.

    c. nothing. They are deleted codes.

    d. items not accepted by Medicaid in any state for any reason.

4. LO 30.1 HCPCS Level II codes are used, most often, to report all except

    a. drugs used for treatment of a patient.

    b. equipment provided to a patient.

    c. anesthesia administered by an anesthesiologist.

    d. dental services.

5. LO 30.3 The acronym DME stands for

    a. determination of medical effectiveness.

    b. durable medical equipment.

    c. donated medical equipment.

    d. diluted medicine equivalent.

6. LO 30.1 HCPCS Level II codes are presented as

    a. five numbers.

    b. one letter followed by four numbers.

    c. four numbers followed by one letter.

    d. five letters.

7. LO 30.1 HCPCS is an acronym that stands for

    a. Health Care Professional Classification Systems.

    b. Health and Caretaker Providers Coding Series.

    c. Home Care Providers Coding System.

    d. Healthcare Common Procedure Coding System.

8. LO 30.3 The code D1110 is an example of a

    a. HCPCS Level I code, also known as a CPT code.

    b. HCPCS Level II code.

    c. HCPCS Level III code.

    d. HCPCS Level IV code.

9. LO 30.3 The D0000–D9999 codes are created and maintained by the
   a. American Medical Association.
   b. American Dental Association.
   c. Centers for Medicare and Medicaid Services.
   d. Department of Health and Human Services.

10. LO 30.2 You can look up key words in the HCPCS Alphabetic Index by using which of the following?
   a. Generic name of the drug
   b. Medical supply item
   c. Orthotic
   d. All of these

11. LO 30.3 The E codes shown in the HCPCS Level II book are
   a. an expansion of the E codes in the ICD-10-CM book.
   b. used to identify DME provided to a patient.
   c. not accepted by Medicaid.
   d. always first listed on a claim form.

12. LO 30.3 An example of DME is
   a. an injection of Demerol.
   b. a prosthetic ankle.
   c. a three-prong cane.
   d. home infusion therapy.

13. LO 30.4 A deleted code in the HCPCS Level II book means
   a. the procedure is obsolete.
   b. the service is no longer reimbursable.
   c. the code is reinstated.
   d. the code is no longer available to represent the service or item.

14. LO 30.3 Alcohol intervention treatment might be coded in the range
   a. H0001–H2037
   b. H5000–H9999
   c. F1000–F9999
   d. G0000–G9999

15. LO 30.4 A code with a capital "A" or A next to it means that
   a. a drug was administered intravenously.
   b. the machine can only be used for infusion therapy.
   c. the service is limited to a specific age group.
   d. the equipment is illegal in some states.

Let's Check It! Symbols and Notations

Part I
Match each HCPCS Level II symbol to the appropriate HCPCS Level II description

1. LO 30.4 The female symbol.
2. LO 30.4 Indicates that it is the first year that the code is included in this code set.
3. LO 30.4 Lets you know that the code's description has been changed or adjusted since last year or that a rule or guideline regarding the code has changed.
4. LO 30.4 Means that the code has been deleted and may no longer be used.
5. LO 30.4 Identifies that the code had been deleted but now has been restored (reinstated).

A. ●
B. ▲
C. ○
D. ⊘

6. LO 30.4 Reminds you that the code describes maternity procedures, services, and equipment that are performed or used on a pregnant female 12–55 years of age.

7. LO 30.4 The male symbol.

8. LO 30.4 Identifies a specific quantity of material or supply. It is a reminder for you to check the detail in the notes and report the code not only for the item it represents but for the amount as well.

9. LO 30.4 Highlights the fact that a code is used only for procedures, services, and equipment that are performed or used on a patient of a certain age group.

10. LO 30.4 Identifies a code that is not covered under the skilled nursing facility (SNF) prospective payment system (PPS).

E. ☑

F. ♂

G. ♀

H. 🅰

I. 🅼

J. ~~Z1111~~

Part II

Match each HCPCS Level II notation to the appropriate notation description.

1. LO 30.4 This notation cross-references this code with another code that may be similar in description. The notation serves as a reminder for you to double-check that you are using the most accurate code.

2. LO 30.4 Refers you to a CPT code for a description that is potentially better and may be more specific for reporting what was actually done or given to the patient.

3. LO 30.4 When one code is to be reported with other codes, a notation to "Report in addition to" (a particular code) will identify those circumstances. It not only tells you the circumstances but also tells you which code to use.

4. LO 30.4 This notation directs you to always report this code with a code for another specific procedure.

5. LO 30.4 This notation indicates when to use or not use the code.

6. LO 30.4 Serves as a warning to you to make certain that there is no better or more specific code in either the CPT or elsewhere in this HCPCS Level II book that correctly reports the services or procedures performed.

7. LO 30.4 This notation warns that you need to go back and double-check the provider's notes carefully. If this is what was actually done, then be certain to attach documentation explaining why that method was used instead of the newer technique because it is surely going to be questioned.

8. LO 30.4 Warns you of circumstances when you are not permitted to use a code.

9. LO 30.4 Provides you with alternative names, brand names, and other terms that are also represented by the code's description.

10. LO 30.4 This notation giving you information about coverage, particularly Medicare and Medicaid coverage.

11. LO 30.4 Warns you up-front that you should include the proper documentation along with the claim the first time you submit it, rather than wait to be asked by the third-party payer, which would delay payment.

A. Always report concurrent to the *xxx* procedure

B. *See also code . . .*

C. Clarifications of coverage

D. *Report in addition to code . . .*

E. *See code(s): . . .*

F. Determine if an alternative HCPCS Level II or a CPT code better describes. . .

G. *Use this code for. . .*

H. Pertinent documentation to evaluate medical appropriateness should be. . .

I. Do not use this code to report. . .

J. Medicare covers . . .

K. *Code with caution*

Let's Check It! Rules and Regulations

Please answer the following questions from the knowledge you have gained after reading this chapter.

1. LO 30.1 List four HCPCS Level II codes specific to aspects for health care services.
2. LO 30.1 Do all insurance carriers accept HCPCS Level II codes? What is the responsibility of the coding specialist with regards to billing third-party payers?
3. LO 30.2 List five ways to look up the key words after abstracting them from the provider's notes.
4. LO 30.3 What HCPCS Level II codes represent Procedures and Professional Services (Temporary)?
5. LO 30.4 What does the notation *"Use this code for . . ."* indicate?

YOU CODE IT! Basics

First, identify the HCPCS Level II main term in the following statements; then code the procedure or service.

Example: Airlift by helicopter, one-way:

a. main term: *Ambulance*   b. procedure: *A0431*

Example: A 5 ml injection, IM, of Robaxin:

a. main term: *Robaxin*   b. procedure: *J2800*

1. A bottle of 50 blood glucose reagent strips:
   a. main term: _____   b. procedure: _____
2. Johannsen Health Care delivered 1000 mL of distilled water for use with nebulizer:
   a. main term: _____   b. procedure: _____
3. Youth-sized disposable incontinence brief, one:
   a. main term: _____   b. procedure: _____
4. Arterial blood tubing:
   a. main term: _____   b. procedure: _____
5. Neonate ambulance transport, one-way, base rate:
   a. main term: _____   b. procedure: _____
6. Ambulance ride with oxygen administered along with other advanced life support (ALS) services:
   a. main term: _____   b. procedure: _____

7. Nonemergency transportation by stretcher van:
   a. main term: _____   b. procedure: _____
8. A 200-mg injection IM of chloroquine hydrochloride:
   a. main term: _____   b. procedure: _____
9. An injection SC of 30 mg of codeine phosphate:
   a. main term: _____   b. procedure: _____
10. Dr. Longwell ordered Fosphenytoin, with an initial dose of 50 mg:
    a. main term: _____   b. procedure: _____
11. A 25-mg injection of lepirudin:
    a. main term: _____   b. procedure: _____
12. A seat attachment for a Starke's walker:
    a. main term: _____   b. procedure: _____
13. One heel protector:
    a. main term: _____   b. procedure: _____
14. Portable noninvasive ventilator:
    a. main term: _____   b. procedure: _____
15. Prostate cancer screening, antigen test:
    a. main term: _____   b. procedure: _____

YOU CODE IT! Practice

Using the techniques described in this chapter, carefully read through the case studies and find the most accurate HCPCS Level II code(s) and modifier(s) if appropriate for each case study.

NOTE: All insurance carriers and third-party payers for the patients accept HCPCS Level II codes and modifiers.

1. Daisha Kurucz, a 23-year-old female, has severe asthma. Dr. Benton ordered a nebulizer, with compressor, for her to use at home. Code for the home health agency that supplied the equipment.

2. Daniel Hair, a 56-year-old male with end-stage renal disease (ESRD), was fitted for a reciprocating peritoneal dialysis system. Code the supply of the equipment.

3. Due to his condition, Daniel Hair (previous case study) had an unscheduled dialysis treatment at the nearest hospital outpatient department; this hospital is not certified as an ESRD facility.

4. Muddy Hambaugh, a 27-year-old female with a history of bipolar disorder, was given an injection IM of Thorazine, 45 mg. Code for the drug.

5. Allen Jeter, a 48-year-old male, was being prepared for his kidney transplant. The nurse administered 100 mg of Zenapax, IV, parenteral. Code the drug.

6. After Allen Jeter (previous case study) received his kidney transplant, the nurse gave him an oral dose of 250 mg of CellCept (mycophenolate mofetil) in the hospital. Code the drug.

7. Shirley Loveichelle, an 82-year-old female, was having trouble eating for such a long period of time that she was exhibiting signs of malnutrition. Therefore, Dr. Milliner ordered enteral formula (Ensure) to be administered through a feeding tube at 500 calories per day. Code for the nutritional supplement only.

8. Keith Pawley, a 34-year-old male, came to see Dr. Praylow, his dentist, for an implant-supported porcelain crown on his back tooth.

9. Johnette Potash, a 13-year-old female, lost her retainer at camp. She is at Dr. Rivera's office to get a replacement.

10. Clifton Beckman, a 15-year-old male, sat in poison ivy while camping in the woods. Dr. Gregg prescribed a portable sitz bath for him to use at home.

11. Roberta Henthorne, a 52-year-old female, was recuperating from surgery to repair a complex fracture of her tibia and a compound fracture of her ankle. To help her be more comfortable, Dr. Locklear ordered a fixed-height hospital bed, without side rails and with a mattress, for her to use at home. Code for the DME only.

12. Kenneth Paynter, a 68-year-old male, was on complete bed rest while recuperating from surgery. Because his skin was very sensitive, he was particularly prone to decubitus ulcers. Dr. Roche prescribed a lamb's wool sheepskin pad to help prevent any ulcers from forming.

13. Dr. Sloan provided a complete set of dentures, maxillary and mandibular, for Cheryl Delaney.

14. Dennis Lederrick, a 39-year-old male, had surgery on his left foot. To enable him to take a shower safely, Dr. Willrodt gave him a tub stool to sit on.

15. Scott Zamcho came home from serving in the Marines a double amputee, having had both legs damaged badly in a suicide bomber's attack. Dr. Lovell supplied him with an amputee wheelchair, desk height, with detachable arms and no footrests or leg rests.

 YOU CODE IT! Application

On the following pages, you will see physicians' notes documenting encounters with patients at our textbook's health care facility, Prader, Bracker, & Associates. Carefully read through the notes, and find the best code or codes from the HCPCS Level II book for each of the cases.

NOTE: All insurance carriers and third-party payers for the patients accept HCPCS Level II codes and modifiers.

PRADER, BRACKER, & ASSOCIATES

A Complete Health Care Facility

159 Healthcare Way • SOMEWHERE, FL 32811 • 407-555-6789

PATIENT: ADDLER, ANNETTE

ACCOUNT/EHR #: ADDLAN001

(continued)

Date: 12/21/19

Representative: Elizabeth Alexander

Attending Physician: Renee O. Bracker, MD

The Pt is a 27-year-old female who recently returned from working in Africa. She was diagnosed with variola and has been on a gastric feeding tube to increase her fluids, electrolytes, and calories because the pharyngeal lesions make swallowing difficult. Nasogastric tubing without a stylet was supplied for this patient.

A: Variola

P: Service number given to caregiver

Elizabeth Alexander

EA/mg   D: 12/21/19 09:50:16   T: 12/22/19 12:55:01

Determine the best, most appropriate HCPCS Level II code(s).

BRACKER DURABLE MEDICAL EQUIPMENT

A Complete Health Care Facility

159 Healthcare Way • SOMEWHERE, FL 32811 • 407-555-6789

PATIENT: CARLYLE, JOY

ACCOUNT/EHR #: CARJAY001

Date: 11/05/19

Representative Technician: LuAnn Hallmark

Attending Physician: Renee O. Bracker, MD

The Pt is a 72-year-old female diagnosed with adult kyphosis caused by poor posture. Dr. Bracker prescribed bed rest on a firm mattress with pelvic traction attached to the footboard. At 5:00 p.m. on this date, I delivered a bed board and the traction frame to Ms. Carlyle's home. I placed the bed board underneath the existing mattress in order to create a firm surface upon which the patient could sleep. I then attached the traction frame to the footboard of the existing bed. I spent 45 minutes instructing the patient, her family, and caretaker on the proper use of the equipment, how to properly get into and out of the traction, and the expected sensations.

A: Adult kyphosis

P: Follow up in 2 weeks to see if patient has any questions or concerns.

LuAnn Hallmark

LH/mg   D: 11/05/19 09:50:16   T: 11/08/19 12:55:01

Determine the best, most appropriate HCPCS Level II code(s).

PRADER ONCOLOGY

A Complete Health Care Facility

159 Healthcare Way • SOMEWHERE, FL 32811 • 407-555-6789

PATIENT: BALMORAL, MARK

ACCOUNT/EHR #: BALMAR001

Date: 10/26/19

Attending Physician: Oscar R. Prader, MD

Pt is a 61-year-old male with metastatic testicular tumors. He comes in today for the administration of cisplatin solution, IV, 20 mg. It is the first of five treatments he will receive this week.

IV infusion given over 7 hours.

Patient reports mild nausea. Refuses any pharmaceutical treatment for that side effect of this treatment.

Patient discharged at 4:15 p.m.

ORP/mg   D: 10/26/19 09:50:16   T: 10/27/19 12:55:01

Determine the best, most appropriate HCPCS Level II code(s).

VICTORS AMBULANCE SERVICE

159 Healthcare Way • SOMEWHERE, FL 32811 • 407-555-6789

PATIENT: CUTTER, WILIMENA

ACCOUNT/EHR #: CUTTWI001

Date: 10/15/19

Attending Physician: Renee O. Bracker, MD

EMT/Attendant: Lance H. Reynoso, EMT

Pt is a 78-year-old female who appears to have suffered a myocardial infarction in her nursing home's day room. Pt complained of numbness and tingling in the left arm and sharp pains in her chest. EKG showed abnormal activity. Pulse and respiration were abnormal.

While preparing the patient for transport, she went into arrest. Defibrillator restored heartbeat. ALS1-emergency services were administered, and patient was transported immediately to Barton Hospital.

Routine disposable supplies were used.

Total Mileage: 4.5

Lance H. Reynoso, EMT

LHR/mg   D: 10/15/19 09:50:16   T: 10/17/19 12:55:01

Determine the best, most appropriate HCPCS Level II code(s).

PRADER, BRACKER, & ASSOCIATES

A Complete Health Care Facility

159 Healthcare Way • SOMEWHERE, FL 32811 • 407-555-6789

PATIENT: VANCE, TOMIKA

ACCOUNT/EHR #: VANTOM001

Date: 12/09/19

Attending Physician: Salvatore L. Bloome, MD

Indications: Ulcerative enterocolitis

Procedure: Colonoscopy

Instrument: Olympus video colonoscope CF 100L

Anesthesia: Versed 4 mg; Demerol 75 mg MAC < 30 min

HISTORY: This is a 71-year-old female admitted to the ambulatory surgical center for a colonoscopy. Due to her chronic enterocolitis, she is at high risk for a malignancy of the colon, and, therefore, this screening is being done. She has been informed of the nature of the procedure, the risks, and the consequences, as well as told of alternative procedures. She consents to the procedure.

PROCEDURE: The patient is placed in the left lateral decubitus position. The rectal exam reveals normal sphincter tone and no masses. A colonoscope is introduced into the rectum and advanced to the distal sigmoid colon. Due to a marked fixation and severe angulation of the rectosigmoid colon, the scope could not be advanced any further and the procedure was aborted. On withdrawal, no masses or polyps are noted, and the mucosa is normal throughout. Retroflexion in the rectal vault is unremarkable.

DISPOSITION: The patient tolerated the procedure and was discharged from the minor operating department in satisfactory condition.

IMPRESSIONS: Normal colonoscopy, only to the distal sigmoid colon

PLAN: Strong recommendation for a barium enema

Salvatore L. Bloome, MD

SLB/mg   D: 12/09/19 09:50:16   T: 12/11/19 12:55:01

Determine the best, most appropriate HCPCS Level II code(s).

Design elements: ©McGraw-Hill

DMEPOS and Transportation Capstone

31

Learning Outcomes

After completing this chapter, the student should be able to:

LO 31.1 Determine the correct codes for these case studies using the HCPCS Level II code set.

The health care team extends beyond the physician's office or hospital. Home care services are on the increase as a greater number of patients prefer care in their residences, whenever possible. The provision of these services enables patients greater comfort and lowers costs, especially for those with chronic conditions.

In addition, transportation of patients should be recorded and reported for reimbursement purposes, as well as the provision of orthotics and prosthetics. And, as you learned in previous chapters about CPT coding, the provision of medication (drugs) by a health care professional also must be recorded and reimbursed.

For each of the following case studies, read through the documentation and determine

- What medical supply, equipment, or other item or service was provided to this patient. Do not code the procedure.

- Whether any modifiers are necessary, and, if so, which modifiers and in what order.

- Whether more than one code is required, and, if so, the sequence in which to report the codes.

Remember, read carefully and completely.

CASE STUDY #1: RHONDA SYNCOWSKI

Rhonda Syncowski is a 64-year-old female with a long-standing history of a seizure disorder. She also has hypertension (high blood pressure) and chronic obstructive pulmonary disease (COPD). She is no stranger to the hospital because of her health issues. At home, she takes a number of medications, including three for her COPD and three—levetiracetam, lamotrigine, and valproate sodium—to help control seizures.

The patient went to see Dr. Bushera, her family physician, last week because she was wheezing and having trouble breathing. Dr. Bushera conducted a physical examination that yielded signs of an acute worsening of her COPD—including FEV1 of less than 50% predicted value plus respiratory failure.

PLAN: Orders written for flunisolide 160 mcg, b.i.d. via nebulizer; portable oxygen (gaseous) with 1-month supply. Follow up with physician in 3 weeks, or PRN.

Joshua Medical Supplies and Equipment was called by the patient to provide the equipment and medications to the patient's home. As per physician's orders:

1. Nebulizer with compressor

2. Flunisolide inhalation solution 1 mg

3. Portable oxygen system (gaseous), rental, cannula

4. Portable O$_2$ contents, gaseous, 1 unit

CASE STUDY #2: RYAN MCNAULTY

Ryan McNaulty, a 6-year-old male with a defect in bowel function, was hospitalized for severe constipation. He was given a dose of neostigmine methylsulfate 0.4 mg, IM. Code for the drug, one date of service, only.

CASE STUDY #3: NADIYA LONGSTEP

Nadiya Longstep was rescued from her apartment building, which was engulfed in a two-alarm fire. The firemen carried her out, and she was handed over to the EMTs, who immediately began to examine the burns on 45% of her body. She was having trouble breathing and was given oxygen. She lost consciousness. CPR was started immediately, followed by external defibrillation at 200 joules until normal sinus rhythm was reestablished. Orders came through to take her to the MacHill Burn Center unit of Mulford Hospital immediately.

CASE STUDY #4: SONIA GRASSO

Sonia Grasso, an 11-year-old female, was diagnosed with idiopathic adolescent scoliosis.

Joshua Medical Supplies and Equipment was referred by Dr. Karpel, her orthopedist, to provide a Milwaukee brace: cervical/thoracic/lumbar/sacral orthotic.

CASE STUDY #5: DANIEL BISHOP

Daniel Bishop, an 18-year-old male, was in an MVA and subsequently diagnosed with whiplash, resulting in pain in C2–C4. Dr. Samman recommended traction for his cervical region, which he could attach to the headboard of his bed at home. Dr. Samman told Daniel to spend at least 5 hours each night in the traction device for 3 weeks. Follow-up appointment in 2 weeks.

CASE STUDY #6: MALIK HUMISTON

Malik Humiston, a 16-year-old male, suffered a displaced (comminuted) fracture of the right tibial shaft during his high school football game. Dr. Peterson prescribed articulating, spring-assisted underarm crutches for him upon postsurgical discharge. Joshua Medical Supplies and Equipment provided him with a pair and spent approximately 30 minutes fitting him and teaching him how to use them properly.

CASE STUDY #7: ZIVAH MASTRIANI

Zivah Mastriani, a 41-year-old female, was diagnosed with type 2 diabetes mellitus, and Dr. Ross wrote a prescription for her to obtain a home glucose disposable monitor. Zivah brought the order to Roxone Home Medical Supplies, where a monitor and test strips were provided. Harold Carter spent about 20 minutes teaching her how to use it correctly.

CASE STUDY #8: VICTOR JEFFRIES

Victor Jeffries, a 71-year-old male, weighs 320 pounds and is currently bedridden due to a fractured hip. In an effort to prevent any pressure ulcers or decubitus ulcer development, Dr. Abreen ordered an air pressure mattress pad for his bed at home.

CASE STUDY #9: ANNA CHENG

Anna Cheng, an 83-year-old female, has been exhibiting dysphagia (problems swallowing), resulting in her no longer wanting to eat. Dr. Baldwin inserted a standard gastrostomy/jejunostomy tube to enable enteral nutrition for 10 days.

CASE STUDY #10: CECIL DENOSO

Cecil Denoso, a 27-year-old male, was admitted to the Masters Behavioral Health Center due to his current manic state. Dr. Levine ordered Haloperidol 5 mg IM t.i.d. Code for the drug, one date of service, only.

CASE STUDY #11: COURTNEE CALLAHAN

SUBJECTIVE FINDINGS: This patient is a 55-year-old white female with pain in her lumbosacral spine, extending into her buttocks bilaterally. She describes the pain as being sharp and sometimes intense. She states it diminishes to an achy feeling. She rates its intensity at 10/10 at its worst. Normally, she states it is 6–7/10. She describes the pain as being ever-present, varying in intensity, increasing with activities and decreasing with rest. She is using pain medications currently and is able to sleep through the night.

HISTORY: This patient initially injured her back by catching a falling bookcase. She had immediate pain that was disabling. The pain was resolved with occasional recurrence. She sought intervention last year from doctors, who diagnosed degenerative disc disease and arthritis. She had a course of physical therapy with some resolution, but recurrence of pain occurred in June secondary to bending over while washing her hands. She was referred here.

OBJECTIVE FINDINGS:

Observation: This patient appears as a normally developed white female of stated age. She reports moving with forward flexed posture and an occasional antalgic gait on the right when the pain is increasing. She currently postures and moves normally.

Palpation: Positive over L5 and S1 and paravertebral muscles at that same level.

Lumbosacral range of motion: Forward flexion 35 degrees with pain at the end of range. Right side bending 30 degrees with pain at the end of range. Left side bending 35 degrees. Extension 0 degree with pain at the end of range.

Resisted motion: Positive in all directions

DTRs: Hyperreflexive bilaterally

Lasègue's sign: Positive at 25 degrees bilaterally

Cram test: Positive at 25 degrees bilaterally

Cervical range of motion:
1. Right side bending: Within normal limits, painful
2. Left side bending: Within normal limits
3. Forward flexion: 45 degrees with pain at the end of range
4. Extension: Within normal limits

Radiculopathy: Positive with pain down the left arm and occasional tingling and numbness

TREATMENT PLAN: We would like to see the patient three times per week to initiate exercises and modalities to decrease pain and increase range of motion and function.

GOALS: The purpose of physical therapy intervention is to

1. Increase range of motion to normal limits.
2. Decrease pain to zero.
3. Increase strength and function to normal.

RECOMMENDATION: I discussed with the patient the benefit of using a transcutaneous electrical nerve stimulation device on her lumbar area. I suggested that she rent the unit from us to give her the opportunity to try it out and see if it helps to reduce pain at L5–S1. She agreed, and we provided her with a 2-lead unit. Instructions were for her to use it every day, 15 minutes, b.i.d., first thing in the morning after getting out of bed and immediately prior to bed. Richard Penuto, my associate, taught her how to apply the leads and use the machine. Appointment made for her to return in 2 weeks for evaluation.

Code for the provision of the transcutaneous electrical nerve stimulation device only.

CASE STUDY #12: ARTHUR PAIGE

HISTORY OF PRESENT ILLNESS: This patient is a 43-year-old male with pain in his cervical spine. He states that the pain extends over the entire posterior neck and into the right shoulder, including the upper trapezius. He rates that at a level of 7–8 on a scale of 10 currently. He states that at its least it is 3–4 on a scale of 10. The patient is using a cervical collar with good results. He also uses ibuprofen at night.

This patient was involved in an MVA 5 years ago resulting in a fracture of C5. He had manipulation approximately 3 years ago resulting in pain for approximately

5 months. He had neck pain develop again approximately 18 months ago resulting in bilateral shoulder surgery. The pain has remained the same, although the numbness is better for approximately 1 year. He currently has complaints of a radial distribution into his left hand, which caused him enough concern to seek intervention from Dr. Furmenn. The patient was then referred here.

PHYSICAL EXAMINATION:

Observation: This patient is a normally developed male of stated age. He gaits normally without apparent guarding or splinting.

Palpation: Positive over the right upper trapezius

Range of motion: Right rotation is 50 degrees, left rotation is 45 degrees, right side bending 30 degrees with pain at the end of range, left side bending 30 degrees, forward flexion 35 degrees, and extension 25 degrees.

Resisted motion: Negative

Radiculopathy: Positive in the left shoulder extending down to the left hand into his thumb and digits 2 and 3.

Sensation: Some decreased sensation over the left hand to pinprick, particularly over the radial digits.

TREATMENT PLAN: We would like to see the patient three times per week as per instructions for cervical traction and exercises.

GOALS: The purpose of physical therapy intervention is to

1. Increase range of motion to normal limits.

2. Increase pain-free function to normal.

3. Decrease pain generally to zero.

RECOMMENDATION: To encourage healing, I discussed with the patient using traction equipment at home, for beneficial outcomes in between appointments. Petra Zoztrev, our trainer, worked with Arthur to show him how to set up the equipment, put it on, and take it off. Instructions for use are every night to sleep in the equipment until we determine he has made sufficient progress. I also gave him a sheet with exercises—diagrammed out, for him to do at home also. Petra helped him carry the box out to his car.

Code for the provision of the traction equipment only.

CASE STUDY #13: WILLETTA FREEDMAN

HISTORY: The patient is a 23-year-old black female professional athlete who, last month, fell on her left elbow while reaching for a ball during a tennis game, sustaining a left distal humerus fracture. The patient states the following day she had surgery to stabilize the fracture. The patient was unsure if the surgery performed was for plates and screws.

PAST MEDICAL HISTORY: The patient fractured her right wrist approximately a year ago.

CHIEF COMPLAINT: The patient reports left elbow pain, currently 8/10, at best 7/10, and at worst 10/10. The patient states she is taking her pain medications, which provide minimal relief but affect her performance on the court. The patient reports she does have numbness in the left upper extremity, along the ulnar nerve distribution. The patient states she does use some ice or heat; it provides minimal relief. The patient is left-hand dominant.

PHYSICAL EXAMINATION: Left elbow AROM 35–120 degrees. Left elbow PROM 30–135 degrees. Left shoulder AROM within normal limits. Left wrist AROM within functional limits. Left elbow strength 3–/5. Left shoulder strength grossly 4/5. Left wrist strength grossly 4/5. Left grip strength is 30 pounds. Right grip strength is 55 pounds.

Palpation: The patient is tender to palpation in the posterolateral aspect of the left elbow. The incision is healed. No signs of infection. No swelling in the left elbow, no bruising.

GOALS:

1. Increase left elbow AROM and PROM to within normal limits.
2. Increase left elbow strength to within normal limits.
3. Eliminate pain.
4. Independent with home exercise program.
5. Return function to normal.

TREATMENT PLAN: We would like to see the patient three times a week to initiate and advance range of motion, stretching, and strengthening program to left elbow; may use modalities as needed for pain control.

RECOMMENDATIONS: To ensure progress to help this patient recover more completely, I recommend a static progressive stretch elbow device with a range of motion adjustment for her use at home. I discussed a workout plan, using the equipment, with Willetta and her coach. They left with the device and instructions. Appointment is made for her to return in 1 week to begin regular treatment.

Code for the provision of the device only.

CASE STUDY #14: GARY ELLIOTT

SUBJECTIVE FINDINGS: The patient said that he slept well last night.

OBJECTIVE FINDINGS:

General: The patient is a well-developed, obese male in no apparent distress.

Vital signs: Temperature 98.6 degrees, pulse 72, respirations 18, and blood pressure 158/80.

HEENT: Head is normocephalic

Neck: Supple to palpation

Extremities: Examination of the extremities shows incision site to be healing well without any sign of infection or skin breakdown. Peripheral pulses are intact. Minimal edema in the left lower extremity. Homans sign is absent.

FUNCTIONAL STATUS: Functionally, the patient is able to demonstrate improvement with full range of motion, –5 to 80 degrees of flexion actively and 86 degrees passively. His functional gait has advanced 200 feet with the use of front-wheel walker with supervision. He is supervised level with his bedside commode transfers and contact guard assistance with shower chair transfers. He is modified independent level with his eating and set up with his grooming skills. He requires moderate assistance with lower body dressing.

IMPRESSION:

1. Polyarthritis
2. Left total knee arthroplasty
3. Status post coronary artery bypass graft
4. Chronic obstructive pulmonary disease

PLAN: We provided the patient with a Continuous Positive Airway Pressure (CPAP) machine with headgear and instructed both Gary and his wife on how to use it properly. Instructions are provided in writing. I emphasized the importance of using the CPAP machine every night. Continue with current treatment program. We will continue to monitor the patient's hypertension, which is still out of control.

Code for the provision of the CPAP machine with headgear.

CASE STUDY #15: PAULA BARKIN

Paula, a 4-year-old female, was referred for speech therapy by her school after discussion about parents' concerns over her difficulties pronouncing certain speech sounds. These irregular pronunciations were making it challenging for those outside her family to understand Paula when she spoke to them. Paula had suffered from hearing loss and had grommets inserted at age 3.

An initial assessment was performed to look at her current speech profile and to provide information as to whether intervention was needed and, if so, what kind. Assessment results revealed that Paula had difficulties with the 't' and 'd' sounds and was replacing these with 'k' and 'g,' so 'letter' was 'lekker' and 'bed' was 'beg'. I explained to the parents that this is called 'backing,' whereby sounds that should be produced at the front of the mouth are produced at the back of the mouth instead. This is not a process found in typically developing speech and therefore would be targeted in therapy.

Paula also showed difficulties with other early developing sounds 's' and 'v.' These sounds that are produced with a long flow of air were being cut short so 'f' was 'p'—therefore, 'fish' was 'pish.' This process is called stopping, which is expected to have resolved by the age of 3 years and so was also targeted in therapy.

Paula was set up for individual therapy sessions at her home, by me, for 30 minutes each visit. The sessions will be focused on developing Paula's awareness and production of the above speech sounds and processes. For each sound, visual materials including a picture card with the grapheme and cued articulation (similar to a gesture/sign) are used to help Paula learn them. Before asking Paula to produce any of the sounds she had difficulties with, Paula was provided with many opportunities to hear these sounds being produced correctly (this is known as auditory bombardment). Paula then completed tasks in which she had to discriminate between a target sound, e.g., 't,' and the sound that she replaced it with, e.g., 'k,' to ensure she could tell the two apart.

Therapy will then move to production. How each of the sounds is produced in the mouth will be explained to Paula using words accompanied by diagrams. The first step is to get Paula to try to produce her new sounds in isolation (e.g., 't') and then combined with a vowel (e.g., 'tee'). The next steps are to practice new sounds at the start of words (e.g., 'tiger'), followed by at the end of words (e.g., 'boat') and then in the middle of words (e.g., 'bottle') and finally onto sentences. These will be incorporated into fun games. Parents will be given activities to practice in between weekly sessions; in addition, advice on how to support Paula's new speech sounds in natural conversations will also be provided. For example, if Paula made an error with one of her new speech sounds, others will be able to provide her with options, e.g., is it a 'kiger' or a 'tiger,' emphasizing the correct sound.

PLAN: In addition to the 30-minute sessions at her home, I supply software with 30 minutes of prerecorded sounds and messages so the parents can work with her in between our sessions.

Code for the one 30-minute home visit by the speech-language pathologist + the speech software.

Design elements: ©McGraw-Hill

PART V

INPATIENT (HOSPITAL) REPORTING

Reporting inpatient (hospital) and outpatient encounters requires the same foundational knowledge and skill: anatomy, physiology, and medical terminology. Part V of this text provides you with the next layer of your learning about coding health care.

In these chapters, you will learn how to employ ICD-10-PCS (International Classification of Diseases–10th revision–Procedure Coding System), the code set used to report the procedures, services, and treatments provided by the acute care facility (hospital) *to inpatients (those who have been admitted).*

32 Introduction to ICD-10-PCS

Key Terms

Approach
Axis of Classification
Body Part
Body System
Device
Qualifier
Root Operation Term

Learning Outcomes

After completing this chapter, the student should be able to:

LO 32.1 Explain the purpose of ICD-10-PCS codes.
LO 32.2 Identify the structure of ICD-10-PCS codes.
LO 32.3 Recognize the proper ways to use the Alphabetic Index and Tables in ICD-10-PCS.
LO 32.4 Discern the general conventions for using ICD-10-PCS.
LO 32.5 Determine the principal ICD-10-PCS code and proper sequencing for multiple procedure codes.

 STOP!   Remember, you need to follow along in your <u>ICD-10-PCS</u> code book for an optimal learning experience.

32.1 The Purpose of ICD-10-PCS

The *International Classification of Diseases–10th revision–Procedure Coding System* (ICD-10-PCS) was implemented in the United States on October 1, 2015, for the reporting of procedures, services, and treatments provided to a patient who has been admitted into an inpatient facility.

Earlier in Part III of this book, you learned how to use the CPT code set to report physician's services in any facility. And you learned that CPT codes are also used to report services provided by an outpatient facility, during the care of the patient. Now, you will learn to use the ICD-10-PCS code set to report the inpatient facility's participation in providing these services.

When patients are provided with room and food, in addition to medical care, and stay overnight in the facility, they are considered "inpatients." This means that acute care hospitals, as well as skilled nursing facilities, long-term care facilities, and short-term care facilities, may use this code set.

The structure of this code set is very different, as you will learn in this and the next few chapters. Rather than looking up the code and determining the correct choice from a list, you will build the code from the details shown in the tables of ICD-10-PCS (see Figure 32-1). Each table contains details about procedures pertaining to that particular type of procedure and that particular body system and body part.

32.2 The Structure of ICD-10-PCS Codes

The main purpose of creating the *International Classification of Diseases–10th Revision–Procedure Coding System* (ICD-10-PCS) was to give you, the professional coder, an easier way to determine the best, most accurate, and most specific code to report procedures, services, and treatments provided to an inpatient (a patient admitted to an

Section	0	Medical and Surgical
Body System	2	Heart and Great Vessels
Operation	4	Creation: Putting in or on biological or synthetic material to form a new body part that to the extent possible replicates the anatomic structure or function of an absent body part

Body Part	Approach	Device	Qualifier
F Aortic Valve	**0** Open	**7** Autologous Tissue Substitute **8** Zooplastic Tissue **J** Synthetic Substitute **K** Nonautologous Tissue Substitute	**J** Truncal Valve
G Mitral Valve **J** Tricuspid Valve	**0** Open	**7** Autologous Tissue **8** Zooplastic Tissue **J** Synthetic Substitute **K** Nonautologous Tissue Substitute	**2** Common Atrioventricular Valve

FIGURE 32-1 An example from the Medical and Surgical Tables of 2019 ICD-10-PCS

acute care hospital or other inpatient facility). That purpose has led to a new structure for the codes. In this code set, you will actually build the code.

Seven Characters

Every ICD-10-PCS code is made up of seven (7) alphanumeric characters, and each character position has its own specific meaning—a specific piece of information relating to the procedure, service, or treatment provided. You must read carefully because each section has its own particular use for the character. As always, in coding, you can never assume!

Let's begin with the first, and largest, section of the ICD-10-PCS code set . . . *Medical and Surgical* section, just as an example. You will learn all the details about this and all of the other code set sections in the chapters that follow this one. In this section, the seven characters describe, in order, the:

1. *Section* of the ICD-10-PCS code set.
2. *Body system* upon which the procedure or service was performed.
3. *Root operation,* which explains the category or type of procedure.
4. *Body part,* which identifies the specific anatomical site involved in the procedure.
5. *Approach,* which reports which method was used to perform the service or treatment.
6. *Device,* which reports, when applicable, the type of device involved in the service or procedure.
7. *Qualifier,* which adds any additional detail.

Let's go through each of these character positions, one by one, to understand what each represents. To help illustrate these data points, we are going to use a snippet from an operative report and build the code as an ongoing example:

Laparoscopic bypass, radial vein to ulnar vein, left, using autologous tissue substitute

CODING BITES

ICD-10-PCS codes may include any letter of the alphabet *except* the letters *O* and *I*. This is done to avoid any confusion between the letter *O* and the number 0 (zero), as well as any mix-up between the letter *I* and the number 1 (one).

Using this short statement as an example to work with, you are going to build the ICD-10-PCS code as you make your way through this chapter. You will learn how each character reports a part of the whole story about the specific procedure or service. This should then help you understand how to build a code on your own.

Section (First Character)

The first character in the seven-character sequence identifies the section of the ICD-10-PCS code set in which the procedure is listed. There are 17 section titles:

0 Medical and Surgical

1 Obstetrics

2 Placement

3 Administration

4 Measurement and Monitoring

5 Extracorporeal or Systemic Assistance and Performance

6 Extracorporeal or Systemic Therapies

7 Osteopathic

8 Other Procedures

9 Chiropractic

B Imaging

C Nuclear Medicine

D Radiation Therapy

F Physical Rehabilitation and Diagnostic Audiology

G Mental Health

H Substance Abuse Treatment

X New Technology

EXAMPLES

An ankle x-ray is an imaging procedure—Section **B**

A breech extraction is an obstetrics procedure—Section **1**

An amputation is a surgical procedure—Section **0**

Body System (Second Character)

Body System
The physiological system, or anatomical region, upon which the procedure was performed.

The second character of the code reports the **body system** upon which the procedure, service, or treatment was performed. The classes you took in anatomy will be very important to your accuracy in determining the correct character to report. Plus, you need to pay careful attention due to greater specificity than typically defined by standard anatomy classifications. There are 31 body systems used for clarification and identification by the second character of codes reporting a medical or surgical procedure or service:

0 Central Nervous System and Cranial Nerves

1 Peripheral Nervous System

2 Heart and Great Vessels

3 Upper Arteries

4 Lower Arteries

5 Upper Veins

6 Lower Veins

7 Lymphatic and Hemic Systems

8 Eye

9 Ear, Nose, Sinus

B Respiratory System

C Mouth and Throat

D Gastrointestinal System

F Hepatobiliary System and Pancreas

G Endocrine System

H Skin and Breast

J Subcutaneous Tissue and Fascia

K Muscles

L Tendons

M Bursae and Ligaments

N Head and Facial Bones

P Upper Bones

Q Lower Bones

R Upper Joints

S Lower Joints

T Urinary System

U Female Reproductive System

V Male Reproductive System

W Anatomical Regions, General

X Anatomical Regions, Upper Extremities

Y Anatomical Regions, Lower Extremities

The other sections of the code set describe the body systems that are appropriate to those services. Take a look at Table 32-1, The Other Sections of ICD-10-PCS and Their Body Systems.

CODING BITES

Using our example . . . *radial vein to ulnar vein*

Remember learning this in anatomy class? Don't worry if you don't; use that anatomy resource now. Then, you will know, for certain, that these veins are located in the arm (upper extremity). Therefore, your second character will report a procedure that was performed on the patient's *upper veins*.

First character   =   0
Second character =   5

0 Medical and Surgical
   5 Upper veins

Root Operation (Third Character)

The third character in the ICD-10-PCS code reports the **root operation term**—the central aspect of the procedure or service being provided. Just as you learned when reporting procedures using CPT, you are essentially looking for the term that describes WHAT the physician did for the patient. You can see that these terms are, for the most part, familiar to you. Notice that once again the *Medical and Surgical* section has 31 different root operations.

Root Operation Term
The category or classification of a particular procedure, service, or treatment.

0 Alteration	J Inspection
1 Bypass	K Map
2 Change	L Occlusion
3 Control	M Reattachment
4 Creation	N Release
5 Destruction	P Removal
6 Detachment	Q Repair
7 Dilation	R Replacement
8 Division	S Reposition
9 Drainage	T Resection
B Excision	U Supplement
C Extirpation	V Restriction
D Extraction	W Revision
F Fragmentation	X Transfer
G Fusion	Y Transplantation
H Insertion	

TABLE 32-1 The Other Sections of ICD-10-PCS and Their Body Systems

SECTION	BODY SYSTEM(S)
1 Obstetrics	0 Pregnancy
2 Placement	W Anatomical Regions Y Anatomical Orifices
3 Administration	0 Circulatory C Indwelling Device E Physiological Systems & Anatomical Regions
4 Measurement and Monitoring	A Physiological Systems B Physiological Devices
5 Extracorporeal or Systemic Assistance and Performance	A Physiological Systems
6 Extracorporeal or Systemic Therapies	A Physiological Systems
7 Osteopathic	W Anatomical Regions
8 Other Procedures	C Indwelling Device E Physiological Systems & Anatomical Regions
9 Chiropractic	W Anatomical Regions
B Imaging	[See *Medical and Surgical* body systems]
C Nuclear Medicine	[See *Medical and Surgical* body systems]
D Radiation Therapy	[See *Medical and Surgical* body systems]
F Physical Rehabilitation and Diagnostic Audiology	0 Rehabilitation* 1 Diagnostic Audiology
G Mental Health	Z None
H Substance Abuse	Z None
X New Technology	2 Cardiovascular Systems H Skin, Subcutaneous Tissue, Fascia and Breast K Muscles, Tendons, Bursae and Ligaments N Bones R Joints W Anatomical Regions Y Extracorporeal

*The **Rehabilitation and Diagnostic Audiology** section identifies the body system with the fourth character rather than the second as with other sections. The same 31 body systems used for the **Medical and Surgical** section apply here, as well.

This is a long list. But don't worry. You will learn about each of these root operation terms, and more used in other sections, in the upcoming chapters. Most importantly, they are in your code book, along with their descriptions. So, no memorization is required . . . just reading carefully and completely.

The other sections may use some of the same terms as the *Medical and Surgical* section in addition to some terms specific to their area. Try not to get overwhelmed by all these terms. You have time to learn about these procedures, look them up in a medical dictionary, and become familiar with them. And remember, they are always right there, at your fingertips, in the ICD-10-PCS code book.

CODING BITES

In ICD-10-PCS, the word *operation* has nothing to do with surgery.

CODING BITES

Using our example . . . *bypass*

Yes, sometimes it really is this easy. The physician uses the same term for the procedure as the ICD-10-PCS code book does.

First character	= 0
Second character	= 5
Third character	= 1

0 Medical and Surgical
  5 Upper veins
    1 Bypass

NOTE: They are not all this easy. More to help you interpret root operation terms in the upcoming chapters.

Body Part (Fourth Character)

The fourth character of the ICD-10-PCS code provides information regarding the specific **body part**, anatomical site, or body region upon which the procedure, service, or treatment was performed. These characters, and what they represent, vary, determined by the section and body system. This is one of the reasons the Alphabetic Index will not usually reach this level of specificity.

Body Part
The anatomical site upon which the procedure was performed.

CODING BITES

Using our example . . . *radial vein to ulnar vein, left*

You can see how the details are built into the code.

The radial and ulnar veins are both specifically grouped into the category of brachial veins. Again, If you did not know this offhand, don't worry. Check your medical dictionary or anatomy reference. This is one of the wonderful aspects of being a coder; you can always use your resources to ensure accuracy.

Character 4 will provide the more specific detail, including laterality (right or left).

First character	= 0
Second character	= 5
Third character	= 1
Fourth character	= A

0 Medical and Surgical
5 Upper veins
1 Bypass
  A Brachial vein, left

Approach (Fifth Character)

The term **approach**, as reported by the fifth character, reports the technique or methodology used during the procedure, such as open or laparoscopic. This character explains how the physician got to the anatomical site upon which the procedure was performed.

NOTE: Other sections use this character position (character 5) to report a different detail, such as single or multiple duration for extracorporeal therapy. The *Imaging* section uses this position to report the use of contrast materials. Again, don't worry; the ICD-10-PCS code book will share this information with you. All you have to do is read carefully and completely.

CODING BITES

Using our example . . . *Laparoscopic*

This detail must be provided by the physician in his or her operative notes. *The words may not be identical, so you will have to understand the meaning so you can interpret.*

A laparoscope is an *endoscope* inserted through an incision in the abdominal wall (*percutaneously*), used to visualize the interior of the peritoneal cavity. Therefore, you would interpret this as a PERCUTANEOUS ENDOSCOPIC approach.

First character   = 0
Second character = 5
Third character   = 1
Fourth character = A
Fifth character   = 4

0 Medical and Surgical
5 Upper veins
1 Bypass
   A Brachial vein, left
      4 Percutaneous endoscopic

More about the specific approaches coming up in the following chapters.

Device (Sixth Character)

Some of the sections use the sixth character to identify a **device** used in the procedure. To some, this term may conjure up pictures of hard, metal equipment. However, in ICD-10-PCS, the term *device* is used in a more general sense to mean any item that will remain in or with the body after the procedure is complete. So it might mean equipment, such as a pacemaker, or it may report the use of a graft.

CODING BITES

Using our example . . . *using autologous tissue substitute*

For the sixth character, you need to read the notes to determine if any devices, substances, or other components were used. First, check your ICD-10-PCS section to familiarize yourself with what type of details this character, in this table, will report. Then, you will know what to look for in the documentation.

Here, in our example code, you have already determined that you are working with the 051 Table in ICD-10-PCS. In this table, the sixth character reports a device, something that will remain in, or with, the patient after the procedure is completed. Look at the options you have for the sixth character in this table: tissue substitutes of various origins. *Autologous tissue substitute* was used during the bypass to support the rerouting of the vein.

(continued)

First character = 0
Second character = 5
Third character = 1
Fourth character = A
Fifth character = 4
Sixth character = 7

0 Medical and Surgical
5 Upper veins
1 Bypass
   A Brachial vein, left
      4 Percutaneous endoscopic
         7 Autologous tissue substitute

Some sections of ICD-10-PCS, such as the ***Administration*** section, will have you report a category of substance, such as anti-inflammatory or antineoplastic, with the sixth character. When you are working in that section, keep your pharmacology reference close at hand.

    More about this in the following chapters.

Qualifier (Seventh Character)

The seventh character of the ICD-10-PCS code, the **qualifier**, is like a wild card, reporting whatever additional information may be needed. Because the coding system is designed for future expansion, there will be cases where a specific procedure does not currently have the details to require all seven characters. In such cases, the letter **Z** is used to indicate that nothing in that position was applicable to the particular procedure.

Qualifier
Any additional feature of the procedure, if applicable.

CODING BITES

Using our example . . . ***to ulnar vein***

In this case, there is one more detail that must be explained . . . <u>to</u> what anatomical site was the radial vein rerouted, or bypassed "to"—a different upper vein.

    As you have seen throughout this textbook, **GUIDANCE CONNECTION** icons direct you to official guidelines that will help you make accurate determinations for each character. For this case, Guideline B3.6a directs you to specify the body part bypassed <u>from</u> for the fourth character and the body part bypassed <u>to</u> for the seventh character. In this table, you only have one choice. However, there may be occasions in the future where this reminder will come in handy. Good thing these guidelines are always right there, in the front of your code book.

First character = 0
Second character = 5
Third character = 1
Fourth character = A
Fifth character = 4
Sixth character = 7
Seventh character = Y

  0 Medical and Surgical
  5 Upper veins
  1 Bypass
    A Brachial vein, left
       4 Percutaneous endoscopic
          7 Autologous tissue substitute
            Y Upper vein

(continued)

Again, you will need to look at the table within the section of ICD-10-PCS first to discover what detail or type of detail this character of this code will report. As you read earlier, sometimes there is nothing left to share, so you will use the letter **Z No Qualifier.**

Don't worry. More about this all coming in the next chapters.

Placeholder Characters

The letter *Z* means "not applicable" or "none." The **Z** placeholder will be used most often as the seventh character; however, it can be used in any of the seven character positions, when needed. It also can be used in multiple positions in one code.

EXAMPLE

Dr. McCoy performed a biopsy on Clark's neck. The ICD-10-PCS code to report this would be 0WB6XZX . . .

    0 = Medical and Surgical
    W = Anatomical regions, general
    B = Excision
    6 = Neck
    X = External
    Z = No device
    X = Diagnostic

There is no device, so there is nothing to report in the sixth character position. But you can't leave that part of the code out. So you put a *Z* in that spot and report that there is no device.

EXAMPLE

Dr. Rothwell used a percutaneous endoscope in an attempt to control post-procedural bleeding in Isaac's colon, after several polyps had been removed. The ICD-10-PCS code to report this would be 0W3P4ZZ . . .

    0 = Medical and Surgical
    W = Anatomical regions, general
    3 = Control
    P = Gastrointestinal tract
    4 = Percutaneous endoscope
    Z = No device
    Z = No qualifier

There is no device, so there is nothing to report in the sixth character position. There is no qualifier, so there is nothing to report in the seventh character position either. By placing a *Z* in both positions, you are explaining exactly that. By the way, this is not a decision you have to make. In this subsection of the ICD-10-PCS tables, **Z No Device** and **Z No Qualifier** are the only choices on the chart for those two character positions.

32.3 The ICD-10-PCS Book

The ICD-10-PCS book is divided into two parts: the Alphabetic Index and the Tables. [*NOTE: Some publishers add a third section, which is a listing of all of the possible ICD-10-PCS codes, similar to the other code books. Therefore, if one does not want to "build" a code from the Tables, it can be looked up.*]

The Alphabetic Index

The Alphabetic Index's entries are primarily sorted by root operation terms.

• Root operation term

A root operation term identifies the specific service or type of treatment that is the basis of the entire procedure.

> **EXAMPLES**
>
> Root operation terms include *bypass, drainage, excision,* and *insertion.*

After you find the root operation term, as stated in the documentation, there are subentries listed by the following:

• Body system

> **EXAMPLES**
>
> Digestive system
>
> Musculoskeletal system

• Body part

> **EXAMPLES**
>
> Arm, leg, hand, foot

• Common procedure names and eponyms

The Alphabetic Index also lists common terms for some procedures and eponyms.

> **EXAMPLES**
>
> *Hysterectomy* is listed and then cross-referenced to *resection* (a root operation term) and *female reproductive system* (body system).
>
> *Roux-en-Y* operation is listed and then cross-referenced to *bypass* (a root operation term) and *gastrointestinal system* or *hepatobiliary system and pancreas* (both are body systems).

The Alphabetic Index will usually give you only the first three or four characters of the seven-character procedure code. You then must go to the Tables to find the additional characters. You won't have to be reminded to *never code from the Alphabetic Index* with ICD-10-PCS. Often, you won't be able to code from the Alphabetic Index alone anymore!

> **EXAMPLE**
>
> Fragmentation
>
> Bladder 0TF8-

For the most part, you will find that the Alphabetic Index will include information relating to the first three characters. This information will enable you to turn to the correct page in the Tables and determine the rest of the characters for the code. As you have seen, virtually all of the sections are consistent with the first three elements. However, as you get to the last four characters, the information represented by these characters may change, depending upon what type of procedure was performed or upon what body system a procedure was performed. This is a major aspect of the flexibility of the ICD-10-PCS system.

The Tables

The Tables are divided by body systems. Of course, like all the other code sets, each section is in order by the first character in the code. Within each section's body system division, the list continues in order by the root operation term for that procedure. Each section of the list has a grid that specifies the assigned meaning to each letter or number along with its position in the seven-character code. (See an example in Figure 32-2.)

Body System
The physiological system, or anatomical region, upon which the procedure was performed.

Root Operation Term
The category or classification of a particular procedure, service, or treatment.

Section	0	Medical and Surgical
Body System	2	Heart and Great Vessels
Operation	7	Dilation: Expanding an orifice or the lumen of a tubular body part

Body Part	Approach	Device	Qualifier
0 Coronary Artery, One Artery **1** Coronary Artery, Two Arteries **2** Coronary Artery, Three Arteries **3** Coronary Artery, Four or More Arteries	**0** Open **3** Percutaneous **4** Percutaneous Endoscopic	**4** Intraluminal Device, Drug-eluting **5** Intraluminal Device, Drug-eluting, Two **6** Intraluminal Device, Drug-eluting, Three **7** Intraluminal Device, Drug-eluting, Four or More **D** Intraluminal Device **E** Intraluminal Device, Two **F** Intraluminal Device, Three **G** Intraluminal Device, Four or More **T** Intraluminal Device, Radioactive **Z** No Device	**6** Bifurcation **Z** No Qualifier
F Aortic Valve **G** Mitral Valve **H** Pulmonary Valve **J** Tricuspid Valve **K** Ventricle, Right **L** Ventricle, Left **P** Pulmonary Trunk **Q** Pulmonary Artery, Right **S** Pulmonary Vein, Right **T** Pulmonary Vein, Left **V** Superior Vena Cava **W** Thoracic Aorta, Descending **X** Thoracic Aorta, Ascending/Arch	**0** Open **3** Percutaneous **4** Percutaneous Endoscopic	**4** Intraluminal Device, Drug-eluting **D** Intraluminal Device **Z** No Device	**Z** No Qualifier
R Pulmonary Artery, Left	**0** Open **3** Percutaneous **4** Percutaneous Endoscopic	**4** Intraluminal Device, Drug-eluting **D** Intraluminal Device **Z** No Device	**T** Ductus Arteriosus **Z** No Qualifier

FIGURE 32-2 Table 027 from the Medical and Surgical Section 2019 ICD-10-PCS

You will go through the grid and construct the correct code based on the physician's notes. As you have already learned, _all_ ICD-10-PCS codes are seven characters. Therefore, you will build the code in this order, as directed by the grid.

- First character: Section (such as _Medical and Surgical, Mental Health_, or _Imaging_)
- Second character: **Body system**
- Third character: **Root operation**
- Fourth character: **Body part** or region
- Fifth character: **Approach**
- Sixth character: **Device**
- Seventh character: **Qualifier**

Therefore, when you review the information in Figure 32-2, you can see that the correct ICD-10-PCS code for _Dilation of one site of a Coronary Artery, using an open approach with an Intraluminal device_ is 02700DZ.

Body Part
The anatomical site upon which the procedure was performed.

Approach
The specific technique used for the procedure.

Device
The identification of any materials or appliances that may remain in or on the body after the procedure is completed.

Qualifier
Any additional feature of the procedure, if applicable.

 LET'S CODE IT! SCENARIO

Jahlil Browne was playing football in the park with his friends. A player on the other team hit him at full force in the chest when he ran to catch a pass. Jahlil was taken to the ED by ambulance and admitted into the hospital with an open fracture of the third rib, right side. Dr. Wolf operated on Jahlil to insert an internal fixation device, using a percutaneous endoscopic approach to secure the fractured bone together with the fourth rib, so it can heal properly.

Let's Code It!

What did the doctor do for Jahlil? Dr. Wolf _inserted an internal fixation device_ on Jahlil's fractured rib. It is always wise to begin with the actual term that the physician used in his or her notes, so let's go to the Alphabetic Index and look up the term _insertion._

Below the main term, _insertion,_ is a list. None of these terms seem to go with this situation. Wait a minute. Right below this is a main term that does fit: _Insertion of device in._ Beneath this is a list of anatomical sites. What anatomical site did the fixation device go onto? _Rib._ Then, check the documentation to identify how many ribs were involved in the procedure. Find

> **Insertion of device in**
>   Rib
>   1 to 2 0PH1
>   3 or more 0PH2

These four characters are a good start. Remember, all ICD-10-PCS codes require seven (7) characters. You must go to the Tables to confirm this is correct.

In the Tables, turn to the _**Medical and Surgical**_ section: 0PH. Look carefully at the second row.

Section	0	Medical and Surgical		
Body System	P	Upper Bones		
Operation	H	Insertion		

Body Region	Approach	Device	Qualifier
1 Ribs, 1 to 2 **2** Ribs, 3 or more **3** Cervical Vertebra **4** Thoracic Vertebra **5** Scapula, Right **6** Scapula, Left	**0** Open **3** Percutaneous **4** Percutaneous Endoscopic	**4** Internal Fixation Device	**Z** No Qualifier

(continued)

OK, let's build a code:

The section:	**0 Medical and Surgical** (Dr. Wolf performed surgery on Jahlil)
The body system:	**P Upper Bones** (the ribs are in the upper half of the body)
The root operation:	**H Insertion** (Dr. Wolf inserted a fixation device)
The body part:	**1 Ribs, 1 to 2** (as per the physician's documentation)
The approach:	**4 Percutaneous Endoscopic** (the documentation states this approach)
	4 Internal Fixation Device (this equipment will stay on Jahlil's rib after the procedure
The device:	until it is healed)
The qualifier:	**Z No Qualifier**

The ICD-10-PCS code to report the repair of Jahlil's rib is **0PH144Z.**
   Good job!

 LET'S CODE IT! SCENARIO

Montell was in a car accident and his right knee hit against the steering column. He was admitted into the hospital, and Dr. Tompkins took a high osmolar x-ray of his knee.

Let's Code It!

What did Dr. Tompkins do for Montell? He *x-rayed his knee.*
   In the Alphabetic Index, look up *x-ray.* The Alphabetic Index suggests

X-ray—see Plain Radiography

OK, so turn to *Plain Radiography* in the Alphabetic Index. Beneath this main term is a long list of anatomical sites, so read down and find

Plain Radiography
   Knee
         Left BQ08
         Right BQ07

The Alphabetic Index provided only four of the seven needed characters of this suggested code, so turn to the Tables to complete the code and confirm its correctness.
   In the Tables, turn to the *Imaging* section: BQ0.

Section	B	Imaging
Body System	Q	Non-Axial Lower Bones
Type	0	Plain Radiology: Planar display of an image developed from the capture of external ionizing radiation on photographic or photoconductive plate

Body Region	Approach	Device	Qualifier
0 Hip, Right **1** Hip, Left	**0** High Osmolar **1** Low Osmolar **Y** Other Contrast	**Z** None	**Z** None
0 Hip, Right **1** Hip, Left	**Z** None	**Z** None	**1** Densitometry **Z** None
3 Femur, Right **4** Femur, Left	**Z** None	**Z** None	**1** Densitometry **Z** None

(continued)

7 Knee, Right **8** Knee, Left **G** Ankle, Right **H** Ankle, Left	**0** High Osmolar **1** Low Osmolar **Y** Other Contrast **Z** None	**Z** None	**Z** None
D Lower leg, Right **F** Lower leg, Left **J** Calcaneus, Right **K** Calcaneus, Left **L** Foot, Right **M** Foot, Left **P** Toe(s), Right **Q** Toe(s), Left **V** Patella, Right **W** Patella, Left	**Z** None	**Z** None	**Z** None
X Foot/Toe Joint, Right **Y** Foot/Toe Joint, Left	**0** High Osmolar **1** Low Osmolar **Y** Other Contrast	**Z** None	**Z** None

OK, let's build the code:

The section:	**B Imaging** (you know that x-rays are a type of imaging)
The body system:	**Q Non-axial lower bones** (*non-axial* means away from the central part of the body, and you know that the knee is a lower bone)
The root operation:	**0 Plain Radiography** (also known as x-ray)
The body part:	**7 Knee, Right** (as per the physician's notes)
The contrast:	**0 High Osmolar** (as per the physician's notes)
The qualifier:	**Z None**
The qualifier:	**Z None**

The ICD-10-PCS code to report the x-ray of Montell's knee is **BQ070ZZ**.
Good work!

Appendices

The information shared in the appendices of your ICD-10-PCS code book can be very valuable as you abstract documentation to interpret to the correct character as you build your code. In addition to the definitions for each of the major components of the ICD-10-PCS code, there are also examples, which may help your understanding. And . . . they are right there in the back of your ICD-10-PCS code book!

Appendices
Components of the Medical and Surgical Approach Definitions
Root Operation Definitions
Comparison of Medical and Surgical Root Operations
Body Part Key
Body Part Definitions
Device Key and Aggregation Table
Device Definitions
Substance Key/Substance Definitions
Sections B-H Character Definitions
Hospital Acquired Conditions
Answers to Coding Exercises
Procedure Combination Tables

Axis of Classification
A single meaning within the code set; providing a detail.

Use the information in these appendices to support your determination of the accurate characters and the correct ICD-10-PCS code.

32.4 ICD-10-PCS General Conventions

The ICD-10-PCS code set has its own set of guidelines, of course. The following list contains the general conventions of how the codes are constructed and how to use the Tables.

Read through these guidelines to get a strong start to accurately reporting inpatient procedures. But don't worry about memorizing them because they are right there, in the front of your code book.

A1. ICD-10-PCS codes are composed of seven characters. Each character is an **axis of classification** that specifies information about the procedure performed. Within a defined code range, a character specifies the same type of information in that axis of classification.

This convention is explaining that all ICD-10-PCS codes must have seven (7) characters—no more, no less—and that each character position (axis of classification) has a specific meaning.

EXAMPLE

The third character of the code specifies the *root operation term.*

A2. One of 34 possible values can be assigned to each axis of classification in the seven-character code: they are the numbers 0 through 9 and the letters of the alphabet (except I and O because they are easily confused with the numbers 1 and 0). The number of unique values used in an axis of classification differs as needed.

When this convention refers to "34 possible values," it is referring to the fact that this code set uses letters of the American alphabet (letters A to Z minus O and I, so 26 letters minus 2 = 24 possible letters) plus 10 possible numbers (0–9) = 34 possibilities for each position in each code. And while there may be 34 possibilities, only what is needed is used at this time. This means that this code set has lots of room to grow and include new codes as they become a part of our standards of care.

EXAMPLE

Where the fifth character specifies the approach, seven different approach values are currently used to specify the approach.

A3. The valid values for an axis of classification can be added to as needed.

This convention means that this code set has lots of room to grow and include new codes as they become a part of our standards of care.

EXAMPLE

If a significantly distinct type of device is used in a new procedure, a new device value can be added to the system.

A4. As with words in their context, the meaning of any single value is a combination of its axis of classification and any preceding values on which it may be dependent.

This convention tells you to interpret each meaning, not only according to each specific character's definition, but also in combination with the meanings of the other characters that are in that table, in that row. It is the total meaning that you must look at, as well as each individual character. So, if once you put all seven characters together, something doesn't make sense, you need to read again.

EXAMPLE

The meaning of a body part value in the **Medical and Surgical** section is always dependent on the body system value. The body part value 0 in the Central Nervous body system specifies Brain; the body part value 0 in the Peripheral Nervous body system specifies Cervical Plexus.

A5. As the system is expanded to become increasingly detailed, over time more values will depend on preceding values for their meaning.

This convention means that they will continue to expand the system and ensure that new characters added will not overlap or duplicate the meanings of characters that already exist in that table, in the row.

EXAMPLE

In the Lower Joints body system:

- Under the root operation *Insertion: Table 0SH*

    Device character 6: value 3 specifies "Infusion Device"

- Under the root operation *Replacement: Table 0SR*

    Device character 6: value 3 specifies "Synthetic Substitute, Ceramic"

A6. The purpose of the Alphabetic Index is to locate the appropriate table that contains all information necessary to construct a procedure code. The PCS Tables should always be consulted to find the most appropriate valid code.

Essentially, this convention is telling you what you may have learned when coding from other code sets. *Never* report a code from the Alphabetic Index. *Always* refer to the tables and double-check the meaning for each and every character in that table, in that row.

A7. It is not required to consult the Index first before proceeding to the tables to complete the code. A valid code may be chosen directly from the tables.

This takes convention A6 a little further in telling you that you are NOT required to ever look in the Alphabetic Index. As you gain more experience, and you are on the job, you may learn your way through this code set. So, if you are coding for the labor and delivery services to a pregnant woman, you can go directly to the **Obstetrics** tables without looking in the Alphabetic Index if you don't need the suggestion. And if you are coding for a psychiatrist providing care to a patient in a behavioral health hospital, you can go directly to the **Mental Health** tables.

A8. All seven characters must be specified to be a valid code. If the documentation is incomplete for coding purposes, the physician should be queried for the necessary information.

Every character in every code must report the facts, as supported by the physician's documentation. If any detail is missing, and you are not able to determine the correct character, then you must query the physician to have the documentation amended. You can *never* assume and never guess.

A9. Within a PCS table, valid codes include all combinations of choices in characters 4 through 7 contained in the same row of the table. In the example below, 0HTWXZZ is a valid code, and 0HTW0ZZ is **not** a valid code.

Section	**0**	Medical and Surgical		
Body System	**H**	Skin and Breast		
Operation	**T**	Resection: Cutting out or off, without replacement, all of a body part		
Body Part		*Approach*	*Device*	*Qualifier*
Q Finger Nail **R** Toe Nail **W** Nipple, Right **X** Nipple, Left		**X** External	**Z** No Device	**Z** No Device
T Breast, Right **U** Breast, Left **V** Breast, Bilateral **Y** Supplemental Breast		**0** Open	**Z** No Device	**Z** No Device

This convention tells you how to read the table to build your code. Once you find the table with the correct first three characters (section, body system, root operation term), then go down the column to find the correct 4th character. Once you determine this accurate character, you can only go across in that one row. If you determine that the procedure was done on the right nipple (character **W** in the first row), then you only have one option for the approach: **X External.** If the documentation states an open approach was used, then you cannot put **0 Open** with **W Nipple, Right** because they are on two different rows. This would highlight to you that you need to go back to the documentation because you can't build this code from more than one row.

A10. "And," when used in a code description, means "and/or," except when used to describe a combination of multiple body parts for which separate values exist for each body part (e.g., Skin and Subcutaneous Tissue used as a qualifier, where there are separate body part values for "Skin" and "Subcutaneous Tissue").

Take a look at an example: *Knee Bursa and Ligament.* You would interpret this as

Knee Bursa and Ligament
Knee Bursa
Knee Ligament

EXAMPLE

Lower Arm and Wrist Muscle means lower arm and/or wrist muscle.

A11. Many of the terms used to construct PCS codes are defined within the system. It is the coder's responsibility to determine what the documentation in the medical record equates to in the PCS definitions. The physician is not expected to use the terms used in PCS code descriptions, nor is the coder required to query the physician when the correlation between the documentation and the defined PCS terms is clear.

This convention tells you, directly, that it is your responsibility to interpret the terms and phrases used by the physician in the documentation. For example, if the physician documents that he performed a *biopsy*, you, as the coder, must interpret that to the ICD-10-PCS root operation term *excision*, and if the physician documents that she manipulated the dislocated shoulder back into position, you, as the coder, must interpret this into the ICD-10-PCS root operation term *reposition*.

> **EXAMPLE**
>
> When the physician documents "cauterization," the coder can independently correlate "cauterization" to the root operation "destruction" without querying the physician for clarification.

32.5 Selection of Principal Procedure

Similar to CPT and HCPCS Level II coding, ICD-10-PCS has its guidelines for determining the sequencing when reporting more than one procedure provided during an encounter. This is always going to be determined in coordination with the diagnosis codes being reported to identify the medical necessity for performing these procedures. Here are the Official Guidelines for ICD-10-PCS code sequencing:

The following instructions should be applied in the selection of principal procedure and clarification on the importance of the relation to the principal diagnosis when more than one procedure is performed:

1. Procedure performed for definitive treatment of both principal diagnosis and secondary diagnosis.
   a. Sequence procedure performed for definitive treatment most related to principal diagnosis as principal procedure.
2. Procedure performed for definitive treatment and diagnostic procedures performed for both principal diagnosis and secondary diagnosis.
   a. Sequence procedure performed for definitive treatment most related to principal diagnosis as principal procedure.
3. A diagnostic procedure was performed for the principal diagnosis and a procedure is performed for definitive treatment of a secondary diagnosis.
   a. Sequence diagnostic procedure as principal procedure, since the procedure most related to the principal diagnosis takes precedence.
4. No procedures performed that are related to principal diagnosis; procedures performed for definitive treatment and diagnostic procedures were performed for secondary diagnosis.
   a. Sequence procedure performed for definitive treatment of secondary diagnosis as principal procedure, since there are no procedures (definitive or nondefinitive treatment) related to principal diagnosis.

Source: ICD-10-PCS *Official Guidelines for Coding and Reporting,* 2019.

As you read through these four guidelines to determine how multiple ICD-10-PCS procedure codes should be sequenced, notice that you must refer to the diagnosis codes, and the sequencing of those codes, as part of your decision-making process. In addition, you must understand why each procedure was performed—not only for the intended outcome, but also to understand if the procedure was done for diagnostic or therapeutic purposes.

CODING BITES

You learned about the different types of procedures in the chapter *Introduction to the Languages of Coding,* the section titled *Procedure Coding.*

 GUIDANCE CONNECTION

Read the **ICD-10-PCS Official Guidelines for Coding and Reporting,** section **Selection of Principal Procedure.**

CODING BITES

Additional information about ICD-10-PCS can be found at:

https://www.cms.gov/Medicare/Coding/ICD10/2019-ICD-10-PCS.html

Chapter Summary

The purpose of this chapter is to provide an overview of ICD-10-PCS, giving you an idea of what to expect, and to help you establish a comfort level so that you are not apprehensive about the new system. This chapter shared with you the distinct benefits of this code set. Then, step by step, the chapter differentiated the way the codes look and are constructed. The notations and explanations, exclusive to ICD-10-PCS, are all reviewed. Examples are provided to illustrate the concepts and elements throughout the chapter.

CHAPTER 32 REVIEW
Introduction to ICD-10-PCS

Mc Graw Hill **connect®**

Enhance your learning by completing these exercises and more at mcgrawhillconnect.com!

Let's Check It! Terminology

Match each key term to the appropriate definition.

1. LO 32.3 The identification of any materials or appliances that may remain in or on the body after the procedure is completed.

2. LO 32.3 The category or classification of a particular procedure, service, or treatment.

3. LO 32.3 The anatomical site upon which the procedure was performed.

4. LO 32.3 Any additional feature of the procedure, if applicable.

5. LO 32.3 The physiological system, or anatomical region, upon which the procedure was performed.

6. LO 32.3 The specific technique used for the procedure.

7. LO 32.4 A single meaning within the code set; providing a detail.

A. Approach
B. Axis of Classification
C. Body Part
D. Body System
E. Device
F. Qualifier
G. Root Operation Term

Let's Check It! Concepts

Choose the most appropriate answer for each of the following questions.

1. LO 32.1 In ICD-10-PCS, the initials *PCS* stand for
   a. Popular Coding System.
   b. Procedure Coding System.
   c. Possible Coding Solutions.
   d. Proper Coding System.

2. LO 32.2 The Alphabetic Index's entries are primarily sorted by
   a. root operation terms.
   b. the approach.
   c. the device.
   d. the body system.

3. LO 32.2 The structure of ICD-10-PCS codes includes
   a. three numbers.
   b. five numbers.
   c. seven characters.
   d. up to nine characters.

4. LO 32.2 ICD-10-PCS codes include
   a. only numbers.
   b. only letters.
   c. one letter followed by numbers.
   d. letters and numbers.

5. LO 32.2 An example of a root operation term is
   a. bypass.
   b. x-ray.
   c. obstetrics.
   d. hysterectomy.

6. LO 32.2 Digestive system is an example of a

   a. body part.

   c. medical procedure.

   b. root operation term.

   d. body system.

7. LO 32.2 The 17 sections of ICD-10-PCS are identified by

   a. numbers 1–17.

   c. letters *A–Z*.

   b. numbers 0–9, then letters *B-H* and *X*.

   d. alphabetic order by the name of the section.

8. LO 32.2 Placeholders are indicated in ICD-10-PCS with

   a. the number 0.

   c. the letter *Z*.

   b. the letter *X*.

   d. the number 9.

9. LO 32.2 An example of an approach is

   a. open.

   c. pacemaker.

   b. ileostomy.

   d. ventricular.

10. LO 32.2 An example of a device, for purposes of ICD-10-PCS coding, is

    a. ablation.

    c. pacemaker.

    b. laparoscopy.

    d. allotransplantation.

11. LO 32.2 The ICD-10-PCS code for the provision of a cesarean section would be found in

    a. Section 2 Placement.

    c. Section B Imaging.

    b. Section 1 Obstetrics.

    d. Section 6 Extracorporeal Therapies.

12. LO 32.2 Coding a chiropractic manipulative treatment would begin in

    a. Section 0 Medical and Surgical.

    b. Section 4 Measurement and Monitoring.

    c. Section 7 Osteopathic.

    d. Section 9 Chiropractic.

13. LO 32.2 What is the letter or number that represents the device in code 2W22X4Z?

    a. 2

    c. 4

    b. W

    d. X

14. LO 32.2 What is the letter or number that represents the approach in code 3E00X3Z?

    a. E

    c. 0

    b. X

    d. Z

15. LO 32.2 What is the letter or number that represents the root operation in code 3E1S38Z?

    a. 1

    c. 8

    b. S

    d. E

16. LO 32.2 What is the letter or number that represents the section in code 2W10X7Z?

    a. 2

    c. 1

    b. W

    d. 0

17. LO 32.2 What is the letter or number that represents the qualifier in code 3E0Y70M?

    a. 0

    c. 7

    b. Y

    d. M

18. LO 32.3 The Alphabetic Index will usually give you only the first _____ or _____ characters of the seven-character procedure code.

    a. one, two

    c. three, four

    b. two, three

    d. five, six

19. **LO 32.4** Which ICD-10-PCS general convention states that within a PCS table, valid codes include all combinations of choices in characters 4 through 7 contained in the same row of the table?

   a. A1   **b.** A3

   c. A6   **d.** A9

20. **LO 32.5** ICD-10-PCS does not have guidelines for determining the sequencing when reporting more than one procedure provided during an encounter.

   a. True   **b.** False

Let's Check It! Rules and Regulations

Please answer the following questions from the knowledge you have gained after reading this chapter.

1. **LO 32.2** ICD-10-PCS codes may include any letter of the alphabet *except* the letter(s) _____; include why these letters are avoided.

2. **LO 32.2** List the related pieces of information for the seven ICD-10-PCS character positions.

3. **LO 32.3** How are the ICD-10-PCS tables divided?

4. **LO 32.4** What are the 11 ICD-10-PCS General Convention guidelines? Include a brief description of each.

5. **LO 32.5** What are the instructions for selection of the principal procedure when more than one procedure is performed?

 YOU CODE IT! Application

The following exercises provide practice in abstracting physicians' notes and learning to work with documentation from our health care facility, Westward Hospital. These case studies are modeled on real patient encounters. Using the techniques described in this chapter, carefully read through the case studies and determine the most accurate answers for each case study.

WESTWARD HOSPITAL

591 Chester Road

Masters, FL 33955

PATIENT: WELLINGTON, ALISHA

DATE OF ADMISSION: 03/13/19

DATE OF SURGERY: 03/13/19

DATE OF DISCHARGE 03/14/19

PREOPERATIVE DX: Right ureteral obstruction secondary to colon cancer

POSTOPERATIVE DX: Same

PROCEDURE: Cystoscopy
         Right retrograde pyelogram
         Removal and replacement of double-J stent

ANESTHESIA: General

HISTORY/INDICATIONS: This is a 39-year-old female with a history of colon cancer and secondary right ureteral obstruction who had a stent inserted a number of months ago. At this time, she is in the hospital and it is time for a stent change. Consequently, the patient presents for the procedure.

(continued)

PROCEDURE: The patient was taken to the operating room and there she was given general anesthetic, positioned in the dorsal lithotomy position, the genitalia scrubbed and prepped with Betadine. Sterile towels and sheets were utilized to drape the patient in the usual fashion. A cystoscope was introduced into the bladder. The ureteral catheter was identified. It was grabbed and removed without any difficulty. Subsequently, the cystoscope was reinserted into the bladder and the right ureteral orifice was identified over a Pollack catheter. A glide wire was inserted into the right collecting system. Some contrast was injected and a hydronephrotic right side was noted. Then, the wire was placed through the Pollack catheter. With the wire in position, over the wire a 7 French 26 cm double-J stent was inserted. Excellent coiling was noted fluoroscopically in the kidney and distally with a cystoscope. The bladder was then drained and again it was inspected prior to removal. There was no evidence of any tumors or lesions in the bladder. The stent was in good position. The cystoscope was removed and the patient was taken to the recovery room awake and in stable condition.

Benjamin Johnston, MD—2222

556839/mt98328: 03/15/19 09:50:16 T: 03/15/19 12:55:01

In Dr. Johnston's documentation of Alisha Wellington's procedure, what is/are the root operation term(s)?

a. Replacement
b. Fluoroscopy
c. Replacement and fluoroscopy
d. Removal

WESTWARD HOSPITAL

591 Chester Road

Masters, FL 33955

PATIENT: FIELDING, STEPHEN

DATE OF ADMISSION: 07/15/19

DATE OF SURGERY: 07/15/19

DATE OF DISCHARGE: 07/16/19

PREOPERATIVE DX: Superior canalicular laceration

POSTOPERATIVE DX: Same

PROCEDURE: Superior canalicular repair

This patient is a 3-year-old male who is admitted into the Pediatric Unit with a dog bite to left side of face.

HPI: Approximately 3 hours ago, patient was playing with a large dog, the pet of a neighbor. Family witnessed the dog make a single lunge at the boy's face. Due to the adults' attempts to intervene, only the top jaw made contact. The dog did not attack further, and the incomplete bite to the left face was the only injury sustained. Ophthalmology called in for consult.

POH/PMH/SH: No past ocular history. No past medical history. No current medications or allergies. Well-adjusted preschool child lives at home with both parents. Childhood immunizations are up-to-date, according to the mother.

OCULAR EXAM:

• VA 20/25 OD and OS without correction

(continued)

- Extraocular motility and IOP were normal, OU

- CVF: Full OD, OS

- Lids: Right side—Normal

- Lids: Left side—2 lacerations on the left upper lid, the larger and deeper of the lacerations passes just medial to the upper punctum. Initial exploration of laceration raises concerns for probable canalicular involvement, but further detailed examination in this anxious pediatric patient was unable to be accomplished.

- Continuation of the examination in the operating suite revealed that the remainder of the anterior segment examination and DFE were normal.

TREATMENT: Primary surgical repair of the lacerated or avulsed canaliculus using pigtail probes is performed immediately. The patient was taken to the operating suite for examination under general anesthesia (EUA) and laceration repair, likely to include canalicular repair.

DX: Superior canalicular laceration

Roxan Kernan, MD—4444

556848/mt98328: 07/17/19 09:50:16 T: 07/17/19 12:55:01

In Dr. Kernan's documentation of the procedure on Stephen Fielding, what is the root operation term?

a. Repair
b. Eyelid
c. Canalicular
d. Bite

WESTWARD HOSPITAL

591 Chester Road

Masters, FL 33955

PATIENT: O'LEARY, KEVIN

DATE OF ADMISSION: 03/05/19

DATE OF DISCHARGE: 03/17/19

PREOPERATIVE DX: Third-degree burn, neck

POSTOPERATIVE DX: Same

PROCEDURE: Skin graft

ANESTHESIA: General

This patient is a 43-year-old male who works as a county firefighter. He is recovering from third-degree burns on his neck. He was admitted today for the first session of skin grafting. Patient is brought into the surgical suite and general anesthesia is administered by Dr. Rambeau. Once the patient is unconscious, he is prepped and draped in the usual, sterile fashion. A split-thickness autograft, which contains the dermis with only a portion of the epidermis, is taken from a donor site on the patient's inner thigh, left. The graft harvested is 11/1000ths of an inch in thickness, using a derma-tome. The graft is carefully spread on the bare area and held in place with surgical staples. Plasmatic imbibition is initiated. The graft is meshed with lengthwise rows of short, interrupted cuts, each a few millimeters long, with each

(continued)

row offset by half a cut length. The area is covered with derma-surgical gauze. Patient is awakened and taken to recovery.

Benjamin Johnston, MD—2222

556839/mt98328: 03/15/19 09:50:16 T: 03/15/19 12:55:01

What is/are the root operation term(s), as documented in Dr. Johnston's procedure notes for Kevin O'Leary?

a. Excision
b. Excision and replacement
c. Replacement and neck
d. Neck

WESTWARD HOSPITAL

591 Chester Road

Masters, FL 33955

PATIENT: SWANSONN, HANS

DATE OF ADMISSION: 05/23/19

DATE OF DISCHARGE: 05/23/19

PREOPERATIVE DX: Rule out bladder tumor

POSTOPERATIVE DX: Same

PROCEDURE: Cystoscopy, biopsy, and fulguration of bladder

ANESTHESIA: Spinal

INDICATIONS: The patient is a 67-year-old male with a history of grade II superficial transitional cell carcinoma of the bladder. Cystoscopy showed a suspicious erythematous area on the right trigone. He presented today for cystoscopy, biopsy, and fulguration. Findings: The urethra was normal; the bladder was 1+ trabeculated; the mid and right trigone areas were slightly erythematous and hypervascular. No papillary tumors were noted; no mucosal abnormalities were noted.

PROCEDURE: The patient was placed on the table in supine position. Satisfactory spinal anesthesia was obtained. He was placed in dorsal lithotomy position and prepped sterilely with Hibiclens and draped in the usual manner. A #22 French cystoscopy sheath was passed per urethra in atraumatic fashion. The bladder was resected with the 70-degree lens with findings as noted above. Cup biopsy forceps were placed and three biopsies were taken of the suspicious areas of the trigone. These areas were fulgurated with the Bugby electrode; no active bleeding was seen. The scope was removed; the patient was returned to recovery having tolerated the procedure well. Estimated blood loss was minimal.

PATHOLOGY REPORT: Chronic cystitis (cystica) with squamous cell metaplasia.

Roxan Kernan, MD—4444

556848/mt98328: 05/24/19 09:50:16 T: 05/24/19 12:55:01

What is the root operation term identified in Dr. Kernan's procedure notes about Hans Swansonn?

a. Diagnostic
b. Excision
c. Bladder
d. Endoscopic

WESTWARD HOSPITAL

591 Chester Road

Masters, FL 33955

PATIENT: ZANDER, MARISSA

DATE OF ADMISSION: 02/16/19

DATE OF DISCHARGE: 02/18/19

PREOPERATIVE DX: Delivery

POSTOPERATIVE DX: Same

PROCEDURE: Cesarean section, classical

In the 40th week of her first pregnancy, a 29-year-old female arrived at labor and delivery at 0830 for a planned induction of labor due to mild, pregnancy-induced hypertension. After intra-vaginal placement of misoprostol, the nurse observed her briefly and, at 1100, discharged her from the unit. She went for a walk with her husband in a park next to the hospital. Patient's membranes spontaneously ruptured and she readmitted to the labor and delivery unit. The nurse admitted the patient, took her vital signs, and checked the fetal heart rate. The mother's blood pressure was 176/95, but the nurse thought this was related to nausea, vomiting, and discomfort from the contractions. The resident examined the mother, determined that her cervix was 5–6 cm, 90 percent effaced, and the vertex was at 0 station. An internal fetal heart monitor was placed because the mother's vomiting and discomfort caused her to move around too much in the bed, making it hard to record the fetal heart rate with an external monitor. The internal monitor revealed a steady fetal heart rate of 120 and no decelerations. The mother continued to complain of pain-ful contractions and requested an epidural. Shortly after placement of the epidural, the monitor recorded a prolonged fetal heart rate deceleration. The heart rate returned slowly to the baseline rate of 120 as the nurse repositioned the mother, increased her intravenous fluids, and administered oxygen by mask. An epidural analgesia infusion pump was started. The fetal heart rate strip indicated another deceleration that recovered to baseline. The nurse informed the resident, who checked the tracing and told her to "keep an eye on things." The primary nurse noted in the labor record that the baseline fetal heart rate was "unstable, between 100–120," but she did not report this to the resident. The nurse recorded that the fetal heart rate was "flat, no variability." As the nurse was documenting this as a non-reassuring fetal heart rate pattern, the patient expressed a strong urge to push and the nurse called for an exam. A resident came to the bedside, examined the mother, and noted that she was fully dilated with the caput at +1. A brief update was written in the chart, but the clinician who had performed the exam was not noted. The mother was repositioned and began pushing. The fetal heart rate suddenly dropped and remained profoundly bradycardic for 11 minutes. The resident was called and attempted a vacuum delivery since the fetal head was at +2 station. The attending then entered and attempted forceps delivery. An emergency classical cesarean delivery was performed; the baby was stillborn. The physician identified a uterine rupture that required significant blood replacement. Whole blood transfusion, nonautologous, was performed, via peripheral vein.

Roxan Kernan, MD—4444

556848/mt98328: 07/17/19 09:50:16 T: 07/17/19 12:55:01

In Dr. Kernan's documentation on the procedure performed on Marissa Zander, identify the root operation term(s).

a. Extraction
b. Transfusion
c. Percutaneous
d. Extraction and transfusion

Design elements: ©McGraw-Hill

ICD-10-PCS Medical and Surgical Section

33

Learning Outcomes

After completing this chapter, the student should be able to:

LO 33.1 Identify the section and body systems used in Medical and Surgical section codes.

LO 33.2 Interpret the procedure to determine the accurate root operation term used in Medical and Surgical section codes.

LO 33.3 Utilize knowledge of anatomy to determine the body part treated to be used in Medical and Surgical section codes.

LO 33.4 Identify the approach used to accomplish the procedure used in Medical and Surgical section codes.

LO 33.5 Distinguish the type of device implanted, when applicable, for Medical and Surgical section codes.

LO 33.6 Select the appropriate qualifier character for Medical and Surgical section codes.

LO 33.7 Determine the correct way to report multiple and discontinued procedures for Medical and Surgical section codes.

LO 33.8 Analyze all of the details to build an accurate seven-character code for Medical and Surgical section codes.

 STOP! Remember, you need to follow along in your ICD-10-PCS code book for an optimal learning experience.

33.1 Medical/Surgical Section/Body Systems: Characters 1 and 2

As you learned earlier, every ICD-10-PCS code has seven characters, and each **character** position has a meaning. While all of these codes have the same number of characters, each section uses each character position differently. So let's review the meanings for the *Medical and Surgical* section characters:

Character
A letter or number component of an ICD-10-PCS code.

Character Position	Character Meaning
1	Section of the ICD-10-PCS book
2	Body system being treated
3	Root operation term
4	Body part (specific anatomical site)
5	Approach used by physician
6	Device
7	Qualifier

Character Position 1: Medical and Surgical Section 0 (Zero)

Character Position	Character Meaning
1	Section of the ICD-10-PCS book
2	Body system being treated
3	Root operation term
4	Body part (specific anatomical site)
5	Approach used by physician
6	Device
7	Qualifier

All of the codes reporting a medical or surgical procedure will begin with a zero. *Medical and Surgical* is the first section of the Tables, after the Alphabetic Index. When you look up a procedure in the Alphabetic Index and see that the suggested code begins with a zero, you will know immediately that you will find the rest of this code in the *Medical and Surgical* Tables.

Character Position 2: Body System

Character Position	Character Meaning
1	Section of the ICD-10-PCS book
2	Body system being treated
3	Root operation term
4	Body part (specific anatomical site)
5	Approach used by physician
6	Device
7	Qualifier

In this code set, the body systems are broken down into further detail than the organ systems you learned in your anatomy and physiology course. The body systems and their corresponding characters are:

0 Central Nervous System and Cranial Nerves

1 Peripheral Nervous System

2 Heart and Great Vessels

3 Upper Arteries

4 Lower Arteries

5 Upper Veins

6 Lower Veins

7 Lymphatic and Hemic Systems

8 Eye

9 Ear, Nose, Sinus

B Respiratory System

C Mouth and Throat

D Gastrointestinal System

F Hepatobiliary System and Pancreas

G Endocrine System

H Skin and Breast

J Subcutaneous Tissue and Fascia

K Muscles

L Tendons

M Bursae and Ligaments

N Head and Facial Bones

P Upper Bones

Q Lower Bones

R Upper Joints

S Lower Joints

T Urinary System

U Female Reproductive System

V Male Reproductive System

W Anatomical Regions, General

X Anatomical Regions, Upper Extremities

Y Anatomical Regions, Lower Extremities

GUIDANCE CONNECTION

Read the ICD-10-PCS Official Guidelines for Coding and Reporting, **Medical and Surgical Section Guidelines (Section 0),** subhead **B2. Body system,** paragraphs **B2.1a** and **B2.1b**.

Notice that, in this list, there is a 0 (zero) and a number 1 (one) but no letter *O* or letter *I*. The creators of this code set did this purposely to avoid confusion.

Take a look at body system **5** Upper Veins and **6** Lower Veins. As explained in the guidelines, the imaginary transverse line is at the diaphragm, dividing the body into top (upper) and bottom (lower). A procedure performed on the brachial vein, located in the arm, will be reported with body system character 5, and a procedure performed on the gastric vein, located in the stomach, is reported with body system character 6. Similarly, the same applies for characters 3 and 4 (Upper and Lower Arteries), P and Q (Upper and Lower Bones), and R and S (Upper and Lower Joints).

Now, let's look at body system characters W, X, and Y, which report anatomical regions instead of a specific body section or system. These should be used only when the documentation identifies that the procedure was performed on an anatomical cavity rather than an individual body part. You must read carefully to distinguish the details. To illustrate this, let's look at a case of a patient diagnosed with ascites (a buildup of fluid in the abdominal cavity). The physician drains this excess fluid from the abdominal cavity; therefore, it will require a character of W for the body system: Anatomical Regions, General.

You do not need to worry about remembering that the liver is part of the hepatobiliary system or that a pacemaker generator is inserted into the subcutaneous tissue and fascia and its leads are inserted into the heart. The Alphabetic Index will help you, as will the listings for body part (character position 4).

EXAMPLES

Dr. Franklin inserted a neurostimulator lead into Matthew Short's cerebrum, during an open procedure.

The Body System is reported: Central Nervous System and Cranial Nerves with a 0 (zero) character.

YOU INTERPRET IT!

Identify which body system this anatomical site would report for the second character.

1. Umbilical artery: _____

2. Cervical lymph node: _____

3. Cornea: _____

4. Pharynx: _____

5. Stomach: _____

6. Deltoid muscle: _____

7. Zygomatic process of frontal bone: _____

8. Coccyx: _____

9. Elbow joint: _____

10. Trachea: _____

33.2 Medical/Surgical Root Operations: Character 3

Character Position	Character Meaning
1	Section of the ICD-10-PCS book
2	Body system being treated
3	**Root operation term**
4	Body part (specific anatomical site)
5	Approach used by physician
6	Device
7	Qualifier

Root Operation Term
The category or classification of a particular procedure, service, or treatment.

The *Medical and Surgical* section uses 31 **root operation terms** to describe what procedure was performed for the patient during this encounter. Don't worry—the definitions are listed in the ICD-10-PCS code book. However, you still need to learn and understand them so that you can abstract the operative report or procedure notes accurately and completely from the documentation. Remember that you are required to use the ICD-10-PCS term definition in its entirety. Also, just as in reporting with CPT procedure codes, it is important that you understand all of the components of a specific root operation or procedure. You don't want to code inclusive components separately or miss a second code because a component is not part of that procedure automatically. Using the root operation term is the most efficient way of using the Alphabetic Index as well.

Alteration

> **Alteration: Modification of a natural anatomic structure of a body part without affecting the function of the body part . . .** Character: **0 (zero)**

GUIDANCE CONNECTION

Read the ICD-10-PCS Official Guidelines for Coding and Reporting, **Medical and Surgical Section Guidelines (Section 0),** subsection **B3. Root Operation,** paragraphs **B3.1a** through **B3.17.**

EXAMPLE

Alteration is a procedure most often performed for cosmetic purposes, to improve the patient's appearance, such as a face lift.

Rhytidectomy (face lift surgery) is a procedure performed to alter the look of the skin on the face. Liposuction and breast augmentation are also examples of this type of procedure.

> 0J013ZZ   Alteration of subcutaneous tissue and fascia, face, percutaneous approach

Bypass

GUIDANCE CONNECTION

Read the ICD-10-PCS Official Guidelines for Coding and Reporting, **Medical and Surgical Section Guidelines (Section 0),** subsection **B3. Root Operation,** subhead **Bypass procedures,** paragraphs **B3.6a, B3.6b,** and **B3.6c.**

> **Bypass: Altering the route of the contents of a tubular body part . . .** Character: **1**

Bypass procedures are coded by identifying the body part bypassed "from," identified by character **4** (Body Part), and the body part bypassed "to," identified by character **7** (Qualifier).

EXAMPLE

A *bypass* can be performed only on a tubular body part, such as a vein or an artery, the esophagus, or the intestines. A colostomy formation is another example of a bypass.

> 02114Z8   Coronary artery bypass, one site, percutaneous endoscopic approach, rerouted to internal mammary, right side

Change

Change: Taking out or off a device from a body part and putting back an identical or similar device in or on the same body part without cutting or puncturing the skin or a mucous membrane . . . Character: **2**

EXAMPLE

Change is a root operation used only when a device is involved in the procedure—a device that stays with the patient after the procedure is complete. A urinary catheter change and a gastronomy tube change are good examples. Often, this term will actually be used in the documentation.

0020X0Z	Changing a drainage device in the brain, external approach

---

Control

Control: Stopping, or attempting to stop, postprocedural or other acute bleeding . . . Character: **3**

The root operation term *Control* is used only when the only action taken during this procedure is the intent to stop the hemorrhage. If this attempt was unsuccessful and another procedure was performed to accomplish this task, such as excision or resection, then report the code for *that* root operation *instead* of Control. You will not report both.

EXAMPLE

Control is a procedure to stop massive bleeding (hemorrhaging).

0W3B0ZZ	Control post-procedural bleeding in the pleural cavity, left side, open approach

---

GUIDANCE CONNECTION

Read ICD-10-PCS Official Guidelines for Coding and Reporting, **Medical and Surgical Section Guidelines (Section 0),** subsection **B3. Root Operation,** subhead **Control vs. more definitive root operations,** paragraph **B3.7.**

Creation

Creation: Putting in or on biological or synthetic material to form a new body part that to the extent possible replicates the anatomic structure or function of an absent body part . . . Character: **4**

This procedure is used when the physician actually makes a new structure, such as creation of an artificial vagina during a male-to-female procedure in a gender reassignment surgery, procedures to correct congenital anomalies, or replacement of a dysfunctional heart valve.

EXAMPLES

Creation of a body part, such as a penis or a heart valve, is reported with this root operation term.

0W4N0J1	Creation of an artificial penis using synthetic substitute, open approach
024G082	Creation of a mitral valve using zooplastic tissue, open approach

---

Destruction

Destruction: Physical eradication of all or a portion of a body part by the direct use of energy, force, or a destructive agent . . . Character: **5**

Several methodologies are reported as destruction, such as fulguration, the application of high-frequency electrical current, also known as electrofulguration, when it is used to destroy tissue (typically malignant neoplasm). Chemical agents, such as salicylic acid, can also be used to destroy tissue.

> **EXAMPLE**
>
> *Destruction* is used to describe when the tissue is no longer in existence, and there is no specimen to send to pathology.
>
> Terms that may be used in the documentation include *fulguration, cauterization,* and *cryosurgery.*
>
> 0U5B8ZZ   Fulguration of endometrium, vaginal endoscopic approach

Detachment

Detachment: Cutting of all or a portion of the upper or lower extremities . . . Character: **6**

This is the root operation term for *amputation* of an arm or a leg, in whole or in part.

> **EXAMPLE**
>
> *Detachment* is only used to report the amputation of an arm or leg, no other body part.
>
> 0Y6J0Z1   Amputation, directly below knee, left leg, open approach

Dilation

Dilation: Expanding an orifice or the lumen of a tubular body part . . . Character: **7**

Remember, an orifice is a natural body opening (such as vagina or anus) and the lumen of a tubular body part (*lumen* = "space within the tube"). Blood vessels are tubular body parts, as are a woman's fallopian tubes.

> **EXAMPLES**
>
> *Dilation* is the process of opening a closed tubular body part.
>
> 037H34Z   Dilation of right common carotid artery, with drug-eluting intraluminal device, percutaneous approach
> 0U7C7ZZ   Dilation of the cervix, via natural opening

Division

Division: Cutting into a body part, without draining fluids and/or gases from the body part, in order to separate or transect a body part . . . Character: **8**

> **EXAMPLE**
>
> *Division* is the separation of body parts.
>
> An episiotomy, an osteotomy, and spinal cordotomy are all good examples.
>
> 0K820ZZ   Division of sternocleidomastoid muscle, right side, open approach

Drainage

Drainage: Taking or letting out fluids and/or gases from a body part . . . Character: 9

> **EXAMPLE**
>
> *Drainage* is, as it sounds, the process of helping gases or fluids escape.
>
> 0W9B30Z   Drainage of excess air from left pleural cavity, percutaneous approach

Excision

Excision: Cutting out or off, without replacement, a portion of a body part . . . Character: B

Pay close attention to this description of excision. This term has a narrower meaning in ICD-10-PCS than it does in CPT and in many physicians' notes. Excision is used in ICD-10-PCS only when a segment is cut out. This includes obtaining a tissue biopsy, performing a lumpectomy, and cutting out a bone spur. However, if the entire organ or body part is removed, the root operation term used is *resection* (even if the physician documents that an organ was excised—you must interpret it).

GUIDANCE CONNECTION

Read the ICD-10-PCS Official Guidelines for Coding and Reporting, **Medical and Surgical Section Guidelines (Section 0),** subsection **B3. Root Operation,** subhead **Excision vs. Resection,** paragraph **B3.8,** and **Excision for Graft,** paragraph **B3.9.**

> **EXAMPLE**
>
> *Excision* is the surgical removal of a *part or portion* of a body part, not the entire organ.
>
> 0FB13ZX   Excision, liver, right lobe, percutaneous approach, diagnostic procedure

Extirpation

Extirpation: Taking or cutting out solid matter from a body part . . . Character: C

This reference to "solid matter" may indicate a blood clot or gallstones when surgically removed.

> **EXAMPLE**
>
> *Extirpation* is the surgical removal of a solid formation from within the body.
>
> Some good examples are thrombectomy (surgical removal of a blood clot attached to the wall of a vein or artery) and cholelithotomy (surgical removal of gallstones).
>
> 04CL0ZZ   Extirpation of thrombus, femoral artery, left side, open approach

Extraction

Extraction: Pulling or stripping out or off all or a portion of a body part by the use of force . . . Character: D

> **EXAMPLE**
>
> *Extraction* may be done by scraping (curettage), pulling, suction, or other process.
>
> Vein stripping, D&C (dilation and curettage), and a cesarean section (extracting a baby from the womb) are all good examples.
>
> 0UDB8ZZ   Suction extraction of endometrium, via natural opening, endoscopic approach

Fragmentation

Fragmentation: Breaking solid matter in a body part into pieces . . . Character: F

An example of fragmentation is lithotripsy—the use of shock waves to break kidney stones (renal lithiasis) into smaller pieces with the hope that the body will be able to pass them naturally.

> ### EXAMPLE
>
> *Fragmentation* is the process of breaking up something in the body into smaller pieces, such as the procedure of lithotripsy.
>
> 0TFCXZZ   Fragmentation of stones in the bladder neck, using external approach

Fusion

Fusion: Joining together portions of an articular body part rendering the articular body part immobile . . . Character: G

Arthrodesis, the surgical immobilization of a joint, such as of the spine, is one type of fusion (*articular* = "joint").

> ### EXAMPLE
>
> *Fusion* is a procedure that is the opposite of *division*.
>
> 0RG40A0   Fusion of cervicothoracic vertebral joint, open procedure, anterior approach, anterior column, using an interbody fusion device

GUIDANCE CONNECTION

Read the ICD-10-PCS Official Guidelines for Coding and Reporting, **Medical and Surgical Section Guidelines (Section 0),** subsection **B3. Root Operation,** subhead **Fusion procedures of the spine,** paragraphs **B3.10a, B3.10b,** and **B3.10c.**

Insertion

Insertion: Putting in nonbiological appliance that monitors, assists, performs, or prevents a physiological function but does not physically take the place of a body part . . . Character: H

This is another opportunity for reading very carefully. In ICD-10-PCS, this root operation applies only to the placement into the body of a medical device, such as a pacemaker, that will remain in the body after the procedure is completed.

> ### EXAMPLE
>
> *Insertion* is the placing of a device into the body.
>
> 05H933Z   Insertion of catheter (infusion device) into right brachial vein, percutaneous approach

Inspection

Inspection: Visually and/or manually exploring a body part . . . Character: J

This root operation term is limited to the physician's looking at the body part.

> ### EXAMPLE
>
> *Inspection* in this case is just like the English word . . . to look at.
>
> 09JEXZZ   Inspection of the left inner ear, external approach

GUIDANCE CONNECTION

Read the ICD-10-PCS Official Guidelines for Coding and Reporting, **Medical and Surgical Section Guidelines (Section 0),** subsection **B3. Root Operation,** subhead **Inspection procedures,** paragraphs **B3.11a, B3.11b,** and **B3.11c.**

Map

Map: Locating the route of passage of electrical impulses and/or locating functional areas in a body part . . . Character: **K**

Cardiac conduction mapping and brain mapping are two illustrations of this root operation. Note that this root operation term reports the examination only.

> **EXAMPLE**
>
> *Map* is a methodology that enables the physician to obtain a record of the function of a specific anatomical part.
>
> 00K03ZZ   Mapping of brain function, percutaneous approach

Occlusion

Occlusion: Completely closing an orifice or lumen of a tubular body part . . .
Character: **L**

There are times when an opening, such as a fistula, or a tubular body part, such as a fallopian tube, is purposely closed off or blocked.

> **EXAMPLE**
>
> *Occlusion* is the opposite of *dilation.*
>
> 0VLH4ZZ   Occlusion of spermatic cords, bilaterally, percutaneous endoscopic approach, no device

Reattachment

Reattachment: Putting back in or on all or a portion of a separated body part to its normal location or other suitable location . . . Character: **M**

This word is the same as the term most often used by physicians for this procedure, such as reattaching a finger after it has been severed during an accident.

> **EXAMPLE**
>
> *Reattachment* is reported for anatomical sites only.
>
> 0XMP0ZZ   Reattachment of left index finger, open approach

Release

Release: Freeing a body part from an abnormal physical constraint by cutting or by use of force . . . Character: **N**

The procedure reported with this root operation term involves cutting or separation only, such as tendon lengthening, in order to free a body part from some type of restriction.

> **EXAMPLE**
>
> *Release* is similar to *division,* so be careful to read the descriptions and the documentation very carefully.
>
> 0LNS0ZZ   Release of right ankle tendon, open approach

GUIDANCE CONNECTION

Read the ICD-10-PCS Official Guidelines for Coding and Reporting, **Medical and Surgical Section Guidelines (Section 0),** subsection **B3. Root Operation,** subhead **Occlusion vs. Restriction for vessel embolization procedures,** paragraph **B3.12.**

GUIDANCE CONNECTION

Read the ICD-10-PCS Official Guidelines for Coding and Reporting, **Medical and Surgical Section Guidelines (Section 0),** subsection **B3. Root Operation,** subhead **Release procedures,** paragraph **B3.13,** and **Release vs. Division,** paragraph **B3.14.**

Removal

Removal: Taking out or off a device from a body part . . . Character: **P**

Read this carefully: As the description specifically states "device," this can be used only for this type of procedure—to remove a previously inserted device. As you abstract the physician's notes, be cautious of the use of this term in documentation. The removal of a mole, for example, is really an excision, not a removal.

> **EXAMPLE**
>
> *Removal* is only used when a <u>device</u> has been removed.
>
> 0QP304Z   Removal of internal fixation device from left pelvic bone, open approach

Repair

Repair: Restoring, to the extent possible, a body part to its normal anatomic structure and function . . . Character: **Q**

> **EXAMPLE**
>
> *Repair* is often the therapeutic process of correcting an abnormality.
>
> 0CQV8ZZ   Repair of left vocal cord, via natural opening, endoscopic approach

Replacement

Replacement: Putting in or on biological or synthetic material that physically takes the place and/or function of all or a portion of a body part . . . Character: **R**

Essentially, this is the placement of a prosthetic device, such as a hip replacement or a prosthetic heart valve.

> **EXAMPLE**
>
> *Replacement* is directly related to the use of internal prosthetics.
>
> 02RG0JZ   Replacement of mitral valve with synthetic prosthesis, open approach

GUIDANCE CONNECTION

Read the ICD-10-PCS Official Guidelines for Coding and Reporting, **Medical and Surgical Section Guidelines (Section 0),** subsection **B3. Root Operation,** subhead **Reposition for fracture treatment,** paragraph **B3.15.**

Reposition

Reposition: Moving to its normal location or other suitable location all or a portion of a body part . . . Character: **S**

> **EXAMPLE**
>
> *Reposition* is the correction that is usually employed with a patient who has a dislocation.
>
> 0PSFXZZ   Reposition humeral shaft, right side, external approach

Resection

Resection: Cutting out or off, without replacement, all of a body part . . . Character: **T**

Remember how this differs from *excision*. When the entire body part is surgically removed, it is reported as a resection. If only a portion of the body part is removed, it is reported as an excision.

GUIDANCE CONNECTION

Read the ICD-10-PCS Official Guidelines for Coding and Reporting, **Medical and Surgical Section Guidelines (Section 0),** subsection **B3. Root Operation,** subhead **Excision vs. Resection,** paragraph **B3.8.**

> **EXAMPLE**
>
> *Resection* is the root operation term used for the surgical removal of an <u>entire</u> organ.
>
> 0FT44ZZ   Resection of gallbladder, percutaneous endoscopic approach

Restriction

> **Restriction: Partially closing an orifice or lumen of a tubular body part . . .**
> Character: **V**

Compare this with the root operation term *occlusion*. Restriction is a partial closure, and occlusion is a complete closure.

> **EXAMPLE**
>
> *Restriction* is a surgical methodology for limiting the function, or malfunction, of an anatomical site.
>
> 0DV44CZ   Restriction of esophagogastric junction, using extraluminal device, percutaneous endoscopic approach

Revision

> **Revision: Correcting, to the extent possible, a portion of a malfunctioning device or the position of a displaced device . . .** Character: **W**

Again, pay careful attention to the word *device*. This root operation term can only be used when a medical device is being fixed.

> **EXAMPLE**
>
> *Revision* is correcting the internal positioning of a device.
>
> 02WA0MZ   Revision of cardiac lead, open approach

Supplement

> **Supplement: Putting in or on biological or synthetic material that physically reinforces and/or augments the function of a portion of a body part . . .**
> Character: **U**

NOTE: In the Tables section, *supplement* is in alphabetic order by its character *U,* not by the term *supplement,* so it falls between *resection* and *restriction.*

> **EXAMPLES**
>
> *Supplement,* just as in English, is something that provides support.
>
> 0TUB4JZ   Supplementation of bladder, percutaneous endoscopic approach, using synthetic mesh
>
> 0YUA47Z   Use of autologous tissue substitute mesh to repair an inguinal hernia laparoscopically, bilateral

GUIDANCE CONNECTION

Read the ICD-10-PCS Official Guidelines for Coding and Reporting, **Medical and Surgical Section Guidelines (Section 0),** subsection **B3. Root Operation,** subhead **Transfer procedures using multiple tissue layers,** paragraph **B3.17.**

Transfer

Transfer: Moving, without taking out, all or a portion of a body part to another location to take over the function of all or a portion of a body part . . .
Character: **X**

> ### EXAMPLE
>
> *Transfer* is the process when the body part transferred still remains connected to its original vascular and nervous supply.
>
> 0JX03ZB Transfer of skin and subcutaneous tissue, scalp, percutaneous approach

Transplantation

Transplantation: Putting in or on all or a portion of a living body part taken from another individual or animal to physically take the place and/or function of all or a portion of a similar body part . . . Character: **Y**

ICD-10-PCS uses this term in the same manner that physicians do. However, this includes more than just organ transplant procedures.

> ### EXAMPLE
>
> *Transplantation* is the implanting of a donor body organ into a recipient.
>
> 0TY00Z0 Transplant of an allogeneic right kidney, open approach

GUIDANCE CONNECTION

Read the ICD-10-PCS Official Guidelines for Coding and Reporting, **Medical and Surgical Section Guidelines (Section 0),** subsection **B3. Root Operation,** subhead **Transplantation vs. Administration,** paragraph **B3.16.**

Adjusting Your Interpretations

As you abstract the physician's documentation, you may need to adjust some of your interpretative processes for reporting procedures using ICD-10-PCS. The root operation term is based on the objective of the procedure. You are seeking the word describing the action, such as *excision* or *drainage.* Combination terms with which you are very familiar, such as *colonoscopy, liver biopsy,* or *appendectomy,* may describe the procedure; however, these terms do not specifically explain the action of the physician, or do they? Let's take a closer look at these terms and interpret them into the root operation terms:

Colonoscopy: *colon* = "large intestine" (anatomical site) + -*oscopy* = "to view"

In ICD-10-PCS, you would use the root operation term *Inspection: Visually and/or manually exploring a body part.*

Liver biopsy: *liver* = anatomical site + *biopsy* = "excision of tissue for diagnostic purposes"

In ICD-10-PCS, you would use the root operation term *Excision: Cutting out or off, without replacement, a portion of a body part.* In just a bit, you will learn about adding a qualifier in the character 7 position to include the detail that this was a diagnostic excision.

Appendectomy: *append* = "appendix" (anatomical site) + -*ectomy* = "surgical removal"

In ICD-10-PCS, you would use the root operation term *Resection: Cutting out or off, without replacement, all of a body part.*

With some procedures, you will use your knowledge of the specific procedure and what it is expected to accomplish. For example, you will need to remember that lithotripsy is performed for *Fragmentation: Breaking solid matter in a body part into pieces,*

CODING BITES

Review *Appendix: Root Operation Definitions* in the back of your ICD-10-PCS code book.

which is done when a patient has kidney stones. Another example is thoracentesis (*thora* = "thorax [chest]" + *-centesis* = "puncture"), performed for *Drainage: Taking or letting out fluids and/or gases from a body part.*

YOU INTERPRET IT!

Practice interpreting from the common procedure terms used to reference the ICD-10-PCS root operation term. The Root Operation Definitions Appendix may help you.

11. Colostomy formation: _____
12. Cautery of skin lesion: _____
13. Transluminal angioplasty: _____
14. Choledocholithotomy: _____
15. Free skin graft: _____
16. Adhesiolysis: _____
17. Fallopian tube ligation: _____
18. Diagnostic arthroscopy: _____
19. Ankle arthrodesis: _____
20. Total nephrectomy: _____
21. Esophagogastric fundoplication: _____

33.3 Medical/Surgical Body Parts: Character 4

Character Position	Character Meaning
1	Section of the ICD-10-PCS book
2	Body system being treated
3	Root operation term
4	**Body part (specific anatomical site)**
5	Approach used by physician
6	Device
7	Qualifier

The fourth character position identifies the specific body part that is the focus of a procedure. The operative report or the procedure notes should be clear about these details. However, sometimes it can be a challenge to match the documentation to the choices offered in the tables. Following are some guidelines to help you determine the accurate code in ICD-10-PCS.

General Guidelines

There may be times when the notes are more specific than the code character specifics. If the physician documents that the procedure was performed on a specific anatomical site, such as the biceps femoris muscle, yet the listing of body parts under Muscles (Body System character K) does not provide this detail, you will need to code to the body part that includes this anatomical site. In this case, you would report Upper Leg Muscle.

Bilateral Procedures

If the documentation identifies that a procedure was performed on both a right body part and a left body part, and a Body Part code character is available to report the bilateral procedure, that is the one code to report. However, if there is no code character available to report a bilateral procedure, then you will need to report two codes: one for each procedure.

EXAMPLES

0HRV3KZ	Replacement of breasts, bilateral, percutaneous approach
0CNT8ZZ	Release of right vocal cord, via natural opening endoscopic
0CNV8ZZ	Release of left vocal cord, via natural opening endoscopic

Coronary Arteries

While the coronary arteries are represented by one code character, there are additional characters to report when more than one site is treated in this one set of arteries.

EXAMPLE

Dr. Forreau performed an angioplasty in the left anterior descending coronary artery in two distinct sites with two intraluminal, drug-eluting stents placed.

02713DZ	Dilation of coronary artery, two sites, percutaneous approach with intraluminal device, drug-eluting

Joints and Muscles

Many body systems provide individual code characters for body parts specific to a joint or a muscle. There are some cases when the Body Part characters may not be as specific as the physician's notes. The guidelines provide direction in determination of a code character to report the body part. When a procedure is performed on the skin, the subcutaneous tissue, or the fascia that is lying over a joint,

- Shoulder is reported as Upper Arm.
- Elbow is reported as Lower Arm.
- Wrist is reported as Lower Arm.
- Hip is reported as Upper Leg.
- Knee is reported as Lower Leg.
- Ankle is reported as Foot.

When a body system does not include a separate Body Part code character for fingers or toes,

- Finger is reported as Hand.
- Toe is reported as Foot.

Gastrointestinal Body System

Certain areas within the gastrointestinal Body System tables group the individual body parts of the intestinal tract into upper and lower. For these cases, the Upper Intestinal Tract includes the esophagus, stomach, and small intestine, up to and including the duodenum. The Lower Intestinal Tract includes the jejunum, ileum, cecum, and large intestine, all the way to and including the anus.

The **Body Part Key Appendix** in ICD-10-PCS also can help you when a specific anatomical site is documented and the Body Part components are not as specific. For instance, Stensen's duct is reported as the parotid duct, and the superior gluteal nerve is described in ICD-10-PCS as the lumbar plexus.

GUIDANCE CONNECTION

Read the ICD-10-PCS Official Guidelines for Coding and Reporting, **Medical and Surgical Section Guidelines (Section 0),** subsection **B4. Body Part,** paragraphs **B4.1a** through **B4.8.**

CODING BITES

Review **Appendix: Body Part Key** and **Appendix: Body Part Definitions** in the back of your ICD-10-PCS code book. Various publishers of ICD-10-PCS code books may present these appendices in a different order, and some may not include all. Don't worry. If your coding manual does not include appendices, you can download the Definitions, included within the file titled *2019 ICD-10-PCS Addendum,* from https://www.cms.gov/Medicare/Coding/ICD10/2019-ICD-10-PCS.html.

Practice using the Body Part Key Appendix and fill in the descriptions used by ICD-10-PCS for coding.

22. Superior olivary nucleus: _____

23. Sigmoid vein: _____

24. Right suprarenal vein: _____

25. Ulnar notch: _____

26. Ventricular fold: _____

27. Sweat gland: _____

28. Optic disc: _____

29. Oropharynx: _____

30. Nasal concha: _____

31. Manubrium: _____

32. Ischium: _____

33.4 Medical/Surgical Approaches: Character 5

Character Position	Character Meaning
1	Section of the ICD-10-PCS book
2	Body system being treated
3	Root operation term
4	Body part (specific anatomical site)
5	Approach used by physician
6	Device
7	Qualifier

GUIDANCE CONNECTION

Read the ICD-10-PCS Official Guidelines for Coding and Reporting, **Medical and Surgical Section Guidelines (Section 0)**, subhead **B5. Approach,** paragraphs **B5.2, B5.3a, B5.3b,** and **B5.4.**

As you continue to build a code, you can see that you are telling a story. The first four characters explain what the physician did and the anatomical site upon which he or she worked. Now, with the fifth character, you are going to explain how the physician got to the anatomical site to perform the procedure. This is known as the **approach**, and seven approaches are used within the *Medical and Surgical* section.

Approach
The path the physician took to access the body part upon which the treatment or procedure was targeted.

Open

Open: Cutting through the skin or mucous membrane and any other body layers necessary to expose the site of the procedure . . . Character: **0**

An open procedure is the traditional approach when the physician makes an incision into the body to access an internal organ. The operative notes should include the details of the incision, providing open access to the internal organ that needs the treatment.

EXAMPLES

You might see documentation that states:

". . . Attention was then turned to the patient's lower abdomen. Incision was made from symphysis pubis to umbilicus, midline. The incision was carried down through the dermis, subcutaneous fat, and linea alba using electrocautery. Preperitoneal fat was incised using electrocautery. Peritoneum was grasped with pickups. . . ."

(continued)

You can see that the physician describes the incision made, cutting through the subcutaneous and adipose layers to the peritoneum (the membrane that lines the abdominal cavity).

". . . The patient was taken to the operating room after being administered an epidural anesthetic, placed in the supine position, prepped and draped in a sterile fashion with a wedge under the right hip. A Pfannenstiel skin incision was made and carried down through layers along the old incision line. . . ."

In this excerpt from an operative report, the physician states this process more simply, but you can still understand that the patient is being cut into.

GUIDANCE CONNECTION

Read the ICD-10-PCS Official Guidelines for Coding and Reporting, **Medical and Surgical Section Guidelines (Section 0),** subsection **B5. Approach,** subhead **Open approach with percutaneous endoscopic assistance,** paragraph **B5.2.**

Percutaneous

Percutaneous: Entry, by puncture or minor incision, of instrumentation through the skin or mucous membrane and any other body layers necessary to reach the site of the procedure . . . Character: **3**

When a percutaneous approach is used, the physician cannot see inside the body. Often, a radiologist will provide imaging guidance (which would be reported separately). A needle aspiration and needle biopsy are good illustrations of a percutaneous approach.

EXAMPLE

You might see documentation that states:

". . . The patient was prepped and draped in the usual fashion. A long, thin needle is inserted through the patient's abdominal wall, periumbilical quadrant, passed into the amniotic sac. Ultrasound guidance is used. When puncture into the sac is confirmed, a small sample of amniotic fluid is extracted and sent to the lab. . . ."

A needle is inserted through the dermis (percutaneously) all the way into the amniotic sac. The fact that ultrasound guidance was used supports the fact that the physician could not see where the point of the needle was going (no scope to see inside; no internal visualization).

Percutaneous Endoscopic

Percutaneous Endoscopic: Entry, by puncture or minor incision, of instrumentation through the skin or mucous membrane and any other body layers necessary to reach and visualize the site of the procedure . . . Character: **4**

In this type of approach, a scope is placed through the incision or puncture. A laparoscopic procedure is a good example.

EXAMPLES

You might see documentation that states:

". . . The patient was positioned supine on the operating room table. . . . A small umbilical incision allowed for introduction of the Veress needle and inflation of the abdomen to 15 cm of water pressure using carbon dioxide gas. The 0 degree, 5-mm laparoscope was introduced through a 5-mm port at the umbilicus and 3 additional ports were placed in the usual anatomic positions. The liver was found to be markedly enlarged. . . ."

> A percutaneous endoscopic approach also can be described as a laparoscopic procedure. This approach also can be recognized by the description of a "small" incision, which only needs to be large enough to fit the endoscope through, typically about one inch long (2.54 cm).

Via Natural or Artificial Opening

<u>Via Natural or Artificial Opening</u>: Entry of instrumentation through a natural or artificial external opening to reach the site of the procedure . . . Character: 7

The natural openings to the body include the nose, mouth, ear, vagina, urethra, and anus. An artificial opening includes a stoma (an opening that has been surgically created).

EXAMPLE

> "... A weighted speculum was placed in the posterior vaginal wall and the right-angle retractor used to visualize the cervix. The cervix was grasped across the anterior lip with a single-toothed tenaculum. . . . The cervix was circumferentially excised with the scalpel. . . ."

This excerpt is from the operative notes for a vaginal hysterectomy. Just the name tells you that the approach was via the patient's vagina, but you know that the name is insufficient upon which to support a code. As you read the description of what the physician did, you know you have the documentation to support the reporting of this hysterectomy being performed using a vaginal (natural opening) approach.

Via Natural or Artificial Opening Endoscopic

<u>Via Natural or Artificial Opening Endoscopic</u>: Entry of instrumentation through a natural or artificial external opening to reach and visualize the site of the procedure . . . Character: 8

Note that the difference between this approach and "via natural or artificial opening" is the use of an endoscope to visualize the anatomical site upon which the procedure will be performed.

EXAMPLES

You might see documentation that states:

> "... The patient was placed in the dorsolithotomy position on a cystoscopy table, prepped and draped in the usual fashion. A #21 French cystoscope was passed through the urethra into the bladder. . . ."

The urethra is the anatomical tube that leads from the urinary bladder to the outside of the body. This is a natural opening into visceral organs, such as the bladder, ureters, and kidneys. The insertion of the cystoscope through the urethra is an endoscope being used to see inside the body via a natural opening.

> "... The patient was brought to the operative suite, placed in the supine position. After satisfactory induction of general endotracheal anesthesia, a flexible Olympus bronchoscope was passed through the endotracheal tube, visualizing the distal trachea, carina, right and left main stem bronchus with primary and secondary divisions. . . ."

Your understanding of anatomy will help you identify this natural opening—the pharynx is the medical term for the throat. The bronchoscope was threaded through the patient's mouth, down the throat, into the bronchi.

Via Natural or Artificial Opening with Percutaneous Endoscopic Assistance

Via Natural or Artificial Opening with Percutaneous Endoscopic Assistance: Entry of instrumentation through a natural or artificial external opening and entry, by puncture or minor incision, of instrumentation through the skin or mucous membrane and any other body layers necessary to aid in the performance of the procedure . . . Character: **F**

This approach is kind of a combination endoscopic (laparoscopic) approach along with the use of a natural or artificial opening.

EXAMPLE

You might see documentation that states:

". . . The endoscope is inserted into the esophagus and down into the esophogastric junction. The anterior aspect of the gastric lining is visualized. A 2.5-cm incision is made into the right lateral aspect of the abdominal wall to allow for the insertion of the gastrostomy tube. . . ."

This excerpt from the documentation of the placement of a feeding tube (also known as a G-tube) uses a percutaneous endoscopic gastrostomy (PEG) approach along with the natural opening approach of the mouth for the esophagogastro-duodenoscope (EGD).

External

External: Procedure performed directly on the skin or mucous membrane and procedures performed indirectly by the application of external force through the skin or mucous membrane . . . Character: **X**

👥 GUIDANCE CONNECTION

Read the ICD-10-PCS Official Guidelines for Coding and Reporting, **Medical and Surgical Section Guidelines (Section 0),** subsection **B5. Approach,** subhead **External approach,** paragraphs **B5.3a** and **B5.3b.**

EXAMPLES

You might see documentation that states:

". . . Used the McIvor mouth gag to retract the tongue and endotracheal tube inferiorly, giving good exposure to the oropharynx. The tonsils were visualized. . . ."

As you read this physician's description, it clearly indicates that the patient's mouth was held open so the *tonsils were visualized* . . . seen by the naked eye. There were no incisions or penetrations through the tissues, neither was any type of scope used.

". . . Upper eyelid incision was performed in the skin with 15 blade scalpel. . . ."

The eyelid is right there, on the outside (external) part of the body. Again, no incisions, penetrations through the tissues, or any type of scope was necessary.

CODING BITES

As you abstract the documentation and interpret the way the physician describes how the procedure was performed, you may find ***Appendix: Components of the Medical and Surgical Approach Definitions*** or ***Approach Table*** in your ICD-10-PCS code book helpful. Various publishers of ICD-10-PCS code books may present these appendices in a different order, and some may not include all. Don't worry. If your coding manual does not include appendices, you can download the Definitions, included within the file titled *2019 ICD-10-PCS Addendum,* from https://www.cms.gov/Medicare/Coding/ICD10/2019-ICD-10-PCS.html.

Practice using the Medical and Surgical Approach Definitions Appendix or the Approach Table and fill in the approach used by ICD-10-PCS for coding.

33. Liposuction: _____

34. Sigmoidoscopy: _____

35. Laparoscopic hysterectomy: _____

36. Fracture manipulation (closed): _____

37. Traditional cholecystectomy: _____

38. Foley catheter placement: _____

39. Lumbar puncture: _____

40. Breast biopsy with guidance: _____

41. Endoscopy: _____

42. Cesarean section: _____

43. Blepharotomy: _____

33.5 Medical/Surgical Devices: Character 6

Character Position	Character Meaning
1	Section of the ICD-10-PCS book
2	Body system being treated
3	Root operation term
4	Body part (specific anatomical site)
5	Approach used by physician
6	Device
7	Qualifier

GUIDANCE CONNECTION

Read the ICD-10-PCS Official Guidelines for Coding and Reporting, **Medical and Surgical Section Guidelines (Section 0),** subsection **B6. Device,** paragraphs **B6.1a, B6.1b, B6.1c,** and **B6.2.**

As you can see, a character placed in the sixth position will identify a device that will remain with the patient after the procedure has been completed. ICD-10-PCS qualifies these generalized types of devices:

- Grafts
- Prostheses
- Implants
- Simple or mechanical appliances
- Electronic appliances

Reading through the *Medical and Surgical* section, with a focus on some of the options for the sixth character, you will find a limited number of descriptors. Let's take a closer look at these:

Grafts
    Autologous Tissue . . . Character: **7**
    Autologous Venous Tissue . . . Character: **9**
    Autologous Arterial Tissue . . . Character: **A**

This refers to a graft made with tissue from the patient's own body.

    Synthetic Substitute . . . Character: **J**

This explains that the graft material may be carbon fibers, polypropylene, or other non-human substance.

Nonautologous Tissue Substitute . . . Character: **K**

This graft is made from materials other than the patient's own tissue.

Zooplastic Tissue . . . Character: **8**

This identifies that the graft was made with tissue from a species other than human.

Simple or Mechanical Appliances

Drainage Device . . . Character: **0**
Monitoring Device . . . Character: **2**
Monitoring Device, Pressure Sensor . . . Character: **0**
Infusion Device . . . Character: **3**
Extraluminal Device . . . Character: **C**
Intraluminal Device . . . Character: **D**
Intraluminal Device, Two . . . Character: **E**
Intraluminal Device, Three . . . Character: **F**
Intraluminal Device, Four or More . . . Character: **G**
Intraluminal Device, Drug-Eluting . . . Character: **4**
Intraluminal Device, Drug-Eluting, Two . . . Character: **5**
Intraluminal Device, Drug-Eluting, Three . . . Character: **6**
Intraluminal Device, Drug-Eluting, Four or More . . . Character: **7**
Bioactive Intraluminal Device . . . Character: **B**
Intraluminal Device, Radioactive . . . Character: **T**

Implants and Electronic Appliances

Stimulator (Cardiac) Lead . . . Character: **M**
Cardiac Lead, Pacemaker . . . Character: **J**
Intracardiac Pacemaker . . . Character: **N**
Implantable Heart Assist System . . . Character: **Q**
External Heart Assist System . . . Character: **R**
Radioactive Element . . . Character: **1**
No Device . . . Character: **Z**

In operative reports and procedure notes, when a device is placed into the patient, the notes will identify the brand name and details, rather than "synthetic substitute" or "intraluminal device." For instance, an AxiaLIF® System is an interbody fusion device used in lower joints, or Ultrapro plug is a synthetic substitute. Don't panic. You don't have to memorize these brand names. Just bookmark *Appendix: Device Key and Aggregation Table* in your ICD-10-PCS code book.

EXAMPLES

How can you determine if a device was implanted into the patient? The documentation will state something like one of these surgical notes excerpts.

". . . A Kapandji technique was also used for intrafocal pinning, taking a 0.062 K-wire in both the radial and ulnar aspects of the distal fragment and elevating it, followed by reducing it, controlling the distal fragment. . . ."

". . . A Palmaz Blue Genesis stent, 6 × 80 mm was used. It was deployed across the left renal artery stenosis in good position. . . ."

". . . A stylet (a thin wire) is inserted inside the center channel of the pacemaker lead to make it more rigid, and the lead-stylet combination is then inserted into the sheath and advanced under fluoroscopy to the appropriate heart chamber. . . ."

Practice using the Device Key Appendix and fill in the device description used by ICD-10-PCS for coding.

44. Bovine pericardial valve: _____

45. Acuity Steerable Lead: _____

46. Embolization coil(s): _____

47. Tissue bank graft: _____

48. Pump reservoir: _____

49. Lap-Band® Adjustable Gastric Banding System: _____

50. Prestige cervical disc: _____

51. Versa: _____

52. Novacor Left Ventricular Assist Device: _____

53. EndoSure® sensor: _____

54. Brachytherapy seeds: _____

33.6 Medical/Surgical Qualifiers: Character 7

Character Position	Character Meaning
1	Section of the ICD-10-PCS book
2	Body system being treated
3	Root operation term
4	Body part (specific anatomical site)
5	Approach used by physician
6	Device
7	**Qualifier**

This seventh character is required. In many cases, there may be no more details to add, so you will use the placeholder **Z** No Qualifier—the equivalent of "not applicable."

You will find that, depending on the procedure provided, you may need to check the documentation for applicable details. For instance, when an excision is performed, you may find a Qualifier character option to explain that this was a biopsy (for diagnostic purposes . . . character **X**).

Earlier in this chapter, in the section that discussed root operation terms, you learned that bypass procedures are coded by identifying the body part bypassed "from," identified by character 4 (Body Part), and the body part bypassed "to," identified by character 7 (Qualifier). This is just a reminder that, in some cases, the Qualifier character will partner with the Body Part character to explain the whole story about the procedure.

EXAMPLE

0D164JA   Gastric bypass, percutaneous endoscopic approach, rerouted from stomach to jejunum

 LET'S CODE IT! SCENARIO

Callie MacDonald, a 2-year-old female, was admitted to the hospital by her ophthalmologist, Dr. Epps. Her right lacrimal duct was occluded. After sedation was administered, Dr. Epps probed her nasolacrimal duct and inserted

(continued)

a transluminal balloon catheter to expand the duct. The balloon was deflated and removed. She tolerated the procedure well.

Let's Code It!

Let's go through the steps of coding for ICD-10-PCS and determine the code or codes that should be reported for this encounter between Dr. Epps, an ophthalmologist, and Callie MacDonald.

> **First character: Section: Medical and Surgical . . . 0**
> **Second character: Body System: Eye . . . 8**

What root operation term would be most accurate? Read through the scenario carefully. Dr. Epps "expanded" the duct. The description of the term "dilation" is to expand an orifice or the lumen of a tubular body part.

> **Third character: Root Operation: Dilation . . . 7**

Now, which "tubular body part" was dilated? The scenario states, "*Her right lacrimal duct . . .*"

You may have been tempted to think "eye"; however, when you get to the table for Eye, Dilation . . . 087, you will see that "eye" is the Body System and not an option for Body Part.

> **Fourth character: Body Part: Lacrimal Duct, Right . . . X**

Dr. Epps inserted the catheter directly into the duct (this opening is how our tears flow from our eyes). Therefore, he used a natural opening.

> **Fifth character: Approach: Via Natural or Artificial Opening . . . 7**

Dr. Epps inserted a *transluminal balloon catheter;* however, then the documentation states, "*The balloon was deflated and removed.*" Therefore, there is no Device reported in this position.

> **Sixth Character: Device: No Device . . . Z**
> **Seventh Character: Qualifier: No Qualifier . . . Z**

The ICD-10-PCS code you will report is

> **087X7ZZ   Dilation, lacrimal duct, right, via natural or artificial opening**

Good job!!

33.7 Multiple and Discontinued Procedures in Medical and Surgical Cases

Multiple Procedures

> **GUIDANCE CONNECTION**
>
> Read the ICD-10-PCS Official Guidelines for Coding and Reporting, **Medical and Surgical Section Guidelines (Section 0),** subsection **B3. Root Operation,** subhead **Multiple procedures,** paragraph **B3.2.**

Just because the physician performs more than one procedure does not necessarily mean you will report more than one code. The Official Guidelines provide four illustrations of cases when you will report multiple procedures:

a. *The same root operation is performed on different body parts as defined by distinct values of the body part character.* Two codes are reported.

b. *The same root operation is repeated at different body sites that are included in the same body part value.* You will report the same code twice. It is recommended that a report to explain is appended.

c. *Multiple root operations with distinct objectives are performed on the same body part.* Two codes are reported, one for each root operation.

d. *The intended root operation is attempted using one approach but is converted to a different approach.* One code will report what was actually accomplished with the first approach, and a second code will report the second approach.

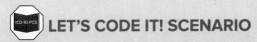 **LET'S CODE IT! SCENARIO**

Ronald Markum, a 21-year-old male, was riding his motorcycle when he skidded out. The bike fell on top of him and his left ankle was dislocated. He was admitted into the hospital, and Dr. Traub tried to manually realign the tarsal bone to its rightful position. Unfortunately, he was unable to accomplish this and had to take Ronald to the OR to perform an open procedure.

Let's Code It!

Let's go through the steps of coding for ICD-10-PCS and determine the code or codes that should be reported for this encounter between Dr. Traub and Ronald Markum.

First code:

First character: Section: Medical and Surgical . . . 0

What is the body system? The documentation states, "*tarsal bone.*"That is in the ankle . . . therefore, **Lower Bones.**

Second character: Body System: Lower Bones . . . Q

What did the physician actually do? The documentation states, "*manually realign the tarsal bone to its rightful position.*" Read the definitions of the root operation terms. This matches **Reposition.**

Third character: Root Operation: Reposition . . . S

What body part was treated? The documentation states, "*his left ankle*" + "*the tarsal bone.*"

Fourth character: Body Part: Tarsal, Left . . . M

What was the approach? Did the physician go into the body? No, treatment was done from the outside.

Fifth character: Approach: External . . . X

Was any device inserted into the patient and left there? There is no mention of this.

Sixth Character: Device: No Device . . . Z

No details left to report.

Seventh Character: Qualifier: No Qualifier . . . Z

The ICD-10-PCS code you will report is

0QSMXZZ   Reposition, left tarsal bone, externally

Remember the guideline about multiple procedures, B3.2, part d. You will need a second code to report the second attempt to realign Ronald's ankle. Notice the differences between the first attempt and the second attempt. The only difference is that the procedure was changed from an EXTERNAL approach to an OPEN approach.

Second code:

First character: Section: Medical and Surgical . . . 0
Second character: Body System: Lower Bones . . . Q
Third character: Root Operation: Reposition . . . S
Fourth character: Body Part: Tarsal, Left . . . M
Fifth character: Approach: Open . . . 0
Sixth character: Device: No Device . . . Z
Seventh character: Qualifier: No Qualifier . . . Z

The ICD-10-PCS code you will report is

0QSM0ZZ   Reposition, left tarsal bone, open approach

Finally, consider in what sequence you will report these two codes. The rule is that the most intense procedure will be reported first, so you should report the open procedure first, followed by the external approach.

0QSM0ZZ   Reposition, left tarsal bone, open approach
0QSMXZZ   Reposition, left tarsal bone, externally

Good job!

Discontinued Procedures

It has happened: The physician begins a procedure and for some reason must stop before accomplishing the goal originally planned. Should this occur, you are directed to report those root operations that were actually done.

> ### 👥➡ GUIDANCE CONNECTION
>
> Read the ICD-10-PCS Official Guidelines for Coding and Reporting, **Medical and Surgical Section Guidelines (Section 0)**, subsection **B3. Root Operation**, subhead **Discontinued or incomplete procedures**, paragraph **B3.3**, for more details.

> ### EXAMPLE
>
> Dr. Zander has planned a laparoscopic cholecystectomy. The incisions are made and the scope is inserted. The gallbladder can be visualized. However, before the organ can be surgically removed, the patient has a seizure. Dr. Zander stops the procedure and closes the incisions.
>
> 0FJ44ZZ   Inspection of gallbladder, percutaneous endoscopic approach

 YOU CODE IT! CASE STUDY

Nita Yessa has been in the hospital with a compound fracture of the leg, and she was brought into the procedure room to have her two-lead pacemaker replaced. Dr. Balthazar was able to remove her current pacemaker easily. However, there was a problem with the new device and he did not want to insert it. He closed the incision and sent Nita back to her room. He told Rita Holsman, his assistant, to notify him as soon as a new pacemaker was available.

You Code It!

Dr. Balthazar intended to replace Nita's pacemaker, but he couldn't complete the procedure. Using your ICD-10-PCS code book, determine the correct code to report this procedure.

Step #1: Read the case carefully and completely.

Step #2: Abstract the scenario. Which key words or terms describe what service the physician provided to the patient during this encounter?

Step #3: Are there any details missing or incomplete for which you would need to query the physician? [If so, ask your instructor.]

Step #4: Build the correct ICD-10-PCS procedure code or codes to explain the details about what was provided to the patient during this encounter.

Step #5: Check for any relevant guidance.

Step #6: Double-check your work.

Answer:

Did you determine this to be the correct code?

    02PA3QZ   **Removal of implantable heart assist system, percutaneous approach**

As Guideline B3.3 directs you, when an intended procedure is discontinued, you need to code for what was actually completed. Dr. Balthazar was able to remove the old pacemaker, so you must code for the removal. You cannot code for the insertion of the new pacemaker because this was not done.

    Good work!

33.8 Medical/Surgical Coding: Putting It All Together

 LET'S CODE IT! SCENARIO

PATIENT: Randolph Joy

HISTORY OF PRESENT ILLNESS: Patient was admitted to the Medical/Surgical floor last evening with acute upper abdominal pain and dyspnea. Blood work results were inconclusive, as was x-ray. Today, we are going to perform an EGD to investigate further.

PROCEDURE PERFORMED: Esophagogastroduodenoscopy

MEDICATIONS: Fentanyl 50 mcg, Versed 4 mg.

DESCRIPTION OF PROCEDURE: Informed consent was obtained. The patient was then placed in the left lateral decubitus position. IV sedation was started in a sequential fashion until the appropriate level of consciousness was achieved. Hurricaine spray was applied to the back of the throat and the endoscope was then advanced under direct visualization over the tongue, the esophagus, stomach, and duodenum. It was slowly withdrawn and the mucosa was carefully evaluated. Duodenal mucosal abnormalities were not visualized. Antegrade and retrograde views of the stomach did demonstrate some mild nonerosive gastritis, predominantly in the antrum. Portal gastropathy was noted throughout the gastric body, cardia, and fundus. Thickened gastric folds were noted and biopsied. Retroflexed view as well demonstrated no signs of a gastric varix; no coffee grounds or red blood was seen in the gastric lumen either. The scope was then withdrawn through the GE junction and careful examination did demonstrate shallow esophageal ulceration distally; biopsies were obtained. The suspicion of Barrett's esophagus noted with two salmon tongues of mucosa emanating 1 cm proximal to the GE junction. Careful examination of the remainder of the esophagus did demonstrate a hyperemic esophagus without further ulceration. The scope was then withdrawn from the patient and the procedure terminated. It was well tolerated and there were no immediate complications.

POST-PROCEDURE DIAGNOSES:
1. Probable Barrett's esophagus
2. Distal esophageal ulceration
3. Thickened hypertrophied gastric folds
4. Portal gastropathy and nonerosive gastritis

IMPRESSION AND PLAN: I suspect this patient's upper GI bleed is likely related to the ulcerations noted on this examination. As we await results of biopsies, I will change his proton pump inhibitor from an IV drip to oral and begin oral feeding as well. Hemoglobin and hematocrit will continue to be followed and, if stable, discharge may take place tomorrow.

Let's Code It!

Dr. Ferrante performed an EGD to visually inspect Randolph's interior stomach to determine the cause of the pain and respiratory issues.

First character: Section: Medical and Surgical . . . 0

(continued)

An esophagogastroduodenoscopy was performed. What body system does this involve? You learned about this in medical terminology class. *Esopha-* = esophagus + *-gastro-* = stomach + *-duoden-* = duodenum. To what body system do these anatomical sites belong?

Second character: System: Gastrointestinal System . . . D

Dr. Ferrante performed an EGD to visually inspect Randolph's interior stomach to determine the cause of the pain. This would point to the root operation term *inspection*. However, then tissue biopsies were taken, which points to the root operation term *excision*. Do you report two ICD-10-PCS codes? Let's analyze this. They are two different reasons for the procedure; however, while an inspection could be done without any excisions, the fact is that the biopsies could not be acquired without the inspection. Therefore, you only need one code, using the root operation term *Excision*.

Third character: Root Operation: Excision . . . B

From what anatomical site were the biopsies taken? The documentation states, "*esophageal ulceration distally; biopsies were obtained.*"

Fourth character: Body Part/Region: Esophagus, Lower . . . 3

How did Dr. Ferrante get to the distal (lower) esophagus? The documentation states, "*the endoscope was then advanced under direct visualization. . . .*"

Fifth character: Approach: Via Natural or Artificial Opening Endoscopic . . . 8
Sixth character: Device: No Device . . . Z

Our last character will explain the essential reason for this procedure. Was it to gather details to support a diagnosis (i.e., diagnostic)? Or was it to repair or fix a problem (i.e., therapeutic)?

Seventh character: Qualifier: Diagnostic . . . X

Now, you can put all of these characters together to report the ICD-10-PCS code, with confidence:

0DB38ZX   **Esophagogastroduodenoscopy, with biopsies, diagnostic**

Good work!

LET'S CODE IT! SCENARIO

PATIENT: Gary Salton

PREOPERATIVE DIAGNOSIS: Subdural hematoma, traumatic

HISTORY OF PRESENT ILLNESS: This is a 17-year-old male, legally blind since birth, admitted after an assault. During the assault, he suffered extensive subarachnoid hemorrhage, LeFort fracture of the face, right arm venous phlebitis, and subdural hematoma. He was maintained on SICU, prophylaxis Dilantin, because of extensive subarachnoid hemorrhage. He went to the OR for facial ORIF. His course was complicated by ventricular tachycardia, but he was ruled out for MI at that time. He was started on amiodarone for the rate control. He also suffered a mandibular fracture so PEG was placed because of his inability to eat. No mention is made of acute seizure in this patient. There is no report of MRIs anywhere in the documentation. Preadmission summary states intracerebral hemorrhage and subdural hematoma, although they do not state where. He had to be emergently intubated due to hypoxemia. Other complications, during his hospital course, include cellulitis around the trach site, FUOs, and sinusitis. He has phlebitis in his right forearm. Repeat head CT showed increased bilateral frontal subdural hygroma and subarachnoid hemorrhage. He also developed hyphema of the right eye.

PAST MEDICAL HISTORY: Hypertension

FAMILY HISTORY: Hypertension and stroke

SOCIAL HISTORY: He smokes a pack a day and occasional alcohol. Otherwise, independent prior to the admission.

(continued)

MEDICATIONS: Prednisone, bacitracin topical cream, amiodarone, vancomycin, methadone b.i.d., dalteparin subcu daily, BuSpar 10 mg b.i.d., metoprolol 50 mg b.i.d., Pepcid, and Percocet.

PROCEDURE: Patient was taken to the OR for excision of frontal subdural hygroma and subarachnoid hemorrhage for evacuation. Once endotracheal administration of anesthesia was accomplished, patient was prepped and draped in the usual fashion, in a supine position. Using the drill, one small hole was made in the skull to relieve pressure and allow blood and fluids to be drained from the anterior cerebral vein. This was accomplished, and suction was applied to ensure the area was cleaned thoroughly. The area was bandaged and the patient was aroused successfully.

Scott Taucher, MD

Let's Code It!

Dr. Taucher drained Gary Salton's anterior cerebral vein. Let's analyze the documentation and build the code.

First character: Section: Medical and Surgical . . . 0

What specific body system was operated upon? The documentation states, "*anterior cerebral vein.*" The body system, therefore, would be the cerebrovascular system. However, there is not one character to cover this. Instead, you have four: **3** Upper Arteries; **4** Lower Arteries; **5** Upper Veins; and **6** Lower Veins. In which of these does the "*anterior cerebral vein*" fit? Cerebral indicates the brain, and, therefore, Upper Veins.

Second character: System: Upper Veins . . . 5

What did Dr. Taucher actually do in this procedure? The documentation states, "*allow blood and fluids to be drained.*"

Third character: Root Operation: Drainage . . . 9

Now, turn to the 059 Table in the Tables section. Read carefully through the options listed for the fourth character. Can you find "*anterior cerebral vein*"? You can see it with a broader descriptor . . .

Fourth character: Body Part: Intracranial Vein . . . L

Do you see the specific type of approach used in this procedure? The documentation states, "*Using the drill, one small hole was made in the skull.*"

Fifth character: Approach: Open . . . 0

Go back to the notes. Was a device placed into the patient and left there after the procedure ended?

Sixth character: Device: No Device . . . Z

Did Dr. Taucher do this to gather information to determine a diagnosis, or was this to fix or repair a problem?

Seventh character: Qualifier: No Qualifier . . . Z

Now you can put all of these characters together to report this ICD-10-PCS code, with confidence:

059L0ZZ   **Drainage of intracranial vein, open approach**

Good work!

 LET'S CODE IT! SCENARIO

PATIENT: Anabelle Preston

DATE OF OPERATION: 10/18/2019

PREOPERATIVE DIAGNOSIS: Bilateral urolithiasis

POSTOPERATIVE DIAGNOSIS: Bilateral urolithiasis

(continued)

OPERATIONS PERFORMED:
1. Cystoscopy
2. Right retrograde pyelogram
3. Right ureteral stent placement
4. Right percutaneous nephrolithotripsy

SURGEON: Sonia Petrosky, MD

ANESTHESIA: Laryngeal mask general

ANESTHESIOLOGIST: Matthew Sorensten, MD

ESTIMATED BLOOD LOSS: Minimal

IV FLUIDS: 2.5 liters crystalloid

DRAINS: A #5-French × 28 cm right double-pigtail ureteral stent and #18-French Foley catheter

COMPLICATIONS: None

INDICATIONS: The patient is a 63-year-old female, admitted last night through the ED with acute right flank pain, who denies prior history of kidney stones. She underwent parathyroidectomy 3 years ago. She stated that over the past few weeks she had intermittent right flank pain. An ultrasound showed mild dilation of the right collecting system with an 11-mm stone. Smaller stones were noted in the left kidney without any hydronephrosis. This was confirmed on her KUB showing an 11-mm stone in the right mid kidney and three stones on the left measuring 3–6 mm. She has had follow-up testing showing a 24-hour urine calcium output of only 90 mg. Her serum calcium level is normal.

DESCRIPTION OF THE PROCEDURE: The patient was brought to the lithotripsy suite. After induction of laryngeal mask general anesthesia, she was placed in dorsal lithotomy position. Perineum and introitus were prepped and draped. A #22-French rigid cystoscope was passed per urethra with obturator. The bladder was drained and then inspected with 12- and 70-degree lenses. She has a central cystocele. Both orifices appear normal. Minimal squamous metaplasia in the bladder neck area and no suspicious mucosal changes elsewhere. No trabeculation noted. Pollack catheter was threaded into the right ureter and dilute contrast was used to perform segmental pyelogram images on the right. Distally, multiple pelvic calcifications are lateral to the ureter consistent with phleboliths. No obvious filling defects seen. There is mild dilation of the majority of the collecting system above the pelvic brim. The stone appeared to be free floating within the renal pelvis.

Sensor guidewire was threaded up into the kidney. The Pollack catheter was inserted over the wire and the ureteral length was estimated. The contrast in the kidney was also allowed to drain to improve visualization of the stone for lithotripsy. The guidewire was then replaced and the Pollack catheter removed. A #5-French × 28-cm Polaris double-pigtail stent was then inserted with good pigtail formation on both ends. Cystoscope was removed and replaced with an #18-French Foley catheter.

Next, we performed a percutaneous nephrolithotripsy on the right kidney stone in the ureteropelvic junction. The stone appeared to fragment well. Periodic AP and oblique fluoroscopy was used. The patient was awakened, extubated, and transported to the recovery room in stable condition.

Let's Code It!

Dr. Petrosky completed two procedures on Annabelle during this session: insertion of a stent + the percutaneous nephrolithotripsy. Let's begin with the nephrolithotripsy:

First character: Section: Medical and Surgical . . . 0

These procedures were performed on Annabelle's kidneys. Therefore, the body system is the

Second character: System: Urinary System . . . T

What exactly does a nephrolithotripsy do? This procedure is performed to remove kidney stones by breaking them up. A good clue is in the documentation, where it states, "The stone appeared to fragment well."

Third character: Root Operation: Fragmentation . . . F

Read the options listed in the Body Part (character 4) column of this Table. The documentation states, "*in the ureteropelvic junction.*" There is an additional descriptor under Kidney Pelvis, which also matches the

(continued)

documentation, which states, "*The stone appeared to be free floating within the renal pelvis*" and "*on the right kidney stone.*"

Fourth character: Body Part/Region: Kidney Pelvis, Right . . . 3

What approach was used to access the kidney stone to fragment it? The documentation states, "*percutaneous.*"

Fifth character: Approach: Percutaneous . . . 3

The options for the sixth and seventh characters are straightforward.

Sixth character: Device: No Device . . . Z
Seventh character: Qualifier: No Qualifier . . . Z

Now, you can put all of these characters together to report this ICD-10-PCS code, with confidence:

0TF33ZZ   Nephrolithotripsy, percutaneous, kidney pelvis, right.

Good work!

Chapter Summary

This chapter showed you that building a code in ICD-10-PCS may require you to become familiar with a different perspective and way of interpreting the physician's notes. However, it all fits together, even though you will be using your knowledge in a slightly different way.

The ICD-10-PCS is used for reporting procedures performed in hospital inpatient health care settings only. And the ***Medical and Surgical Section*** code components are necessary for the largest percentage of procedures provided to patients while admitted to a hospital.

CODING BITES

Medical and Surgical Section character positions and their meanings:

Character Position	Character Meaning
1	Section of the ICD-10-PCS book
2	Body system being treated
3	Root operation term
4	Body part (specific anatomical site)
5	Approach used by physician
6	Device
7	Qualifier

You Interpret It! Answers

1. Lower Arteries, **2.** Lymphatic and Hemic Systems, **3.** Eye, **4.** Mouth and Throat, **5.** Gastrointestinal System, **6.** Muscles, **7.** Head and Facial Bones, **8.** Lower Bones, **9.** Upper Joints, **10.** Respiratory System, **11.** Bypass, **12.** Destruction, **13.** Dilation, **14.** Extirpation, **15.** Replacement, **16.** Release, **17.** Occlusion, **18.** Inspection, **19.** Fusion, **20.** Resection, **21.** Restriction, **22.** Pons, **23.** Inferior Mesenteric Vein, **24.** Inferior Vena Cava, **25.** Radius, **26.** Larynx, **27.** Skin, **28.** Retina, **29.** Pharynx, **30.** Nasal Turbinate,

31. Sternum, **32.** Pelvic Bone, **33.** Percutaneous, **34.** Via Natural or Artificial Opening Endoscopic, **35.** Via Natural or Artificial Opening with Percutaneous Endoscopic Assistance, **36.** External, **37.** Open, **38.** Via Natural or Artificial Opening, **39.** Percutaneous, **40.** Percutaneous, **41.** Via Natural or Artificial Opening Endoscopic, **42.** Open, **43.** External, **44.** Zooplastic Tissue, **45.** Cardiac Lead, **46.** Intraluminal Device, **47.** Nonautologous Tissue Substitute, **48.** Infusion Device, Pump, **49.** Extraluminal Device, **50.** Synthetic Substitute, **51.** Pacemaker, Dual Chamber, **52.** Implantable Heart Assist System, **53.** Monitoring Device, Pressure Sensor, **54.** Radioactive Element

CHAPTER 33 REVIEW
ICD-10-PCS Medical and Surgical Section

Enhance your learning by completing these exercises and more at mcgrawhillconnect.com!

Let's Check It! Terminology

Match each key term to the appropriate definition.

1. LO 33.1 A letter or number component of an ICD-10-PCS code.
2. LO 33.4 The path the physician took to access the body part upon which the treatment or procedure was targeted.
3. LO 33.2 The term used to describe the function or purpose of the procedure.

A. Approach
B. Character
C. Root Operation Term

Let's Check It! Concepts

Choose the most appropriate answer for each of the following questions.

1. LO 33.1 Character position 4 represents which of the following?
   a. The body system being treated
   b. The approach used by the physician
   c. The body part (specific anatomical site)
   d. A device

2. LO 33.1 Character position 2: Body Systems: The endocrine system is identified by what number or letter?
   a. 2
   b. G
   c. 7
   d. S

3. LO 33.1 What letters are *not* found in the list of body systems?
   a. B and H
   b. C and W
   c. K and Q
   d. O and I

4. LO 33.2 According to the Official Guidelines for Coding and Reporting paragraph B2.1a, the example "Control of postoperative hemorrhage" is coded to the _____ "Control" found in the general anatomical regions body systems.
   a. root operation
   b. approach
   c. device
   d. qualifier

5. LO 33.1 According to the Official Guidelines for Coding and Reporting paragraph B2.1b, the example "Vein body parts above the diaphragm" is found in the _____ body system.
   a. Heart and Great Vessels
   b. Upper Veins
   c. Anatomical Regions, Upper Extremities
   d. Upper Arteries

6. LO 33.2 Which character position does the root operation term represent?
   a. 1
   b. 3
   c. 5
   d. 7

7. LO 33.2 Creation of a vagina in male perineum with nonautologous tissue substitute, open approach, would be coded with which of the following?

a. 0W4M070

b. 0W4N071

c. 0W4M0K0

d. 0W4N0K1

8. LO 33.2 According to the Official Guidelines for Coding and Reporting paragraph B3.7, the example "Resection of spleen to stop post-procedural bleeding" is coded to

a. resection.

b. control.

c. excision.

d. incision.

9. LO 33.2 Extraction of the right cornea, external approach, would be coded with which of these?

a. 08D9XZX

b. 08D83ZZ

c. 08DKXZX

d. 08D8XZZ

10. LO 33.2 The complete closing of an orifice or a lumen of a tubular body part is known as

a. map.

b. occlusion.

c. fusion.

d. detachment.

11. LO 33.2 According to the Official Guidelines for Coding and Reporting paragraph B3.14, the example "Severing a nerve root to relieve pain" is coded to the root operation term

a. release.

b. reposition.

c. division.

d. restriction.

12. LO 33.2 A diagnostic arthroscopy would be interpreted as

a. bypass.

b. extirpation.

c. resection.

d. inspection.

13. LO 33.2 An esophagogastric fundoplication would be interpreted as

a. fusion.

b. restriction.

c. resection.

d. dilation.

14. LO 33.1 The ileum is part of which body system?

a. Upper Intestinal Tract

b. Upper Leg

c. Lower Intestinal Tract

d. Lower Leg

15. LO 33.3 The appendix that helps you when a specific anatomical site is documented and the body part components are not as specific is entitled

a. *Definition Key.*

b. *Body Part Key.*

c. *Device Key.*

d. *Device Aggregation Table.*

16. LO 33.4 The approach to a procedure was entry, by puncture or minor incision, of instrumentation through the skin or mucous membrane and any other body layers necessary to reach the site of the procedure and is identified with the character 3. What type of approach was used?

a. Open

b. External

c. Percutaneous

d. Via natural or artificial opening

17. LO 33.4 Endoscopic repair of the urethra via natural opening would be coded with which of these?

a. 0TQC8ZZ

b. 0TQD7ZZ

c. 0TQD4ZZ

d. 0TQD8ZZ

18. LO 33.5 A cardiac lead, pacemaker implant device is represented by what sixth character?

a. M

b. J

c. K

d. R

19. LO 33.6 A diagnostic qualifier is identified by what letter?

a. X

b. Z

c. B

d. F

20. LO 33.5 Single upper tooth drainage device implant, open approach, would be coded with which of the following?

a. 0C9W000

b. 0C9XX02

c. 0C9W0Z1

d. 0C9W001

Let's Check It! Guidelines

Refer to the Official ICD-10-PCS Medical and Surgical Section Guidelines and fill in the blanks accordingly.

only	Open	Percutaneous
root operations	overlapping	Release
Inspection	device	coded
after	deepest	not
Reposition	separate	autograft
fused	freed	External
indirectly	drainage	bypassed

1. Biopsy procedures are coded using the _____ Excision, Extraction, or Drainage and the qualifier Diagnostic.

2. If the root operations Excision, Repair or Inspection are performed on _____ layers of the musculoskeletal system, the body part specifying the _____ layer is coded.

3. If multiple coronary arteries are _____, a separate procedure is coded for each coronary artery that uses a different device and/or qualifier.

4. If an _____ is obtained from a different procedure site in order to complete the objective of the procedure, a separate procedure is coded.

5. If multiple vertebral joints are _____, a separate procedure is coded for each vertebral joint that uses a different device and/or qualifier.

6. _____ of a body part(s) performed in order to achieve the objective of a procedure is not coded separately.

7. In the root operation _____, the body part value coded is the body part being _____ and not the tissue being manipulated or cut to free the body part.

8. Reduction of a displaced fracture is coded to the root operation _____ and the application of a cast or splint in conjunction with the Reposition procedure is _____ coded separately.

9. If a body system does not contain a _____ body part value for fingers, procedures performed on the fingers are coded to the body part value for the hand.

10. Procedures performed using the open approach with percutaneous endoscopic assistance are coded to the approach _____.

11. Procedures performed _____ by the application of external force through the intervening body layers are coded to the approach _____.

12. Procedures performed percutaneously via a _____ placed for the procedure are coded to the approach _____.

13. A device is coded only if a device remains _____ the procedure is completed.

14. Procedures performed on a device _____ and not on a body part are specified in the root operations Change, Irrigation, Removal and Revision, and are _____ to the procedure performed.

15. A separate procedure to put in a _____ device is coded to the root operation Drainage with the device value Drainage Device.

Let's Check It! Rules and Regulations

Please answer the following questions from the knowledge you have gained after reading this chapter.

1. **LO 33.1** List the seven character positions of an ICD-10-PCS Medical and Surgical section code; include each character's meaning.

2. **LO 33.3** If the notes state a bilateral procedure was performed and there is no code character available to report a bilateral procedure, how would you report this procedure accurately?

3. **LO 33.3** What is the title of the appendix that helps you when a specific anatomical site is documented and the body part components are not as specific?

4. **LO 33.4** List the seven approaches used within the Medical and Surgical section; explain each approach.

5. **LO 33.7** The Official Guidelines provide four illustrations of cases when you will report multiple procedures. What are the four cases?

Let's Check It! Anatomical Term: ICD-10-PCS Value

Refer to the ICD-10-PCS Appendix entitled "Body Part Key" and identify the ICD-10-PCS value for each anatomical term.

Example: *Abdominal aortic plexus:*

    a. ICD-10-PCS value: <u>*Abdominal Sympathetic Nerve*</u>

1. Apneustic center:
    a. ICD-10-PCS value: _____

2. Columella:
    a. ICD-10-PCS value: _____

3. Dural venous sinus:
    a. ICD-10-PCS value: _____

4. Fifth cranial nerve:
    a. ICD-10-PCS value: _____

5. Gastroduodenal artery:
    a. ICD-10-PCS value: _____

6. Genitofemoral nerve:
    a. ICD-10-PCS value: _____

7. Inferior cardiac nerve:
    a. ICD-10-PCS value: _____

8. Mammillary body:
    a. ICD-10-PCS value: _____

9. Palatine gland:
    a. ICD-10-PCS value: _____

10. Recurrent laryngeal nerve:
    a. ICD-10-PCS value: _____

11. Stylopharyngeus muscle:
    a. ICD-10-PCS value: _____

12. Tympanic nerve:

    a. ICD-10-PCS value: _____

13. Ventricular fold:

    a. ICD-10-PCS value: _____

14. Xiphoid process:

    a. ICD-10-PCS value: _____

15. Zygomaticus muscle:

    a. ICD-10-PCS value: _____

 YOU CODE IT! Practice

Using the techniques described in this chapter, carefully read through the case studies and determine the most accurate ICD-10-PCS code(s) for each case study.

1. Theron Patel, a 12-year-old male, is experiencing obstructive sleep apnea. Dr. Pascal admits Theron to the hospital and performs an adenoidectomy, open approach.

2. Juanita Keane, a 38-year-old female, was admitted to Westwood Hospital yesterday. Dr. Chavez performs a laparoscopic cholecystectomy today.

3. Tom Gilbert, a 29-year-old male, is admitted to Weston Hospital due to severe hypertension. Dr. Benton notes left kidney atrophy and performs an endoscopic left renal artery biopsy.

4. Bella Cable, a 62-year-old female, has severe pain in her right foot when she walks. Upon examination her right big toe has turned toward the second toe. Bella is admitted to the hospital, where Dr. Meltzer performs a bunionectomy, open approach, with a soft tissue correction.

5. Richard McMillan, a 26-year-old male, has had a bad cough for the last 3 months. Therefore, Dr. Skenes admitted him into the hospital and performed a diagnostic fiberoptic bronchoscopy with hopes of determining the cause of the irritation.

6. Merle Sims, a 34-year-old female, is a professional runner and has won three marathons. Today, she is admitted to the hospital for a total arthroplasty (replacement) of her right knee, nonautologous tissue substitute, open approach.

7. Carolyn Bulwark, a 21-year-old female, feels she has "big ears." Carolyn was admitted to the hospital, where her external ears were altered bilaterally, percutaneous approach.

8. Harry Matthews, a 48-year-old male, was admitted to Westwood Hospital yesterday. Harry was diagnosed with esophageal cancer. A middle esophagus bypass, percutaneous endoscopic approach, rerouted to stomach, was performed today.

9. John Andrews, a 46-year-old male, was admitted to the hospital, where he underwent urinary bladder surgery 2 days ago. Today, John's urinary bladder drainage device is changed, external approach.

10. Annie Campbell, a 28-year-old female, was admitted to Westwood Hospital. The patient closed the car door on her foot and severely injured her left foot. Annie's left 5th toe is completely amputated.

11. Wilburn Backwinkel, a 54-year-old male, has had left upper quadrant pain radiating to his back. Dr. Dix admits Wilburn to Westwood Hospital, where he performs an endoscopic (via natural opening) inspection of the pancreatic duct.

12. Lynda Dibble, a 39-year-old female, gave birth to her fourth child 6 months ago. The patient presents today requesting tubal ligation. Lynda is admitted to Westwood Hospital, where Dr. Connell performs a bilateral fallopian tube ligation, percutaneous endoscopic approach.

13. Mike Raval, a 53-year-old male, underwent an abdominal procedure this morning at Westwood Hospital. After the procedure was completed, Mike began to hemorrhage. Dr. Scott performed a control of postoperative bleeding in the abdominal wall, open approach.

14. Lee Spigner, an 83-year-old male, cannot swallow his food and has lost a substantial amount of weight. Lee is admitted to the hospital, where Dr. Ubaldo inserts a feeding device in Lee's stomach, percutaneous endoscopic approach.

15. Vickie Turner, a 24-year-old female, has a history of uncontrolled motor movements and some uncontrolled eye movement. Vickie is admitted to the hospital, where Dr. Allen performs a mapping of Vickie's basal ganglia signals, percutaneous approach.

 # YOU CODE IT! Application

The following exercises provide practice in abstracting physicians' notes and learning to work with documentation from our health care facility, Westward Hospital. These case studies are modeled on real patient encounters. Using the techniques described in this chapter, carefully read through the case studies and determine the most accurate ICD-10-PCS code(s), if appropriate, for each case study.

WESTWARD HOSPITAL

591 Chester Road

Masters, FL 33955

OPERATIVE REPORT

PATIENT: FASCHEL, MARTIN

DATE OF ADMISSION: 11/15/19

DATE OF SURGERY: 11/16/19

DATE OF DISCHARGE: 11/19/19

ADMITTING DIAGNOSIS: Uncontrolled epilepsy

DISCHARGE DIAGNOSIS: Uncontrolled epilepsy

PROCEDURE PERFORMED: Left vagal nerve stimulator insertion.

SURGEON: Kevin Mulford, MD

ASSISTANT: Denny Granger, MD

ANESTHESIA: General endotracheal

ESTIMATED BLOOD LOSS: Less than 10 mL

COMPLICATIONS: None

DRAINS: None

OPERATIVE FINDINGS: A model 102 generator with 2-mm electrodes was utilized.

INDICATION FOR PROCEDURE: The patient is a 6-year-old child who was found to have progressive epilepsy. It was recommended that a vagal nerve stimulator be placed. We discussed the options, the risks, and benefits with the child's parents, and their questions were welcomed and answered. The procedure and potential risks of surgery include, but are not limited to, vagal nerve injury, vascular damage,

(continued)

---

stroke, inoperability, malfunction, the need for continuous monitoring and evaluations, the possible need for further surgical interventions, among others. With the family's understanding and permission, the child was brought to the operating room for this procedure.

DESCRIPTION OF PROCEDURE: After suitable general endotracheal anesthesia was obtained, the patient was placed in the supine position and the head immobilized in a donut. The skin was prepared using Betadine scrub and solution and a suitable surgical drape. Marcaine with epinephrine was infiltrated.

Initially, we made a 2.5-cm incision along the neck crease, and the platysma muscle was divided. The sternocleidomastoid muscle was retracted and dissected medially, and we identified the carotid sheath. The carotid sheath was opened and we identified the vagal nerve. This was then isolated with vessel loops.

We then attached the two electrodes in the grounding mechanism using 2-mm size coils. These were found to be securely placed and a small loop was left for anchoring.

We then prepared the pocket while making a 6-cm curvilinear incision just medial to the axilla. A subcutaneous pocket was created over the pectoralis muscle, and the area was irrigated.

We then used the tunneling device from the cervical to the chest incisions, and the electrodes were placed in the subcutaneous tunnel. The model 102 generator was then connected to the electrodes. An impedance test was done and was found to be 1.

The electrode in the subclavian was left with a small loop for growth, and this was anchored to the fascia using a Vicryl suture.

Subsequently, the generator was turned on at the 0.25 mA at 30 Hz, on 30 seconds, off for 5 minutes, with a magnet strength of 0.5 for 60 seconds.

The wounds were then irrigated and subsequently painted with Betadine solution. They were then closed using 3-0 Vicryl sutures for the deep layer. The skin was approximated using 4-0 Vicryl suture in a running subcuticular fashion. Steri-Strips were applied, and the patient was awakened and transported to the recovery room, having tolerated the procedure well.

We discussed the operation, the findings, and the potential implications and complications with the patient's family. Their questions were welcomed and answered, and they expressed understanding of the situation.

556839/mt98328: 06/01/19 09:50:16   T: 06/01/19 12:55:01

Determine the most accurate ICD-10-PCS code(s).

WESTWARD HOSPITAL

591 Chester Road

Masters, FL 33955

OPERATIVE REPORT

PATIENT: TUTTLE, BARBIE

DATE OF ADMISSION: 05/07/19

DATE OF SURGERY: 05/08/19

DATE OF DISCHARGE: 05/11/19

ADMITTING DIAGNOSIS: Avascular necrosis with severe collapse, total head involvement, left hip.

DISCHARGE DIAGNOSIS: Avascular necrosis with severe collapse, total head involvement, left hip.

OPERATION PERFORMED: Left total hip arthroplasty.

(continued)

SURGEON: Gerard Brighton, MD

ASSISTANT: Peter Alfredson, MD

ANESTHESIA: General.

INDICATIONS FOR OPERATION: This 55-year-old female was noted to have progressively worsening hip pain. She was noted to have on x-ray avascular necrosis with severe collapse and loss of sphericity of the femoral head, Ficat grade 4. The risks and benefits of total hip arthroplasty were discussed in detail, and the patient signed surgical consent.

DESCRIPTION OF OPERATION: The surgical site was signed. The patient was prepped and draped in a routine sterile manner. The IV antibiotics were given prior to the procedure. The surgical team used space suits for added sterility. A posterolateral approach to the hip was made. The fascia was identified and split in line of its fibers. The short external rotators were identified. A T-capsulotomy was performed. The hip was dislocated. The femoral neck was cut using a reciprocating saw. The cut was made based on intraoperative and preoperative templating.

Once the neck was cut, the patient's anteversion was noted, and bone wax was placed on the neck cut to decrease bleeding. The acetabular retractors were placed, a cobra retractor anteriorly, and a posterior-inferior retractor placed into the obturator foramen after an inferior radial capsulotomy. The acetabulum was exposed. The soft tissues, including the labrum and pulvinar, were removed from the acetabulum, and then the acetabulum was progressively reamed from a size 50 up to a size 56. Using a Zimmer M/L Taper Hip Prosthesis, 16.5 mm, ceramic on polyethylene, with a Zimmer head diameter of 12/14 internal taper, a 57-mm Converge cup was then impacted into place at position of 45 degrees of abduction and 20 degrees of anteversion. The overhanging osteophytes were removed. The 38-mm liner was snapped into the cup. A lap sponge was used to protect the cup.

The acetabular retractors were removed. A proximal femoral retractor was placed. The proximal femur was machined first with a cookie cutter osteotome, then a lateralizing reamer, and then progressive broaches. The broaches were taken up to a size 13.5. This initially had good fit. X-rays were taken with a 13.5-mm stem and a neutral ball.

Of note, intraoperative x-rays did note that there was residual room at the lateral aspect of the femur. This was likely secondary to scarred bone from her prior cord decompression. The trial stem was then removed, and using a large curette, the lateral bone was removed. We then again machined from a size 13.5 up to a size 16.25 stem. The 16.25 had excellent fit, kept the equal leg length at the same level as the intraoperative x-ray, taken with the 13.5, but had better canal fill. The real stem was then placed. A neutral ball was placed.

The hip was then tested for range of motion, noted to be quite stable with flexion to 90 degrees, internal rotation to 70, and no instability with extension, external rotation. The capsule was then repaired with #2 FiberWire. The short external rotators were repaired with #2 FiberWire to the trochanter. The fascia was closed with 0 PDS, the subcutaneous tissue was closed with 0 Vicryl, a running 3-0 Monocryl was placed at the subcuticular region. Dermabond was placed at the skin.

The patient was taken to recovery room in stable condition. Estimated blood loss was 150 mL. Sponge and needle counts were correct.

556848/mt98328: 08/01/19 09:50:16   T: 08/01/19 12:55:01

Determine the most accurate ICD-10-PCS code(s).

WESTWARD HOSPITAL

591 Chester Road

Masters, FL 33955

OPERATIVE REPORT

(continued)

PATIENT: LATCHMAN, VICTOR

DATE OF ADMISSION: 03/05/19

DATE OF DISCHARGE: 03/17/19

ADMITTING DIAGNOSIS: Dislocation, right humeroulnar joint

PROCEDURE: Open repair

Patient is a 31-year-old male, admitted via the ED with acute pain in his right arm. Patient is a landscaper and tree trimmer and was hit by a falling tree limb. X-rays show dislocation of the humeroulnar joint, right side.

Patient was taken into the operating room and placed in the supine position. General anesthesia was administered. The area was opened with a 9-cm incision point to the distal aspect of the joint. Once the dislocation was visualized, manipulation was employed to reconfigure the tendons, muscles, and bones back to normal position.

The incision was closed using 4.0 silk; bandage and cast were applied. The patient was taken into the recovery room, having tolerated the procedure well.

Benjamin Johnston, MD—2222

556845/mt98328: 03/17/19 09:50:16   T: 03/17/19 12:55:01

Determine the most accurate ICD-10-PCS code(s).

WESTWARD HOSPITAL

591 Chester Road

Masters, FL 33955

OPERATIVE REPORT

PATIENT: MAGGUIOTT, FELIX

DATE OF ADMISSION: 01/15/19

DATE OF DISCHARGE: 01/17/19

ADMITTING DIAGNOSIS: Inguinal hernia, left

PROCEDURE: Herniorrhaphy, with synthetic substitute

OPERATION: Left inguinal hernia repair with mesh

DESCRIPTION OF OPERATION: The patient was taken to the operating room and placed supine on the operating room table. After general anesthesia was induced, the left inguinal area was prepped with Betadine solution and sterilely draped in the usual manner for procedure in this area. The skin and subcutaneous tissues of the left inguinal area were anesthetized, and an incision beginning at the left pubic tubercle and extending laterally along natural skin lines was created. The incision was extended through the subcutaneous tissues to the aponeurosis of the external oblique. Hemostasis was obtained with the Bovie cautery. The subaponeurotic tissues were anesthetized.

The aponeurosis of the external oblique was incised along the length of its fibers. Care was taken to avoid the ilioinguinal nerve. At the level of the pubic tubercle, the spermatic cord was bluntly dissected from its surrounding structures and encircled with a 0.25-inch Penrose drain. The direct hernia sac was dissected off of the cord structures and invaginated into the preperitoneal space. A search for an indirect component proved fruitless.

(continued)

A large Marlex mesh "plug" was placed in the preperitoneal space, reducing the direct inguinal hernia. It was anchored to the conjoint tendon and the shelving edge of the Poupart's ligament and the pubic tubercle with 2-0 PDS sutures. The onlay portion was placed over the floor of the inguinal canal, while it was anchored to the shelving edge of the Poupart's ligament to the conjoint tendon and laterally to the internal oblique with interrupted 2-0 PDS sutures. The Marlex mesh plug was attached to the onlay portion with a 3-0 Prolene suture. The aponeurosis of the external oblique was closed with a running suture of 3-0 PDS. Subcutaneous tissues were approximated with interrupted sutures of 3-0 PDS. The skin was closed with subcuticular suture of 4-0 PDS. A 0.5-inch Steri-Strip tape was applied. A sterile occlusive dressing was applied over this.

The patient tolerated the procedure well and was transferred to the recovery room in stable condition. Estimated blood loss was 5 cc. Sponge, needle, and instrument counts were correct.

Kenzi Bloomington, MD—7777

556839/mt98328: 01/17/19 09:50:16   T: 01/17/19 12:55:01

Determine the most accurate ICD-10-PCS code(s).

WESTWARD HOSPITAL

591 Chester Road

Masters, FL 33955

OPERATIVE REPORT

PATIENT: KENSINGTON, LOUIS

DATE OF ADMISSION: 10/07/19

DATE OF DISCHARGE: 10/09/19

ADMITTING DIAGNOSIS: Chronic anal fissure and anal stenosis.

DISCHARGE DIAGNOSIS: Chronic anal fissure and anal stenosis.

OPERATIONS:
1. V-Y anoplasty.
2. Lateral internal sphincterotomy with fissurectomy.
3. Flexible sigmoidoscopy.

ESTIMATED BLOOD LOSS: 30 mL.

SPECIMENS: No specimens.

DRAINS: A 0.25-inch Penrose to the flap.

COMPLICATIONS: None.

DESCRIPTION OF OPERATION: After informed consent was obtained, the patient was taken to the OR. He was placed in the prone jackknife position and IV sedation was given by the anesthesiologist. The buttocks were taped laterally, exposing the perianal area. I began with the lubricated scope. The videoscope was inserted into the rectum and advanced through the colon to about 40 cm. At 40 cm, there was some angulation and some looping of the scope, and I elected not to proceed beyond this point. I then began to slowly withdraw the scope, carefully inspecting the lumen. The prep was adequate up to this point. I withdrew the scope. I noted no tumors or polyps. There was no evidence of colitis or proctitis and no diverticular disease was noted. I then desufflated the colon and rectum and removed the scope.

(continued)

The perianal area was then prepped with Betadine and draped in the usual fashion. I then used a solution of 0.5% Marcaine with epinephrine and injected about 30 mL perianally as well as intramuscularly to achieve some relaxation of the sphincter muscles. After adequate analgesia was obtained, the small Ferguson retractor was inserted and the anal canal was inspected. The anterior fissure was very chronic appearing and measured about 1 × 0.5 cm in size. The anal canal was rather small and there seemed to be spasm of the distal edge of the internal sphincter muscle.

I then inserted the Buie retractor and opened it to expose the right lateral anal canal. An incision was made over the anoderm in the right lateral position and then I dissected down to the distal edge of the internal sphincter muscle, which was easily palpable as a tight band. I used a hemostat to dissect underneath it and elevated and divided it for a length of less than 1 cm. This did achieve relaxation of the sphincter muscle.

Then at this point, I was able to remove the Buie retractor and inserted the Chelsea-Eaton retractor. There was a definite release of the spasm of the sphincter muscle. However, there was also now obvious evidence of stenosis of the anal canal and there was no way to bring the mucosal edges together to cover the sphincterotomy wound without putting tension on the anal canal. Because of this, I did elect to go ahead with the anoplasty.

I used a marking pen to outline a house-shaped flap on the perianal skin in the right lateral position. I then anesthetized this area. I used a #15 blade scalpel to incise the skin edges. I then mobilized the flap by dissecting laterally to give the flap a very broad base. With the lateral dissection, I was then able to mobilize the flap down into the anal canal to cover up the lateral internal sphincterotomy wound.

The area was irrigated. Then the flap was sewed into place using interrupted sutures, using combination of #3-0 Vicryl and #4-0 Vicryl sutures, using the #3-0 Vicryl primarily on the tension points of the flap. Once the proximal edge of the flap was sewed to the dentate line, I then came up the anterior and posterior sides of the flap, suturing again in an interrupted fashion to the cut mucosal edges. I then used a scalpel to make a small incision in the right posterior position about 1 centimeter or 2 away from the flap and then used the stab incision to bring a 0.25-inch Penrose through the skin and positioned it underneath the flap. It was sutured to the skin with a single #3-0 Vicryl suture. The excess drain was then cut away, leaving about 2 or 3 cm protruding and the remainder positioned underneath the flap. I then used #2-0 Vicryl and a mattress suture to perform the long portion of the Y of the flap. This was done on the distal edge of the incision, bringing the two skin edges together with two of these mattress sutures to form the Y.

At this point, I now just had the remainder of the bottom of the Y portion of the flap to close and this was done again using a combination of interrupted #3-0 and #4-0 Vicryl sutures. At this point, I had good hemostasis throughout the flap and the flap appeared to be viable. There was no tension on it. There was a good color with no blanching noted.

I then directed my attention back toward the anal fissure in the anterior position. The small anterior tag was excised. That was a small hypertrophied anal papilla. I then mobilized the mucosal side of the fissure, elevating the mucosa, and a very small amount of muscle as well and then used a #4-0 Vicryl suture to bring this mucosal edge about halfway up the fissure to partially cover it and facilitate the healing process. There was a small amount of bleeding that was controlled with the #3-0 Vicryl figure-of-eight suture.

At this point, I had good release of the anal stenosis and good hemostasis throughout. On further examination, there was a very small posterior anal fissure, which was simply coagulated with the electrocautery. At this point, the retractor was removed. A roll of Gelfoam was placed in the anal canal and then a fluffy gauze dressing was placed over the Gelfoam.

The patient was then returned to the supine position and taken to the recovery area in stable condition.

Phillip Carlsson, MD—1111

556845/mt98328: 10/09/19 09:50:16   T: 10/09/19 12:55:01

Determine the most accurate ICD-10-PCS code(s).

Design elements: ©McGraw-Hill

Obstetrics Section

34

Key Terms

Abortifacient
Laminaria
Products of Conception

 STOP! Remember, you need to follow along in your ICD-10-PCS code book for an optimal learning experience.

34.1 Obstetrics Section/Body System: Characters 1 and 2

Obstetrics is the medical specialty that focuses on the care of pregnant women. The relationship between the physician—the obstetrician—and the patient often begins prior to conception and lasts all the way through gestation through delivery to the postpartum period. The entire scope of this care is *not* an issue for coders in a hospital. However, there will be times when a pregnant woman might be admitted into a hospital requiring acute care. These are the procedures and services reported from this section.

So let's review the meanings for the **Obstetrics** section characters:

GUIDANCE CONNECTION

Read the ICD-10-PCS Official Guidelines for Coding and Reporting, **Obstetrics Section Guidelines (Section 1),** subsection **C. Obstetrics Sections,** paragraphs **C1** and **C2**.

Character Position	Character Meaning
1	Section of the ICD-10-PCS book
2	Body system being treated (Pregnancy)
3	Root operation term
4	Body part (Products of Conception)
5	Approach used by physician
6	Device
7	Qualifier

At this time, there are only two Official Guidelines to support your reporting from the *Obstetrics* section in ICD-10-PCS. You should become familiar with them both.

Character Position 1: Obstetrics Section 1

Character Position	Character Meaning
1	**Section of the ICD-10-PCS book**
2	Body system being treated (Pregnancy)
3	Root operation term
4	Body part (Products of Conception)
5	Approach used by physician
6	Device
7	Qualifier

All of the codes reporting an obstetrics procedure provided to a pregnant woman who has been admitted into a hospital will begin with the number one (1).

Character Position 2: Body System: 0

Character Position	Character Meaning
1	Section of the ICD-10-PCS book
2	**Body system being treated (Pregnancy)**
3	Root operation term
4	Body part (Products of Conception)
5	Approach used by physician
6	Device
7	Qualifier

In this section there is only one body system, that is, the gestational term:

Pregnancy . . . Character: **0**

From conception to delivery, procedures, services, and treatments provided to the products of conception within a woman who is pregnant and has been admitted into a hospital are reported with codes from this section to report the hospital (facility) care. Before conception or after the baby is born, the services will be reported from a different section of this code set.

34.2 Obstetrics Root Operations: Character 3

Character Position	Character Meaning
1	Section of the ICD-10-PCS book
2	Body system being treated (Pregnancy)
3	**Root operation term**
4	Body part (Products of Conception)
5	Approach used by physician
6	Device
7	Qualifier

The *Obstetrics* section uses 12 root operation terms to describe the specific procedure provided during this encounter. Some interpretation may be necessary so you can understand what terms to abstract from the operative report or procedure notes accurately and completely. Using the root operation term is the most efficient way of using the Alphabetic Index, as well.

As you learned in previous chapters, the root operation term is based on the objective of the procedure. You are seeking the word describing the action, such as *extraction* or *delivery*. Terms with which you are very familiar, such as cesarean section (c-section) or amniocentesis, may name the procedure; however, these terms do not specifically explain the action of the physician, or do they? Let's take a closer look at these two terms, as examples, and interpret them into the root operation terms:

Cesarean section: What precisely is this procedure? The extraction of the baby via surgical incision. This explanation leads you to the root operation term used in ICD-10-PCS, *extraction.*

Amniocentesis: What specifically is done during this procedure? Using a needle, the physician takes out (drains) some of the amniotic fluid. Understanding this, you can interpret that the root operation term *drainage* describes this perfectly.

With some procedures, you will use your knowledge of the specific procedure and what it is expected to accomplish. For example, you will need to remember that the physician supporting the natural process of a vaginal delivery is reported with the root operation term *delivery.* That one works very well in translation, doesn't it?

Now, let's go over each of the 12 root operation terms used in this section of ICD-10-PCS and look at some examples, to help you understand what each reports.

Abortion

Abortion: Artificially terminating a pregnancy . . . Character: **A**

Note, this is not typically reporting a voluntary abortion. Those are most often performed on an *out*patient basis. This root operation term refers to a procedure performed for medical necessity only.

GUIDANCE CONNECTION

Read the ICD-10-PCS Official Guidelines for Coding and Reporting, **Obstetrics Section Guidelines (Section 1),** subsection **C. Obstetrics Section,** subhead **Procedures following delivery or abortion,** paragraph **C2.**

> **EXAMPLES**
>
> Deena Wolff has been in a coma for a week, as a the result of being raped and beaten. Blood work shows she is pregnant and her injuries make the pregnancy not viable. Dr. Owens performed an abortion, vaginal approach, using a vacuum method.
>
> 10A07Z6   Abortion of products of conception via natural or artificial opening using vacuum
>
> The patient was pregnant with monochorionic twins (twins that share a common placenta) and there was a problem. Evidence of unbalanced flow of blood from one twin to the other twin caused twin–twin transfusion syndrome. Because she was only at 13 weeks, a pregnancy termination was determined to be the best option for the mother's health and a future opportunity to get pregnant again. He performed a dilation and curettage.
>
> 10A08ZZ   Abortion of products of conception via natural or artificial opening

Change

Change: Taking out or off a device from a body part and putting back an identical or similar device in or on the same body part without cutting or puncturing the skin or a mucous membrane . . . Character: **2**

> ### EXAMPLE
>
> Two days ago, Dr. Conners inserted a fetal scalp electrode on Jenna's 27-gestational-week-old fetus. Today, Jenna is admitted into the hospital to monitor her and the fetus, and to change the current electrode to a new one.
>
> 102073Z   Changing a monitoring device for the products of conception via natural or artificial opening

GUIDANCE CONNECTION

Read the ICD-10-PCS Official Guidelines for Coding and Reporting, **Obstetrics Section Guidelines (Section 1),** subsection **C. Obstetrics Section,** subhead **Procedures following delivery or abortion,** paragraph **C2.**

Delivery

> **Delivery: Assisting the passage of the products of conception** from the genital canal . . . Character: **E**

> ### EXAMPLE
>
> The patient is a 31-year-old G2, P0 female at 38 weeks and 5 days estimated gestational age who presented in labor. On vaginal examination, the patient was found to be 4 cm dilated, 70% effaced, and −3 station, and the fetal heart tracing at that time was in the 140s with minimal long-term variability. She was admitted to Labor and Delivery for Pitocin augmentation and amniotomy. She continued to have a good labor pattern and proceeded to deliver a viable 6-pound, 12-ounce male infant over an intact perineum with Apgars of 8 and 9 at 1 and 5 minutes. There were no nuchal cords and no true knots, and the number of vessels in the cord was three. Her postpartum course was uncomplicated, and the patient was discharged to home in stable and satisfactory condition.
>
> 10E0XZZ   Delivery of a neonate (products of conception), external approach
>
> *NOTE:* The administration of the Pitocin, IV, would be reported separately (you will learn about these codes in the *Placement through Chiropractic Sections* chapter, section *Reporting Services from the Administration Section.*

Drainage

> **Drainage: Taking or letting out fluids and/or gases from a body part** . . . Character: **9**

> ### EXAMPLES
>
> Maria Lettio was 39 years old when Dr. Platt confirmed she was pregnant. Today, she has been admitted into the hospital for a gastroesophageal fundoplication. While here, Dr. Lowenthal performed an amniocentesis to check the fetus for genetic abnormalities.
>
> 10903ZU   Drainage of amniotic fluid, percutaneous approach, for diagnostic purposes
>
> Concern for the existence of alloimmune thrombocytopenia, fetal blood sampling to assess the baby's platelet count is performed.
>
> 10903Z9   Drainage, fetal blood sampling, percutaneously
>
> The patient's uterus is compressing due to an overabundance of amniotic fluid. Therefore, today we will perform an amnioreduction to decompress the womb to prevent preterm delivery. A needle is inserted into the amniotic cavity and the excess fluid is removed.
>
> 10903ZC   Drainage of amniotic fluid, percutaneous approach, for therapeutic purposes

Extraction

> **Extraction: Pulling or stripping out or off all or a portion of a body part by the use of force** . . . Character: **D**

A great example of an extraction is a cesarean section, which is not a separate root operation because the intention is to *extract* the baby from the mother's body. However, it is not the only type of procedure reported with this root operation.

GUIDANCE CONNECTION

Read the ICD-10-PCS Official Guidelines for Coding and Reporting, **Obstetrics Section Guidelines (Section 1),** subsection **C. Obstetrics Section,** subhead **Procedures following delivery or abortion,** paragraph **C2.**

EXAMPLES

Dr. Traucher determined that Petricka's pregnancy was ectopic. He used an endoscopic method, via her vagina, to remove the fertilized egg from her fallopian tube.

10D28ZZ	Extraction of ectopic products of conception via natural or artificial opening, endoscopic

The patient was admitted on the morning of her scheduled surgery. Detailed informed consent was again reobtained. All consents were signed. Under spinal anesthesia, uncomplicated repeat low transverse cesarean section was performed. A viable male infant with Apgars of 9 and 9 with birth weight of 8 pounds 6 pounds was delivered. The patient's postoperative course was uneventful.

10D00Z1	Extraction of products of conception, open approach, using a low cervical incision

Insertion

> **Insertion: Putting in nonbiological appliance that monitors, assists, performs, or prevents a physiological function but does not physically take the place of a body part** . . . Character: **H**

This is another opportunity for reading very carefully. In ICD-10-PCS, this root operation, *insertion,* applies only to the placement into the body of a medical device, such as a monitoring device, that will remain in the body after the procedure is completed.

EXAMPLE

Concerned about the fetus's sustainability, Dr. Franklin placed a scalp electrode while Mei Lynn was still in the hospital for another issue.

10H073Z	Insertion of monitoring electrode via natural or artificial opening

Inspection

> **Inspection: Visually and/or manually exploring a body part** . . . Character: **J**

This root operation term is limited to the physician's looking.

EXAMPLE

Using a scope via a percutaneous incision, Dr. Klotzky viewed the fetus's position using an operative fetoscopy.

10J04ZZ	Inspection of productions of conception, percutaneous endoscopic approach

Removal

> **Removal: Taking out or off a device from a body part** . . . Character: **P**

Read this carefully: As the description specifically states "device," this can only be used for this type of procedure, to remove a previously inserted device. As you abstract the physician's notes, be cautious of the use of this term in documentation. The removal of a mole, for example, is really an excision, not a removal.

> **EXAMPLE**
>
> After gathering the data he needed, Dr. Abernathy removed the electrode that had been placed on the fetus's scalp.
>
> 10P003Z   Removal of monitoring electrode, open approach

Repair

Repair: Restoring, to the extent possible, a body part to its normal anatomic structure and function . . . Character: **Q**

> **EXAMPLES**
>
> Dr. Atlante determined that Geena Simpson's fetus has indications of spina bifida. He performed a repair of the skin over the spinal opening, in utero, with hopes of enabling the child to be born without disability.
>
> 10Q03ZQ   Repair of skin, percutaneous approach
>
> Aortic stenosis may be relieved in utero by performing an aortic balloon valvuloplasty. This is accomplished by inserting a needle into the fetal heart through which the balloon catheter is passed.
>
> 10Q03ZF   Repair of cardiovascular system, percutaneous approach

Reposition

Reposition: Moving to its normal location or other suitable location all or a portion of a body part . . . Character: **S**

> **EXAMPLE**
>
> Rae-Ann was in the last stage of labor and ready to deliver when Dr. Bornstine realized the baby was breech. Externally, he manually manipulated the position of the baby, and a 7 lb. 3 oz. boy was delivered a short time later.
>
> 10S0XZZ   Reposition of fetus, external approach

Resection

Resection: Cutting out or off, without replacement, all of a body part . . . Character: **T**

Remember how this differs from excision. When the entire body part is surgically removed, it is reported as a resection. If only a portion of the body part is removed, it is reported as an excision.

> **EXAMPLE**
>
> Dr. Peterson determined that Ursula's fertilized egg was stuck in her left fallopian tube and was growing. He had to surgically remove the fallopian tube before it burst.
>
> 10T28ZZ   Resection of fallopian tube for ectopic products of conception, via natural or artificial opening, endoscopic

Transplantation

Transplantation: Putting in or on all or a portion of a living body part taken from another individual or animal to physically take the place and/or function of all or a portion of a similar body part . . . Character: Y

ICD-10-PCS uses this term in the same manner that physicians do, when a donor organ is placed in lieu of a natural organ that is malformed or dysfunctional. Technology has enabled some organ transplants to be performed on a fetus (in utero).

> ### EXAMPLE
>
> A percutaneous bone marrow transplant was performed on a 25-gestational-week-old fetus.
>
> 10Y03ZG   Transplantation, percutaneous, lymphatics and hemic

YOU INTERPRET IT!

Practice interpreting from the common term used to reference the ICD-10-PCS root operation term.
   1. Amniocentesis: _____
   2. Chorionic villus sampling: _____
   3. Surgical treatment of ectopic pregnancy: _____
   4. Cerclage of cervix during pregnancy: _____
   5. Intrauterine cordocentesis (percutaneous umbilical cord blood sampling): _____
   6. Fetal shunt placement: _____
   7. Induced abortion, by dilation and curettage: _____
   8. Uterine evacuation and curettage: _____
   9. In utero fetal kidney transplant: _____
  10. Vaginal delivery: _____
  11. Hysterorrhaphy: _____

34.3 Obstetrics Body Parts: Character 4

Character Position	Character Meaning
1	Section of the ICD-10-PCS book
2	Body system being treated (Pregnancy)
3	Root operation term
4	**Body part (Products of Conception)**
5	Approach used by physician
6	Device
7	Qualifier

The only procedures reported from this section are those performed on the **products of conception**: zygote, embryo, or fetus, as well as the amnion, umbilical cord, and placenta.

When a sperm fertilizes an oocyte (egg), a zygote is created. Two weeks later (after fertilization), the zygote becomes an embryo. At week 8, the embryo, about 1 inch in length, is considered a fetus.

Products of Conception
The zygote, embryo, or fetus, as well as the amnion, umbilical cord, and placenta.

The *Obstetrics* section focuses on three body parts, which are not specific anatomical sites with which you are familiar:

Products of conception . . . Character: **0 (zero)**
Products of conception, retained . . . Character: **1**
Products of conception, ectopic . . . Character: **2**

In the simplest terms, the products of conception are fertilized ova (zygote, embryo, or fetus) along with the components that accompany, including amnion (the inmost membrane, also known as the *amniotic sac,* that encloses the fetus in utero and the amniotic fluid), umbilical cord, and placenta. The change in the character will designate if these components are ectopic (outside of the uterus) or retained (still inside).

There are times when placental tissue remnants or fetal tissue may remain inside the uterus after a miscarriage, planned pregnancy termination, or a successful delivery. This is known as retained products of conception (RPOC).

A zygote (fertilized egg) usually travels through the fallopian tube and plants itself into the wall of the uterus to begin to grow. When there is a narrowing or other blockage preventing the completion of the journey into the uterus, the zygote may begin to develop outside the uterus. This condition can be life-threatening to the mother and is known as an ectopic pregnancy.

34.4 Obstetrics Approaches: Character 5

Character Position	Character Meaning
1	Section of the ICD-10-PCS book
2	Body system being treated (Pregnancy)
3	Root operation term
4	Body part (Products of Conception)
5	Approach used by physician
6	Device
7	Qualifier

As you continue to build a code, you can see that you are telling a story. The first four characters explain what the physician did and the anatomical site upon which he or she worked. Now, with the fifth character, you are going to explain how the physician got to the anatomical site to perform the procedure. You learned in previous chapters that this is known as the *approach.*

Open

Open: Cutting through the skin or mucous membrane and any other body layers necessary to expose the site of the procedure . . . Character: **0**

An open procedure is the traditional approach when the physician makes an incision into the body to access an internal organ.

> **EXAMPLE**
>
> 10D00Z1   Cesarean section, low cervical, open incision

Percutaneous

Percutaneous: Entry, by puncture or minor incision, of instrumentation through the skin or mucous membrane and any other body layers necessary to reach the site of the procedure . . . Character: **3**

GUIDANCE CONNECTION

Read the ICD-10-PCS Official Guidelines for Coding and Reporting, **Obstetrics Section Guidelines (Section 1),** subsection **C. Obstetrics Section,** subhead **Products of conception,** paragraph **C1.**

Percutaneous Endoscopic

Percutaneous Endoscopic: Entry, by puncture or minor incision, of instrumentation through the skin or mucous membrane and any other body layers necessary to reach and visualize the site of the procedure . . . Character: **4**

CODING BITES

In utero procedures can be performed on the fetus by percutaneous endoscopic approach using a fetoscope.

Via Natural or Artificial Opening

Via Natural or Artificial Opening: Entry of instrumentation through a natural or artificial external opening to reach the site of the procedure . . . Character: **7**

Via Natural or Artificial Opening Endoscopic

Via Natural or Artificial Opening Endoscopic: Entry of instrumentation through a natural or artificial external opening to reach and visualize the site of the procedure . . . Character: **8**

External

External: Procedure performed directly on the skin or mucous membrane and procedures performed indirectly by the application of external force through the skin or mucous membrane . . . Character: **X**

YOU INTERPRET IT!

Interpret these statements from physicians' documentation on the approach used to determine the ICD-10-PCS approach term.

12. Endoscope was inserted into vagina and into the uterus:_____

13. Needle aspiration of amniotic fluid: _____

14. Transverse incision: _____

15. Vaginal delivery: _____

16. Laparoscopic entry into uterus for in vitro surgery: _____

34.5 Obstetrics Devices: Character 6

Character Position	Character Meaning
1	Section of the ICD-10-PCS book
2	Body system being treated (Pregnancy)
3	Root operation term
4	Body part (Products of Conception)
5	Approach used by physician
6	Device
7	Qualifier

As you can see, a character placed in the sixth position will identify a device that will remain with the patient after the procedure has been completed. Remember, the patient for whom the device is involved in care—in this section of ICD-10-PCS—is the fetus . . . *not* the mother.

Monitoring Electrode . . . Character: **3**
Other Device . . . Character: **Y**
No Device . . . Character: **Z**

Fetal monitoring can be performed either internally or externally. When done internally, the physician will place an electrode (electronic transducer) directly onto the scalp of the fetus, typically using a natural opening approach (through the vagina/cervix), with the intention of directly and continuously evaluating the fetal heart rate as well as its variability between beats, particularly in relation to the uterine contractions of labor. Another device, called an internal uterine pressure monitor (IUPM), may be used in conjunction with internal fetal heart rate monitoring. Using a catheter inserted via the vagina/cervix, an IUPM is placed inside the uterus, next to the fetus, to transmit the readings of the contraction pressure to a nearby monitor.

External fetal heart rate monitoring can be accomplished with a handheld electronic Doppler ultrasonic device, most often used at outpatient prenatal visits. Continuous electronic fetal heart monitoring, typically used during labor and delivery, consists of placing an ultrasound transducer on the mother's abdomen, where it can transfer the sounds of the fetal heart to a computer. The computer is able to show the heart pattern on a screen as well as print it out on paper similar to that used during an EKG.

34.6 Obstetrics Qualifiers: Character 7

Character Position	Character Meaning
1	Section of the ICD-10-PCS book
2	Body system being treated (Pregnancy)
3	Root operation term
4	Body part (Products of Conception)
5	Approach used by physician
6	Device
7	Qualifier

The seventh character is required. In some cases, there may be no more details to add, so you will use the placeholder letter Z No Qualifier—the equivalent of "not applicable."

Extraction Procedures

During a delivery, if the physician uses forceps or another assisting mechanism, this delivery becomes an *extraction,* and the additional detail will be reported with a Qualifier character:

Low Forceps . . . Character: **3**
Mid Forceps . . . Character: **4**
High Forceps . . . Character: **5**
Vacuum . . . Character: **6**
Internal Version . . . Character: **7**
Other . . . Character: **8**

- *Low forceps:* The physician uses forceps to help the neonate the last short way out of the birth canal; the baby's head is visible from the outside.
- *Mid forceps:* Forceps are used to help the baby before the head has reached the lower part of the birth canal.
- *High forceps:* A very unusual situation where forceps are used to delivery the baby through the birth canal prior to engagement.
- *Vacuum:* The physician places a cup, attached to a vacuum pump, on the baby's head to guide the neonate through the birth canal.
- *Internal version:* The physician manually turns the fetus using his hand or fingers through the dilated cervix.

Earlier you learned that a cesarean delivery is reported in ICD-10-PCS using the root operation term *extraction.* For this procedure, the Qualifier character will report

High (Classical c-section incision) . . . Character: 0
Low Cervical . . . Character: 1
Extraperitoneal . . . Character: 2

- *High:* Incision is made vertically, from the naval to the pubic line.
- *Low:* Incision is made transversely just above the pubic line; also known as the bikini cut.
- *Extraperitoneal:* Incision is made into the lowest part of the anterior aspect of the uterus.

EXAMPLES

You may read these words in the physician's documentation:

"*. . . low transverse cesarean section . . .*"
"*. . . Lower uterine segment was then scored in a curvilinear fashion . . .*" [extraperitoneal]
"*. . . A vertical incision was made in the umbilicus . . .*" [classical]

Drainage Procedures

During amniocentesis, or any other drainage procedure performed on a pregnant woman, the Qualifier character will explain exactly <u>what</u> was drained:

Fetal Blood . . . Character: **9**
Fetal Cerebrospinal Fluid . . . Character: **A**
Fetal Fluid, Other . . . Character: **B**
Amniotic Fluid, Therapeutic . . . Character: **C**
Fluid, Other . . . Character: **D**
Amniotic Fluid, Diagnostic . . . Character: **U**

CODING BITES

Read carefully! There are two different characters available to report the drainage of amniotic fluid . . . therapeutic or diagnostic. Check the documentation to determine why the amniocentesis was done.

Abortive Procedures

When the artificial termination of a pregnancy (abortion) is performed, the Qualifier character will report the methodology:

Vacuum ... Character: **6**
Laminaria ... Character: **W**
Abortifacient ... Character: **X**

Laminaria
Thin sticks of kelp-related seaweed, used to dilate the cervix, that can induce abortive circumstance during the first 3 months of pregnancy.

Abortifacient
A drug used to induce an abortion.

- *Vacuum:* The use of aspiration using a cannula (tube) inserted into the uterus; also known as suction curettage.
- *Laminaria:* A small rod, created of dehydrated types of kelp, is inserted into the cervix for the purposes of dilation.
- *Abortifacient:* A substance, using a pharmaceutical, used to induce expulsion of the products of conception.

In Utero Procedures

The Qualifier character will report the body system that was repaired or transplanted during an in utero procedure performed on the fetus (root operation *repair* or *transplantation*).

Nervous System ... Character: **E**	**Hepatobiliary and Pancreas** ... **N**
Cardiovascular System ... **F**	**Endocrine System** ... **P**
Lymphatics and Hemic ... **G**	**Skin** ... **Q**
Eye ... **H**	**Musculoskeletal System** ... **R**
Ear, Nose, and Sinus ... **J**	**Urinary System** ... **S**
Respiratory System ... **K**	**Female Reproductive System** ... **T**
Mouth and Throat ... **L**	**Male Reproductive System** ... **V**
Gastrointestinal System ... **M**	**Other Body System** ... **Y**

 LET'S CODE IT! SCENARIO

PATIENT: Elicia Moralise

DATE OF DELIVERY: 05/29/2019

HISTORY OF PRESENT ILLNESS: The patient is a 26-year-old G1, P0 at 39-3/7 weeks with an EDD of 06/01/2019 based on a 6-week ultrasound. The patient presented to labor and delivery with complaints of contractions every 3 minutes and leaking of fluid since 0400 on 05/28/2019. The patient reports positive fetal movement and denies vaginal bleeding. Prenatal care began at 9 weeks × 15 visits. Total weight gain was 37 pounds. The patient is A positive, rubella immune, GBS positive. She has no known drug allergies.

(continued)

Upon admission, vaginal exam was 1, 80%, and −1 station per the RN. Fetal heart tones were 124, positive long-term variability, positive acceleration, and no decelerations. Uterine contractions every 2 to 3 minutes, 60 to 80 seconds and moderate to palpation.

PLAN: Admit the patient to the labor and delivery unit. Dr. Lorrantz informed and agrees with plan. GBS protocol, ampicillin. The patient encouraged to ambulate, shower, use the birth ball. Reassess in 3 to 4 hours or p.r.n.

LABOR PROGRESS: At 0900, the patient was pushing with contractions. She was feeling pressure but was still comfortable with the epidural. The patient stated that she was exhausted. The Pitocin was restarted at 2 mU as the RN realized that the catheter had come loose from the patient's IV and the Pitocin was not being delivered to the patient. Pitocin currently now at 18 mU per minute. Contractions were every 2 to 6 minutes, 50 to 60 seconds long. Fetal heart tones were 125, average variability, 15 × 15 accelerations with mild variable decelerations with good return to baseline. Vaginal exam at 0830 hours was complete, 100%, with the head at the 0 station and the caput at +2 station. The patient appeared to be making some progress with pushing; however, Dr. Lorrantz was consulted and was asked by the CNM to assess the patient after leaving an OR case. The plan was that the patient would continue pushing provided fetal heart tones remained stable until Dr. Lorrantz was able to get out of the OR to evaluate her. The plan was to consider vacuum extraction.

DELIVERY NOTE: The patient pushed extremely well and through excellent maternal efforts and frequent position changes, the infant rotated and descended and normal spontaneous vaginal delivery occurred at 0950 hours in the LOA position over intact perineum. Meconium-stained fluid was noted as the head came over the perineum and Neonatology was called to the room. The mouth and nose were bulb suctioned on the perineum by the CNM. The shoulders delivered easily and a nuchal cord loose x1 was noted and reduced with the delivery of the body. The cord was immediately clamped x2 and cut by the father of the baby and the infant was taken to the warmer for evaluation by Neonatology. The placenta delivered spontaneously at 0958 hours, was complete, had a 3-vessel cord, and was in the Schultz fashion. Estimated blood loss was 200 mL. Pitocin was run open after the delivery of the placenta. The vagina was inspected and a first-degree vaginal and left first-degree labial laceration were repaired with 2-0 chromic and 3-0 Vicryl respectively. The fundus was firm, midline, and −2. There was light lochia. Infant's Apgars were 6, 8, and 9. Weight was 6 pounds 9 ounces. The mother and the infant were left in stable condition.

Let's Code It!

Congratulations! A healthy baby was born. Now, let's determine the accurate ICD-10-PCS code for the delivery.

From which section would you report the delivery of this baby? The baby is a product of conception, therefore, **Obstetrics**.

First character: Section: Obstetrics . . . 1

Only one option for the body system . . .

Second character: System: Pregnancy . . . 0

This is also straightforward. The documentation states, "*normal spontaneous vaginal delivery.*"

Third character: Root Operation: Delivery . . . E

The rest of this code will come together easily because there is only one option for each of the last four characters:

Fourth character: Body Part: Products of Conception . . . 0
Fifth character: Approach: External . . . X
Sixth character: Device: No Device . . . Z
Seventh character: Qualifier: No Qualifier . . . Z

Now put it all together and report, with confidence, this ICD-10-PCS code:

10E0XZZ Natural, spontaneous vaginal delivery

Good job!

34.7 Obstetrics Coding: Putting It All Together

Throughout this chapter, you have learned about each of the seven components of an ICD-10-PCS code used to report a procedure, service, or treatment on a pregnant woman. Now, let's put it all together and determine some codes all the way through.

 LET'S CODE IT! SCENARIO

LaToya Donner, a 37-year-old female, is pregnant, G1 P0, second trimester (15 weeks, 3 days), and has been admitted to have some tests, including an amniocentesis. Because she is categorized as eldergravida, Dr. Brummel is performing this test to determine the health and well-being of the fetus.

Let's Code It!

Let's go through the steps of coding for ICD-10-PCS and determine the code or codes that should be reported for this encounter between Dr. Brummel and LaToya Donner.

> **First character: Section: Obstetrics . . . 1**
> **Second character: Body System: Pregnancy . . . 0**
> **Third character: Root Operation: Drainage . . . 9**

Remember the meaning and purpose of this procedure: amniocentesis (puncturing of the amnion) to drain amniotic fluid.

> **Fourth character: Body Part: Products of Conception . . . 0**
> **Fifth character: Approach: Percutaneous . . . 3**
> **Sixth character: Device: No Device . . . Z**
> **Seventh character: Qualifier: Amniotic Fluid, Diagnostic . . . U**

What is being drained? Amniotic fluid. Why? To test (diagnostics).

The ICD-10-PCS code you will report is

> **10903ZU   Amniocentesis for prenatal testing**

Good job!

 LET'S CODE IT! SCENARIO

PATIENT NAME: Yessina Catina

PHYSICIAN: Travis Jonquin, MD

DATE OF ADMISSION: 05/28/2019

DATE OF DISCHARGE: 05/29/2019

ADMITTING DIAGNOSIS: Intrauterine pregnancy at 38 weeks and 5 days. Presented with contractions, leakage of fluid, and decreased fetal movements that day.

HISTORY OF PRESENT ILLNESS/HOSPITAL COURSE: The patient is a 31-year-old G2, P0 female at 38 weeks and 5 days estimated gestational age who presented in labor. On vaginal examination, the patient was found to be 4 cm dilated, 70% effaced, and −3 station, and the fetal heart tracing at that time was in the 140s with minimal long-term variability. She was admitted to Labor and Delivery for Pitocin augmentation and amniotomy. She continued to have a good labor pattern and proceeded to deliver a viable 6-pound, 12-ounce male infant over an intact perineum with Apgars of 8 and 9 at 1 and 5 minutes. There were no nuchal cords and no true knots, and the number of vessels in the cord was three. Her postpartum course was uncomplicated, and the patient was discharged to home in stable and satisfactory condition.

(continued)

PROCEDURES PERFORMED: Normal spontaneous delivery and Pitocin augmentation.

COMPLICATIONS: None.

FINAL DIAGNOSIS: Status post normal spontaneous vaginal delivery at 38 weeks and 5 days.

DISCHARGE INSTRUCTIONS: Call for increased pain, fever, or increased bleeding.

DIET: Advance as tolerated.

ACTIVITY: Advance as tolerated. Pelvic rest for 6 weeks. Nothing to be inserted into the vagina for 6 weeks, i.e., no tampons, douche, or sex.

Code for the delivery.

Let's Code It!

Let's go through the steps of ICD-10-PCS coding and determine the code to report for Dr. Jonquin's support in the delivery of Yessina's baby.

> **First character: Section: Obstetrics . . . 1**
> **Second character: Body System: Pregnancy . . . 0**

This was documented as a vaginal delivery.

> **Third character: Root Operation: Delivery . . . E**

The neonate was delivered, and this boy is a product of conception.

> **Fourth character: Body Part: Products of Conception . . . 0**

There is only one option for each of the following three characters.

> **Fifth character: Approach: External . . . X**
> **Sixth character: Device: No Device . . . Z**
> **Seventh character: Qualifier: None . . . Z**

Put the seven characters together to get the code to report:

> **10E0XZZ   Delivery of products of conception, vaginally**

Good work!

 LET'S CODE IT! SCENARIO

PATIENT: Isabelle Calaveri

DATE: 11/15/19

PROCEDURE: Primary low segment transverse cesarean section

DESCRIPTION OF OPERATION: Due to concern that the umbilical cord was around the fetus's neck, the patient was brought to the operating room and placed on the table in supine position, and after adequate epidural anesthesia, she was prepped and draped in the usual sterile fashion.

A Pfannenstiel incision was made with a clean scalpel. The incision was taken down the fascial layer with a clean second knife. The fascial layer was incised transversely to the full length of the primary incision. The underlying muscle bellies were dissected with blunt and sharp dissection. The muscle belly was split in the midline. The peritoneum was then grasped between 2 Kelly clamps and elevated. After ensuring no adherent bowel or bladder, the peritoneum was nicked between clamps. The abdominal cavity was thus entered. The bladder flap was formed with blunt and sharp dissection and then the uterus was scored in the lower uterine segment in transverse fashion, and

(continued)

the incision was enlarged in elliptical fashion with bandage scissors. The infant was found to be in face presentation with nuchal cord x1. Mouth and nose were suctioned prior to delivery of rest of the body. The cord was slipped over the shoulders and then the infant was delivered. It was a living female with Apgars of 8 and 9. There was meconium, but it was not thick. Cord pH was 7.30. The cord was doubly clamped, cut between the clamps, and the infant was handed away to the pediatrician, Dr. Toliver. Cord bloods were taken.

The placenta was then manually separated. The edges of the uterine incision were then reapproximated with continuous running suture of #1 chromic catgut. The second imbricating layer was also sewn using #1 chromic catgut. Good hemostasis was noted. The abdomen was cleaned of blood and clots. Tubes and ovaries were inspected and found to be normal. Then, the abdomen was closed in layers after correct sponge, needle, and instrument counts. The peritoneum was closed with continuous running suture of 0 chromic catgut. The muscle bellies were closed with interrupted sutures of 0 chromic catgut. The fascia was closed with 2 continuous running sutures of 0 Vicryl beginning at either angle of the incision intermittently overlapping the midline. The subcutaneous tissue was closed with continuous running suture of 3-0 plain catgut, and the skin was closed with surgical staples. A sterile pressure dressing was applied. Sponge, needle, and instrument counts were correct at the end of the procedure.

Matthew Ansara, MD

Let's Code It!

Dr. Ansara performed a c-section to deliver Isabelle's baby.

First character: Section: Obstetrics . . . 1
Second character: Body System: Pregnancy . . . 0

This was documented as a c-section. You have learned that ICD-10-PCS uses the term *extraction*.

Third character: Root Operation: Extraction . . . D

What has been extracted? The fetus, which is a *product of conception.*

Fourth character: Body Part: Products of Conception . . . 0

What was the approach the physician used? The documentation states, "*A Pfannenstiel incision was made with a clean scalpel.*" This tells you the approach was *open.*

Fifth character: Approach: Open . . . 0

Was there a device involved in this procedure? No.

Sixth character: Device: No Device . . . Z

The Qualifier will report the type of incision used by the physician. The documentation states, "*The fascial layer was incised transversely.*" You learned about the different incisions, and that this is known as a "low cervical."

Seventh character: Qualifier: Low Cervical . . . 1

Put all seven characters together to get the code to report:

10D00Z1   Extraction of products of conception, open approach using low cervical incision

Good job!

Chapter Summary

The services, procedures, and treatments reported with codes from the **Obstetrics Section** of ICD-10-PCS are all provided in a pregnant inpatient. The most important thing to remember is that, for these procedures, the patient is the product of conception—what is inside a pregnant patient.

You Interpret It! Answers

1. Drainage, **2.** Extraction, **3.** Resection, **4.** Insertion, **5.** Drainage, **6.** Insertion, **7.** Abortion, **8.** Extraction, **9.** Transplantation, **10.** Delivery, **11.** Repair, **12.** Via natural or artificial opening endoscopic, **13.** Percutaneous, **14.** Open, **15.** Via natural or artificial opening, **16.** Percutaneous endoscopic

CHAPTER 34 Obstetrics Section

Let's Check It! Terminology

Match each key term to the appropriate definition.

1. LO 34.6 A drug used to induce an abortion.

2. LO 34.3 The zygote, embryo, or fetus, as well as the amnion, umbilical cord, and placenta.

3. LO 34.6 Thin sticks of special seaweed used to dilate the cervix that can induce abortive circumstance during the first 3 months of pregnancy.

A. Abortifacient

B. Laminaria

C. Products of Conception

Let's Check It! Concepts

Choose the most appropriate answer for each of the following questions.

1. LO 34.4 Within the Obstetric Section, character position 5 represents which of the following?

   a. Body system
   b. Root operation term
   c. Approach
   d. Device

2. LO 34.1 All of the codes reporting an Obstetrics procedure will begin with which section number?

   a. 5
   b. 4
   c. 2
   d. 1

3. LO 34.3 The products of conception include

   a. zygote and embryo.
   b. amnion and umbilical cord.
   c. placenta.
   d. all of these.

4. LO 34.2 All of the following are root operation terms in the Obstetrics Section *except*

   a. abortion.
   b. delivery.
   c. irrigation.
   d. inspection.

5. LO 34.2 Within the Obstetrics Section, character position 5 Approach, the approach to an intrauterine cordocentesis would be which of the following?

   a. Via natural or artificial opening

   b. Percutaneous endoscopic

   c. External

   d. Open

6. LO 34.4 Inspection of retained products of conception, vaginal approach, would be coded

   a. 10J17ZZ

   b. 10J18ZZ

   c. 10J12ZZ

   d. 10J00ZZ

7. LO 34.5 Within the Obstetrics Section, character position 6 represents

   a. body system being treated.

   b. root operation.

   c. device.

   d. qualifier.

8. LO 34.6 During a delivery, the physician uses mid forceps for the extraction. This will be reported with the qualifier character

   a. 6

   b. 4

   c. 5

   d. 3

9. LO 34.6 The qualifier character that reports on an in utero procedure performed on the fetus's eye is

   a. E.

   b. N.

   c. M.

   d. H.

10. LO 34.1 Within the Obstetrics Section, what is the one body system that is the gestational term?

    a. 1

    b. 0

    c. 3

    d. 5

Let's Check It! Root Operation Definitions—Obstetrics

Refer to the ICD-10-PCS Appendix entitled "Root Operation Definitions." Look for Root Operation Definitions for Other Sections, Obstetrics, and match the ICD-10-PCS value for each Operation, Character 3, to its definition.

1. Delivery	**A.** A
2. Removal	**B.** D
3. Resection	**C.** E
4. Abortion	**D.** H
5. Inspection	**E.** J
6. Insertion	**F.** P
7. Repair	**G.** Q
8. Reposition	**H.** S
9. Transplantation	**I.** T
10. Extraction	**J.** Y

Let's Check It! Guidelines

Refer to the Official ICD-10-PCS Obstetrics Section Guidelines and fill in the blanks accordingly.

Amniocentesis	retained	obstetric
all	therapeutic	pregnant
Obstetrics	Medical and Surgical	postpartum
delivery	Endometrium	Extraction

1. Procedures performed on the products of conception are coded to the _____ section.

2. Procedures performed on the _____ female other than the products of conception are coded to the appropriate root operation in the _____ section.

3. _____ is coded to the products of conception body part in the Obstetrics section. Repair of _____ urethral laceration is coded to the urethra body part in the Medical and Surgical section.

4. Procedures performed following a _____ or abortion for curettage of the endometrium or evacuation of _____ products of conception are _____ coded in the Obstetrics section, to the root operation _____ and the body part Products of Conception, Retained.

5. Diagnostic or _____ dilation and curettage performed during times other than the _____ or post-abortion period are all coded in the Medical and Surgical section, to the root operation Extraction and the body part _____ .

Let's Check It! Rules and Regulations

Please answer the following questions from the knowledge you have gained after reading this chapter.

1. LO 34.2 Explain the difference between delivery and extraction; include the character that represents each.

2. LO 34.3 The Obstetrics section character position 4 focuses on three body parts, which are not specific anatomical sites. List the three body parts; include the character that identifies each.

3. LO 34.4 List the six approaches used in the Obstetrics section of ICD-10-PCS, explain each approach, and include the character that identifies each approach.

4. LO 34.6 What does the Obstetrics section seventh character position present, and is it required?

5. LO 34.6 Explain what a cesarean section procedure is and include the root operation term used in ICD-10-PCS.

YOU CODE IT! Practice

Using the techniques described in this chapter, carefully read through the case studies and determine the most accurate ICD-10-PCS code(s) for each case study.

1. Candy Moss, a 31-year-old female, is G1 P0, 8-weeks gestation. Candy requests an abortion due to genetic problems in the fetus. She is admitted to the hospital, where a vacuum abortion is performed, via natural opening.

2. Keren Medlin, a 29-year-old female, is admitted to Westward Hospital at 12-weeks gestation. Dr. Hanks performs a repair to the fetus's urinary system endoscopically, via natural opening.

3. Annie Charles, a 23-year-old female, G2 P1, at 40-weeks gestation in active labor, is admitted to Westward Hospital. Dr. Downs assisted in a vaginal delivery, low forceps over midline episiotomy.

4. Loretta Smith, a 36-year-old female, G3 P2 at 38-weeks gestation, is admitted to Westward Hospital. Dr. McWhirter changes a monitor electrode, vaginal approach.

5. Debbie Slay, a 29-year-old female, G1 P0, is admitted to Westward Hospital in labor. Dr. Atkinson inserts an intrauterine pressure catheter, vaginal approach, to evaluate contractions.

6. Rhonda Hart, a 19-year-old female, is admitted to Westward Hospital in labor at 41-weeks gestation, G1 P0. AROM is performed and spontaneous vaginal delivery with intact perineum occurs 1 hour later, manually assisted delivery.

7. Laura McMillan, a 28-year-old female, at 39-weeks gestation, is admitted to Westward Hospital in labor; a vaginal delivery occurs 6 hours later, vacuum assisted.

8. Latoya Medlin, an 18-year-old female, G1 P0, is admitted to Westward Hospital at 18-weeks gestation. Latoya is requesting termination of pregnancy due to confirmed fetal anencephaly. Pregnancy was terminated by a luminaria stick, which produced a complete abortion.

9. Sherry Moore, a 29-year-old female, is admitted to Westward Hospital for an open in utero fetal mouth repair.

10. Janie Knight, a 16-year-old female, G1 P0, is admitted to Westward Hospital, and Dr. Gifford performs an amniotic fluid test for therapeutic purposes.

11. Sharon Heyward, a 24-year-old female, G2 P1 at 40-weeks gestation, is admitted to Westward Hospital. Dr. Jessup performs a pelvic examination revealing an open, soft cervix.

12. Kristi Williams, a 31-year-old female, is admitted to Westward Hospital in active labor at 41-weeks gestation. Dr. Gerald assisted with a vaginal delivery, with high forceps, 4 hours later.

13. Keyana Haulbrook, a 17-year-old female, G1 P0, 12-weeks gestation, is admitted to Westward Hospital to terminate pregnancy due to a genetic defect in the fetus. Abortion was performed by hysterotomy technique.

14. Natalie Phillips, a 32-year-old female, 37.5-weeks gestation, G2 P1, is admitted to Westward Hospital for a fetal spinal tap, percutaneous.

15. Eleanor Coaxum, a 26-year-old female, G1 P0, 32-weeks gestation, is admitted to Westward Hospital for a fetal skin transplantation, via natural opening.

 ## YOU CODE IT! Application

The following exercises provide practice in abstracting physicians' notes and learning to work with documentation from our health care facility, Westward Hospital. These case studies are modeled on real patient encounters. Using the techniques described in this chapter, carefully read through the case studies and determine the most accurate ICD-10-PCS code(s) for each case study.

WESTWARD HOSPITAL

591 Chester Road

Masters, FL 33955

DISCHARGE SUMMARY

PATIENT: ALBERTS, SERITA

DATE OF ADMISSION: 03/05/19

DATE OF DISCHARGE: 03/17/19

ADMITTING DIAGNOSIS: 1. Intrauterine pregnancy at 40 plus weeks.
                     2. Active labor.
                     3. History of two previous cesarean sections.

DISCHARGE DIAGNOSIS: 1. Intrauterine pregnancy at 40 plus weeks.
                     2. Active labor.
                     3. History of two previous cesarean sections.

OPERATION: Repeat low transverse cesarean section.

FLUIDS: 2,500 mL lactated Ringer.

ESTIMATED BLOOD LOSS: 300 mL.

URINE OUTPUT: 125 mL, clear and yellow.

DESCRIPTION OF OPERATION: The patient was identified and taken to the operating room. Appropriate anesthesia was administered. The patient was placed in the dorsal supine position with a leftward tilt and prepped and draped in the usual sterile fashion. Following that, a low Pfannenstiel skin incision was made with a #10 scalpel. This incision was carried down to the underlying layer of fascia with

(continued)

the scalpel. The fascia was then nicked in the midline with the scalpel. This fascial incision was then extended laterally with the Mayo scissors and pickups with teeth.

Following that, the superior aspect of the fascial incision was grasped with straight Kocher clamps x2, tented up from the rectus muscles below and dissected away sharply with the scalpel and Mayo scissors. This was repeated similarly to the inferior aspect of the fascial incision. Following that, the peritoneum was identified below, grasped with hemostat x2, and entered sharply with Metzenbaum scissors. After appropriate visualization of the bowel and bladder, the peritoneal incision was extended superiorly and inferiorly. The bladder blade was then placed inferiorly and the vesicouterine peritoneum tented up with the smooth pickups, incised with the Metzenbaum scissors, and this incision was extended laterally.

Following that, the bladder blade was replaced deflecting the bladder anteriorly and inferiorly. The #10 scalpel was taken in hand again, and a 3-cm low transverse area incision was then made. This incision was then extended laterally. Following that, the infant's vertex was mobilized and delivered through the incision in a direct OP position. The infant's nasopharynx was suctioned with the bulb syringe and then the rest of the infant was delivered along with fundal pressure.

Following that, the infant's cord was clamped and cut and the infant was handed off to the awaiting pediatricians. Following that, the placenta was spontaneously expressed. The uterus was then exteriorized and cleared of all clots and debris. The uterine incision was repaired with #1 chromic in a running-locking fashion. The uterus was then returned to the abdominal cavity, and the abdominal cavity was cleared of all clots and debris.

The uterine incision and the pelvic cavity were reinspected and excellent hemostasis was noted overall. The fascial incision was reapproximated with #0 Vicryl in a running fashion x2. Following that, the skin was reapproximated with staples. The instrument, needle, and sponge counts were correct x2.

Benjamin Johnston, MD—2222

556845/mt98328: 03/17/19 09:50:16 T: 03/17/19 12:55:01

Determine the most accurate ICD-10-PCS code(s) for the c-section.

WESTWARD HOSPITAL

591 Chester Road

Masters, FL 33955

OPERATIVE REPORT

PATIENT: HUDSON, LYNN

ACCOUNT/EHR #: HUDSLY001

DATE OF ADMISSION: 17 March 2019

ATTENDING PHYSICIAN: Denny Stewart, MD

ANESTHESIA: EPIDURAL TYPE OF DELIVERY: NSVD

CONDITION OF PERINEUM: MLE

EPISIOTOMY: Midline performed

VAGINA/CERVIX: Intact

DELIVERED: Live, single-born female, weight 7 lb. 2 oz. @ 02:17

TYPE OF STIMULATION: Mouth suction

(continued)

CONDITION: Good

BIRTH INJURY: None

APGAR RATING: 1 min. = 9 . . . 5 min. = 9

Denny Stewart, MD-1234

558645/mt98328: 03/17/19 09:50:16 T: 03/17/19 12:55:01

Determine the most accurate ICD-10-PCS code(s) for the delivery.

WESTWARD HOSPITAL

591 Chester Road

Masters, FL 33955

OPERATIVE REPORT

PATIENT: CARROLL, DAWN

ACCOUNT/EHR #: CARRDA001

DATE OF ADMISSION: 21 March 2019

ATTENDING PHYSICIAN: Steven Phifer, MD

In the 40th week of her first pregnancy, a 34-year-old woman arrived at Labor and Delivery at 5:00 a.m. for a planned induction of labor due to mild, pregnancy-induced hypertension. After intravaginal placement of misoprostol, the nurse observed her briefly and, at 9:00 a.m., discharged her from the unit. She went for a walk with her husband in a park next to the hospital.

Patient's membranes spontaneously ruptured, and she returned to the Labor and Delivery unit. Patient's vital signs were taken, and the fetal heart rate checked. The mother's blood pressure was 182/97, but the nurse thought this was related to nausea, vomiting, and discomfort from the contractions.

The resident examined the mother, determined that her cervix was 5–6 cm, 90 percent effaced, and the vertex was at 0 station. An internal fetal heart monitor was placed because the mother's vomiting and discomfort caused her to move around too much in the bed, making it hard to record the fetal heart rate with an external monitor. The internal monitor revealed a steady fetal heart rate of 120 and no decelerations.

The mother continued to complain of painful contractions and requested an epidural. Shortly after placement of the epidural, the monitor recorded a prolonged fetal heart rate deceleration. The heart rate returned slowly to the baseline rate of 120 as the nurse repositioned the mother, increased her intravenous fluids, and administered oxygen by mask.

An epidural analgesia infusion pump was started. The fetal heart rate strip indicated another deceleration that recovered to baseline. The nurse informed the resident, who checked the tracing and told her to "keep an eye on things."

The primary nurse noted in the labor record that the baseline fetal heart rate was "unstable, between 100–120," but she did not report this to the resident.

The nurse recorded that the fetal heart rate was "flat, no variability." As the nurse was documenting this as a nonreassuring fetal heart rate pattern, the patient expressed a strong urge to push and the nurse called for an exam.

A resident came to the bedside, examined the mother, and noted that she was fully dilated with the caput at +1. A brief update was written in the chart, but the clinician who had performed the exam was not noted.

(continued)

The mother was repositioned and began pushing.

The fetal heart rate suddenly dropped and remained profoundly bradycardic for 11 minutes. The resident was called and attempted a vacuum delivery because the fetal head was at +2 station. The attending then entered and attempted forceps delivery.

An emergency cesarean delivery was performed; the baby was stillborn. The physician identified a uterine rupture that required significant blood replacement.

Steven Phifer, MD-4321

558645/mt98328: 03/21/19 1:50:16 T: 03/22/19 12:55:01

Determine the most accurate ICD-10-PCS code(s) for the c-section.

WESTWARD HOSPITAL

591 Chester Road

Masters, FL 33955

OPERATIVE REPORT

PATIENT: FAULDS, MAGGIE

ACCOUNT/EHR #: FAULMA001

DATE OF ADMISSION: 25 March 2019

ATTENDING PHYSICIAN: Sandra Lindler, MD

ANESTHESIA: General

Patient is in her 12th week of pregnancy. She presented to the emergency department with severe cramping and vaginal bleeding. After examination the patient was diagnosed with an incomplete early spontaneous abortion and a D&C was recommended. The patient was fully counseled as to the risks and benefits of the D&C and admitted to the hospital. The patient agreed to the procedure.

The patient was then taken to the operating room and placed in a supine position on the operating room table. General endotracheal anesthesia was administered, and once adequate anesthesia was demonstrated, the patient's legs were then placed in candy cane stirrups. The patient was then prepped and draped in the standard D&C surgical fashion.

The patient was placed in 10 degrees of Trendelenburg. The patient was given 100 mg of doxycycline. The bladder was then decompressed and approximately 45 mL of urine was produced. A weighted speculum was placed in the posterior vagina and the cervix was grasped with single-tooth tenaculum. Uterus sounded to 8.2 cm. The cervix was then serially dilated with Hanks dilator. An 8-cm straight suction curette was then introduced and a suction curettage was performed. Once all products of conception were evacuated, a sharp curettage was performed until a gritty surface was appreciated on all four quadrants of the uterus. No further bleeding was noted. Products of conception were then examined on the back table, which was grossly consistent with products of conception.

The patient tolerated the procedure and anesthesia well, was awakened from anesthesia without complications, and was transported to the recovery room in stable condition.

Sandra Lindler-6789

558645/mt98328: 03/25/19 09:50:16 T: 03/26/19 12:55:01

Determine the most accurate ICD-10-PCS code(s) for the extraction.

(continued)

WESTWARD HOSPITAL

591 Chester Road

Masters, FL 33955

OPERATIVE REPORT

PATIENT: HOFFMEIER, KATHLEEN

ACCOUNT/EHR #: HOFFKA001

DATE OF ADMISSION: 28 March 2019

ADMITTING DIAGNOSIS: Right tubal ectopic pregnancy

PROCEDURE: Operative laparoscopy, right salpingectomy

SURGEON: William G. Cohen, MD

ANESTHESIA: General

This 28-year-old female presents to the emergency room with vaginal bleeding and belly pain that gets worse with movement. Patient states she is pregnant at approximately 8-weeks gestation, G1 P0. Ultrasound report showed a mass near the cul-de-sac. The patient denies any medical or surgical history. No known allergies. Family history is noncontributory. The patient was admitted to the hospital.

The patient was taken to the OR, where general anesthesia was easily obtained. The patient was then prepped and draped in a sterile fashion and placed in dorsal lithotomy position. A weighted speculum was introduced into the patient's vagina for cervical visualization. Once the cervix was visualized, a single-toothed tenaculum was applied to the upper lip of the cervix, and acorn manipulator was introduced into the patient's cervix.

Attention was then drawn to the abdomen, where a 10-mm horizontal incision was done below the umbilicus and carried down all the way to the fascia. Under direct visualization, a 10-mm trocar was introduced into the patient's abdomen. Once intraperitoneal placement was confirmed, pneumoperitoneum was started. Opening pressure was 3 mmHg; pneumoperitoneum was obtained.

Once pneumoperitoneum was obtained, a second port was put two fingerbreadths above the pubic symphysis, and under direct visualization, a 5-mm trocar was then introduced into the patient's abdomen. The patient was placed in Trendelenburg position. Pelvic structures were revealed; ampullary ectopic was noted on the right side with some amount of hemoperitoneum and moderate amount of free fluid.

Attention was focused on the right fallopian tube, which initially was incised where the ectopic pregnancy was and products of conception were removed. Since no hemostasis was able to be obtained from the incision site from the salpingostomy and due to the amount of dense adhesions on that fallopian tube, decision was then made to proceed with right salpingectomy, so the IP ligament was identified and fallopian tube was then grasped by the fimbria and incised from the mesosalpinx. Good hemostasis was noted from the fallopian tube sites and the operative site. Specimen was then removed from the patient's abdomen. Copious irrigation was done and all clots and debris were removed from the patient's abdomen. Once good hemostasis was noted from the patient's abdomen, pneumoperitoneum was deflated and all trocars were removed. Infraumbilical fascia was closed with 0 Vicryl and interrupted suture. The skin was closed with 4-0 Vicryl. The right infrapubic and suprapubic ports were closed with 0 Vicryl in running fashion, and third port, which was introduced two fingerbreadths above the pubis symphysis and 6 cm in the midaxillary line, under direct visualization, was also closed with 4-0 Monocryl. Sponge, lap, and needle counts were correct x2. The patient was taken to the recovery room in stable condition.

(continued)

DIET: As tolerated.

PHYSICAL ACTIVITY: No heavy lifting. Pelvic rest.

William G. Cohen, MD-6543

558645/mt98328: 03/28/19 09:50:16 T: 03/29/19 12:55:01

Determine the most accurate ICD-10-PCS code(s) for the salpingectomy.

35 Placement through Chiropractic Sections

Key Terms

Administration
Extra-articular
Extracorporeal
Measurement
Placement
Somatic

Learning Outcomes

After completing this chapter, the student should be able to:

LO 35.1 Recognize the details reported in the Placement—Anatomical Regions section and Placement—Anatomical Orifices section.

LO 35.2 Evaluate the details to determine the services reported from the Administration section.

LO 35.3 Determine the specifics required to build a code from the Measurement and Monitoring section.

LO 35.4 Interpret the documentation to report a service from the Extracorporeal or Systemic Assistance and Performance section.

LO 35.5 Abstract the documentation to determine a code for a service reported from the Extracorporeal or Systemic Therapies section.

LO 35.6 Utilize knowledge to report a code from the Osteopathic section.

LO 35.7 Identify the details necessary to build a code from the Other Procedures section.

LO 35.8 Distinguish the services provided to determine reporting a code from the Chiropractic section.

LO 35.9 Analyze the documentation to build a complete and accurate code(s) in ICD-10-PCS for sections 2–9.

 STOP! Remember, you need to follow along in your ICD-10-PCS code book for an optimal learning experience.

35.1 Reporting Services from the Placement Section

Character Definitions

The meanings for the *Placement* section characters are in the following table:

Character Position	Character Meaning
1	Section of the ICD-10-PCS book
2	Anatomical region/orifices
3	Root operation term
4	Body region/orifice
5	Approach used by physician
6	Device
7	Qualifier

You might have noticed that these are slightly different meanings for characters 2 and 4 than those in the *Medical and Surgical* and *Obstetrics* sections.

Character Position 1: Placement Section 2

Character Position	Character Meaning
1	Section of the ICD-10-PCS book
2	Anatomical region/orifices
3	Root operation term
4	Body region/orifice
5	Approach used by physician
6	Device
7	Qualifier

The procedures reported with codes from this section explain the location of a device either in or on a body region for protection, immobilization, stretching, compression, or packing. These procedures are some that you are familiar with, such as application of a splint to immobilize or a traction device to stretch a muscle. For the most part, the devices in this section are "off the shelf," so to speak, and not customized fabrications. (More about these devices will be discussed when we get to that character position.)

Character Position 2: Anatomical Region/Orifices

Character Position	Character Meaning
1	Section of the ICD-10-PCS book
2	Anatomical region/orifices
3	Root operation term
4	Body region/orifice
5	Approach used by physician
6	Device
7	Qualifier

> **CODING BITES**
>
> Remember, an anatomical orifice is a natural opening into the body; for example, mouth, nose, urethra.

There are only two body system options:

Anatomical Regions . . . Character: **W**
Anatomical Orifices . . . Character: **Y**

Character Position 3: Root Operation

Character Position	Character Meaning
1	Section of the ICD-10-PCS book
2	Anatomical region/orifices
3	Root operation term
4	Body region/orifice
5	Approach used by physician
6	Device
7	Qualifier

The codes from the *Placement* section only report procedures that are noninvasive, meaning that the outer layer of the skin is not punctured and no incision is made.

Change

> <u>Change</u>: Taking out or off a device from a body part and putting back an identical or similar device in or on the same body part without cutting or puncturing the skin or a mucous membrane . . . Character: **0**

Caution! This root operation term means the same as it does in the *Medical and Surgical* and the *Obstetrics* sections; however, the character used to report this in the *Placement* section is different.

> ### EXAMPLE
>
> 2W05X3Z   Change external back brace

Compression

> <u>Compression</u>: Putting pressure on a body region . . . Character: **1**

> ### EXAMPLE
>
> 2W1RX7Z   Placement of intermittent pressure device on lower left leg

Dressing

> <u>Dressing</u>: Putting material on a body region for protection . . . Character: **2**

> ### EXAMPLE
>
> 2W2EX4Z   Placement of bandage on right hand

Immobilization

> <u>Immobilization</u>: Limiting or preventing motion of an external body region . . . Character: **3**

> ### EXAMPLES
>
> 2W3KX1Z   Application of a splint to a left finger
> 2W35X3Z   Back brace placed on patient

Packing

> <u>Packing</u>: Putting material in a body region or orifice . . . Character: **4**

> ### EXAMPLES
>
> 2W48X5Z   Packing to wound on right upper extremity
> 2Y41X5Z   Packing of nasal cavities due to epistaxis

Removal

> <u>Removal</u>: Taking out or off a device from a body part . . . Character: **5**

Read this carefully: As the description specifically states "device," this can be used only for this type of procedure—to remove a previously placed device. As you abstract the physician's notes, be cautious of the use of this term in documentation.

Caution! This root operation term means the same as it does in the *Medical and Surgical* and the *Obstetrics* sections; however, the character used to report this in the *Placement* section is different.

<table>
<tr><td colspan="2">EXAMPLES</td></tr>
<tr><td>2W5MX3Z</td><td>Removal, G3 XL post-op knee brace, left leg</td></tr>
<tr><td>2W5TX0Z</td><td>Removal of traction apparatus from left foot</td></tr>
</table>

Traction

Traction: Exerting a pulling force on a body region in a distal direction . . .
Character: **6**

Notice that *Traction* is presented as a root operation term as well as traction apparatus that is offered as an option for the device used.

<table>
<tr><td colspan="2">EXAMPLE</td></tr>
<tr><td>2W62X0Z</td><td>Traction apparatus placed at neck</td></tr>
</table>

Character Position 4: Body Region/Orifice

Character Position	Character Meaning
1	Section of the ICD-10-PCS book
2	Anatomical region/orifices
3	Root operation term
4	**Body region/orifice**
5	Approach used by physician
6	Device
7	Qualifier

The two body systems in this section (Anatomical Regions and Anatomical Orifices) each has a list of applicable body regions and their characters.

Anatomical Regions

Head . . . Character: **0**	Upper Arm, Right . . . A	Lower Extremity, Right . . . L
Face . . . 1	Upper Arm, Left . . . B	Lower Extremity, Left . . . M
Neck . . . 2	Lower Arm, Right . . . C	Upper Leg, Right . . . N
Abdominal Wall . . . 3	Lower Arm, Left . . . D	Upper Leg, Left . . . P
Chest Wall . . . 4	Hand, Right . . . E	Lower Leg, Right . . . Q
Back . . . 5	Hand, Left . . . F	Lower Leg, Left . . . R
Inguinal Region, Right . . . 6	Thumb, Right . . . G	Foot, Right . . . S
Inguinal Region, Left . . . 7	Thumb, Left . . . H	Foot, Left . . . T
Upper Extremity, Right . . . 8	Finger, Right . . . J	Toe, Right . . . U
Upper Extremity, Left . . . 9	Finger, Left . . . K	Toe, Left . . . V

Anatomical Orifices

Mouth and Pharynx . . . 0	Ear . . . 2	Female Genital Tract . . . 4
Nasal . . . 1	Anorectal . . . 3	Urethra . . . 5

Character Position 5: Approach

Character Position	Character Meaning
1	Section of the ICD-10-PCS book
2	Anatomical region/orifices
3	Root operation term
4	Body region/orifice
5	**Approach used by physician**
6	Device
7	Qualifier

This one is easy; there is only one choice. Remember that all procedures reported from the *Placement* section do not involve incisions or punctures. This means all of these devices are external.

External Approach . . . Character: **X**

Character Position 6: Device

Character Position	Character Meaning
1	Section of the ICD-10-PCS book
2	Anatomical region/orifices
3	Root operation term
4	Body region/orifice
5	Approach used by physician
6	**Device**
7	Qualifier

It makes sense that there are several options for the character to report a device because that is really the primary activity of this section: **placement** of a device.

Placement
To put a device in or on an anatomical site.

Traction Apparatus . . . Character: **0**
Splint . . . Character: **1**
Cast . . . Character: **2**
Brace . . . Character: **3**
Bandage . . . Character: **4**
Packing Material . . . Character: **5**
Pressure Dressing . . . Character: **6**
Intermittent Pressure Device . . . Character: **7**
Wire . . . Character: **9**
Other Device . . . Character: **Y**
No Device . . . Character: **Z**

EXAMPLES

You might see phrases such as these in the documentation:

"*. . . and a short arm splint, right side, was applied. . . .*"

2W38X1Z   Immobilization using a splint, upper extremity, right

"*. . .The new Philadelphia collar was removed. . . .* "

2W52X3Z   Removal of neck brace

Character Position 7: Qualifier

Character Position	Character Meaning
1	Section of the ICD-10-PCS book
2	Anatomical region/orifices
3	Root operation term
4	Body region/orifice
5	Approach used by physician
6	Device
7	Qualifier

There are no details reported by the Qualifier position, so the only option is **Z** No Qualifier.

 LET'S CODE IT! SCENARIO

Michael Shinto, a 31-year-old male, was in a fight at a bar and was punched in the face. Along with other injuries, Michael's lower jaw was dislocated. Dr. Northrop admitted Michael into the hospital due to internal bleeding. Once in his room, Dr. Northrop took Michael to the procedure room to wire his jaw to immobilize it and permit it to heal.

Let's Code It!

Let's go through the steps of coding for ICD-10-PCS and determine the code or codes that should be reported for this encounter between Dr. Northrop and Michael Shinto.

Which section will provide you with the details to report this procedure? Let's think this through. Dr. Northrop wired Michael's jaw. Therefore, he placed wire . . . the **Placement** section.

First character: Section: Placement . . . 2

You have two choices for body system: Anatomical Regions or Anatomical Orifices. The jaw is not an orifice, so the decision is straightforward.

Second character: Body Region: Anatomical Regions . . . W

What was the purpose of placing the wire? The documentation states, *"to immobilize it."*

Third character: Root Operation: Immobilization . . . 3

Read the options in the Body Region column carefully. Which anatomical site comes closest because *jaw* is not listed? Yes, the jaw is a part of the head, but it is also part of the face. Hmm. In this circumstance, we need to read ahead a little bit to the list shown in the column to the right for Device. You know for certain that *wire* was used, and there is only an option for Wire on the row with Face, not Head. Therefore, you can tell which to report.

Fourth character: Body Region: Face . . . 1

It is logical that the wire was placed externally, and this is the only option you have for the fifth character. Nice.

Fifth character: Approach: External . . . X

You know that the device is Wire because the documentation states, *"wire his jaw."*

Sixth character: Device: Wire . . . 9

There is only one option for the qualifier for this row on this Table.

Seventh character: Qualifier: No Qualifier . . . Z

The ICD-10-PCS code you will report is

2W31X9Z   **Wire jaw**

Good job!

35.2 Reporting Services from the Administration Section

Character Definitions

The meanings for the *Administration* section characters are shown in the following table:

Character Position	Character Meaning
1	Section of the ICD-10-PCS book
2	Physiological system or anatomical region
3	Root operation term
4	Body system or region
5	Approach used by physician
6	Substance
7	Qualifier

For the most part, these character positions have different meanings than the other sections you have already learned about.

Character Position 1: Administration Section 3

Character Position	Character Meaning
1	Section of the ICD-10-PCS book
2	Physiological system or anatomical region
3	Root operation term
4	Body system or region
5	Approach used by physician
6	Substance
7	Qualifier

Procedures reported from the *Administration* section will all begin with the number **3**.

Character Position 2: Physiological System/ Anatomical Region

Character Position	Character Meaning
1	Section of the ICD-10-PCS book
2	Physiological system or Anatomical region
3	Root operation term
4	Body system or region
5	Approach used by physician
6	Substance
7	Qualifier

There are only three options for the second character:

Circulatory . . . Character: **0** [*This is used for transfusion procedures.*]
Indwelling Device . . . Character: **C**
Physiological Systems and Anatomical Regions . . . Character: **E**

> **EXAMPLE**
>
> Roy Shearmann, a 47-year-old male, was diagnosed with myelodysplastic syndrome several months ago when he presented with progressive pancytopenia. Since admission, he has undergone treatment with antibiotics and has received transfusion of nonautologous packed RBCs, administrated via peripheral vein, IV. The patient continues on weekly Procrit. Code for the blood transfusion.
>
> 30233N1   Transfusion, nonautologous red blood cells, peripheral vein, percutaneously

Character Position 3: Root Operation

Character Position	Character Meaning
1	Section of the ICD-10-PCS book
2	Physiological system or anatomical region
3	**Root operation term**
4	Body system or region
5	Approach used by physician
6	Substance
7	Qualifier

There are only three root operation terms used to report procedures in this section:

Introduction: Putting in or on a therapeutic, diagnostic, nutritional, physiological, or prophylactic substance except blood or blood products . . . Character: **0**
Irrigation: Putting in or on a cleansing substance . . . Character: **1**
Transfusion: Putting in blood or blood products . . . Character: **2**

> **EXAMPLE**
>
> Illanya Sibgame, a pleasant 55-year-old female patient, is admitted to undergo treatment for a non-Hodgkin lymphoma. While admitted, intrathecal chemotherapy, DepoCyt 50 mg (a low-dose interleukin-2 drug), was administered. She did tolerate all treatments well with no complication noted, and once stable, was made ready for discharge home.
>
> 3E0R303   Introduction of low-dose interleukin-2 antineoplastic, intrathecal

Character Position 4: Body System/Region

Character Position	Character Meaning
1	Section of the ICD-10-PCS book
2	Physiological system or anatomical region
3	Root operation term
4	**Body system or region**
5	Approach used by physician
6	Substance
7	Qualifier

Specifically for this section, the fourth character position will report the anatomical site into which the substance is administered. Be careful. This may be different from the site expected to benefit from the ultimate effect of this substance. For example, if the substance is administered intradermally (such as an intradermal patch), the body system/region would be skin and mucous membrane, whereas an IM (intramuscular) injection would be reported as the muscle in this character position. IA (intra-arterial) or IV (intravenous) **administrations** would be reported to the peripheral artery or peripheral vein, respectively. However, if a catheter is used—for example, to travel to administer the substance directly to a clot—this would be reported as a central artery or central vein, per the documentation.

Oddly, there is an exception. When an irrigating substance (such as saline solution) is administered into an indwelling device (reported as body system **C** Indwelling Device), the body system/region will be **Z** None.

Character Position 5: Approach

Character Position	Character Meaning
1	Section of the ICD-10-PCS book
2	Physiological system or anatomical region
3	Root operation term
4	Body system or region
5	**Approach used by physician**
6	Substance
7	Qualifier

The approaches for this section are those you have come to know: **0** Open, **3** Percutaneous, **4** Percutaneous Endoscopic, **7** Via Natural or Artificial Opening, **8** Via Natural or Artificial Opening Endoscopic, and **X** External.

Character Position 6: Substance

Character Position	Character Meaning
1	Section of the ICD-10-PCS book
2	Physiological system or anatomical region
3	Root operation term
4	Body system or region
5	Approach used by physician
6	**Substance**
7	Qualifier

In this character position, you will identify the substance being administered. Be careful! The Substance characters reported for Circulatory (second character 0) and those reported for Physiological Systems and Anatomical Regions (second character E) have different meanings for the same letters. This is a great example of why it is so important to read each table carefully and completely and to avoid assuming that the same letter means the same from table to table, even in the same section.

EXAMPLES

30***G*	Administration, Circulatory, ***, Bone marrow, *
3E***G*	Administration, Physiological Systems, ***, Other Therapeutic Substance, *

Character Position 7: Qualifier

Character Position	Character Meaning
1	Section of the ICD-10-PCS book
2	Physiological system or anatomical region
3	Root operation term
4	Body system or region
5	Approach used by physician
6	Substance
7	Qualifier

This character will provide additional detail about the substance, if necessary.

EXAMPLES

Autologous . . . Character: **0**
Nonautologous . . . Character: **1**
Oxazolidinones . . . Character: **8**
No Qualifier . . . Character: **Z**

 LET'S CODE IT! SCENARIO

Sean McRoyale, a 41-year-old male, was admitted into McGraw Hospital. Dr. Toller administered nonautologous pancreatic islet cells, intravenously.

Let's Code It!

Let's go through the steps of coding for ICD-10-PCS and determine the code or codes that should be reported for this encounter between Dr. Toller and Sean McRoyale.

From which section will you report this? The documentation actually tells you, where it states, "*administered.*"

First character: Section: Administration . . . 3

There are three choices, as you learned, for body system in this section. While it might make sense to think that Circulatory would be correct when the documentation states, "*intravenously,*" as you read the Table, however, you can see that there is only one Root Operation Term under this body system, and this is Transfusion [Putting in blood or blood products], and this does not fit at all. Next is Indwelling Device, and that does not fit either. Therefore, the only realistic option is Physiological Systems and Anatomical Regions.

Second character: Physiological Systems and Anatomical Regions . . . E

You have only two options for a Root Operation Term for this body system in the ***Administration*** section: Introduction and Irrigation. You know Irrigation [Putting in or on a cleansing substance] does not fit. And the following details will help you confirm this decision.

Third character: Root Operation: Introduction . . . 0

The documentation states, "*intravenously.*" This means this substance was administered into a vein. This narrows down the options to Central Vein or Peripheral Vein. Venipuncture is typically done in the cubital fossa (inside the elbow), which includes three peripheral veins. Of course, in real life, when you are on the job, you must confirm this with additional documentation or the provider. For now, we will accept this was done via a peripheral vein.

(continued)

Fourth character: Body Region: Peripheral Vein . . . 3

Venipuncture is performed percutaneously, directly into the vein.

Fifth character: Approach: Percutaneous . . . 3

There are many, many choices in this sixth character column. The documentation states "*pancreatic islet cells*" as the substance. Find it, and make certain it is on the same row as Peripheral Vein.

Sixth character: Substance: Pancreatic Islet Cells . . . U

What type of cells? The documentation states, "*nonautologous.*"

Seventh character: Qualifier: Nonautologous . . . 1

The ICD-10-PCS code you will report is

3E033U1   Introduction of nonautologous pancreatic islet cells, percutaneous, to peripheral vein

Good job!

35.3 Reporting Services from the Measurement and Monitoring Section

Character Definitions

The meanings for the *Measurement and Monitoring* section characters are shown in the following table:

Character Position	Character Meaning
1	Section of the ICD-10-PCS book
2	Physiological system
3	Root operation term
4	Body system
5	Approach used by physician
6	Function/device
7	Qualifier

For the most part, these character positions have different meanings than those in the other sections you have already learned about.

Character Position 1: Measurement and Monitoring Section 4

Character Position	Character Meaning
1	Section of the ICD-10-PCS book
2	Physiological system
3	Root operation term
4	Body system
5	Approach used by physician
6	Function/device
7	Qualifier

Procedures reported from the *Measurement and Monitoring* section will all begin with the number **4**.

Character Position 2: Physiological System

Character Position	Character Meaning
1	Section of the ICD-10-PCS book
2	**Physiological system**
3	Root operation term
4	Body system
5	Approach used by physician
6	Function/device
7	Qualifier

There are only two options for the second character:

Physiological Systems . . . Character: **A**
Physiological Devices . . . Character: **B**

Character Position 3: Root Operation

Character Position	Character Meaning
1	Section of the ICD-10-PCS book
2	Physiological system
3	**Root operation term**
4	Body system
5	Approach used by physician
6	Function/device
7	Qualifier

There are only two root operation terms used to report procedures in this section.

<u>Measurement:</u> **Determining the level of a physiological or physical function at a point in time** . . . Character: **0**
<u>Monitoring:</u> **Determining the level of a physiological or physical function repetitively over a period of time** . . . Character: **1**

> **EXAMPLE**
>
> An ECG measures the electrical activity of the heart at one point in time, whereas a Holter monitor continuously monitors the heart's rhythms over 24–48 hours.
>
> 1. ECG reported with **4A02X4Z Measurement of cardiac electrical activity, external**
> 2. Holter reported with **4A12XFZ Monitoring cardiac rhythms, externally**

Character Position 4: Body System

Character Position	Character Meaning
1	Section of the ICD-10-PCS book
2	Physiological system
3	Root operation term
4	**Body system**
5	Approach used by physician
6	Function/device
7	Qualifier

Measurement
To determine a level of a
physiological or physical
function.

The specific body system being measured or monitored is identified by the character in the fourth position. Note that this section includes **measurement** or monitoring of a patient's metabolism, temperature, or sleep. These are reported with a body system of **Z** None.

> ### EXAMPLES
>
> **Central Nervous System . . .** Character: **0**
> **Cardiac System . . .** Character: **2**
> **Respiratory System . . .** Character: **9**

Character Position 5: Approach

Character Position	Character Meaning
1	Section of the ICD-10-PCS book
2	Physiological system
3	Root operation term
4	Body system
5	**Approach used by physician**
6	Function/device
7	Qualifier

The approaches for this section are those you have come to know: **0** Open, **3** Percutaneous, **4** Percutaneous Endoscopic, **7** Via Natural or Artificial Opening, **8** Via Natural or Artificial Opening Endoscopic, and **X** External.

Character Position 6: Function/Device

Character Position	Character Meaning
1	Section of the ICD-10-PCS book
2	Physiological system
3	Root operation term
4	Body system
5	Approach used by physician
6	**Function/device**
7	Qualifier

In this character position, you will identify the specific body function being measured or monitored, such as rhythm (**F**) of the heart or pressure (**B**) of the blood within the veins. This character may also report a device, such as a pacemaker (**S**) or defibrillator (**T**).

Characters are available for measuring and/or monitoring a patient's metabolism (**6**), temperature (**K**), or sleep (**Q**), such as a sleep study. These three functions use a body system character of **Z** None.

> ### EXAMPLES
>
> 4A0HXCZ   External measurement of fetal heart rate
> 4A1ZXQZ   48 hour sleep study, external monitoring

Character Position 7: Qualifier

Character Position	Character Meaning
1	Section of the ICD-10-PCS book
2	Physiological system
3	Root operation term
4	Body system
5	Approach used by physician
6	Function/device
7	Qualifier

This character will provide additional detail about either the body part or system or the procedure performed.

EXAMPLES

4A10X4G	Monitoring of central nervous system activity, intraoperatively, external
4A143J1	Monitoring of peripheral pulse, venous, external

 LET'S CODE IT! SCENARIO

Katrina Vales is a 17-year-old female with a history of asthma who was admitted with status asthmaticus. Once they were able to stop the current attack, Dr. Giffen measures her respiratory volume using a spirometer.

Let's Code It!

Let's go through the steps of coding for ICD-10-PCS and determine the code or codes that should be reported for this encounter between Dr. Giffen and Katrina Vales.

Which section? The documentation states, "*Dr. Giffen measures. . . .*"

First character: Section: Measurement and Monitoring . . . 4

Now, you have two choices for the body system: Physiological Systems or Physiological Devices. The measurement was of Katrina's respiratory function.

Second character: Body Region: Physiological Systems . . . A

You have two options for the root operation term: Measurement or Monitoring. The documentation states, "*Dr. Giffen measures. . . .*"

Third character: Root Operation: Measurement . . . 0

What body system is being measured? The documentation states, "*respiratory.*"

Fourth character: Body System: Respiratory . . . 9

The documentation states, "*using a spirometer,*" meaning that you must know how a spirometer works to determine the next character. Use your medical dictionary or Google to find the facts about this method.

Fifth character: Approach: External . . . X

(continued)

The documentation states, "*measures her respiratory volume. . . .*"

Sixth character: Function/Device: Volume . . . L

On this row, there is only one option for the seventh character.

Seventh character: Qualifier: No Qualifier . . . Z

The ICD-10-PCS code you will report is

4A09XLZ   Measurement of respiratory volume

Good job!

35.4 Reporting Services from the Extracorporeal or Systemic Assistance and Performance Section

Character Definitions

The meanings for the *Extracorporeal or Systemic Assistance and Performance* section characters are shown in the following table:

Character Position	Character Meaning
1	Section of the ICD-10-PCS book
2	Physiological system
3	Root operation term
4	Body system
5	Duration
6	Function
7	Qualifier

For the most part, the character positions for the *Extracorporeal or Systemic Assistance and Performance* section have similar meanings as in the other sections about which you have already learned.

Character Position 1: Extracorporeal or Systemic Assistance and Performance Section 5

Character Position	Character Meaning
1	Section of the ICD-10-PCS book
2	Physiological system
3	Root operation term
4	Body system
5	Duration
6	Function
7	Qualifier

Procedures reported from the *Extracorporeal or Systemic Assistance and Performance* section will all begin with the number **5.**

Character Position 2: Physiological System

Character Position	Character Meaning
1	Section of the ICD-10-PCS book
2	Physiological system
3	Root operation term
4	Body system
5	Duration
6	Function
7	Qualifier

There is only one option for the second character:

Physiological Systems . . . Character: **A**

Character Position 3: Root Operation

Character Position	Character Meaning
1	Section of the ICD-10-PCS book
2	Physiological system
3	Root operation term
4	Body system
5	Duration
6	Function
7	Qualifier

There are only three root operation terms used to report procedures in this section:

<u>Assistance</u>: **Taking over a portion of a physiological function by extracorporeal means . . .** Character: **0**

<u>Performance</u>: **Completely taking over a physiological function by extracorporeal means . . .** Character: **1**

<u>Restoration</u>: **Returning, or attempting to return, a physiological function to its original state by extracorporeal means . . .** Character: **2**

EXAMPLE

5A05221 Hyperbaric oxygenation of a wound, continuous (an example of assistance because this is done to improve—or assist—the healing of the wound)

Character Position 4: Body System

Character Position	Character Meaning
1	Section of the ICD-10-PCS book
2	Physiological system
3	Root operation term
4	Body system
5	Duration
6	Function
7	Qualifier

The specific body systems being supported by these procedures are

Cardiac System . . . Character: **2**
Circulatory System . . . Character: **5**
Respiratory System . . . Character: **9**
Biliary System . . . Character: **C**
Urinary System . . . Character: **D**

> **EXAMPLE**
>
> 5A1D00Z   Filtration of a single period of duration, urinary system (hemodialysis takes over the physiological function of the urinary system by extracorporeal means)

Character Position 5: Duration

Character Position	Character Meaning
1	Section of the ICD-10-PCS book
2	Physiological system
3	Root operation term
4	Body system
5	**Duration**
6	Function
7	Qualifier

The fifth character position will report the length of time, or the number of times, the patient received this treatment:

Single . . . Character: **0** [*one time or one session*]
Intermittent . . . Character: **1** [*occasionally*]
Continuous . . . Character: **2** [*nonstop ongoing*]
Less than 24 Consecutive Hours . . . Character: **3** [*nonstop for a period of time*]
24–96 Consecutive Hours . . . Character: **4** [*nonstop for a period of time*]
Greater than 96 Consecutive Hours . . . Character: **5** [*nonstop for a period of time*]
Multiple . . . Character: **6** [*more than one time or one session*]
Intermittent, Less than 6 hours per day . . . Character: **7**
Prolonged Intermittent, 6–18 hours per day . . . Character: **8**
Continuous, Greater than 18 hours per day . . . Character: **9**

> **EXAMPLE**
>
> After the surgery, Brandon was kept on a ventilator for 31 hours.
>
> 5A1945Z   Respiratory ventilator, 24–96 consecutive hours

Character Position 6: Function

Character Position	Character Meaning
1	Section of the ICD-10-PCS book
2	Physiological system
3	Root operation term
4	Body system
5	Duration
6	**Function**
7	Qualifier

In this character position, you will identify the specific physiological function occurring during this procedure:

Filtration . . . Character: **0**
Output . . . Character: **1**
Oxygenation . . . Character: **2**
Pacing . . . Character: **3**
Rhythm . . . Character: **4**
Ventilation . . . Character: **5**

EXAMPLE

5A2204Z   Restoration of heart rhythm, single event (performing CPR)

Character Position 7: Qualifier

Character Position	Character Meaning
1	Section of the ICD-10-PCS book
2	Physiological system
3	Root operation term
4	Body system
5	Duration
6	Function
7	Qualifier

When a device or piece of equipment is used in the provision of the **extracorporeal** assistance or performance, the Qualifier will specify what was used:

Extracorporeal
Outside of the body.

Balloon Pump . . . Character: **0**
Hyperbaric . . . Character: **1**
Manual . . . Character: **2**
Membrane . . . Character: **3**
Nonmechanical . . . Character: **4**
Pulsatile Compression . . . Character: **5**
Other Pump . . . Character: **6**
Continuous Positive Airway Pressure (CPAP) . . . Character: **7**
Intermittent Positive Airway Pressure (IPAP) . . . Character: **8**
Continuous Negative Airway Pressure (CNAP) . . . Character: **9**
Intermittent Negative Airway Pressure (INAP) . . . Character: **B**
Supersaturated . . . Character: **C**
Impeller Pump . . . Character: **D**
Membrane, Central . . . Character: **F**
Membrane, Peripheral Veno-arterial . . . Character: **G**
Membrane, Peripheral Veno-venous . . . Character: **H**
No Qualifier . . . Character: **Z**

 LET'S CODE IT! SCENARIO

Linus Garza, a 63-year-old male, was in the hospital for surgery on his leg. During Linus's admission, Dr. Reagan ordered a CPAP machine to treat Linus's obstructive sleep apnea, only at night.

(continued)

Let's go through the steps of coding for ICD-10-PCS and determine the code or codes that should be reported for this encounter between Dr. Reagan and Linus Garza for the CPAP treatment.

You already learned that *extracorporeal* means "outside of the body." You also need to know how a CPAP machine works.

First character: Section: Extracorporeal or Systemic Assistance and Performance . . . 5

There is only one body system option for this section.

Second character: Body System: Physiological Systems . . . A

A CPAP machine helps the body's breathing; it does not breathe for the patient. Therefore, assistance is the appropriate root operation term.

Third character: Root Operation: Assistance . . . 0

The CPAP assists the patient's breathing, so this is the Respiratory system.

Fourth character: Body System: Respiratory . . . 9

How long was Linus to be using the CPAP continuously? The documentation states, "*only at night,*" therefore, less than 24 hours.

Fifth character: Duration: Less than 24 Consecutive Hours . . . 3

There is only one option for the sixth character, but it fits because *ventilation,* in health care, is breathing.

Sixth character: Function: Ventilation . . . 5

What does CPAP stand for?

Seventh character: Qualifier: Continuous Positive Airway Pressure . . . 7

The ICD-10-PCS code you will report is:

5A09357   **CPAP ventilation, less than 24 consecutive hours**

Good job!

35.5 Reporting Services from the Extracorporeal or Systemic Therapies Section

Character Definitions

The meanings for the *Extracorporeal or Systemic Therapies* section characters are shown in the following table:

Character Position	Character Meaning
1	Section of the ICD-10-PCS book
2	Physiological systems
3	Root operation
4	Body system
5	Duration
6	Qualifier
7	Qualifier

For the most part, the character positions for the *Extracorporeal or Systemic Therapies* section have similar meanings as in the other sections about which you have already learned. The difference between the procedures reported from this section and those from the *Extracorporeal or Systemic Assistance and Performance* section is that these therapies do not involve the process of assisting a physiological function or performing that function for the body.

Character Position 1: Extracorporeal or Systemic Therapies Section 6

Character Position	Character Meaning
1	Section of the ICD-10-PCS book
2	Physiological systems
3	Root operation
4	Body system
5	Duration
6	Qualifier
7	Qualifier

Procedures reported from the *Extracorporeal or Systemic Therapies* section will all begin with the number **6.**

Character Position 2: Physiological Systems

Character Position	Character Meaning
1	Section of the ICD-10-PCS book
2	Physiological systems
3	Root operation
4	Body system
5	Duration
6	Qualifier
7	Qualifier

There is only one option for the second character:

Physiological Systems . . . Character: **A**

Character Position 3: Root Operation

Character Position	Character Meaning
1	Section of the ICD-10-PCS book
2	Physiological systems
3	Root operation
4	Body system
5	Duration
6	Qualifier
7	Qualifier

There are 11 root operation terms used to report procedures in this section.

Atmospheric Control: Extracorporeal control of atmospheric pressure and composition . . . Character: **0**

Decompression: Extracorporeal elimination of undissolved gas from body fluids . . . Character: **1**

Electromagnetic Therapy: Extracorporeal treatment by electromagnetic rays . . . Character: **2**

Hyperthermia: Extracorporeal raising of body temperature . . . Character: **3**

Hypothermia: Extracorporeal lowering of body temperature . . . Character: **4**

Pheresis: Extracorporeal separation of blood products . . . Character: **5**

Phototherapy: Extracorporeal treatment by light rays . . . Character: **6**

Ultrasound Therapy: Extracorporeal treatment by ultrasound . . . Character: **7**

Ultraviolet Light Therapy: Extracorporeal treatment by ultraviolet light . . . Character: **8**

Shock Wave Therapy: Extracorporeal treatment by shock waves . . . Character: **9**

Perfusion: Extracorporeal treatment by diffusion of therapeutic fluid . . . Character: **B**

- The root operation term *decompression* is specific to a hyperbaric chamber used for treating decompression sickness, also known as the bends.
- When a *hyperthermic* procedure is used to treat a temperature imbalance, this is the section from which to report the code. However, if hyperthermia is used as an adjunct radiation treatment for a malignancy, this procedure is reported from the *Radiation Therapy* section (character **D**).
- The procedure *pheresis* is used primarily for two purposes: (1) to treat a condition during which too much of a specific blood component is produced by the body (such as leukemia) and (2) to remove a blood product from donor blood for purposes of transfusion to another patient, such as platelets.
- The *phototherapy* process removes blood from the patient into a machine that exposes that blood to light rays, recirculates it, and then returns this blood to the body.
- Note that *Shock Wave Therapy* is placed in the Tables section in numeric order (following table 8, Ultraviolet Light Therapy) and not in alphabetic order.

Character Position 4: Body System

Character Position	Character Meaning
1	Section of the ICD-10-PCS book
2	Physiological systems
3	Root operation
4	**Body system**
5	Duration
6	Qualifier
7	Qualifier

The specific body systems being supported by these procedures are

Skin . . . Character: **0**
Urinary . . . Character: **1**
Central Nervous . . . Character: **2**
Musculoskeletal . . . Character: **3**
Circulatory . . . Character: **5**
Respiratory System . . . Character: **B**

Hepatobiliary System and Pancreas . . . Character: **F**
Urinary System . . . Character: **T**
None . . . Character: **Z**

Therapies such as atmospheric control, hyperthermia, and hypothermia are performed on the entire body and, therefore, have a body system of **Z** None.

Character Position 5: Duration

Character Position	Character Meaning
1	Section of the ICD-10-PCS book
2	Physiological systems
3	Root operation
4	Body system
5	**Duration**
6	Qualifier
7	Qualifier

The fifth character position will report the length of time, or the number of times, the patient received this treatment:

Single . . . Character: **0** [*one time or one session*]
Multiple . . . Character: **1** [*more than one time or one session*]

Character Position 6: Qualifier

Character Position	Character Meaning
1	Section of the ICD-10-PCS book
2	Physiological systems
3	Root operation
4	Body system
5	Duration
6	**Qualifier**
7	Qualifier

In this character position, there is one option for the 6AB Perfusion Table:

Donor Organ . . . Character: **B**

For all other Tables in this section, you have one option:

No Qualifier . . . Character: **Z**

Character Position 7: Qualifier

Character Position	Character Meaning
1	Section of the ICD-10-PCS book
2	Physiological systems
3	Root operation
4	Body system
5	Duration
6	Qualifier
7	**Qualifier**

When *pheresis* is performed, the Qualifier will specify what was used:

Erythrocytes . . . Character: **0**
Leukocytes . . . Character: **1**
Platelets . . . Character: **2**
Plasma . . . Character: **3**
Stem Cells, Cord Blood . . . Character: **T**
Stem Cells, Hematopoietic . . . Character: **V**

Ultrasound therapies performed on the circulatory system will utilize a Qualifier character to identify which specific vessels are being treated, when applicable:

Head and Neck Vessels . . . Character: **4**
Heart . . . Character: **5**
Peripheral Vessels . . . Character: **6**
Other Vessels . . . Character: **7**
No Qualifier . . . Character: **Z**

All other root operation terms (therapies) reported from this section have only one option:

No Qualifier . . . Character: **Z**

 LET'S CODE IT! SCENARIO

Nathan Teeger, a 17-year-old male, was out walking near the ski resort where he was vacationing. He fell into a soft bed of snow and could not get out. The ski patrol took 5 hours to find him. At the hospital, Dr. Golden used hyperthermia to warm his body gently back to normal temperature. A single treatment was sufficient.

Let's Code It!

Let's go through the steps of coding for ICD-10-PCS and determine the code or codes that should be reported for this encounter between Dr. Golden and Nathan Teeger for this therapy.

Hyperthermia, from outside of Nathan's body, was used to help improve Nathan's health. You learned that this means it is a therapeutic procedure. Therefore, ***Extracorporeal or Systemic Therapies*** will be the section from which you will report the code for this procedure.

First character: Section: Extracorporeal or Systemic Therapies . . . 6

There is only one option for body system in this section.

Second character: Body Region: Physiological Systems . . . A

The documentation states, "*used hyperthermia.*"

Third character: Root Operation: Hyperthermia . . . 3
Fourth character: Body System: None . . . Z

How many times did Dr. Golden use hyperthermia to treat Nathan? The documentation states, "*A single treatment. . . .*"

Fifth character: Duration: Single . . . 0
Sixth character: Qualifier: None . . . Z
Seventh character: Qualifier: None . . . Z

The ICD-10-PCS code you will report is

6A3Z0ZZ   **Hyperthermia for temperature imbalance**

Good job!

35.6 Reporting Osteopathic Services

Character Definitions

The meanings for the *Osteopathic* section characters are shown in the following table:

Character Position	Character Meaning
1	Section of the ICD-10-PCS book
2	Anatomical regions
3	Root operation term
4	Body region
5	Approach
6	Method
7	Qualifier

The *Osteopathic* section is very direct and straightforward.

Character Position 1: Osteopathic Section 7

Character Position	Character Meaning
1	Section of the ICD-10-PCS book
2	Anatomical regions
3	Root operation term
4	Body region
5	Approach
6	Method
7	Qualifier

Procedures reported from the *Osteopathic* section will all begin with the number **7**.

Character Position 2: Anatomical Regions

Character Position	Character Meaning
1	Section of the ICD-10-PCS book
2	Anatomical regions
3	Root operation term
4	Body region
5	Approach
6	Method
7	Qualifier

There is only one option for the second character:

Anatomical Regions . . . Character: **W**

Character Position 3: Root Operation

Character Position	Character Meaning
1	Section of the ICD-10-PCS book
2	Anatomical regions
3	**Root operation term**
4	Body region
5	Approach
6	Method
7	Qualifier

There is only one root operation used when reporting osteopathic services:

Treatment: Manual treatment to eliminate or alleviate somatic dysfunction and related disorders . . . Character: **0**

EXAMPLE

7W03X2Z   General mobilization of the lumbar region

Character Position 4: Body Region

Character Position	Character Meaning
1	Section of the ICD-10-PCS book
2	Anatomical regions
3	Root operation term
4	**Body region**
5	Approach
6	Method
7	Qualifier

The specific body regions supported by osteopathic services are

Head . . . Character: **0**
Cervical . . . Character: **1**
Thoracic . . . Character: **2**
Lumbar . . . Character: **3**
Sacrum . . . Character: **4**
Pelvis . . . Character: **5**
Lower Extremities . . . Character: **6**
Upper Extremities . . . Character: **7**
Rib Cage . . . Character: **8**
Abdomen . . . Character: **9**

EXAMPLE

7W06X8Z   Isotonic muscle energy application to lower extremities

Character Position 5: Approach

Character Position	Character Meaning
1	Section of the ICD-10-PCS book
2	Anatomical regions
3	Root operation term
4	Body region
5	**Approach**
6	Method
7	Qualifier

All osteopathic services use an *external* approach, reported with character **X**.

Character Position 6: Method

Character Position	Character Meaning
1	Section of the ICD-10-PCS book
2	Anatomical regions
3	Root operation term
4	Body region
5	Approach
6	**Method**
7	Qualifier

In this character position, you will identify the specific method used by the doctor during this session:

Articulatory-Raising . . . Character: **0**
Facial Release . . . Character: **1**
General Mobilization . . . Character: **2**
High Velocity–Low Amplitude . . . Character: **3**
Indirect . . . Character: **4**
Low Velocity–High Amplitude . . . Character: **5**
Lymphatic Pump . . . Character: **6**
Muscle Energy—Isometric . . . Character: **7**
Muscle Energy—Isotonic . . . Character: **8**
Other Method . . . Character: **9**

EXAMPLE

7W05X4Z	Indirect treatment of the pelvic region

Character Position 7: Qualifier

Character Position	Character Meaning
1	Section of the ICD-10-PCS book
2	Anatomical regions
3	Root operation term
4	Body region
5	Approach
6	Method
7	**Qualifier**

There is only one option for this character in the *Osteopathic* section:

No Qualifier . . . Character: Z

 LET'S CODE IT! SCENARIO

Diane DeLucca, a 39-year-old female, was admitted due to a nerve condition in her face. After the results of the tests were analyzed, Dr. Slack diagnosed her with Bell's palsy. Dr. Slack, an osteopath, performed a facial release.

Let's Code It!

Let's go through the steps of coding for ICD-10-PCS and determine the code or codes that should be reported for this encounter between Dr. Slack and Diane DeLucca for this treatment.

There is nothing related to *facial release* in the Alphabetic Index. The best clue you have here is that Dr. Slack is an osteopath. For this section, you will find only one option presented for each of the first three characters.

First character: Section: Osteopathic . . . 7
Second character: Anatomical Regions . . . W
Third character: Root Operation: Treatment . . . 0

The treatment was applied to Diane's face; however, this is not one of the options provided for the fourth character. There is one option that is close.

Fourth character: Body System: Head . . . 0

There is only one option for the fifth character.

Fifth character: Approach: External . . . X

What method did Dr. Slack use? The documentation states, "*a facial release.*"

Sixth character: Method: Facial Release . . . 1
Seventh character: Qualifier: None . . . Z

The ICD-10-PCS code you will report is

7W00X1Z   Facial release

Good job!

35.7 Reporting from the Other Procedures Section

Character Definitions

The meanings for the *Other Procedures* section characters are shown in the following table:

Character Position	Character Meaning
1	Section of the ICD-10-PCS book
2	Body system
3	Root operation term
4	Body region
5	Approach
6	Method
7	Qualifier

For the most part, the character positions for the *Other Procedures* section have similar meanings as in the other sections about which you have already learned.

Character Position 1: Other Procedures Section 8

Character Position	Character Meaning
1	Section of the ICD-10-PCS book
2	Body system
3	Root operation term
4	Body region
5	Approach
6	Method
7	Qualifier

Procedures reported from the *Other Procedures* section all begin with the number **8.**

Character Position 2: Body System

Character Position	Character Meaning
1	Section of the ICD-10-PCS book
2	Body system
3	Root operation term
4	Body region
5	Approach
6	Method
7	Qualifier

There are only two options for the second character:

Indwelling Device . . . Character: **C**
Physiological Systems and Anatomical Regions . . . Character: **E**

Character Position 3: Root Operation

Character Position	Character Meaning
1	Section of the ICD-10-PCS book
2	Body system
3	Root operation term
4	Body region
5	Approach
6	Method
7	Qualifier

There is just one root operation term used to report procedures in this section.

<u>Other Procedures</u>: Methodologies that attempt to remediate or cure a disorder or disease . . . Character: **0**

Character Position 4: Body Region

Character Position	Character Meaning
1	Section of the ICD-10-PCS book
2	Body system
3	Root operation term
4	**Body region**
5	Approach
6	Method
7	Qualifier

There are several body regions represented in this section.

Character Position 5: Approach

Character Position	Character Meaning
1	Section of the ICD-10-PCS book
2	Body system
3	Root operation term
4	Body region
5	**Approach**
6	Method
7	Qualifier

The fifth character position, reporting the approach, will provide you with options with which you have become familiar: **0** Open, **3** Percutaneous, **4** Percutaneous Endoscopic, **7** Via Natural or Artificial Opening, **8** Via Natural or Artificial Opening Endoscopic, and **X** External.

Character Position 6: Method

Character Position	Character Meaning
1	Section of the ICD-10-PCS book
2	Body system
3	Root operation term
4	Body region
5	Approach
6	Method
7	Qualifier

In this character position, you will identify the method employed during this procedure:

Acupuncture . . . Character: **0**
Therapeutic Massage . . . Character: **1**
Collection . . . Character: **6**
Computer Assisted Procedure . . . Character: **B**
Robotic Assisted Procedure . . . Character: **C**
Near Infrared Spectroscopy . . . Character: **D**
Other Method . . . Character: **Y**

Character Position 7: Qualifier

Character Position	Character Meaning
1	Section of the ICD-10-PCS book
2	Body system
3	Root operation term
4	Body region
5	Approach
6	Method
7	Qualifier

The Qualifier will provide additional details as available or necessary.

You can see from this list, the Qualifier options range from anesthesia to in vitro fertilization to the use of imaging.

Anesthesia . . . Character: **0**
In Vitro Fertilization . . . Character: **1**
Breast Milk . . . Character: **2**
Sperm . . . Character: **3**
Yoga Therapy . . . Character: **4**
Meditation . . . Character: **5**
Isolation . . . Character: **6**
Examination . . . Character: **7**
Suture Removal . . . Character: **8**
Piercing . . . Character: **9**
Prostate . . . Character: **C**
Rectum . . . Character: **D**
With Fluoroscopy . . . Character: **F**
With Computerized Tomography . . . Character: **G**
With Magnetic Resonance Imaging . . . Character: **H**
No Qualifier . . . Character: **Z**

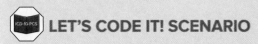

LET'S CODE IT! SCENARIO

Gillian Petrovic, a 31-year-old female, just gave birth via c-section. The nurse provided a pump so that Gillian could collect breast milk for the baby.

Let's Code It!

Let's go through the steps of coding for ICD-10-PCS and determine the code or codes that should be reported for this procedure.

This is not a typical type of hospital procedure, so that might give you a good hint to start with this section, *Other Procedures.*

> **First character: Section: Other Procedures . . . 8**

There are two options for the second character: Indwelling Device or Physiological Systems and Anatomical Regions. Gillian does not have an indwelling device related to this service, so this leaves one option.

> **Second character: Physiological Region: Physiological System and Anatomic Regions . . . E**

There is only one option for the third character.

> **Third character: Root Operation: Other procedures . . . 0**

Don't decide too quickly for the body region. A woman's breast is considered part of the integumentary system, not the female reproductive system.

> **Fourth character: Body Region: Integumentary System and Breast . . . H**

Pumping breast milk is done from outside of the body.

> **Fifth character: Approach: External . . . X**

The pump "collects" the milk.

> **Sixth character: Method: Collection . . . 6**

The qualifier explains what is being collected.

> **Seventh character: Qualifier: Breast Milk . . . 2**

The ICD-10-PCS code you will report is

> **8E0HX62   Collection of breast milk**

Good job!

35.8 Reporting Inpatient Chiropractic Services

Character Definitions

The meanings for the *Chiropractic* section characters are shown in the following table:

Character Position	Character Meaning
1	Section of the ICD-10-PCS book
2	Anatomical regions
3	Root operation term
4	Body region
5	Approach
6	Method
7	Qualifier

The *Chiropractic* section is very direct and straightforward.

Character Position 1: Chiropractic Section 9

Character Position	Character Meaning
1	Section of the ICD-10-PCS book
2	Anatomical regions
3	Root operation term
4	Body region
5	Approach
6	Method
7	Qualifier

Procedures reported from the *Chiropractic* section will all begin with the number **9.**

Character Position 2: Anatomical Regions

Character Position	Character Meaning
1	Section of the ICD-10-PCS book
2	**Anatomical regions**
3	Root operation term
4	Body region
5	Approach
6	Method
7	Qualifier

There is only one option for the second character:

Anatomical Regions . . . Character: **W**

Character Position 3: Root Operation

Character Position	Character Meaning
1	Section of the ICD-10-PCS book
2	Anatomical regions
3	**Root operation term**
4	Body region
5	Approach
6	Method
7	Qualifier

There is only one root operation used when reporting chiropractic services:

<u>Manipulation:</u> **Manual procedure that involves a directed thrust to move a joint past the physiological range of motion, without exceeding the anatomical limit . . .** Character: **B**

EXAMPLE

9WB1XBZ   Non-manual manipulation of the cervical region

Character Position 4: Body Region

Character Position	Character Meaning
1	Section of the ICD-10-PCS book
2	Anatomical regions
3	Root operation term
4	**Body region**
5	Approach
6	Method
7	Qualifier

The specific body regions supported by chiropractic services are:

Head . . . Character: **0**
Cervical . . . Character: **1**
Thoracic . . . Character: **2**
Lumbar . . . Character: **3**
Sacrum . . . Character: **4**
Pelvis . . . Character: **5**
Lower Extremities . . . Character: **6**
Upper Extremities . . . Character: **7**
Rib cage . . . Character: **8**
Abdomen . . . Character: **9**

EXAMPLE

9WB7XKZ   Manipulation of upper extremities, externally, with mechanical assistance

Character Position 5: Approach

Character Position	Character Meaning
1	Section of the ICD-10-PCS book
2	Anatomical regions
3	Root operation term
4	Body region
5	**Approach**
6	Method
7	Qualifier

All chiropractic services use an *external* approach, reported with character **X.**

Character Position 6: Method

Character Position	Character Meaning
1	Section of the ICD-10-PCS book
2	Anatomical regions
3	Root operation term

Character Position	Character Meaning
4	Body region
5	Approach
6	Method
7	Qualifier

In this character position, you will identify the specific method used by the doctor during this session:

Non-Manual . . . Character: **B**
Indirect Visceral . . . Character: **C**
Extra-articular . . . Character: **D**
Direct Visceral . . . Character: **F**
Long Lever Specific Contact . . . Character: **G**
Short Lever Specific Contact . . . Character: **H**
Long and Short Lever Specific Contact . . . Character: **J**
Mechanically Assisted . . . Character: **K**
Other Method . . . Character: **L**

Extra-articular
Located outside a joint.

EXAMPLE

9WB4XFZ   Manipulation of sacrum, external direct visceral method

Character Position 7: Qualifier

Character Position	Character Meaning
1	Section of the ICD-10-PCS book
2	Anatomical regions
3	Root operation term
4	Body region
5	Approach
6	Method
7	Qualifier

There is only one option for this character in the *Chiropractic* section:

No Qualifier . . . Character: **Z**

 LET'S CODE IT! SCENARIO

Ethan Logan, a 49-year-old male, works in a warehouse and hurt his back. He was admitted into the hospital for tests to determine the extent of the injury. While in the hospital, Dr. Maggun, a chiropractor, performed mechanically assisted manipulation on his lumbar region.

You Code It!

Let's go through the steps of coding for ICD-10-PCS and determine the code or codes that should be reported for this encounter between Dr. Maggun and Ethan Logan.

The documentation tells you that Dr. Maggun is a chiropractor, so this is a good reason to turn to the *Chiropractic* section of ICD-10-PCS.

(continued)

You will find only one option for each of the first three characters in this section.

First character: Section: Chiropractic . . . 9
Second character: Body Region: Anatomical Regions . . . W
Third Character: Root Operation: Manipulation . . . B

What region of Ethan's body did Dr. Maggun treat?

Fourth character: Body Region: Lumbar . . . 3

There is only one option here for the fifth character, and it works because chiropractic treatments are done from outside the body.

Fifth character: Approach: External . . . X

What method did Dr. Maggun use on Ethan? The documentation states, "*mechanically assisted. . . .*"

Sixth character: Method: Mechanically Assisted . . . K
Seventh character: Qualifier: None . . . Z

The ICD-10-PCS code you will report is

9WB3XKZ   Chiropractic manipulation of the lumbar region using mechanical assistance

Good job!

35.9 Sections 2–9: Putting It All Together

Throughout this chapter, you have learned about each of the seven components of an ICD-10-PCS code used to report a procedure, service, or treatment from these sections. Now, let's put it all together and determine some codes all the way through.

 LET'S CODE IT! SCENARIO

PATIENT: Alex Renetta

DATE OF ADMISSION: 06/14/2019

ADMITTING DIAGNOSIS: Crush fracture of left lower leg and foot

PAIN MANAGEMENT: The patient has stated that he is in severe pain. However, he is a recovering drug addict, clean 7 years, and will not accept any narcotics.

   Dr. Donnatelli, an acupuncture physician, came in and used acupuncture methodologies to result in anesthesia effect for the left extremity. The patient was relieved by the treatment and the orthopedic surgeon was able to manipulate and cast the leg.
   Code for Dr. Donnatelli.

Let's Code It!

Dr. Donnatelli used acupuncture to administer anesthesia so Alex could have his injury treated. As per the ICD-10-PCS Alphabetic Index, this is reported from the *Other Procedures* section.

First character: Section: Other Procedures . . . 8
Second character: Physiological Systems and Anatomical Regions . . . E
Third character: Root Operation: Other Procedures . . . 0

Remember that anesthesia is a process that uses needles in the skin to accomplish its goal . . .

(continued)

Fourth character: Body Region: Integumentary System and Breast . . . H

Acupuncture is performed by inserting tiny needles gently into the epidermis.

Fifth character: Approach: Percutaneous . . . 3
Sixth character: Method: Acupuncture . . . 0
Seventh character: Qualifier: Anesthesia . . . 0

Put it all together and report code . . .

8E0H300   Anesthesia administered using acupuncture methodologies

Good job!

 LET'S CODE IT! SCENARIO

PATIENT: Travis Clayton

PREOPERATIVE DIAGNOSES:
1. C5–6 facet fracture
2. Left C6 radiculitis

POSTOPERATIVE DIAGNOSES:
1. C5–6 facet fracture
2. Left C6 radiculitis

OPERATIONS PERFORMED:

Attempted closed reduction of vertebral fracture and subluxation with traction.

OPERATION: The patient was taken to the OR and placed in the supine position. Using 1% lidocaine and antibiotic ointment, Gardner-Wells tongs were placed in line with the external auditory meatus approximately a centimeter above the ear. The anesthesiologist, Dr. Mastrioni, administered conscious sedation. The patient tolerated the placement of tongs very well.

Ten pounds of traction were then added and a lateral C-arm image obtained, which showed persistent subluxation. Manual traction was then applied and maneuvers attempted with rotation as well as flexion and extension in an attempt to reduce the fracture. However, persistent subluxation was noted, and the decision was made to proceed with open reduction.

The patient was then administered general anesthetic with use of in-line traction. SSEP and EMG monitoring leads were placed. A Foley catheter was in place. Preoperative antibiotics were administered. SCDs were applied. The patient's arms were tucked to the side. The cervical spine and the left anterior iliac crests were prepped and draped in the standard sterile fashion.

Let's Code It!

Read the documentation of this procedure, and let's take it step by step, one character at a time, to build the correct code:

Traction is . . . placed onto the body, so . . .

First character: Section: Placement . . . 2

The neck is not an orifice, so you have one choice:

Second character: Anatomical Regions . . . W
Third character: Root Operation: Traction . . . 6

In this case, it may be easiest to look at the diagnosis to identify the specific body region being treated. The documentation states, "*C5–6 facet fracture*," which is in the neck.

(continued)

Fourth character: Body Region: Neck . . . 2
Fifth character: Approach: External . . . X
Sixth character: Device: Traction Apparatus . . . 0
Seventh character: Qualifier: No Qualifier . . . Z

Now, put it all together and report this ICD-10-PCS code:

2W62X0Z   Traction apparatus, neck

Good job!

 ## LET'S CODE IT! SCENARIO

Bruce Diaz, a 73-year-old male, was in a car accident and was admitted into the hospital with a concussion and a fractured shoulder. His recent medical history reveals reduced renal function, so Dr. Wester ordered a session of 5 hours of dialysis daily, to be done bedside. Teena Strunk came up to his room with a mobile unit and performed the hemodialysis.

Let's Code It!

Bruce had one hemodialysis session provided to him, bedside. Hemodialysis is when a machine does the job of filtering the blood because the kidneys are not functioning properly. Turn to the ICD-10-PCS Alphabetic Index and find

Hemodialysis *see* Performance, Urinary, 5A1D

The Alphabetic Index has provided you with the first four characters; therefore, you need to check in the Tables section to determine the last three. Turn to the 5A1 Table:

First character: Section: Extracorporeal or Systemic Assistance and Performance . . . 5
Second character: Physiological Systems . . . A

The machine is taking over the function of the kidney, so this is the root operation term: Performance.

Third character: Root Operation: Performance . . . 1
Fourth character: Body System: Urinary . . . D
Fifth character: Duration: Intermittent, less than 6 hours per day . . . 7
Sixth character: Function: Filtration . . . 0
Seventh character: Qualifier: No Qualifier . . . Z

Now put it all together and report this code, with confidence:

5A1D70Z   External filtration of the urinary system, single session

Good work!

Chapter Summary

This chapter has given you the opportunity to walk through the *Placement* (2), *Administration* (3), *Measurement and Monitoring* (4), *Extracorporeal or Systemic Assistance and Performance* (5), *Extracorporeal or Systemic Therapies* (6), *Osteopathic* (7), *Other Procedures* (8), and *Chiropractic* (9) sections of ICD-10-PCS. You have seen how each character position is important to reporting all of the pertinent details of a procedure, service, or treatment. You have learned that, in each section, the same character can have a different meaning. However, you always have the tables there to provide the options and their meanings to build the accurate code.

CHAPTER 35 REVIEW
Placement through Chiropractic Sections

Enhance your learning by completing these exercises and more at connect.mheducation.com!

Let's Check It! Terminology

Match each key term to the appropriate definition.

1. LO 35.4 Outside of the body.
2. LO 35.1 To place a device in or on an anatomical site.
3. LO 35.3 To determine a level of a physiological or physical function.
4. LO 35.6 Related to the body, especially separate from the brain or mind.
5. LO 35.8 Located outside a joint.
6. LO 35.2 To introduce a therapeutic, prophylactic, protective, diagnostic, nutritional, or physiological substance.

A. Administration
B. Extra-articular
C. Extracorporeal
D. Measurement
E. Placement
F. Somatic

Let's Check It! Concepts

Part I: Placement (2), Administration (3), Measurement & Monitoring (4)

Choose the most appropriate answer for each of the following questions.

1. LO 35.1 Within the Placement section, character position 2 Anatomical Region/Orifices, Anatomical Orifices is identified by which character?

   a. Y   b. W   c. X   d. Z

2. **LO 35.1** Within the Placement section, character position 3 Root Operation, Putting pressure on a body region (identified with number 1), is which of the following?

   a. Dressing   **b.** Immobilization

   c. Compression   **d.** Traction

3. **LO 35.1** Within the Placement section, character position 4 Body Region/Orifice, the upper extremity, right, is identified by which character or number?

   a. A   **b.** 8

   c. C   **d.** 9

4. **LO 35.1** Within the Placement section, character position 5 Approach, which is the correct approach?

   a. Open   **b.** Percutaneous

   c. Via natural or artificial opening   **d.** External

5. **LO 35.1** Johnny was playing at school and fractured his left arm. Dr. Keller applied a cast to Johnny's left arm. Within the Placement section, character position 6 Device, what number identifies the cast?

   a. 1   **b.** 2

   c. 3   **d.** 4

6. **LO 35.2** All procedures reported from the Administration section will begin with which section number?

   a. 1   **b.** 2

   c. 3   **d.** 4

7. **LO 35.2** Within the Administration section, character position 2 Physiological System/Anatomical Region, an indwelling device would be identified with which character or number?

   a. 0   **b.** C

   c. E   **d.** X

8. **LO 35.2** A blood transfusion would be reported from which section?

   a. Obstetrics   **b.** Placement

   c. Administration   **d.** Measurement and Monitoring

9. **LO 35.2** Within the Administration section, character position 4 Body System/Region, when an irrigating substance (such as saline solution) is administered into an indwelling device (reported as body system Indwelling Device . . . C), the body system/region will be reported with which character?

   a. Z   **b.** X

   c. C   **d.** G

10. **LO 35.2** Within the Administration section, character position 7 Qualifier, Oxazolidinones is reported with which character or number?

   a. 1   **b.** Z

   c. 8   **d.** X

11. **LO 35.3** Within the Measurement and Monitoring section, character position 6 represents which of the following?

   a. Physiological system   **b.** Body system

   c. Function/device   **d.** Qualifier

12. **LO 35.3** Within the Measurement and Monitoring section, character position 2, a physiological device would be represented by which of the following characters or numbers?

   a. A   **b.** 1

   c. B   **d.** 2

13. LO 35.3 Within the Measurement and Monitoring section, character position 3 Root Operation, determining the level of a physiological or physical function repetitively over a period of time (identified by number 1) is known as

a. an abortifacient.

b. monitoring.

c. measurement.

d. laminaria.

14. LO 35.3 Within the Measurement and Monitoring section, character position 6, measuring a patient's temperature would be reported with which character?

a. F

b. S

c. Q

d. K

15. LO 35.3 Within the Measurement and Monitoring section, character position 6, a sleep study would be reported with which character?

a. B

b. Q

c. X

d. Z

Part II: Extracorporeal or Systemic Assistance and Performance (5), Extracorporeal or Systemic Therapies (6), Osteopathic (7), Other Procedures (8), and Chiropractic (9) Sections

1. LO 35.4 Within the Extracorporeal or Systemic Assistance and Performance section, character position 6 represents which of the following?

a. Body system

b. Root operation term

c. Duration

d. Function

2. LO 35.4 Which of these is a term meaning "outside the body"?

a. Phototherapy

b. Extracorporeal

c. Extra-articular

d. Somatic

3. LO 35.4 All of the Extracorporeal or Systemic Assistance and Performance procedures will begin with which section number?

a. 5

b. 4

c. 2

d. 1

4. LO 35.4 Within the Extracorporeal or Systemic Assistance and Performance section, character position 3 Root Operation, all of the following are root operation terms *except*

a. assistance.

b. performance.

c. manipulation.

d. restoration.

5. LO 35.5 Within the Extracorporeal or Systemic Therapies section, character position 5 represents which of the following?

a. Body system

b. Root operation term

c. Duration

d. Function

6. LO 35.5 Within the Extracorporeal or Systemic Therapies section, character position 3 Root Operation, which of the following is/are a root operation term(s)?

a. Atmospheric control

b. Hypothermia

c. Pheresis

d. All of these

7. LO 35.5 Within the Extracorporeal or Systemic Therapies section, character position 4 Body System, number 3 represents which of the following?

a. Urinary

b. Central nervous

c. Musculoskeletal

d. Circulatory

8. LO 35.5 Within the Extracorporeal or Systemic Therapies section, character position 7 Qualifier, ultrasound therapies performed on the circulatory system, peripheral vessels, would be reported with which character or number?

   a. 6   b. X

   c. 5   d. Z

9. LO 35.6 Within the Osteopathic section, character position 6 represents which of the following?

   a. Anatomical region   b. Method

   c. Body region   d. Qualifier

10. LO 35.6 All of the Osteopathic section procedures will begin with which section number?

   a. 5   b. 4

   c. 7   d. 1

11. LO 35.6 Within the Osteopathic section, which of the following is an option for character position 3 Root Operation?

   a. Treatment   b. Manipulation

   c. Phototherapy   d. Electromagnetic therapy

12. LO 35.6 Within the Osteopathic section, character position 6, which number identifies low velocity–high amplitude?

   a. 0   b. 3

   c. 5   d. 8

13. LO 35.7 All of the Other Procedures section procedures will begin with which section number?

   a. 5   b. 8

   c. 7   d. 9

14. LO 35.7 Within the Other Procedures section, character position 2 Body System, an indwelling device is identified with which of the following characters?

   a. H   b. E

   c. Y   d. C

15. LO 35.7 Within the Other Procedures section, character position 5 Approach, a procedure performed via natural or artificial opening is identified with which character or number?

   a. 7   b. 3

   c. 8   d. X

16. LO 35.7 Within the Other Procedures section, character position 6 Method, acupuncture would be identified with which character or number?

   a. B   b. 6

   c. 0   d. D

17. LO 35.8 All of the Chiropractic section procedures will begin with which section number?

   a. 5   b. 8

   c. 7   d. 9

18. LO 35.8 Within the Chiropractic section, character position 2 Anatomical Regions, you have one option for the character. Which of the following represents the anatomical regions?

   a. B   b. W

   c. X   d. Z

19. LO 35.8 Within the Chiropractic section, character position 5 Approach, you have one option for the character. Which of the following represents the approach?

   a. Open   b. Percutaneous

   c. Via natural or artificial opening   d. External

20. LO 35.8 Within the Chiropractic section, character position 6 Method, a long and short lever specific contact will be reported with which character?

a. G

b. F

c. J

d. L

Let's Check It! Rules and Regulations

Please answer the following questions from the knowledge you have gained after reading this chapter.

1. LO 35.1 List the seven root operation terms used in the Placement section, character position 3; explain each root operation term, and include the character that identifies each term.

2. LO 35.2 Within the Administration section, character position 4, Body System/Region, there is an exception. What is that exception?

3. LO 35.3 Within the Measurement and Monitoring section, character position 3, Root Operation, what are the root operation terms? Include the description and character identifier.

4. LO 35.4 List the seven Extracorporeal or Systemic Assistance and Performance section character positions; include each character's meaning.

5. LO 35.8 Within the Chiropractic section, character position 1 is identified by what section number?

 YOU CODE IT! Practice

Using the techniques described in this chapter, carefully read through the case studies and determine the most accurate ICD-10-PCS code(s) for each case study.

1. Marvin Dunham, a 68-year-old male, is admitted to the hospital with a deep laceration to the forehead. Dr. Wallace applies a pressure dressing to his head to control the bleeding.

2. Tony Botnet, a 62-year-old male, has a nose bleed that will not stop bleeding. Tony's hemoglobin has dropped, so he is admitted to the hospital. Dr. Caulkins packed his nasal cavity, external approach, to control the bleeding.

3. Harry Watson, a 32-year-old male, is admitted to the hospital with a hemoglobin of 5.6 g/dL. Dr. Hanks performs a red blood cell transfusion, peripheral vein, percutaneous, nonautologous.

4. Angela Niles, a 58-year-old female, has been in the hospital for 3 days with a peritoneal cavity indwelling device. Dr. Adams performs an irrigation of the device with irrigation substance, percutaneous approach.

5. Cynthia Yackey, a 9-year-old female, is admitted to Westward Hospital with an unexplained high fever. Dr. Hamilton measures Cynthia's temperature.

6. Steven Wallace, an 18-year-old male, wanted to join his college's football team. The team physical examination revealed a cardiac abnormality. Steven is admitted to Westward Hospital, where Dr. Jefferson monitors Steven's total cardiac activity under stress.

7. Meagan Garrison, a 43-year-old female, presents today with shortness of breath and a dry cough. Dr. Mansfield admits Meagan to the hospital and monitors her respiratory capacity, external approach.

8. Mason Dugan, a 57-year-old male, has been hospitalized for a week. Mason's lungs were not performing; he was placed on a respiratory ventilator 5 days ago.

9. Kwakita Sumwalt, a 39-year-old female, presents today in cardiac dysrhythmia. Dr. Tumbokon admits Kwakita to Westward Hospital and restores Kwakita's normal sinus rhythm.

10. Barbara Bell, a 33-year-old female, has been in the hospital for 4 days. Barbara has been complaining of right foot pain, so Dr. Harrison performs extracorporeal shockwave therapy, right heel, single treatment.

11. Duncan Bowens, a 64-year-old male, has been hospitalized with diabetic polyneuropathy. He has also been diagnosed with urinary incontinence. Today Duncan receives a single treatment of electromagnetic therapy for his incontinence. Code today's treatment.

12. Kimberly Morgan, a 59-year-old female, was in a car accident and has been hospitalized for 2 days. She is currently having lower back pain. Today she receives an osteopathic treatment, lumbar region, low velocity–high amplitude, external approach, to relieve the pain. Code today's treatment.

13. Twanda Walters, a 34-year-old female diagnosed with trigeminal neuralgia, was admitted to Westward Hospital for stereotacic radiosurgery, which is scheduled for later in the week. Today Twanda is in pain and receives an acupuncture treatment, integumentary system, percutaneous approach, no qualifier. Code today's treatment.

14. Robert Thompson, a 16-year-old male, is admitted to the hospital with severe neck pain. Dr. Bell performs a chiropractic manipulation of the cervical region, mechanically assisted, external approach, to try and relieve the pain.

15. Susan Chapman, a 37-year-old female, is having chronic hip pain and has been admitted to Westward Hospital. Dr. Dugan performs a chiropractic manipulation of the pelvic region with long and short lever specific contact, external approach.

 # YOU CODE IT! Application

The following exercises provide practice in abstracting physicians' notes and learning to work with documentation from our health care facility, Westward Hospital. These case studies are modeled on real patient encounters. Using the techniques described in this chapter, carefully read through the case studies and determine the most accurate ICD-10-PCS code(s) for each case study.

WESTWARD HOSPITAL

591 Chester Road

Masters, FL 33955

DISCHARGE SUMMARY

PATIENT: NATHANSON, MYRA

DATE OF ADMISSION: 05/30/19

DATE OF DISCHARGE: 06/01/19

ADMITTING DIAGNOSIS: Status asthmaticus

DISCHARGE DIAGNOSIS: 1. Status asthmaticus.
2. Bronchiolitis, empirically treated.

CONSULTANTS: None.

BRIEF HISTORY: The patient is a 17-year-old white female with known history of asthma since infancy, possible environmental allergies, who presented with progressive wheezing and respiratory distress for the past 2 days. The patient had been doing well on only p.r.n. medications per family's report. However, just previous to admission, the patient was exposed to dust and other particles after moving into a new house. After conservative treatment at home, the patient was brought into the emergency room, where she did not improve on albuterol, Atrovent treatments, or intravenous steroids immediately. Initial examination showed tachycardia of 128, rest tachypnea of about 35–40, and inspiratory and expiratory wheezes and rhonchi on lung examination. The patient was referred for admission for evaluation of worsening asthma and possible pneumonia.

(continued)

STUDIES: The admission chest x-ray showed clear lungs. Clean catch urine culture showed only mixed skin flora.

HOSPITAL COURSE:

1. Status asthmaticus: The patient was admitted to the pediatric intensive care unit in moderate to severe respiratory distress with continuous albuterol treatments, Atrovent treatments q.4 h., Decadron intravenously, and empiric treatment of respiratory infection with azithromycin intravenously. The patient responded to this aggressive treatment and within 1 day was transferred to the regular pediatric medical floor. The patient was afebrile with normal oxygen saturations and appearing much better. Before discharge, she received asthma education and social counseling along with the family and was connected with social work to help provide a home nebulizer for use.

2. Empiric respiratory infection treatment: The patient did not show any specific indications of pneumonia or bronchitis by lab work; however, her initial physical examination showed possible pneumonia. She was started on intravenous antibiotics and was transferred to oral antibiotics before discharge.

DISCHARGE DISPOSITION: To home.

DISCHARGE INSTRUCTIONS

ACTIVITY: Ad lib.

DIET: Regular, as appropriate for age.

MEDICATIONS: Zithromax for 2 remaining days, albuterol one dose nebulizer treatment q.i.d. and p.r.n., and Flovent 110mcg two puffs b.i.d.

FOLLOW-UP: Follow up with primary care physician in 1 week.

Benjamin Johnston, MD—2222

556839/mt98328: 06/01/19 09:50:16   T: 06/01/19 12:55:01

Determine the most accurate ICD-10-PCS code(s) for the administration of the medications.

WESTWARD HOSPITAL

591 Chester Road

Masters, FL 33955

DISCHARGE SUMMARY

PATIENT: WARTTEL, JUDITH

DATE OF ADMISSION: 07/15/19

DATE OF SURGERY: 07/29/19

DATE OF DISCHARGE: 08/01/19

ADMITTING DIAGNOSIS: Peripheral vascular disease

DISCHARGE DIAGNOSIS: Peripheral vascular disease, status post right above-knee amputation

PROCEDURES:
1. Hyperbaric oxygen therapy.
2. Hemodialysis
3. Lower extremity arterial Doppler.

(continued)

4. A 2D echocardiogram with left ventricular hypertrophy, inferior septal hypokinesis and mildly impaired left ventricular function, sclerotic aortic valve, moderate mitral and severe tricuspid insufficiency.
5. Lower extremity Doppler negative for deep venous thrombosis. Initial lower extremity Doppler positive for calf deep venous thrombosis in the right lower extremity.

DISCHARGE DIAGNOSES:

1. Peripheral vascular disease, status post right above-knee amputation.
2. End-stage renal disease.
3. Non-insulin diabetes mellitus.
4. Hypertension.
5. Atrial fibrillation.
6. Mild congestive heart failure.
7. Protein depletion.
8. Anemia of chronic disease and postoperative anemia.
9. Hypothyroidism.

HOSPITAL COURSE: The patient was initially admitted with right lower extremity calf thrombosis and cellulitis of the right calf. The patient was seen by renovascular surgery and infectious disease. At that time, she was started on IV antibiotics. She was continued with hyberbaric oxygen therapy (HBO), which had been performed as an outpatient. The patient had a repeat lower extremity Doppler, which did not reveal DVT; anticoagulation was discontinued at that time. The patient was seen by the pain management service. The patient was seen by cardiology for wide complex tachycardia that was self-limiting. No further workup was warranted by cardiology other than echo at this time. The patient's Coumadin was stopped and she was placed on Plavix due to bleeding. The patient continued on IV antibiotics and wound care. The patient's family requested a second opinion on above-knee amputation, as they were wishing for a below-knee amputation. Dr. Gerald saw the patient and advised the same. The patient underwent an AKA by Dr. Gerald without significant complications.

The patient was somewhat weak after surgery. She will continue with HBO and antibiotics. She was transferred to the floor from the PCU. She will continue with good pulmonary toilet. She was started back on Plavix and Coumadin was not restarted. She continued on hemodialysis, intermittent, 4 hours per day. Accu-Chek and sliding scale insulin were performed. The patient was arranged for skilled nursing facility (SNF) placement; however, prior to SNF placement, she slipped out of the bed and fell on her stump. Initial x-ray showed possible fracture. CT showed no fracture. The patient also had a full spinal x-ray and right shoulder x-ray performed without significant abnormalities. There was an area seen on the right shoulder x-ray, in the right parotid region, that appeared calcified; however, the patient does wear a bridge and had it on at the time of the x-ray, most likely representing these findings. I would recommend follow-up x-ray in 1 month of the right mandibular area to ensure this is unchanged.

The patient is discharged to skilled nursing facility at this time. She has finished HBO at this time. She will continue with hemodialysis as an outpatient. She is no longer on antibiotics. She will continue with blood sugar control. I still recommend a follow-up right mandibular x-ray in 3 to 4 weeks to ensure there are no changes and this definitely was the patient's bridge. She will follow with renovascular surgery, ID, cardiology, and skilled nursing facility MD once discharged.

Roxan Kernan, MD—4444

556848/mt98328: 08/01/19 09:50:16   T: 08/01/19 12:55:01

Determine the most accurate ICD-10-PCS code(s) for the hyperbaric oxygen therapy and hemodialysis.

WESTWARD HOSPITAL

591 Chester Road

Masters, FL 33955

PATIENT: SHEPARD, JANIS

DATE OF ADMISSION: 01/14/19

ADMITTING DIAGNOSIS: Staghorn calculi

ATTENDING PHYSICIAN: Julio Yearlin, MD

Pt is a 69-year-old female who was admitted to the hospital with hematuria, nausea, and vomiting. A routine ECG is taken today in preparation for the surgical removal of the stones, which is scheduled for tomorrow.

Julio Yearlin, MD—9513

556848/mt98328: 01/14/19 09:50:16   T: 01/15/19 12:55:01

Determine the most accurate ICD-10-PCS code(s) for the EKG.

WESTWARD HOSPITAL

591 Chester Road

Masters, FL 33955

DISCHARGE SUMMARY

PATIENT: KENSINGTON, CHARLES

DATE OF ADMISSION: 01/15/19

DATE OF DISCHARGE: 01/17/19

ADMITTING DIAGNOSIS: Confusion, staring

DISCHARGE DIAGNOSIS: Possible TIA

This is an outpatient 58-year-old right-handed white male with a history of episodes of confusion and staring. He had an abnormal EEG in the past.

Routine 18-channel digital EEG was obtained to rule out any seizure activity or focal abnormalities.

FINDINGS: Background rhythm during awake stage shows well-organized, well-developed, average voltage 8 to 9 Hertz alpha activity in the posterior regions. It blocks with eye opening and it is bilaterally synchronous and symmetrical. No spike-and-wave discharges or any lateralizing abnormalities are seen. Photic stimulation did not produce any abnormalities. Hyperventilation was performed for 3 minutes. No abnormalities were found during the procedure. Intermittent EMG artifacts were seen. Stage II sleep was not achieved.

IMPRESSION: Normal awake study. No epileptiform discharges or any other paroxysmal activities or focal abnormalities seen. Clinical correlation is recommended.

Kenzi Bloomington, MD—7777

556839/mt98328: 01/17/19 09:50:16   T: 01/17/19 12:55:01

Determine the most accurate ICD-10-PCS code(s) for the EEG.

WESTWARD HOSPITAL

591 Chester Road

Masters, FL 33955

DISCHARGE SUMMARY

PATIENT: HELMSLEY, GRAYSON

DATE OF ADMISSION: 10/07/19

DATE OF DISCHARGE: 10/09/19

ADMITTING DIAGNOSIS: Abnormal liver function, weight loss

DISCHARGE DIAGNOSIS: Metastatic pancreatobiliary carcinoma and metastatic disease to the peritoneal wall and the dome of the bladder

The patient is a 57-year-old male who was recently admitted to the hospital with significant weight loss associated with abnormal liver function tests. A CAT scan of the abdomen and pelvis noted a large mass in the tail of the pancreas and multiple hypodensities in the liver. He was seen in consultation and was subjected to a CAT scan–guided liver biopsy. He was also subjected to tumor markers that included a CEA and a CA19-9. He was noted to have markedly elevated CA19-9 at 2050. His CEA was 4.3 and his alfa-fetoprotein was less than 1.2.

The CAT-guided liver biopsy noted a high-grade infiltrating adenocarcinoma that was CK-7 and CAM 5.2 positive. The hepar antigen was negative. Based on this immunohistochemical staining, he was noted to have a metastatic pancreatobiliary carcinoma. His staging workup with CAT scan of the chest noted nonspecific mediastinal and axillary lymphadenopathy. The bone scan was essentially negative for metastatic disease. The CAT scan of the pelvis noted an enlarged prostate with questionable inflammatory changes on the dome of the bladder. Based on this evaluation, he was diagnosed with metastatic pancreatobiliary carcinoma and metastatic disease to the peritoneal wall and the dome of the bladder.

Following his diagnosis, he was referred to me and has been started on palliative chemotherapy with Gemzar. He has been tolerating Gemzar without much adverse effects. He was admitted to the hospital early this morning with uncontrolled blood sugars. The most likely etiology of his uncontrolled blood sugars is prednisone therapy.

Phillip Carlsson, MD—1111

556845/mt98328: 10/09/19 09:50:16   T: 10/09/19 12:55:01

Determine the most accurate ICD-10-PCS code(s) for the administration of the chemotherapy.

Design elements: ©McGraw-Hill

Imaging, Nuclear Medicine, and Radiation Therapy Sections

36

Learning Outcomes

After completing this chapter, the student should be able to:

LO 36.1 Recognize the details reported from the Imaging section.

LO 36.2 Evaluate the details to determine the correct code reported from the Nuclear Medicine section.

LO 36.3 Determine the specifics required to build a code from the Radiation Therapy section.

LO 36.4 Analyze all of the details to build an accurate seven-character code for sections B, C, and D.

Key Terms

Densitometry
High Osmolar
Intravascular Optical Coherence
Low Osmolar

 STOP! Remember, you need to follow along in your ICD-10-PCS code book for an optimal learning experience.

36.1 Reporting from the Imaging Section

Character Definitions

The meanings for the *Imaging* section characters are shown in the following table:

Character Position	Character Meaning
1	Section of the ICD-10-PCS book
2	Body system
3	Root type
4	Body part (specific anatomical site)
5	Contrast
6	Qualifier
7	Qualifier

You might have noticed that character positions here have many of the same meanings as for those in the *Medical and Surgical* section. You learned a lot about imaging services when you learned about coding from the *Radiology* section of CPT, so you have a bit of a head start for these procedures.

Character Position 1: Imaging Section B

Character Position	Character Meaning
1	Section of the ICD-10-PCS book
2	Body system
3	Root type
4	Body part (specific anatomical site)
5	Contrast
6	Qualifier
7	Qualifier

All of the codes from this section will begin with the letter **B**.

Character Position 2: Body System

Character Position	Character Meaning
1	Section of the ICD-10-PCS book
2	Body system
3	Root type
4	Body part (specific anatomical site)
5	Contrast
6	Qualifier
7	Qualifier

The body systems of the *Imaging* section are very similar to those you learned about for the *Medical and Surgical* section:

Central Nervous System . . . Character: **0**
Heart . . . Character: **2**
Upper Arteries . . . Character: **3**
Lower Arteries . . . Character: **4**
Veins . . . Character: **5**
Lymphatic system . . . Character: **7**
Eye . . . Character: **8**
Ears, Nose, Mouth and Throat . . . Character: **9**
Respiratory System . . . Character: **B**
Gastrointestinal System . . . Character: **D**
Hepatobiliary System . . . Character: **F**
Endocrine System . . . Character: **G**
Skin, Subcutaneous Tissue and Breast . . . Character: **H**
Connective Tissue . . . Character: **L**
Skull and Facial Bones . . . Character: **N**
Non-Axial Upper Bones . . . Character: **P**
Non-Axial Lower Bones . . . Character: **Q**
Axial Skeleton, Except Skull and Facial Bones . . . Character: **R**
Urinary System . . . Character: **T**
Female Reproductive System . . . Character: **U**
Male Reproductive System . . . Character: **V**
Anatomical Regions . . . Character: **W**
Fetus and Obstetrical . . . Character: **Y**

Two things to remember:

- The dividing line between *upper* and *lower* is the diaphragm.
- The *axial skeleton* is the torso (the body) and the *appendicular (non-axial) skeleton* is comprised of the extremities.

Character Position 3: Root Type

Character Position	Character Meaning
1	Section of the ICD-10-PCS book
2	Body system
3	**Root type**
4	Body part (specific anatomical site)
5	Contrast
6	Qualifier
7	Qualifier

The root type describes the type of imaging technology being used:

Plain Radiography (X-ray) . . . Character: **0**
Fluoroscopy . . . Character: **1**
Computerized Tomography (CT Scan) . . . Character: **2**
Magnetic Resonance Imaging (MRI) . . . Character: **3**
Ultrasonography . . . Character: **4**

- *Plain Radiography (X-ray):* Radiography is the use of electromagnetic radiation to visualize the visceral aspects (internal structures) of the human body.
- *Fluoroscopy:* Fluoroscopy is the emission of continuous x-ray beams to produce a real-time, dynamic image. High-density contrast agents, such as barium, might be administered to enable comparative data.
- *Computerized Tomography (CT Scan):* An x-ray beam is emitted, aimed through the anatomical site being studied, and then recorded by detectors. Then, the emissions are reconstructed to create a two- or three-dimensional image—a cross-sectional slice through the patient at a specific point. Each consecutive image is acquired at a slightly different angle, providing a more complete picture of the internal aspects.
- *Magnetic Resonance Imaging (MRI):* Three-dimensional views of internal body organs are created in real time, with greater visibility of variations within soft tissues. This technique makes visualization of brain, spine, muscles, joints, and other structures more detailed.
- *Ultrasonography:* Ultrasound, also known as ultrasonography, uses high-frequency sound waves to capture cross-sectional images of visceral organs, including the arteries, veins, and lymph nodes.

Character Position 4: Body Part

Character Position	Character Meaning
1	Section of the ICD-10-PCS book
2	Body system
3	Root type
4	**Body part (specific anatomical site)**
5	Contrast
6	Qualifier
7	Qualifier

From the brain to the toes, each body part is listed, specific to the body system in conjunction with the root type.

Character Position 5: Contrast

Character Position	Character Meaning
1	Section of the ICD-10-PCS book
2	Body system
3	Root type
4	Body part (specific anatomical site)
5	**Contrast**
6	Qualifier
7	Qualifier

As you learned earlier in this textbook, there are several types of imaging procedures performed with contrast materials. These materials may be barium or an iodine dye that is injected to highlight or make the visceral organs and body parts more clearly seen in the image.

High Osmolar
An ionic water-soluable iodinated contrast medium.

Low Osmolar
A non-ionic water-soluble iodinated contrast medium.

High Osmolar . . . Character: **0**
Low Osmolar . . . Character: **1**
Other Contrast . . . Character: **Y**
None . . . Character: **Z**

- *High Osmolar:* Also known as ionic contrast media. Examples include diatrizoate, metrizoate, and iothalamate.
- *Low Osmolar:* Also known as organic or non-ionic contrast media. Examples include iopamidol, ioxilan, and ioversol.

EXAMPLE

You might see something like this in the documentation about an MRI taken:

". . . Multiplanar sagittal, coronal and axial images were obtained through the left forearm prior to and following contrast administration using diatrizoate. Markers have been placed near the patient's indicated site of swelling, which includes the dorsum of the distal left forearm and also over the wrist. . . ."

Multiplanar imaging typically refers to Magnetic Resonance Imaging (MRI). Never assume. Query the radiologist once and then you will know for certain going forward.

Character Position 6: Qualifier

Character Position	Character Meaning
1	Section of the ICD-10-PCS book
2	Body system
3	Root type
4	Body part (specific anatomical site)
5	Contrast
6	Qualifier
7	Qualifier

As you can see, a character placed in the sixth position will identify an additional detail specific to that table.

Unenhanced and Enhanced . . . Character: **0**
Laser . . . Character: **1**
Intravascular Optical Coherence . . . Character: **2**
None . . . Character: **Z**

Character Position 7: Qualifier

Character Position	Character Meaning
1	Section of the ICD-10-PCS book
2	Body system
3	Root type
4	Body part (specific anatomical site)
5	Contrast
6	Qualifier
7	Qualifier

The seventh character is required and may enable you to share additional details about this specific imaging procedure:

Intraoperative . . . Character: **0**
Densitometry . . . Character: **1**
Intravascular . . . Character: **3**
Transesophageal . . . Character: **4**
Guidance . . . Character: **A**
None . . . Character: **Z**

Intravascular Optical Coherence
A high-resolution, catheter-based imaging modality used for the optimized visualization of coronary artery lesions.

Densitometry
The process used to measure bone density, most often done to assess the patient's risk for osteopenia or osteoporosis.

> **EXAMPLE**
>
> You might see something like this in the operative report:
>
> *". . . The wire was then passed down to the superior vena cava without difficulty under direct fluoroscopy. . . ."*
> *". . . With fluoroscopy, the catheter was then checked. It was noted to be in the superior vena cava just above the right atrium. . . ."*
>
> As you read the first snippet, you can see that the fluoroscopy is providing guidance so the wire could be placed accurately. So, this code's 7th character should be **A** Guidance.
>
> In the second snippet, the fluoroscopy was used during a procedure on the patient's heart, directing you to report a 7th character of **0** Interoperative.

LET'S CODE IT! SCENARIO

Belinda Crandel, a 59-year-old female, has a family history of osteoporosis and was admitted into the hospital with a hairline fracture of the right hip. Dr. Franklin took a plain radiographic densitometry of her right hip to see if osteoporosis was an underlying cause of the fracture.

Let's Code It!

Let's go through the steps of coding for ICD-10-PCS and determine the code or codes that should be reported for the procedure that was performed.

First character: Section: Imaging . . . B

What body system was imaged? The documentation states, "*her right hip,*" which is a non-axial (not the head or torso) lower bone.

Second character: Body System: Non-Axial Lower Bones . . . Q

What type of imaging was used? The documentation states, "*plain radiographic.*"

Third character: Root Operation: Plain Radiography . . . 0 (as in Zero)

Which specific body part was imaged? The documentation states, "*her right hip.*"

Fourth character: Body Part: Hip, Right . . . 0

There is no mention of any contrast being used, and there is only one option for the sixth character.

Fifth character: Contrast: None . . . Z
Sixth character: Qualifier: None . . . Z

The documentation does provide the detail for you to determine the accurate seventh character, where it states, "*densitometry.*"

Seventh character: Qualifier: Densitometry . . . 1

The ICD-10-PCS code you will report is

BQ00ZZ1   Plain radiography densitometry, right hip

Good job!

36.2 Reporting from the Nuclear Medicine Section

Character Definitions

The meanings for the *Nuclear Medicine* section characters are shown in the following table:

Character Position	Character Meaning
1	Section of the ICD-10-PCS book
2	Body system
3	Root type
4	Body part
5	Radionuclide
6	Qualifier
7	Qualifier

Character Position 1: Nuclear Medicine Section C

Character Position	Character Meaning
1	Section of the ICD-10-PCS book
2	Body system
3	Root type
4	Body part
5	Radionuclide
6	Qualifier
7	Qualifier

The procedures reported with codes from the *Nuclear Medicine* section describe the use of radioactive material administered into the patient's body to enable the creation of an image for further study. This modality is beneficial as a diagnostic tool for the assessment of metabolic functions and/or a therapeutic tool for the treatment of pathologic conditions.

NOTE: When radioactive materials are used to treat malignancies, the procedure is reported from the *Radiation Therapy* section, discussed later in this chapter.

Character Position 2: Body System

Character Position	Character Meaning
1	Section of the ICD-10-PCS book
2	Body system
3	Root type
4	Body part
5	Radionuclide
6	Qualifier
7	Qualifier

The character descriptors of body systems in this section are those with which you have become familiar in this code set.

> **EXAMPLES**
>
> **Central nervous system . . .** Character: **0**
>
> **Lymphatic and Hematologic System . . .** Character: **7**
>
> **Respiratory System . . .** Character: **B**
>
> **Urinary System . . .** Character: **T**

Character Position 3: Root Type

Character Position	Character Meaning
1	Section of the ICD-10-PCS book
2	Body system
3	Root type
4	Body part
5	Radionuclide
6	Qualifier
7	Qualifier

The codes from the *Nuclear Medicine* section only report procedures that are noninvasive, meaning that the outer layer of the skin is not punctured and no incision is made.

Planar Nuclear Medicine Imaging: Introduction of radioactive materials into the body for single-plane display of images developed from the capture of radioactive emissions . . . Character: **1**

Tomographic (Tomo) Nuclear Medicine Imaging: Introduction of radioactive materials into the body for three-dimensional display of images developed from the capture of radioactive emissions . . . Character: **2**

Positron Emission Tomographic (PET) Imaging: Introduction of radioactive materials into the body for three-dimensional display of images developed from the simultaneous capture, 180 degrees apart, of radioactive emissions . . . Character: **3**

Nonimaging Nuclear Medicine Uptake: Introduction of radioactive materials into the body for measurements of organ function, from the detection of radioactive emissions . . . Character: **4**

Nonimaging Nuclear Medicine Probe: Introduction of radioactive materials into the body for the study of distribution and fate of certain substances by the detection of radioactive emissions; or alternatively, measurement of absorption of radioactive emissions from an external source . . . Character: **5**

Nonimaging Nuclear Medicine Assay: Introduction of radioactive materials into the body for the study of body fluids and blood elements, by the detection of radioactive emissions . . . Character: **6**

Systemic Nuclear Medicine Therapy: Introduction of unsealed radioactive materials into the body for treatment . . . Character: **7**

Character Position 4: Body Part

Character Position	Character Meaning
1	Section of the ICD-10-PCS book
2	Body system
3	Root type
4	**Body part**
5	Radionuclide
6	Qualifier
7	Qualifier

The list of body parts or systems for this section is similar to the list shown in the *Imaging* section. Combination descriptors—such as Ear, Nose, Mouth and Throat—as well as regions—such as Lower Extremity Veins, Right—are included along with specific body parts, such as thyroid gland and spleen.

Character Position 5: Radionuclide

Character Position	Character Meaning
1	Section of the ICD-10-PCS book
2	Body system
3	Root type
4	Body part
5	**Radionuclide**
6	Qualifier
7	Qualifier

The options in this list include the descriptors of radioactive materials—the source of the radiation. Be careful—some of these are very similar.

Technetium 99m (Tc-99m) . . . Character: **1**
Cobalt 58 (Co-58) . . . Character: **7**
Samarium 153 (Sm-153) . . . Character: **8**
Krypton (Kr-81m) . . . Character: **9**
Carbon 11 (C-11) . . . Character: **B**
Cobalt 57 (Co-57) . . . Character: **C**
Indium 111 (In-111) . . . Character: **D**
Iodine 123 (I-123) . . . Character: **F**
Iodine 131 (I-131) . . . Character: **G**
Iodine 125 (I-125) . . . Character: **H**
Fluorine 18 (F-18) . . . Character: **K**
Gallium 67 (Ga-67) . . . Character: **L**
Oxygen 15 (O-15) . . . Character: **M**
Phosphorus 32 (P-32) . . . Character: **N**
Strontium 89 (Sr-89) . . . Character: **P**
Rubidium 82 (Rb-82) . . . Character: **Q**
Nitrogen 13 (N-13) . . . Character: **R**
Thallium 201 (Tl-201) . . . Character: **S**
Xenon 127 (Xe-127) . . . Character: **T**
Xenon 133 (Xe-133) . . . Character: **V**
Chromium (Cr-51) . . . Character: **W**
Other Radionuclide . . . Character: **Y**
None . . . Character: **Z**

CODING BITES

If the documentation shows that more than one radiopharmaceutical is used during one encounter, report a separate code for each identified substance.

The **Y** Other Radionuclide option is available to report any newly approved radionuclides. It is recommended to append documentation to the claim using this character to explain the specific radiation source utilized on the patient. And you may need to report a HCPCS Level II code, if available, to specify the radionuclide.

Character Position 6: Qualifier

Character Position	Character Meaning
1	Section of the ICD-10-PCS book
2	Body system
3	Root type
4	Body part
5	Radionuclide
6	Qualifier
7	Qualifier

This section has only one option for the character reported in the sixth position:

None . . . Character: **Z**

Character Position 7: Qualifier

Character Position	Character Meaning
1	Section of the ICD-10-PCS book
2	Body system

(continued)

CHAPTER 36 | IMAGING, NUCLEAR MEDICINE, AND RADIATION THERAPY SECTIONS   **1097**

Character Position	Character Meaning
3	Root type
4	Body part
5	Radionuclide
6	Qualifier
7	Qualifier

There are no details reported by this Qualifier position, so the only option is . . .

None . . . Character: **Z**

 LET'S CODE IT! SCENARIO

Oscar Farrell, an 83-year-old male, was admitted into the hospital with dyspnea and chest pain. Dr. Lowenthal did a PET imaging of his lungs and bronchi, using Fluorine 18.

Let's Code It!

Let's go through the steps of coding for ICD-10-PCS and determine the code or codes that should be reported for this encounter between Dr. Lowenthal and Oscar Farrell.

If you don't know, you can find PET imaging in the Alphabetic Index of ICD-10-PCS, which will direct you to the *Nuclear Medicine* section.

First character: Section: Nuclear Medicine . . . C

What body system was imaged? The documentation states, "*his lungs and bronchi,*" which are parts of the respiratory system.

Second character: Body System: Respiratory System . . . B

What type of imaging was performed? The documentation states, "*PET imaging.*"

Third character: Root Type: Positron Emission Tomographic (PET) Imaging . . . 3

What specific body parts were imaged? The documentation states, "*his lungs and bronchi.*"

Fourth character: Body Part: Lungs and Bronchi . . . 2

What radionuclide was used? The documentation states, "*Fluorine 18.*"

Fifth character: Radionuclide: Fluorine 18 . . . K

No additional details are required, and you only have one option for each of the last two characters.

Sixth character: Qualifier: None . . . Z
Seventh character: Qualifier: None . . . Z

The ICD-10-PCS code you will report is this:

CB32KZZ   PET imaging of lungs and bronchi, with Fluorine 18

Good job!

36.3 Reporting from the Radiation Therapy Section

Character Definitions

The meanings for the *Radiation Therapy* section characters are shown in the following table:

Character Position	Character Meaning
1	Section of the ICD-10-PCS book
2	Body system
3	Root type (Modality)
4	Treatment site
5	Modality qualifier
6	Isotope
7	Qualifier

Character Position 1: Radiation Therapy Section D

Character Position	Character Meaning
1	**Section of the ICD-10-PCS book**
2	Body system
3	Root type (Modality)
4	Treatment site
5	Modality qualifier
6	Isotope
7	Qualifier

Procedures reported from the *Radiation Therapy* section will all begin with the letter **D**.

Character Position 2: Body System

1	Section of the ICD-10-PCS book
2	**Body system**
3	Root type (Modality)
4	Treatment site
5	Modality qualifier
6	Isotope
7	Qualifier

Again, the list for body system character descriptors in this section is very similar to other sections' lists for body systems.

Character Position 3: Root Type

Character Position	Character Meaning
1	Section of the ICD-10-PCS book
2	Body system
3	**Root type (Modality)**
4	Treatment site
5	Modality qualifier
6	Isotope
7	Qualifier

There are only four root types used to describe the modality of these procedures:

Beam Radiation . . . Character: **0**
Brachytherapy . . . Character: **1**
Stereotactic Radiosurgery . . . Character: **2**
Other Radiation . . . Character: **Y**

- *Beam Radiation:* Also known as external beam therapy (EBT), it uses one or more beams of high-energy x-rays directed at a patient's tumor.
- *Brachytherapy:* This method uses radioactive seeds that are placed in, or near, the tumor (internally). These seeds produce a high radiation dose in a limited manner, directly to the tumor. Use of this process controls the radiation exposure to surrounding, healthy tissues.
- *Stereotactic Radiosurgery:* This radiation methodology uses a focused high-power energy on a small area of the body, sometimes using a tool known as a CyberKnife. *NOTE:* Radiosurgery is not a surgical procedure; it is a treatment with no incisions made into the body.

Character Position 4: Treatment Site

Character Position	Character Meaning
1	Section of the ICD-10-PCS book
2	Body system
3	Root type (Modality)
4	**Treatment site**
5	Modality qualifier
6	Isotope
7	Qualifier

Consistent with other sections, these anatomical sites are very specific. *NOTE:* The same character is used to identify different body parts throughout this section. It changes from body system to body system.

> **EXAMPLES**
>
> **Brain Stem** . . . Character: **1**, under Central and Peripheral Nervous System
>
> **Thymus** . . . Character: **1**, under Lymphatic and Hematologic System
>
> **Nose** . . . Character: **1**, under Ear, Nose, Mouth and Throat
>
> **Bronchus** . . . Character: **1**, under Respiratory System

Character Position 5: Modality Qualifier

Character Position	Character Meaning
1	Section of the ICD-10-PCS book
2	Body system
3	Root type (Modality)
4	Treatment site
5	**Modality qualifier**
6	Isotope
7	Qualifier

This character will provide additional detail about the modality.

Photons <1 MeV . . . Character: **0**
Photons 1–10 MeV . . . Character: **1**
Photons >10 MeV . . . Character: **2**
Electrons . . . Character: **3**
Heavy Particles (Protons, Ions) . . . Character: **4**
Neutrons . . . Character: **5**
Neutron Capture . . . Character: **6**
Contact Radiation . . . Character: **7**
Hyperthermia . . . Character: **8**
High Dose Rate (HDR) . . . Character: **9**
Low Dose Rate (LDR) . . . Character: **B**
Intraoperative Radiation Therapy (IORT) . . . Character: **C**
Stereotactic Other Photon Radiosurgery . . . Character: **D**
Plaque Radiation . . . Character: **F**
Isotope Administration . . . Character: **G**
Stereotactic Particulate Radiosurgery . . . Character: **H**
Stereotactic Gamma Beam Radiosurgery . . . Character: **J**
Laser Interstitial Thermal Therapy . . . Character: **K**

Character Position 6: Isotope

Character Position	Character Meaning
1	Section of the ICD-10-PCS book
2	Body system
3	Root type (Modality)
4	Treatment site
5	Modality qualifier
6	Isotope
7	Qualifier

In this character position, you will identify the specific radioactive substance used during this procedure.

Cesium 137 (Cs-137) . . . Character: **7**
Iridium 192 (Ir-192) . . . Character: **8**
Iodine 125 (I-125) . . . Character: **9**
Palladium 103 (Pd-103) . . . Character: **B**
Californium 252 (Cf-252) . . . Character: **C**
Iodine 131 (I-131) . . . Character: **D**
Phosphorus 32 (P-32) . . . Character: **F**
Strontium 89 (Sr-89) . . . Character: **G**
Strontium 90 (Sr-90) . . . Character: **H**
Other Isotope . . . Character: **Y**
None . . . Character: **Z**

EXAMPLES

You may read something like these in the documentation:

". . . *Palladium 103 radioactive seeds were implanted according to the pre-planned computer calculation—a total of 56 seeds through 16 needles, each seed containing 1.04 mCi per seed. . . .*"

". . . *We implanted a total of 54 iodine-125 radioactive seeds through 12 needles with each seed containing 0.373 millicurie per seed. . . .*"

Character Position 7: Qualifier

Character Position	Character Meaning
1	Section of the ICD-10-PCS book
2	Body system
3	Root type (Modality)
4	Treatment site
5	Modality qualifier
6	Isotope
7	Qualifier

This character will report that this radiation treatment was provided during a surgical procedure—or not.

Intraoperative . . . Character: **0**
No Qualifier . . . Character: **Z**

 LET'S CODE IT! SCENARIO

Richard Raddison has been having severe pain in his stomach and was admitted into the hospital for tests. It was determined that Richard had malignant lesions in the fundus and pylorus areas of his stomach. Dr. Benjamin performed brachytherapy on Richard Raddison's stomach using Cesium 137, high dose rate.

Let's Code It!

Let's go through the steps of coding for ICD-10-PCS and determine the code or codes that should be reported for this encounter between Dr. Benjamin and Richard Raddison.

Brachytherapy was provided, and you already know this is a type of radiation therapy.

First character: Section: Radiation Therapy . . . D

What body system was being treated? The documentation states, "*his stomach,*" which is a part of the gastrointestinal system.

Second character: Body System: Gastrointestinal System . . . D

What type of radiation therapy was used? The documentation states, "*brachytherapy.*"

Third character: Root Type: Brachytherapy . . . 1

What specific body part was treated? The documentation states, "*his stomach.*"

Fourth character: Treatment Site: Stomach . . . 1

What was the modality qualifier? The documentation states, "*high dose rate.*"

Fifth character: Modality Qualifier: High Dose Rate . . . 9

What isotope was used? The documentation states, "*Cesium 137.*"

Sixth character: Isotope: Cesium 137 (Cs-137) . . . 7

There is only one option to report for the seventh character.

Seventh character: Qualifier: None . . . Z

The ICD-10-PCS code you will report is this:

DD1197Z   Brachytherapy, stomach, high dose rate, Cs-137

Good job!

36.4 Sections B, C, and D: Putting It All Together

 LET'S CODE IT! SCENARIO

PATIENT: Carl Bergeron

ORDERING PHYSICIAN: Elias Madison, MD

HPI: Patient was admitted yesterday after falling in his office with no apparent reason. A 5 cm laceration on his scalp confirms that he hit his head on the desk as he fell.

IMAGING: *MRI OF THE HEAD*

The MRI of the head shows diffuse atrophy. There is no abnormality of the craniocervical junction. There is a small probable mucus retention cyst in the inferior right maxillary sinus. The brainstem is grossly intact. There is a slight increase in atrophy with regards to the left temporal lobe in comparison to the right. This is mild asymmetry, however. No large territorial defects are noted.

There is, however, noted on both the T2 and FLAIR images an area of very vague high signal along the left mid lateral ventricle region. This area of white matter suggests some probable demyelination. This is brought up in particular because, when contrast was given, there was a very vague sliver of enhancement directly in that area. This is seen on coronal imaging as well. This could be related to some collateral vessels and they are seen with contrast. Collateral vessels will be necessary due to the absence of good flow to the left MCA and ICA distribution on the left on the MRA, which will be described further following this report. Therefore, that is felt the most likely etiology. Other etiologies on this very vague and subtle enhancement would be tumor or luxury blood flow around a recent small ischemic insult. I would recommend that this simply be followed up over time in approximately 6 to 9 months or sooner if symptoms change.

There is no other area of enhancement of concern that is noted. We do see some asymmetry to the vascular venous drainage pattern with the gadolinium on the axial images in the posterior fossa and around the temporal lobe region on the left, which most likely again is related to the change in collateral flow to the left cerebral hemisphere.

The IAC and cerebellopontine angle regions do not show masses. No enhancing abnormality is noted to suggest an acoustic tumor. The inner ear and mastoid air cells are well aerated.

IMPRESSION:

1. *Diffuse atrophy.*
2. *FLAIR and T2 weighted images suggest some ischemic high signal changes in the white matter adjacent to the left lateral ventricle. In this area, with gadolinium, a small sliver of enhancement persists on both axial and coronal images. This sliver of enhancement may be related to collateral blood flow or luxury perfusion or recent ischemic insult. It could, though felt less likely, be related to mild enhancement of an underlying tumor. I feel this is less likely, and in light of no change in clinical symptoms, I would recommend simply a repeat MRI with gadolinium in approximately 6 to 9 months.*
3. *No other abnormal enhancement is noted.*
4. *There is a mild increase in atrophy with regards to the left temporal lobe when compared to the right; however, this is diffuse and subtle.*
5. *The internal auditory canal and cerebellopontine angle regions are normal in appearance.*

Lawrence Katenberg, MD, Radiology

Let's Code It!

According to the documentation, Dr. Katenberg is interpreting an MRI done of Carl's head. Let's determine the seven characters needed to build this code.

> **First character: Section: Imaging . . . B**
> **Second character: Anatomical Regions . . . W**

(continued)

Third character: Root Operation: Magnetic Resonance Imaging (MRI) . . . 3
Fourth character: Body Part: Head . . . 8

Was contrast used? The documentation states, *"when contrast was given."* There is only one choice to report that contrast was used.

Fifth character: Contrast: Other Contrast . . . Y
Sixth character: Qualifier: Unenhanced and Enhanced . . . 0
Seventh character: Qualifier: None . . . Z

Now, put it all together and report, with confidence, this code:

BW38Y0Z   MRI, head, unenhanced and enhanced

Good work!

 LET'S CODE IT! SCENARIO

The patient is a 71-year-old female who was admitted last night due to subacute progressive spasticity over the last 7 months, increased difficulty walking, increased difficulty moving her right arm and hand, as well as increased rigidity. Her primary care physician has taken multiple MRIs, which included contrast, and there did not seem to be any abnormalities on his review.

She was given a provisional diagnosis of cerebral palsy, which does not fit with the natural course of this disease, as she was normal when she was a child. There seems to be an extrapyramidal as well as pyramidal component on examination today, but I do not appreciate spastic paraparesis as she was previously evaluated to have. The time course and progression of symptoms suggest a degenerative process with pyramidal and extrapyramidal component that could be part of secondary parkinsonian spectrum disease. Perhaps there is a hereditary component to this.

I ordered lab work today to include ferritin, ceruloplasmin, copper, and liver function tests and Wilson disease screening. Also, as per my earlier order, she has just had a PET imaging with C-11 of her brain.

Let's Code It!

For this case, you are going to code for the PET imaging only. Remember, or use your medical dictionary, to confirm that PET stands for Positron Emission Tomographic (PET) imaging, and find it in the ICD-10-PCS Alphabetic Index:

Positron Emission Tomographic (PET) Imaging
    Brain C030

Terrific! Turn to the C03 Table in your ICD-10-PCS code book and let's determine the seven characters to build a correct code:

First character: Nuclear Medicine . . . C

What body system includes the brain? The *central nervous system* . . . that's right!

Second character: Central Nervous System . . . 0
Third character: Root Operation: Positron Emission Tomographic (PET) Imaging . . . 3
Fourth character: Body Part: Brain . . . 0

What radionuclide was used during this patient's imaging? The documentation states, *"with C-11."*

Fifth character: Radionuclide: Carbon 11 (C-11) . . . B
Sixth character: Qualifier: None . . . Z
Seventh character: Qualifier: None . . . Z

Now, you can put it all together and report, with confidence, this ICD-10-PCS code:

C030BZZ   PET imaging, brain, with Carbon 11 (C-11)

LET'S CODE IT! SCENARIO

PATIENT: Eric Periquinn

DATE OF PROCEDURE: 12/03/2019

PREOPERATIVE DIAGNOSIS: Adenocarcinoma of the prostate

POSTOPERATIVE DIAGNOSIS: Adenocarcinoma of the prostate

PROCEDURE PERFORMED: Prostate brachytherapy

SURGEON: Gerald Crenshaw, MD

ANESTHESIA: General anesthesia via laryngeal mask airway (LMA)

DRAINS: One 18-French Foley catheter per urethra

INDICATIONS FOR PROCEDURE: This patient has a recent diagnosis of adenocarcinoma of the prostate diagnosed due to a very slowly rising PSA. His current PSA level is only 2.1, but prostate ultrasound biopsies were performed showing adenocarcinoma of the prostate at the left base of the prostate, and two biopsies were positive out of eight with a Gleason score of 6. Treatment options have been discussed, and he wishes to proceed with prostate brachytherapy. Informed consent has been obtained.

DESCRIPTION OF PROCEDURE: The patient was placed on the operating table in the supine position. General anesthesia was administered via laryngeal mask airway. He was then placed in the dorsal lithotomy position and sterilely prepped and draped in the usual fashion. The prostate ultrasound was inserted. The prostate was visualized using the preplanned study as a guide. Low dose prostate brachytherapy was performed. The patient tolerated the procedure well and had no immediate intraoperative or postoperative complications.

We implanted a total of 54 iodine-125 radioactive seeds through 12 needles with each seed containing 0.373 millicurie per seed. During the procedure, the patient received 4 mg of Decadron IV and 400 mg of Cipro IV. Subsequent fluoroscopy showed good distribution of the seeds throughout the prostate. The patient will have a CAT scan of the pelvis and simulation for his seed localization. Total target dose is 14,500 cGy.

The patient will be discharged with prescriptions for Cardura 1 mg a day for a month with two refills and Tylenol No. 3 one t.i.d. p.r.n. for pain, a total of 20, Pyridium Plus one b.i.d. for 10 days, Cipro 500 mg b.i.d. for 5 days, and prednisone 10 mg t.i.d. for a week.

Discharge instructions were explained to the patient and his wife. He will return to see me in my office in 3 weeks for a follow-up.

Let's Code It!

Dr. Crenshaw performed brachytherapy, which is radiation therapy, on Eric. Turn in the ICD-10-PCS Alphabetic Index to:

> **Brachytherapy** [*read down the long list until you get to . . .*]
> Prostate DV10

Turn to the DV1 Table to complete this code:

> **First character: Section: Radiation Therapy . . . D**
> **Second character: Male Reproductive System . . . V**
> **Third character: Root Operation: Brachytherapy . . . 1**
> **Fourth character: Treatment Site: Prostate . . . 0**

Was this high dose or low dose rate? The documentation states, "*Low dose prostate brachytherapy.*"

> **Fifth character: Modality Qualifier: Low Dose Rate . . . B**

What isotope was used? The documentation states, "*iodine-125 radioactive seeds.*"

(continued)

Sixth character: Isotope: Iodine 125 . . . 9
Seventh character: Qualifier: None . . . Z

Now, put it all together and, with confidence, report this code:

DV10B9Z   Low dose brachytherapy, prostate, with iodine **125**

Really good work!

Chapter Summary

Imaging is a wonderful way for a physician to see inside the body to help determine a diagnosis. Nuclear medicine techniques enable the assessment of metabolic functions and can be used for either diagnostic or therapeutic purposes. And radiation therapies provide an efficacious way to treat malignancy. When provided to a patient who has been admitted into the hospital, these services and treatments are reported with a code from one of these sections.

CODING BITES

For those *Imaging, Nuclear Medicine,* and *Radiation Therapy* services that use pharmaceuticals, you will need an additional code to report more details about the specific contrast material. You can find these drug codes in your HCPCS Level II code book.

Examples

(Contrast) High Osmolar contrast material, up to 149 mg/ml iodine concentration, per ml . . . code **Q9958**

(Contrast) Low Osmolar contrast material, 400 or greater mg/ml iodine concentration, per ml . . . code **Q9951**

(Radionuclide) Technetium 99m arcitumomab, diagnostic, per study dose, up to 45 millicuries . . . code **A9568**

(Isotope) Iodine I-125 serumalbumin, diagnostic, per 5 microcuries . . . code **A9532**

CHAPTER 36 REVIEW
Imaging, Nuclear Medicine, and Radiation Therapy Sections

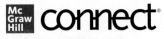

Enhance your learning by completing these exercises and more at mcgrawhillconnect.com!

Let's Check It! Terminology

Match each key term to the appropriate definition.

1. LO 36.1 A non-ionic water-soluble iodinated contrast medium.

2. LO 36.1 A high-resolution, catheter-based imaging modality used for the optimized visualization of coronary artery lesions.

3. LO 36.1 The process used to measure bone density, most often done to assess the patient's risk for osteopenia or osteoporosis.

4. LO 36.1 An ionic water-soluble iodinated contrast medium.

A. Densitometry

B. High Osmolar

C. Intravascular Optical Coherence

D. Low Osmolar

Let's Check It! Concepts

Choose the most appropriate answer for each of the following questions.

1. LO 36.1 Within the Imaging section, character position 5 represents which of the following?
   - **a.** Body system
   - **b.** Contrast
   - **c.** Device
   - **d.** Qualifier

2. LO 36.1 All of the codes reporting an Imaging section procedure will begin with what section letter?
   - **a.** A
   - **b.** B
   - **c.** D
   - **d.** F

3. LO 36.1 All of the following would be found within the Imaging section, character position 3, Root Type, *except*
   - **a.** x-ray.
   - **b.** CT scan.
   - **c.** PET.
   - **d.** MRI.

4. LO 36.1 Within the Imaging section, character position 6 Qualifier, which of the following are available options?
   - **a.** Unenhanced and enhanced
   - **b.** Laser
   - **c.** Intravascular optical coherence
   - **d.** All of these

5. LO 36.2 Within the Nuclear Medicine section, character position 1 is identified by which of the following section letters?
   - **a.** E
   - **b.** B
   - **c.** D
   - **d.** C

6. LO 36.2 Within the Nuclear Medicine section, which character position represents the radioactive materials—the source of the radiation being used?
   - **a.** 5
   - **b.** 4
   - **c.** 3
   - **d.** 2

7. LO 36.2 Introduction of radioactive materials into the body for three-dimensional display of images developed from the capture of radioactive emissions, identified by the character 2, is known as
   - **a.** positron emission tomographic (PET) imaging.
   - **b.** planar nuclear medicine imaging.
   - **c.** nonimaging nuclear medicine uptake.
   - **d.** tomographic (tomo) nuclear medicine imaging.

8. LO 36.3 Within the Radiation Therapy section, which character position describes the modality of the procedure?
   - **a.** 5
   - **b.** 4
   - **c.** 3
   - **d.** 2

9. LO 36.3 Californium would be classified as
   - **a.** a treatment site.
   - **b.** an isotope.
   - **c.** a modality.
   - **d.** a qualifier.

10. LO 36.3 Within the Radiation Therapy section, character position 7 Qualifier, which of the following characters represents the radiation treatment provided during a surgical procedure?
    - **a.** Z
    - **b.** 0
    - **c.** X
    - **d.** 1

Let's Check It! Rules and Regulations

Please answer the following questions from the knowledge you have gained after reading this chapter.

1. LO 36.1 List the five root types found within the Imaging section, character position 3, including the character that identifies each.

2. LO 36.1 List the types of qualifiers found in the Imaging section, character position 7, Qualifier; include the character that identifies each.

3. **LO 36.3** When radioactive materials are used to treat malignancies, the procedure is reported from which ICD-10-PCS section?

4. **LO 36.2** List five types of radionuclides found within the Nuclear Medicine section, character position 5; include the character that identifies each.

5. **LO 36.3** There are only four root types used to describe the modality in the Radiation Therapy section, character position 3. What are they? Include the character that identifies each.

 YOU CODE IT! Practice

Using the techniques described in this chapter, carefully read through the case studies and determine the most accurate ICD-10-PCS code(s) for each case study.

1. Edward Baker, a 26-year-old male, was riding his dirt bike and fell off, hurting his left ankle. Ed presents to Wynguard Hospital, where Dr. Dyson takes an x-ray, without contrast, of the ankle. Dr. Dyson also notes hemarthrosis and admits Ed to Wynguard Hospital. Code the x-ray.

2. Phoebe Eaddy, a 16-year-old female, complains of urinary dribbling and feels like her bladder is still full after voiding. Phoebe was diagnosed with type 1 diabetes 3 years ago. Dr. Barbato admits Phoebe to Weston Hospital and performs an ultrasound of Phoebe's urethra, which reveals nerve damage caused by her diabetes. Code the ultrasound.

3. Hugo Abbott, a 49-year-old male, has been diagnosed with osteosarcoma of his right knee. Hugo has been having difficulty, so Dr. Simmons admits Hugo to Westward Hospital, where an MRI, without contrast, of his right knee is performed.

4. Gregg Huggins, a 25-year-old male diagnosed with Graves' disease, is admitted to the hospital for a planar nuclear medicine imaging procedure of his thyroid gland, iodine 123 (I-123).

5. Hazel Baker, a 51-year-old female, is admitted to the hospital for a tomographic nuclear medicine imaging procedure of her parathyroid glands, radionuclide—technetium 99m (Tc-99m).

6. Susan Gibbons, a 43-year-old female, is admitted to Westward Hospital for a positron emission tomographic (PET) imaging procedure of the lungs and bronchi, radionuclide—fluorine 18 (F-18).

7. Glenda McMahon, a 41-year-old female, is admitted to the hospital due to severe abdominal pain. Dr. Harmon performed a liver and spleen tomography.

8. Joe Jefferson, a 72-year-old male, is admitted to the hospital with heart palpitations and edema of his legs and feet. Dr. Moss performs a heart positron emission tomographic (PET) scan.

9. Frank Ogburn, a 48-year-old male, has unexplained skeletal pain and is admitted to Westward Hospital so Dr. Cannon can perform a systemic nuclear medicine therapy whole body scan, strontium 89 (Sr-89).

10. Ozie Lewis, a 73-year-male, has been diagnosed with esophageal cancer. Ozie was admitted to Westward Hospital for beam radiation therapy to the esophagus, photons 1–10 MeV.

11. Jeff McCord, a 37-year-old male, was admitted to Westward Hospital 3 days ago and has been diagnosed with lymphatic cancer. Today Jeff receives his first treatment of brachytherapy of the inguinal lymphatic nodes, low dose rate, iridium 192 (Ir-192).

12. Harry Glover, a 38-year-old male, was admitted to Westward Hospital for stereotactic gamma beam radiosurgery on his eye.

13. Alna Lindsay, a 68-year-old female, was admitted to Westward Hospital today for brachytherapy of the hypopharynx, low dose rate, iodine 125 (I-125) treatment.

14. Charles Medlin, a 31-year-old male, has been diagnosed with a lung tumor and was admitted to Westward Hospital for stereotactic particulate radiosurgery.

15. Brandon Russell, a 37-year-old female, was admitted to Westward Hospital 2 days ago and has been diagnosed with osteosarcoma. Today she receives beam radiation therapy to the femur, photons >10 MeV.

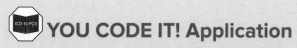 **YOU CODE IT! Application**

The following exercises provide practice in abstracting physicians' notes and learning to work with documentation from our health care facility, Westward Hospital. These case studies are modeled on real patient encounters. Using the techniques described in this chapter, carefully read through the case studies and determine the most accurate ICD-10-PCS code(s) for each case study.

WESTWARD HOSPITAL

591 Chester Road

Masters, FL 33955

PATIENT: ALTERMANN, AMANDA

DATE OF ADMISSION: 8/01/19

DIAGNOSIS: Concussion

REFERRING PHYSICIAN: Jacob Huffman, MD

Pt is a 52-year-old female who presented to the emergency room accompanied by her husband, Ron. Pt is complaining of a severe headache and seeing stars. Her husband said she was standing on a ladder when she fell off, striking her head; she lost consciousness for approximately 3 minutes. Dr. Huffman notes some disorientation, slurred speech, and a delay in response to his questions. Amanda is admitted to the hospital with a concussion. A skull x-ray without contrast and brain MRI without contrast are both performed.

Benjamin Johnston, MD—2222

556848/mt98328: 08/01/19 09:50:16   T: 08/01/19 12:55:01

Determine the most accurate ICD-10-PCS code(s) for the imaging procedure(s).

WESTWARD HOSPITAL

591 Chester Road

Masters, FL 33955

RADIOLOGIST REPORT

PATIENT: GRIFFTH, KERRAN

DATE OF ADMISSION: 08/19/19

DATE OF DISCHARGE: 08/23/19

PREOP DIAGNOSIS: Right ureteral obstruction secondary to colon cancer

POSTOP DIAGNOSIS: Right ureteral obstruction secondary to colon cancer

SURGEON: Roger Abernathy, MD

ANESTHESIA: Moderate sedation

(continued)

Operation:
1. Cystoscopy
2. Right retrograde pyelogram with contrast
3. Removal and replacement of double-J stent

HISTORY/INDICATIONS: This is a 32-year-old female with a history of colon cancer of the cecum and secondary right ureteral obstruction who had a stent inserted a number of months ago. At this time, she is in the hospital and it is time for a stent change. Consequently, the patient presents for the procedure.

PROCEDURE: The patient was taken to the operating room and there she was given midazolam, 0.5 mg, positioned in the dorsal lithotomy position, and the genitalia scrubbed and prepped with Betadine. Sterile towels and sheets were utilized to drape the patient in the usual fashion. A cystoscope was introduced into the bladder. The ureteral catheter was identified. It was grabbed and removed without any difficulty. Subsequently, the cystoscope was reinserted into the bladder and the right ureteral orifice was identified over a Pollack catheter. A glide wire was inserted into the right collecting system. Some contrast was injected and a hydronephrotic right side was noted. Then, the wire was placed through the Pollack catheter. With the wire in position, over the wire a 7 French 26-cm double-J stent was inserted. Excellent coiling was noted fluoroscopically in the kidney and distally with a cystoscope. The bladder was then drained and again it was inspected prior to removal. There was no evidence of any tumors or lesions in the bladder. The stent was in good position. The cystoscope was removed and the patient was taken to the recovery room awake and in stable condition.

Roger Abernathy, MD

556848/mt98328: 08/23/19 09:50:16   T: 08/23/19 12:55:01

Determine the most accurate ICD-10-PCS code(s) for the pyelogram.

WESTWARD HOSPITAL

591 Chester Road

Masters, FL 33955

RADIOLOGY SUMMARY

PATIENT: LACTANA, LAVINIA

DATE OF ADMISSION: 03/05/19

DATE OF DISCHARGE: 03/17/19

ADMITTING DIAGNOSIS: Bilateral breast asymmetry and ptosis, status post left lumpectomy and radiation therapy for cancer.

DISCHARGE DIAGNOSIS: Bilateral breast asymmetry and ptosis, status post left lumpectomy and radiation therapy for cancer.

This 41-year-old single female is status post surgery cleared for bilateral high dose brachytherapy with palladium 103.

Patient tolerated her first treatment and was returned to her room.

Jennell Goren, MD

556845/mt98328: 03/17/19 09:50:16   T: 03/17/19 12:55:01

Determine the most accurate ICD-10-PCS code(s) for brachytherapy.

WESTWARD HOSPITAL

591 Chester Road

Masters, FL 33955

PATIENT: HARRINGTON, ROSA

DATE OF ADMISSION: 01/15/19

DATE OF DISCHARGE: 01/17/19

DIAGNOSIS: Appendicitis

ATTENDING PHYSICIAN: Dennis Beckham, MD

HISTORY OF PRESENT ILLNESS: This is a 39-year-old previously healthy female. She awoke this morning with pain in her abdomen. Her pain continued, periumbilical, and apparently now has traversed to the right lower quadrant. On a 1 to 10 pain scale she states a 7 for pain. She has had some nausea and vomiting. No history of inflammatory bowel disease, colon cancer, abdominal operations, or bleeding. No urinary tract symptomatology.

PAST MEDICAL HISTORY: Noncontributory.

MEDICATIONS: None.

ALLERGIES: None.

SOCIAL HISTORY: No smoking.

FAMILY HISTORY: Unremarkable.

REVIEW OF SYSTEMS: As per ER intake chart.

PHYSICAL EXAMINATION:

HEENT: No scleral icterus.
NECK: Unremarkable.
HEART: No findings.
LUNGS: No findings.
ABDOMEN: Exquisite right lower quadrant tenderness. Positive focal rebound. No masses.
RECTAL: Unremarkable.
EXTREMITIES: Unremarkable.

LABORATORY AND DIAGNOSTIC STUDIES: White blood count is 25, otherwise unremarkable. An ultrasound of the appendix was performed. The patient has clear-cut possible retrocecal appendicitis.

RECOMMENDATIONS/PLAN: The patient has received antibiotics. The patient has consented to a laparoscopic, possible open, appendectomy. She was counseled concerning the benefits and risks of the surgery, including but not limited to bleeding, infection, death, and injury. All questions were answered and she agreed to the procedure. We will place bilateral sequential compression devices and call the operating room to have her scheduled as soon as possible.

Dennis Beckham, MD

556839/mt98328: 01/17/19 09:50:16   T: 01/17/19 12:55:01

Determine the most accurate ICD-10-PCS code(s) for the ultrasonography.

WESTWARD HOSPITAL

591 Chester Road

Masters, FL 33955

HISTORY OF PRESENT ILLNESS ADMISSION

PATIENT: WAYFIELD, PORTER

DATE OF ADMISSION: 10/07/19

DATE OF DISCHARGE: 10/09/19

ADMITTING DIAGNOSIS: Cervical sprain C1–C7; lumbar strain L4–L5; multiple subluxation of cervical spine.

ATTENDING PHYSICIAN: Joanne Stafford, MD

This 31-year-old male was admitted after being involved in a two-car MVA 2 weeks ago. He saw his family physician, Dr. Ashley Proctor, after experiencing constant neck pain radiating into the shoulders. Pain medication and rest (no movement) provided temporary relief. Dr. Proctor suggested admission for further evaluation.

In addition to neck pain, Pt states pain radiating across the lower back area beginning approximately 2 hours after the MVA. He states it hurts to move, bend, and walk. Pt denies similar pain in back or neck before.

BP 122/85, P60. After review of patient history questionnaire, PE indicates general appearance is age appropriate with average build and a protective gait. Normal lymph nodes: cervical; axillae; groin. Upper and lower extremities appear normal with the exception of muscle strength in both arms and left leg. Toe-walk exam rates 3 of 5. Limited-to-no ROM with pain C1–C7 and L4–L5. Pt exhibits spinal tenderness: cervical, dorsal, and lumbar. Evidence of edema: cervical and lumbar regions. Muscle spasms evident: scalenes, traps, lat, and paraspinal.

Patient sent to Radiology for x-rays: cervical and lumbar. Radiologic results show multiple subluxations of the cervical vertebrae with pain on movement. Dens and spinous process are intact. No breaks or fractures. Lumbar spine is intact with no breaks or fractures.

JOANNE STAFFORD, MD

556845/mt98328: 10/09/19 09:50:16 T: 10/09/19 12:55:01

Determine the most accurate ICD-10-PCS code(s) for the imaging procedure(s).

Physical Rehabilitation and Diagnostic Audiology through New Technology Sections

37

 STOP! Remember, you need to follow along in your ICD-10-PCS code book for an optimal learning experience.

37.1 Reporting Services from the Physical Rehabilitation and Diagnostic Audiology Section

Character Definitions

The meanings for the *Physical Rehabilitation and Diagnostic Audiology* section characters are shown in the following table:

Character Position	Character Meaning
1	Section of the ICD-10-PCS book
2	Section qualifier
3	Root type
4	Body system & region
5	Type qualifier
6	Equipment
7	Qualifier

For the most part, these character positions have different meanings than in the other sections you have already learned about.

Character Position 1: Physical Rehabilitation and Diagnostic Audiology Section F

Character Position	Character Meaning
1	Section of the ICD-10-PCS book
2	Section qualifier
3	Root type
4	Body system & region
5	Type qualifier
6	Equipment
7	Qualifier

Procedures reported from the *Physical Rehabilitation and Diagnostic Audiology* section begin with the letter **F**.

Character Position 2: Section Qualifier

Character Position	Character Meaning
1	Section of the ICD-10-PCS book
2	Section qualifier
3	Root type
4	Body system & region
5	Type qualifier
6	Equipment
7	Qualifier

There are only two options for the second character:

Rehabilitation . . . Character: **0**
Diagnostic Audiology . . . Character: **1**

Character Position 3: Root Type

Character Position	Character Meaning
1	Section of the ICD-10-PCS book
2	Section qualifier
3	Root type
4	Body system & region
5	Type qualifier
6	Equipment
7	Qualifier

The root type terms are unique to report procedures in this section.

Rehabilitation
Health care that is committed to improving, maintaining, or returning physical strength, cognition, and mobility.

Audiology
The study of hearing, balance, and related disorders.

Under *Rehabilitation,* you will find these third character options:

Speech Assessment . . . Character: **0**
Motor and/or Nerve Function Assessment . . . Character: **1**
Activities of Daily Living Assessment . . . Character: **2**
Speech Treatment . . . Character: **6**
Motor Treatment . . . Character: **7**
Activities of Daily Living Treatment . . . Character: **8**
Hearing Treatment . . . Character: **9**
Cochlear Implant Treatment . . . Character: **B**
Vestibular Treatment . . . Character: **C**
Device Fitting . . . Character: **D**
Caregiver Training . . . Character: **F**

Under *Diagnostic Audiology,* you will find these third character options:

Hearing Assessment . . . Character: **3**
Hearing Aid Assessment . . . Character: **4**
Vestibular Assessment . . . Character: **5**

Character Position 4: Body System & Region

Character Position	Character Meaning
1	Section of the ICD-10-PCS book
2	Section qualifier
3	Root type
4	**Body system & region**
5	Type qualifier
6	Equipment
7	Qualifier

The specific body system being assessed or rehabilitated will be identified in this character position. In some cases, these may not be specified, such as with some speech assessment procedures or caregiver training. These are reported with a body system of **Z** None.

EXAMPLES

Neurological System—Whole Body . . . Character: **3**
Circulatory System—Upper Back/Upper Extremity . . . Character: **5**
Genitourinary System . . . Character: **N**

Character Position 5: Type Qualifier

Character Position	Character Meaning
1	Section of the ICD-10-PCS book
2	Section qualifier
3	Root type
4	Body system & region
5	Type qualifier
6	Equipment
7	Qualifier

The character placed in this position will provide additional detail about the root type.

> **EXAMPLES**
>
> Under Root Type **Speech Assessment,** the fifth character may identify
>   Motor Speech (**B**) or Fluency (**D**)
> while under Root Type **Activities of Daily Living,** the fifth character may report
>   Feeding/Eating (**2**) or Home Management (**4**)

Character Position 6: Equipment

Character Position	Character Meaning
1	Section of the ICD-10-PCS book
2	Section qualifier
3	Root type
4	Body system & region
5	Type qualifier
6	**Equipment**
7	Qualifier

In this character position, you will report any equipment that was used during the assessment or treatment.

> **EXAMPLES**
>
> F06Z9PZ   Orofacial myofunctional speech treatment using a computer
> F13ZC1Z   Hearing assessment pure tone Stenger, with audiometer

Character Position 7: Qualifier

Character Position	Character Meaning
1	Section of the ICD-10-PCS book
2	Section qualifier
3	Root type
4	Body system & region
5	Type qualifier
6	Equipment
7	**Qualifier**

The only option in this position is

None . . . Character: **Z**

 LET'S CODE IT! SCENARIO

Elias Garmine, a 67-year-old male, was admitted after having a stroke (CVA). Anita Cohen, a certified physical therapist, is working with him on functional ambulation due to right-side hemiplegia.

(continued)

Let's go through the steps of coding for ICD-10-PCS and determine the code or codes that should be reported for this encounter between Anita Cohen and Elias Garmine.

The documentation states that a certified physical therapist is performing the treatment, so this will lead you to the **Physical Rehabilitation** section.

> **First character: Section: Physical Rehabilitation & Diagnostic Audiology . . . F**
> **Second character: Section Qualifier: Rehabilitation . . . 0**

What is the type of treatment, or for what purpose is this being done? The documentation states, "*functional ambulation*," which addresses motor function. Read carefully. This is *motor treatment,* not *assessment.*

> **Third character: Root Type: Motor Treatment . . . 7**

Read the long list of body system/region options. You will note that none of them actually fits this circumstance.

> **Fourth character: Body Region: None . . . Z**

What type of treatment is Anita providing to Elias? The documentation states, "*functional ambulation.*"

> **Fifth character: Type Qualifier: Gait Training/Functional Ambulation . . . 9**

Did Anita use any equipment in her work with Elias? None is documented.

> **Sixth character: Equipment: None . . . Z**

There is only one option for the seventh character.

> **Seventh character: Qualifier: None . . . Z**

The ICD-10-PCS code you will report is this:

> **F07Z9ZZ   Gait training/functional ambulation**

Good job!

37.2 Reporting Services from the Mental Health Section

Character Definitions

The meanings for the *Mental Health* section characters are shown in the following table:

Character Position	Character Meaning
1	Section of the ICD-10-PCS book
2	Body system
3	Root type
4	Type qualifier
5	Qualifier
6	Qualifier
7	Qualifier

Character Position 1: Mental Health Section G

Character Position	Character Meaning
1	Section of the ICD-10-PCS book
2	Body system
3	Root type
4	Type qualifier
5	Qualifier
6	Qualifier
7	Qualifier

Procedures reported from the *Mental Health* section will begin with the letter **G**.

Character Position 2: Body System

Character Position	Character Meaning
1	Section of the ICD-10-PCS book
2	**Body system**
3	Root type
4	Type qualifier
5	Qualifier
6	Qualifier
7	Qualifier

There is only one option for the second character:

None . . . Character: **Z**

Character Position 3: Root Type

Character Position	Character Meaning
1	Section of the ICD-10-PCS book
2	Body system
3	**Root type**
4	Type qualifier
5	Qualifier
6	Qualifier
7	Qualifier

There are 12 root types used in this section.

Psychological Tests: Include developmental, intellectual, psychoeducational, neurobehavioral, cognitive, neuropsychological, personality, and/or behavioral testing . . . Character: **1**

Crisis Intervention: Includes defusing, debriefing, counseling, psychotherapy, and/or coordination of care with other providers or agencies . . . Character: **2**

Medication Management: Analyzing and varying the dosage of medication to find the most efficacious balance, especially when the patient is taking several different pharmaceuticals . . . Character: **3**

Individual Psychotherapy: Includes behavior, cognitive, interactive, interpersonal, psychoanalysis, psychodynamic, psychophysiological, and/or supportive . . . Character: **5**

Counseling: Exploration of vocational interest, aptitudes, and required adaptive behavior skills to develop and carry out a plan for achieving a successful vocational placement, enhancing work-related adjustment, and/or pursuing viable options in training education or preparation . . . Character: **6**

Family Psychotherapy: Remediation of emotional or behavioral problems presented by one or more family members when psychotherapy with more than one family member is indicated . . . Character: **7**

Electroconvulsive Therapy: Includes appropriate sedation and other preparation of the individual . . . Character: **B**

Biofeedback: Includes electroencephalogram (EEG), blood pressure, skin temperature, or peripheral blood flow, electrocardiogram (ECG), electrooculogram, electromyogram (EMG), respirometry or capnometry, galvanic skin response (GSR) or electrodermal response (EDR), perineometry to monitor and regulate bowel or bladder activity and electrogastrogram to monitor and regulate gastric motility . . . Character: **C**

Hypnosis: Induction of a state of heightened suggestibility by auditory, visual, and tactile techniques to elicit an emotional or behavioral response . . . Character: **F**

Narcosynthesis: Administration of intravenous barbiturates in order to release suppressed or repressed thoughts . . . Character: **G**

Group Psychotherapy: Treatment of two or more individuals with a mental health disorder by behavioral, cognitive, psychoanalytic, psychodynamic, or psychophysiological means to improve functioning or well-being . . . Character: **H**

Light Therapy: Application of specialized light treatments to improve functioning or well-being . . . Character: **J**

Psychotherapy
The treatment of mental and emotional disorder through communication or psychologically rather than medical means.

Biofeedback
Training to gain voluntary control of automatic bodily functions.

Character Position 4: Type Qualifier

Character Position	Character Meaning
1	Section of the ICD-10-PCS book
2	Body system
3	Root type
4	Type qualifier
5	Qualifier
6	Qualifier
7	Qualifier

This character will explain whether the procedure was educational or vocational, providing more detail about the encounter. The descriptors presenting these additional details will be represented by the same characters, but they change by the root type.

EXAMPLES

Developmental . . . Character: **0,** under Psychological Tests

Interactive . . . Character: **0,** under Individual Psychotherapy

Educational . . . Character: **0,** under Counseling

Unilateral-Single Seizure . . . Character: **0,** under Electroconvulsive Therapy

Character Position 5: Qualifier

Character Position	Character Meaning
1	Section of the ICD-10-PCS book
2	Body system
3	Root type
4	Type qualifier
5	**Qualifier**
6	Qualifier
7	Qualifier

The only option in this position is

None . . . Character: **Z**

Character Position 6: Qualifier

Character Position	Character Meaning
1	Section of the ICD-10-PCS book
2	Body system
3	Root type
4	Type qualifier
5	Qualifier
6	**Qualifier**
7	Qualifier

The only option in this position is

None . . . Character: **Z**

Character Position 7: Qualifier

Character Position	Character Meaning
1	Section of the ICD-10-PCS book
2	Body system
3	Root type
4	Type qualifier
5	Qualifier
6	Qualifier
7	**Qualifier**

The only option in this position is

None . . . Character: **Z**

 LET'S CODE IT! SCENARIO

While in the hospital for repair of a stomach ulcer, Carlos Weiner, a 53-year-old male, was behaving oddly. Dr. Albessi performed some neuropsychological testing.

(continued)

Let's go through the steps of coding for ICD-10-PCS and determine the code or codes that should be reported for this encounter between Dr. Albessi and Carlos Weiner.

Psychological testing brings us to the **Mental Health** section.

First character: Section: Mental Health . . . G

There is only one option for the body region in this section.

Second character: Body Region: None . . . Z

What was done? The documentation states, "*neuropsychological testing.*"

Third character: Root Type: Psychological Tests . . . 1

Specifically . . .

Fourth character: Type Qualifier: Neuropsychological . . . 3

There are no more details to be reported with the last three characters.

Fifth character: Qualifier: None . . . Z
Sixth character: Qualifier: None . . . Z
Seventh character: Qualifier: None . . . Z

The ICD-10-PCS code you will report is

GZ13ZZZ   Neuropsychological testing

Good job!

37.3 Reporting from the Substance Abuse Treatment Section

Character Definitions

The meanings for the *Substance Abuse* section characters are shown in the following table:

Character Position	Character Meaning
1	Section of the ICD-10-PCS book
2	Body systems
3	Root type
4	Type qualifier
5	Qualifier
6	Qualifier
7	Qualifier

Character Position 1: Substance Abuse Section H

Character Position	Character Meaning
1	Section of the ICD-10-PCS book
2	Body systems
3	Root type
4	Type qualifier
5	Qualifier

(continued)

Character Position	Character Meaning
6	Qualifier
7	Qualifier

Substance Abuse
Regular consumption of a substance with manifestations.

Procedures reported from the **Substance Abuse** *Treatment* section will all begin with the letter **H**.

Character Position 2: Body Systems

Character Position	Character Meaning
1	Section of the ICD-10-PCS book
2	**Body systems**
3	Root type
4	Type qualifier
5	Qualifier
6	Qualifier
7	Qualifier

There is only one option for the second character:

None . . . Character: **Z**

Character Position 3: Root Type

Character Position	Character Meaning
1	Section of the ICD-10-PCS book
2	Body systems
3	**Root type**
4	Type qualifier
5	Qualifier
6	Qualifier
7	Qualifier

There are seven root operation terms used to report procedures in this section:

Detoxification
The process of removing toxic substances or qualities.

Detoxification Services: Not a treatment modality but helps the patient stabilize physically and psychologically until the body becomes free of drugs and the effects of alcohol . . . Character: **2**

Individual Counseling: Comprising several techniques, which apply various strategies to address drug addiction . . . Character: **3**

Group Counseling: Provides structured group counseling sessions and healing power through the connection with others . . . Character: **4**

Individual Psychotherapy: Treatment of an individual with addictive behavior by behavioral, cognitive, psychoanalytic, psychodynamic, or psychophysiological means . . . Character: **5**

Family Counseling: Provides support and education for family members of addicted individuals. Family member participation seen as critical to substance abuse treatment . . . Character: **6**

Medication Management: Monitoring or adjusting the use of replacement medications for the treatment of addiction . . . Character: **8**

Pharmacotherapy: The use of replacement medications for the treatment of addiction . . . Character: **9**

Character Position 4: Type Qualifier

Character Position	Character Meaning
1	Section of the ICD-10-PCS book
2	Body systems
3	Root type
4	**Type qualifier**
5	Qualifier
6	Qualifier
7	Qualifier

This character will add detail to the description of the root type.

> **EXAMPLES**
>
> **12-Step** . . . Character: **3,** under Individual Counseling
>
> **Interactive** . . . Character: **5,** under Individual Psychotherapy
>
> **Nicotine Replacement** . . . Character: **0,** under Pharmacotherapy

Character Position 5: Qualifier

Character Position	Character Meaning
1	Section of the ICD-10-PCS book
2	Body systems
3	Root type
4	Type qualifier
5	**Qualifier**
6	Qualifier
7	Qualifier

In this character position, the only option is

None . . . Character: **Z**

Character Position 6: Qualifier

Character Position	Character Meaning
1	Section of the ICD-10-PCS book
2	Body systems
3	Root type
4	Type qualifier
5	Qualifier
6	**Qualifier**
7	Qualifier

In this character position, the only option is

None . . . Character: **Z**

Character Position 7: Qualifier

Character Position	Character Meaning
1	Section of the ICD-10-PCS book
2	Body systems
3	Root type
4	Type qualifier
5	Qualifier
6	Qualifier
7	Qualifier

In this character position, the only option is

None . . . Character: **Z**

 LET'S CODE IT! SCENARIO

Harrison Argan has been in the New Horizons Substance Abuse Rehabilitation Hospital for 2 weeks now. Today, Dr. Lerner meets with Harrison for medication management with his methadone maintenance treatment plan.

Let's Code It!

Let's go through the steps of coding for ICD-10-PCS and determine the code or codes that should be reported for this encounter between Dr. Lerner and Harrison Argan.

For a patient that has been admitted to a Substance Abuse Rehabilitation Hospital, the section choice is clear.

First character: Section: Substance Abuse . . . H

There is only one option for the second character.

Second character: Body System: None . . . Z

What was Dr. Lerner doing for Harrison at this session? The documentation states, "*for medication management.*"

Third character: Root Type: Medication Management . . . 8

What specifics were focused on? The documentation states, "*methadone maintenance.*"

Fourth character: Type Qualifier: Methadone Maintenance . . . 1

There are no additional details to be reported with the last three characters.

Fifth character: Qualifier: None . . . Z
Sixth character: Qualifier: None . . . Z
Seventh character: Qualifier: None . . . Z

The ICD-10-PCS code you will report is

HZ81ZZZ   **Medication management for methadone maintenance**

Good job!

37.4 Reporting from the New Technology Section

Character Definitions

As you learned earlier, every ICD-10-PCS code has seven characters, and each character position has a meaning. While all of these codes have the same number of characters, each section uses each character position differently. So, let's review the meanings for the *New Technology* section characters:

Character Position	Character Meaning
1	Section of the ICD-10-PCS book
2	Body system being treated
3	Root operation term
4	Body part (specific anatomical site)
5	Approach used by physician
6	Device/Substance/Technology
7	Qualifier, if applicable

You might have noticed that these are different meanings from those used in the *Medical and Surgical* and other sections.

Character Position 1: New Technology Section X

Character Position	Character Meaning
1	Section of the ICD-10-PCS book
2	Body system being treated
3	Root operation term
4	Body part (specific anatomical site)
5	Approach used by physician
6	Device/Substance/Technology
7	Qualifier

GUIDANCE CONNECTION

Read the ICD-10-PCS Official Guidelines for Coding and Reporting, **New Technology Section Guidelines (Section X),** subsection **D. New Technology Section,** subhead **General guidelines,** paragraph **D1.**

The codes reported from the *New Technology* section (beginning with the character **X**) are used to identify a specific procedure. They are not to be used to add detail or information about a procedure reported from another section, nor do they require any additional codes to supplement their meaning. They are complete in and of themselves to explain what was provided to the patient.

Character Position 2: Body System Being Treated

Character Position	Character Meaning
1	Section of the ICD-10-PCS book
2	Body system being treated
3	Root operation term
4	Body part (specific anatomical site)
5	Approach used by physician
6	Device/Substance/Technology
7	Qualifier

Currently, in this section, the body systems from which to choose are:

Cardiovascular System . . . Character: **2**
Skin, Subcutaneous Tissue, Fascia, and Breast . . . Character: **H**
Muscles, Tendons, Bursae and Ligaments . . . Character: **K**
Bones . . . Character: **N**
Joints . . . Character: **R**
Urinary System . . . Character: **T**
Male Reproductive System . . . Character: **V**
Anatomical Regions . . . Character: **W**
Physiological Systems . . . Character: **X**
Extracorporeal . . . Character: **Y**

Character Position 3: Root Operation

Character Position	Character Meaning
1	Section of the ICD-10-PCS book
2	Body system being treated
3	**Root operation term**
4	Body part (specific anatomical site)
5	Approach used by physician
6	Device/Substance/Technology
7	Qualifier

The options are limited for the choice of this character, as well:

Assistance: Taking over a portion of a physiological function by extracorporeal means . . . Character: **A**

Destruction: Physical eradication of all or a portion of a body part by the direct use of energy, force, or a destructive agent . . . Character: **5**

Dilation: Expanding an orifice or the lumen of a tubular body part . . . Character: **7**

Extirpation: A procedure where the physician is cutting out or taking out solid matter from a body part . . . Character: **C**

Fusion: Joining together portions of an articular body part rendering the articular body part immobile . . . Character: **G**

Introduction: The process of putting in, or on, a substance for therapeutic, diagnostic, nutritional, physiological, or prophylactic purposes. Blood and blood products are excluded . . . Character: **0**

Measurement: Determining the level of a physiological or physical function at a point in time . . . Character: **E**

Monitoring: Monitoring is described in ICD-10-PCS as the determination, repeatedly over a period of time, of the level(s) of a physiological or a physical function . . . Character: **2**

Replacement: Putting in or on biological or synthetic material that physically takes the place and/or function of all or a portion of a body part . . . Character: **R**

Reposition: Moving to its normal location, or other suitable location, all or a portion of a body part . . . Character: **S**

Character Position 4: Body Part

Character Position	Character Meaning
1	Section of the ICD-10-PCS book
2	Body system being treated
3	Root operation term
4	**Body part (specific anatomical site)**
5	Approach used by physician
6	Device/Substance/Technology
7	Qualifier

The options for the body part that is the objective of this procedure are also limited in number:

Cardiovascular System

Coronary Artery, One Artery . . . Character: **0**
Coronary Artery, Two Arteries . . . Character: **1**
Coronary Artery, Three Arteries . . . Character: **2**
Coronary Artery, Four or More Arteries . . . Character: **3**

Innominate Artery and Left Common Carotid Artery . . . Character: **5**
Aortic Valve . . . Character: **F**

Skin, Subcutaneous Tissue, Fascia, and Breast
Skin . . . Character: **P**

Muscles, Tendons, Bursae and Ligaments
Muscle . . . Character: **2**

Bones
Lumbar Vertebra . . . Character: **0**
Cervical Vertebra . . . Character: **3**
Thoracic Vertebra . . . Character: **4**

Joints
Knee Joint, Right . . . Character: **G**
Knee Joint, Left . . . Character: **H**
Occipital-Cervical Joint . . . Character: **0**
Cervical Vertebral Joint . . . Character: **1**
Cervical Vertebral Joints, 2 or more . . . Character: **2**
Cervicothoracic Vertebral Joint . . . Character: **4**
Thoracic Vertebral Joint . . . Character: **6**

Thoracic Vertebral Joints, 2 to 7 . . . Character: **7**
Thoracic Vertebral Joints, 8 or more . . . Character: **8**
Thoracolumbar Vertebral Joint . . . Character: **A**
Lumbar Vertebral Joint . . . Character: **B**
Lumbar Vertebral Joints, 2 or more . . . Character: **C**
Lumbosacral Joint . . . Character: **D**

Male Reproductive System
Prostate . . . Character: **0**

Anatomical Regions
Peripheral Vein . . . Character: **3**
Central Vein . . . Character: **4**
Mouth and Pharynx . . . Character: **D**

Extracorporeal
Vein Graft . . . Character: **4**

Character Position 5: Approach

Character Position	Character Meaning
1	Section of the ICD-10-PCS book
2	Body system being treated
3	Root operation term
4	Body part (specific anatomical site)
5	**Approach used by physician**
6	Device/Substance/Technology
7	Qualifier

This position's character options should be familiar to you, at this point.

Open: An open approach is one that uses cutting through the skin or mucous membrane and any other body layers necessary to expose the site of the procedure . . . Character: **0**

Percutaneous: A percutaneous approach is described by ICD-10-PCS as entry, by puncture or minor incision, of instrumentation through the skin or mucous membrane and any other body layers necessary to reach the site of the procedure . . . Character: **3**

Percutaneous Endoscopic: Entry, by puncture or minor incision, of instrumentation through the skin or mucous membrane and any other body layers necessary to reach and visualize the site of the procedure . . . Character: **4**

Via Natural or Artificial Opening Endoscopic: Entry of instrumentation through a natural or artificial external opening to reach the site of the procedure . . . Character: **8**

External: Procedures performed directly on the skin or mucous membrane and procedures performed indirectly by the application of external force through the skin or mucous membrane . . . Character: **X**

Character Position 6: Device/Substance/Technology

Character Position	Character Meaning
1	Section of the ICD-10-PCS book
2	Body system being treated
3	Root operation term
4	Body part (specific anatomical site)
5	Approach used by physician
6	Device/Substance/Technology
7	Qualifier

The devices described in this column's options are new and different from those most of us have encountered. They are listed by the body system being treated.

Cardiovascular System

Cerebral Embolic Filtration, Dual Filter: Cerebral embolic dual-filtration units are designed to protect the brain from injury caused by embolic debris, specifically in patients diagnosed with aortic stenosis having a transcatheter aortic valve replacement (TAVR) procedure . . . Character: **1**

Orbital Atherectomy Technology: Orbital atherectomy is used to treat patients with severely calcified coronary lesions as well as symptomatic peripheral arterial disease (PAD) within the major and branch arteries of the leg. The FDA also cleared the orbital atherectomy system (OAS) to treat stenosis in synthetic arteriovenous shunts that are often used to provide vascular access for dialysis patients . . . Character: **6**

Zooplastic Tissue, Rapid Deployment Technique: The use of zooplastic tissue with rapid deployment technique on an aortic valve can now be reported . . . Character: **3**

Skin, Subcutaneous Tissue, Fascia, and Breast

Skin Substitute, Porcine Liver Derived: The use of porcine liver skin substitute can now be reported accurately . . . Character: **L**

Muscles, Tendons, Bursae and Ligaments

Concentrated Bone Marrow Aspirate: . . . Character: **0**

Bones

Magnetically Controlled Growth Rod(s): Magnetically controlled growth rods are new innovations, especially for children requiring spinal surgery for scoliosis. Instead of sequential surgical procedures to adjust the rods as children grow, the surgeon can use a magnetic device, in the office, to lengthen the rods, in just minutes . . . Character: **3**

Joints

Intraoperative Knee Replacement Sensor: Intraoperative sensors are a disposable tibial insert used to aid orthopedic surgeons in placing prosthetic joint components during knee replacement surgery . . . Character: **2**

Interbody Fusion Device, Nanotextured Surface: The fusion of vertebral joints is not new, but the use of the nanotextured surface is now reported with a code built from this new table . . . Character: **9**

Interbody Fusion Device, Radiolucent Porous: . . . Character: **F**

Male Reproductive System

Robotic Waterjet Ablation: This is a new method, used as an alternative to TURP (transurethral resection of the prostate) as a treatment for BPH (benign prostate hyperplasia) . . . Character: **A**

Anatomical Regions

Ceftazidime-Avibactam Anti-infective: This is provided for the treatment of adult patients with complicated intra-abdominal infections and complicated urinary tract infections including pyelonephritis caused by designated susceptible bacteria, including certain *Enterobacteriaceae* and *Pseudomonas aeruginosa* . . . Character: **2**

Idarucizumab, Dabigatran Reversal Agent: Idarucizumab is an antibody fragment that was developed to reverse the anticoagulant effects of dabigatran (Pradaxa) . . . Character: **3**

Isavuconazole Anti-infective: This is used for the treatment of invasive aspergillosis and treatment of invasive mucormycosis in patients 18 years and older . . . Character: **4**

Blinatumomab Antineoplastic Immunotherapy: This is used for the treatment of patients with Philadelphia chromosome-negative relapsed or refractory B-cell precursor acute lymphoblastic leukemia . . . Character: **5**

Andexanet Alfa, Factor Xa Inhibitor Reversal Agent: Andexanet Alfa is a new drug that reverses the blood-thinning reactions caused by Factor Xa inhibitors (an anticoagulant that directly works on Factor X of the coagulation cascade in the blood), when a Factor Xa has been administered in the wrong dosage or in error . . . Character: **7**

Uridine Triacetate: Uridine triacetate is a new drug that, when taken orally, combats the adverse effects of chemotherapy overdoses, as well as helps those who manifest life-threatening toxicities within four days of having chemotherapy administered. Currently, this treatment is effective when fluorouracil or capecitabine is the drug causing this adverse effect . . . Character: **8**

Defibrotide Sodium Anticoagulant: Defibrotide Sodium anticoagulant is administered as a therapeutic treatment for patients diagnosed with hepatic veno-occlusive disease (VOD) after having a hematopoietic stem cell transplantation (HSCT) [also known as a bone marrow transplant] . . . Character: **9**

Bezlotoxumab Monoclonal Antibody: Bezlotoxumab is a version of human monoclonal antibody designed to neutralize the toxin produced by the *C. diff* bacteria that is known to possibly damage the patient's intestinal walls . . . Character: **A**

Cytarabine and Daunorubicin Liposome Antineoplastic: Liposomal daunorubicin may be helpful in overcoming multidrug resistance in high-risk acute leukemia . . . Character: **B**

Engineered Autologous Chimeric Antigen Receptor T-cell Immunotherapy: Chimeric antigen receptor (CAR) therapy can be compared to autologous bone marrow transplantation. T cells are collected by apheresis, and then expanded and genetically modified . . . Character: **C**

Other New Technology Therapeutic Substance: . . . Character: **F**

Plazomicin Anti-infective: This is an aminoglycoside antibacterial for the treatment of complicated urinary tract infections (UTI) . . . Character: **G**

Synthetic Human Angiotensin II: A solution administered to patients with sepsis or distributive shock to support increase of blood pressure . . . Character: **H**

Extracorporeal

Endothelial Damage Inhibitor: Endothelial dysfunction describes manifestations of cardiovascular risk including diminished production and reduced availability of nitric oxide as well as the possible imbalance in the relative contribution of endothelium-derived relaxing and contracting factors . . . Character: **8**

Character Position 7: Qualifier

Character Position	Character Meaning
1	Section of the ICD-10-PCS book
2	Body system being treated
3	Root operation term
4	Body part (specific anatomical site)
5	Approach used by physician
6	Device/Substance/Technology
7	Qualifier

Each year, this character changes for the new codes added to this specific section. So, for 2019, the seventh character options are

New Technology Group 1 . . . Character: **1**
New Technology Group 2 . . . Character: **2**
New Technology Group 3 . . . Character: **3**
New Technology Group 4 . . . Character: **4**
New Technology Group 5 . . . Character: **5**

The next year that innovations are approved and added to the code set, they will be identified with a qualifier of 5. This will continue each year, as new details are placed into the code set.

 LET'S CODE IT! SCENARIO

Carl Terrosa, a 45-year-old male, has been trying to lower his cholesterol; however, he was diagnosed with two severely calcified coronary lesions. He was admitted to the hospital so Dr. Garrison could perform orbital atherectomy, a new technology to remove the calcification in two sites. Unlike some previous methodologies, this is performed percutaneously, reducing the risk and Carl's length of stay.

Let's Code It!

Let's go through the steps of coding for ICD-10-PCS and determine the code or codes that should be reported for the procedure that was performed.
    In the Alphabetic Index, look up

Orbital Atherectomy Technology X2C

Turn to the ICD-10-PCS Table beginning X2C

First character: Section: New Technology . . . X

The notes state the patient has "coronary lesions," which are part of the cardiovascular system.

Second character: Body System: Cardiovascular System . . . 2

The removal of the calcification fits the definition of extirpation.

Third character: Root Operation: Extirpation . . . C

An "atherectomy" is the surgical removal of fatty deposits located in an artery.

Fourth character: Body Part: Coronary Arteries, Two Arteries . . . 1

The notes state the procedure was performed percutaneously.

Fifth character: Approach: Percutaneous . . . 3

(continued)

The notes state that an orbital atherectomy system was used.

Sixth character: Device: Orbital Atherectomy Technology . . . 6
Seventh character: Qualifier: New Technology Group 1 . . . 1

The ICD-10-PCS code you will report is this:

X2C1361   Orbital Atherectomy Technology, extirpation, coronary arteries, two sites

37.5 Sections F–X: Putting It All Together

 LET'S CODE IT! SCENARIO

PATIENT NAME: Alfredo Sugerman

DATE OF EVALUATION: 11/16/2019

ATTENDING PHYSICIAN: Oscar Clarice, MD

HISTORY OF PRESENT ILLNESS: This is a 71-year-old male with a history of end-stage COPD, previous CVA, seizure disorder, chronic headaches, and chronic pain syndrome who was admitted to the hospital yesterday for increasing pain all over the body. He has also expressed feelings of severe depression, and a psychiatric consultation was requested for evaluation of the same. The patient reports that he had been going through a lot for the past few months. He was referring to his medical problems, chronic obstructive pulmonary disease, especially the pain all over the body for which no clear organic reason has been found so far. He says that he is in pain all the time, constantly. He is tired of it. He cannot take care of himself, and he was recently in a nursing home but had a bad experience over there. He does not want to go back to the nursing home. He was living with a woman for 15 years, but she is not able to take care of him. He was very helpless and hopeless, and he voices passive death wishes but denies any active intentions. He says that he will never do that to himself. Patient admits to having insomnia and extremely depressed crying episodes and reports very poor energy level, motivation, loss of interest, and feeling sad and unhappy all the time. He had some depression symptoms in the past, related to the medical problems, and was placed on Lexapro and Seroquel for sleep for the past few weeks, but it is not helping. Seroquel helped for his sleep, but he does not want this medication as he knows this is an antipsychotic. He denies any delusions or hallucinations.

PAST PSYCHIATRIC HISTORY: No history of any psychiatric illness or psychiatric hospitalization or any suicidal attempts in the past.

CURRENT MEDICATIONS: On admission, Protonix, Synthroid, Nitro-Dur patches, Tenormin 25 mg once a day, Ditropan, Atrovent, Nasonex, multivitamins, Os-Cal, Bumex, Imdur, Micro-K, Lexapro 10 mg daily, magnesium oxide, Klonopin 0.25 mg every 12 hours, Seroquel 100 mg nightly, Phenergan p.r.n., and Pulmicort inhaler.

ALLERGIES: Nonsteroidal anti-inflammatory drugs and sulfa drugs.

PSYCHIATRIC MENTAL STATUS EXAMINATION: The patient is a thinly built male who appears to be in moderate distress from pain. He is generally cooperative and pleasant; he shows significant psychomotor retardation but no agitation. He speaks in a very low volume voice. He is alert and oriented in all three spheres. Memory grossly intact in all modalities. Speech is coherent. Mood is depressed, tearful, constricted affect. No evidence of any overt psychosis or hypomania. He does have passive death wishes; however, he denies any active suicidal intentions or thoughts. Insight and judgment questionable. Intellectual abilities in average normal range.

IMPRESSIONS: Neurobehavioral and cognitive status tests along with my observations lead to these impressions:

Axis I: Major depression, single episode, moderate to severe with anxiety component.
Axis II: Deferred.
Axis III: Chronic pain syndrome, narcotic dependence, chronic obstructive pulmonary disease, status post cerebrovascular accident, and seizure disorder.

(continued)

RECOMMENDATIONS: The patient does not appear to be responding to his current psychotropic medications, so we will discontinue the Lexapro and Seroquel. Instead, we will use Effexor XR 37.5 mg once a.m. and also Desyrel 50 mg nightly. We will continue to monitor the patient closely.

Let's Code It!

Dr. Clarice performed neurobehavioral and cognitive status psychological tests as a part of his evaluation of Mr. Sugerman. Let's work our way through the **Mental Health** section . . . because this was a psychological evaluation.

> **First character: Section: Mental Health . . . G**
> **Second character: System: None . . . Z**

What did Dr. Clarice actually do? The documentation states, "*Psychiatric mental status examination.*"

> **Third character: Root Operation: Psychological Tests . . . 1**

Review the options for the fourth character in Table GZ1. The documentation states, "*Neurobehavioral and cognitive status tests.*"

> **Fourth character: Type Qualifier: Neurobehavioral and Cognitive Status . . . 4**
> **Fifth character: Qualifier: None . . . Z**
> **Sixth character: Qualifier: None . . . Z**
> **Seventh character: Qualifier: None . . . Z**

Now, you can report this ICD-10-PCS code with confidence:

> **GZ14ZZZ Neurobehavioral and cognitive status psychological tests**

 LET'S CODE IT! SCENARIO

PATIENT: Francis Fredericks

The patient had been seen by this department for a clinical swallowing evaluation. At that time, he had reported 3 to 4 months of coughing with liquids, approximately one time per week. He had a barium swallow, which showed one episode of aspiration with appropriate cough response. Given the patient's complaints of coughing with thin liquids and possible reflux-related symptoms, an objective swallowing evaluation was recommended. However, the patient chose not to follow up for further objective testing at that time.

   Admitted today for left side weakness, he is reporting that dysphagia has persisted, and now he feels as though he can cough or choke several times a day with either liquids or solids. He is on a regular diet. He takes his pills with water without difficulty. He has a reported 5- to 10-pound weight loss over the past several months that has been unexplained. His physician has asked him to gain some weight to improve his nutritional status. He has no recent history of pneumonia. The patient does complain of feeling as though he has sluggish passage of his meals and sometimes this will cause him to stop eating early. He has a feeling of increased mucus with frequent throat clearing throughout the day, and he complains of frequent heartburn. He is not on any proton pump inhibitor regimen at this time.

PAST MEDICAL HISTORY: Coronary artery disease requiring LAD stent placement, hypertension, hyperlipidemia, asymptomatic right carotid stenosis, chronic anemia due to renal disease, chronic renal insufficiency that is stable.

CLINICAL OBSERVATIONS: I am performing this swallow dysfunction study at the request of Dr. King. He uses a walker due to knee trouble and the weakness, but he is brought to our office by an orderly in a wheelchair. He is fully alert and oriented, slightly hard of hearing. He is able to provide a comprehensive history. Good speech intelligibility. Vocal quality is slightly raspy, although otherwise within normal limits for age and gender.

ORAL PERIPHERAL EXAM: The patient has naturally present dentition, in poor condition. There is bilateral palatal elevation, good lingual and labial strength and range of motion, and good ability to maintain intraoral pressure. Cough is strong and unproductive. There is good hyolaryngeal elevation and excursion to palpation.

SWALLOWING EVALUATION: Administered p.o. trials of ice chips, thin puree, and particulate solid.

(continued)

ORAL PHASE: The patient is able to self-feed appropriately. He has good bolus containment and timely anterior to posterior transit with mildly delayed trigger of pharyngeal swallow overall. Question premature spillage with multiple sips of thin liquids.

PHARYNGEAL PHASE: Audible and question slightly discoordinated swallowing pattern for multiple sips of thin liquids. One swallow required for single sips of thin, puree, and particulate solids. No overt clinical signs or symptoms of aspiration after any p.o. trial, although the patient reports that he had slight difficulty with the initial sip of water, feeling like it might head down the wrong pipe.

SUMMARY AND IMPRESSION: The patient is an 87-year-old male with a several-year history of reported dysphagia to solids and liquids. This can happen several times per day. Clinically, he does not show significant overt clinical signs of aspiration, although question discoordinated swallowing pattern for thin liquids, especially when given larger quantities. This is likely consistent with the one incidence of symptomatic aspiration on a barium swallow in the past. The patient also complains of multiple symptoms that appear consistent with laryngopharyngeal reflux, and these include increased mucus, throat clearing, and globus sensation. He reports frequent heartburn and sensation of slow esophageal passage. At this time, would recommend objective testing to further evaluate oropharyngeal swallowing mechanism to determine if coordination of swallowing pattern has been affected over time. Further differential diagnosis would be considerable reflux in current complaints. The patient may benefit from a proton pump inhibitor regimen if deemed appropriate by his physicians. At today's session, discussed aspiration precautions, especially given that the patient self-reported drinks multiple sips at a time. In addition, reflux precautions were recommended, including sitting upright 90 degrees with all p.o. and for 1 hour after meals. The patient was also counseled to monitor his nutritional intake. If he is indeed shortening meals due to sensation of sluggish passage, would recommend multiple smaller meals a day rather than three large ones to allow for adequate nutritional intake. The patient understands all given recommendations and is in agreement for a follow-up with an objective swallowing test.

RECOMMENDATIONS:
1. Regular diet with thin liquids.
2. Medications one at a time with water.
3. Further objective testing via modified barium swallow.
4. Upright 90 degrees with all p.o. and for 1 hour after meals.
5. Decrease bolus size and rate of presentation.
6. Single bites and single sips.
7. Consideration of proton pump inhibitor regimen if reflux is deemed by the patient's physicians to be playing a role in the patient's current symptoms.
8. Further recommendations will be made pending outcome of objective study.

Gail Robbins
Speech-Language Pathologist

Let's Code It!

This assessment contains a speech evaluation and a swallow study. Look in the ICD-10-PCS Alphabetic Index; there is no listing for *swallow* or *swallow study*. Let's try this:

> **Speech Assessment F00**

At least it is a place to start, so turn to the F00 Table:

> **First character: Section: Physical Rehabilitation and Diagnostic Audiology . . . F**

This makes sense. The category of speech and swallow studies is considered part of *physical rehabilitation*.

> **Second character: System: Rehabilitation . . . 0**
> **Third character: Root Operation: Speech Assessment . . . 0**

You may be thinking that this cannot be correct because this was really a swallow study. That's good thinking, but let's continue to review the options in this Table before we go looking elsewhere.

> **Fourth character: Body System/Region: None . . . Z**

(continued)

Read carefully all of the options for the fifth character. Bedside Swallowing and Oral Function sounds close, except the documentation states, "*he is brought to our office by an orderly in a wheelchair.*" This tells us this was not done bedside. The next row has a good possibility that works:

Fifth character: Type Qualifier: Instrumental Swallowing and Oral Function . . . J

Review the options for the sixth character. This is straightforward.

Sixth character: Equipment: Swallowing . . . W

Seventh character: Qualifier: None . . . Z

When we take this coding process one step at a time, it is not as confusing as one might perceive. You can now put this all together and, with confidence, report this code:

F00ZJWZ Instrumental swallowing and oral function assessment

 LET'S CODE IT! SCENARIO

George is a 19-year-old male, self-referred for inpatient treatment due to drug and alcohol abuse. He is currently unemployed and homeless, and has charges pending due to a number of "bounced" checks written over the past several months. George reports that both of his parents were drug addicts, and he experienced physical, sexual, and emotional abuse throughout childhood at their hands. His father died of liver disease at the age of 37.

George also reports that, at the age of 12, he was kicked out of his family's home because his father suspected that he was gay. Although they live in the same town, he has not had any contact with either parent for 7 years. George describes his relationship with his younger sister as "fair." He is not presently involved in a steady relationship but does have a network of friends in the local gay community with whom he has been staying off and on. At the time that he left home, George survived by becoming involved in sexual relationships with older men, many of whom were also abusive. He has had numerous sexual partners (both male and female) over the past 7 years, has traded sex for drugs and money, has had sex under the influence of drugs and alcohol, and has been made to have sex against his will. George identifies himself as bisexual, not gay.

George first used alcohol at age 11, when he had his first sexual encounter with a man. He began using other drugs, including inhalants and marijuana, by age 16 and amphetamines and cocaine by age 17. At 18, 3 months prior to entering treatment, he began using crack.

This first individual counseling session was focused on this basic, interpersonal foundation to enable us to establish an efficacious treatment plan. George is strong in his desire to get clean, and I have assured him that we can help him here.

Let's Code It!

George has admitted himself into a substance abuse inpatient treatment program, and this is documentation of his first individual counseling session. Turn to the *Substance Abuse Treatment* section and let's build an ICD-10-PCS code:

First character: Section: Substance Abuse Treatment . . . H
Second character: System: None . . . Z
Third character: Root Operation: Individual Counseling . . . 3
Fourth character: Type Qualifier: Interpersonal . . . 4
Fifth character: Qualifier: None . . . Z
Sixth character: Qualifier: None . . . Z
Seventh character: Qualifier: None . . . Z

Now, put it all together and, with confidence, report this code:

HZ34ZZZ   Interpersonal-based individual counseling for substance abuse treatment

Chapter Summary

This chapter has given you the opportunity to walk through the *Physical Rehabilitation and Diagnostic Audiology* (**F**), *Mental Health* (**G**), *Substance Abuse Treatment* (**H**), and *New Technology* (**X**) sections of ICD-10-PCS. You have seen how each character position is important to reporting all of the pertinent details of a procedure, service, or treatment. You have learned that, in each section, the same character can have a different meaning. However, you always have the Tables there to provide the options and their meanings to build the accurate code.

CODING BITES

More Information:
Physical Medicine and Rehabilitiation
   https://medlineplus.gov/ency/article/007448.htm
National Alliance on Mental Illness (NAMI)
   https://www.nami.org/Learn-More/Treatment
Substance Abuse and Mental Health Services Administration
   http://www.samhsa.gov/treatment

CHAPTER 37 REVIEW
Physical Rehabilitation and Diagnostic Audiology through New Technology Sections

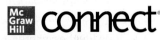

Enhance your learning by completing these exercises and more at mcgrawhillconnect.com!

Let's Check It! Terminology

Match each key term to the appropriate definition.

1. LO 37.2 Training to gain voluntary control of automatic bodily functions.

2. LO 37.2 The treatment of mental and emotional disorder through communication or psychologically rather than medical means.

3. LO 37.3 Regular consumption of a substance with manifestations.

4. LO 37.1 Health care that is committed to improving, maintaining, or returning physical strength, cognition, and mobility.

5. LO 37.1 The study of hearing, balance, and related disorders.

6. LO 37.3 The process of removing toxic substances or qualities.

A. Abuse

B. Audiology

C. Biofeedback

D. Detoxification

E. Psychotherapy

F. Rehabilitation

Let's Check It! Concepts

Choose the most appropriate answer for each of the following questions.

1. LO 37.1 Within the Physical Rehabilitation and Diagnostic Audiology section, character position 6 represents which of the following?

   a. Section qualifier

   b. Type qualifier

   c. Equipment

   d. Qualifier

2. LO 37.1 Within the Physical Rehabilitation and Diagnostic Audiology section, character position 2 Section Qualifier, which of the following characters represents diagnostic audiology?

   a. 0   **b.** 1   **c.** 2   **d.** 3

3. LO 37.1 Within the Physical Rehabilitation and Diagnostic Audiology section, character position 3 Root Type, which of the following characters represents a hearing aid assessment?

a. B **b.** 2 **c.** D **d.** 4

4. LO 37.2 All of the codes reporting a Mental Health section procedure will begin with which section letter?

a. G **b.** H **c.** I **d.** J

5. LO 37.2 Within the Mental Health section, character position 3 Root Type, the encounter documents *Includes behavior, cognitive, interactive, interpersonal, psychoanalysis, psychodynamic, psychophysiological, and/or supportive,* identified by the character 5. This encounter is known as

a. psychological tests. **b.** individual psychotherapy.

c. counseling. **d.** crisis intervention.

6. LO 37.2 Within the Mental Health section, which character position identifies whether the procedure was educational or vocational?

a. 2 **b.** 3 **c.** 4 **d.** 5

7. LO 37.3 All of the codes reporting a Substance Abuse Treatment section procedure will begin with which section letter?

a. F **b.** H **c.** J **d.** K

8. LO 37.3 Within the Substance Abuse Treatment section, the encounter documents *Not a treatment modality but helps the patient stabilize physically and psychologically until the body becomes free of drugs and the effects of alcohol,* represented by the character 2. This is known as

a. individual psychotherapy. **b.** medication management.

c. pharmacotherapy. **d.** detoxification services.

9. LO 37.3 Within the Substance Abuse Treatment section, what character position adds detail to the description of the Root Type?

a. 4 **b.** 5 **c.** 6 **d.** 7

10. LO 37.4 All of the codes reporting a New Technology procedure will begin with the section letter

a. Z **b.** X **c.** Y **d.** W

Let's Check It! Rules and Regulations

Please answer the following questions from the knowledge you have gained after reading this chapter.

1. LO 37.1 List the Physical Rehabilitation and Diagnostic Audiology section, character position 2, Section Qualifier, options, including the character that identifies each.

2. LO 37.1 Within the Physical Rehabilitation and Diagnostic Audiology section, character position 4, Body System and Region, if the encounter is for caregiver training, what would be the character assignment to represent the encounter?

3. LO 37.2 List six Mental Health section, character position 3, Root Type, options; include the description and the character that identify each.

4. LO 37.3 Within the Mental Health section, what does the character position 4, Type Qualifier, explain?

5. LO 37.4 List six options from the New Technology section, character position 6, Device/Substance/Technology; include the description and the character that identify each.

(ICD-10-PCS) YOU CODE IT! Practice

Using the techniques described in this chapter, carefully read through the case studies and determine the most accurate ICD-10-PCS code(s) for each case study.

1. Bennie Hallmon, a 67-year-old male, has been in Westward Hospital for a week and is showing signs of deteriorating speech. Dr. Lindler performs a bedside swallowing and oral function speech assessment, no equipment.

2. Merry Gilbert, a 22-year-old female, was hospitalized 7 days ago due to an automobile accident resulting in left hemiplegia. Dr. Tarrant performs an ADL home management assessment using assistive, adaptive, supportive, and protective equipment.

3. Fred Copeland, a 14-month-old male, was admitted to Westward Hospital because he does not react to sudden loud noises and has not begun to use simple words. Fred is diagnosed with severe sensorineural hearing loss and has a multiple channel cochlear implant. Today, Dr. Cantey performs a cochlear implant rehabilitation treatment. Code today's session.

4. Patricia Swartzenturber, a 23-year-old female, has been experiencing recurring episodes of vertigo and some hearing loss. Dr. Wooton admits Patricia to Westward Hospital, where she is diagnosed with Ménière's disease. Pat complains of ringing in her ears. Dr. Wooton fits a tinnitus masker, no equipment used.

5. Vickie Fulmer, a 61-year-old female, presents to Dr. Derry with trembling and twitchy motions she states are involuntary. Dr. Derry also notes diaphoresis and admits Vickie to the hospital, where she is later diagnosed with generalized anxiety disorder. Today, while in the hospital, Vickie participates in an individual interpersonal psychotherapy session. Code today's session.

6. Ralph Canopus, a 37-year-old male, was very agitated and restless and threatened suicide. Dr. Patterson admitted Ralph to Westward Hospital, where he was diagnosed with major depression. Today, while in the hospital, Ralph and his family participate in a family psychotherapy session led by Dr. Patterson. Code today's session.

7. AKA: Grover Humphrey, age unknown, male, was found wondering the streets with no memory or ability to reason. A card with a name was found in one of his pockets. He was admitted to Westward Hospital, where Dr. Hatfield performed a cognitive status psychological test.

8. Hugo Parsons, a 15-year-old male, is brought to Westward Hospital by his parents. Hugo's parents have noticed a dramatic personality change recently as well as unexplained anger. Dr. Smyth completes a physical examination and finds Hugo has a substance abuse issue. Dr. Smyth admits Hugo to Westward Hospital and begins detoxification treatment.

9. Jessica Abbott, a 41-year-old female, has been admitted to Westward Hospital for esophageal cancer. Jessica has been smoking cigarettes since she was 16 years old. Dr. Barbato manages her nicotine replacement medication.

10. Eloise Baker, a 56-year-old female, had been diagnosed as an alcoholic and is having severe delirium tremens and seizures. Dr. Hewitt admits Eloise to Westward Hospital. Today, while in the hospital, Eloise participated in a 12-step individual psychotherapy session.

11. Edward Skipper, a 24-year-old male, has been diagnosed with human immunodeficiency virus (HIV). Ed attends a post-test group counseling session held by Dr. Dyson at Westward Hospital.

12. Rinika Simms, a 72-year-old female, was admitted to Westward Hospital for a percutaneous cerebral embolic filtration, dual filter, left common carotid artery, new technology group 2.

13. Thomas Balakrishnan, a 59-year-old male, has severe back pain. He was admitted to Westward Hospital for disc fusion: lumbosacral, interbody fusion device, Nanotextured surface, open approach.

14. Margie Lewis, a 49-year-old female, was admitted to Westward Hospital and was diagnosed with invasive aspergillosis. Dr. Marten administers Isavuconazole anti-infective enzyme, peripheral vein, percutaneous, new technology group 1.

15. John Hook, a 9-month-old male, was diagnosed with early onset scoliosis. John is admitted to Westward Hospital for reposition of a thoracic, magnetically controlled growth rod, open approach, new technology group 2.

 # YOU CODE IT! Application

The following exercises provide practice in abstracting physicians' notes and learning to work with documentation from our health care facility, Westward Hospital. These case studies are modeled on real patient encounters. Using the techniques described in this chapter, carefully read through the case studies and determine the most accurate ICD-10-PCS code(s) for each case study.

(continued)

WESTWARD HOSPITAL

591 Chester Road

Masters, FL 33955

PROGRESS NOTES

PATIENT: HOUGH, BETH

DATE OF ADMISSION: 05/30/19

DATE OF DISCHARGE: 06/01/19

ADMITTING DIAGNOSIS: Acute pyelonephritis caused by *E. coli*

DISCHARGE DIAGNOSIS: Acute pyelonephritis caused by *E. coli*

The patient is a 29-year-old female suffering with burning on urination. She stated she also noticed a fishy odor after urination. The urinalysis and culture lab results showed positive for acute pyelone-phritis caused by *E. coli*. She was referred to me. I then admitted her to the hospital for treatment with Ceftazidime-Avibactam Anti-infective, peripheral vein introduction.

Benjamin Johnston, MD—2222

556839/mt98328: 06/01/19 09:50:16   T: 06/01/19 12:55:01

Determine the most accurate ICD-10-PCS code(s) for the Ceftazidime-Avibactam Anti-infective.

WESTWARD HOSPITAL

591 Chester Road

Masters, FL 33955

DISCHARGE SUMMARY

PATIENT: GILLINS, MARTIN

DATE OF ADMISSION: 07/15/19

DATE OF SURGERY: 07/29/19

DATE OF DISCHARGE: 08/01/19

DIAGNOSIS: Left below-knee amputation

DISCHARGE DIAGNOSIS: Pt is a 67-year-old male with a history of peripheral arterial disease and lower extremity bypass surgeries who was admitted with gangrene of left foot. The patient underwent left below-knee amputation.

PAST MEDICAL HISTORY: Hyperlipidemia and hypertension.

SOCIAL HISTORY: Lives with wife.

FAMILY HISTORY: Noncontributory.

PHYSICAL EXAMINATION: At the time of admission, the patient was afebrile. Vital signs are stable. Temperature 97.7. Blood pressure 131/71. Oral mucosa was moist. Sclerae anicteric. Lungs: Bilaterally clear to auscultation. Heart: Regular. Abdomen: Scaphoid. Right foot intact. Minimal erythema. Minimal edema.

(continued)

HOSPITAL COURSE: Dr. Norcross notes patient is medically stable. Compression was not used due to the significant ischemia. The patient was placed on Avelox. Bowels moved on a regular basis. The patient responded to rehabilitation well. Appetite is improving. Albumin was 2.7. Hemoglobin was 11.4. The patient was able to perform all ADLs with supervision. Good range of motion was noted to the left knee. No dehiscence was found. Wife will act as caregiver and was trained in wound care management. The patient was discharged to wife.

MEDICATIONS: Avelox 400 mg daily, aspirin one tablet daily, Roxicodone 5–10 mg every 6 hours as needed for pain, Cardizem 60 mg three times a day, Nitro-Dur patch daily, and Lanoxin 0.25 mg daily.

The patient will follow up with Dr. Norcross on Wednesday. A dry dressing, wrapping with Kling and stockinette, no compression is to be maintained. The patient was prescribed front-wheel walker, 3-in-1 commode, shower chair, and ADL kit. The patient was prescribed home health nursing, physical therapy, occupational therapy, and aide. The patient was also given a wheelchair. All instructions were given.

Karen Norcross, MD

556848/mt98328: 08/01/19 09:50:16   T: 08/01/19 12:55:01

Determine the most accurate ICD-10-PCS code(s) for the caregiver training.

WESTWARD HOSPITAL

591 Chester Road

Masters, FL 33955

PATIENT: WRIGHT, ROBBIN

DATE OF ADMISSION: 03/05/19

DATE OF DISCHARGE: 03/17/19

ADMITTING DIAGNOSIS: Marijuana abuse

ATTENDING PHYSICIAN: Jennell Goren, MD

Robbin Wright, a 16-year-old female, presented to Dr. Goren complaining of a cough and a sore throat, lasting about 1 week. She and her mother deny fever, nasal congestion, or runny nose. She says she feels more tired than usual and her mom states that she hasn't been getting out of bed to go to camp or any other activities. Mom seems most worried that she is much less active than she usually is and that she has been hanging out with her friends until late at night. Patient states that her "mom won't get off my back." She admits that her grades had been dropping before summer break, and she quit the baseball team. Mom leaves the room, and patient admits to smoking pot every day, usually several times a day, for the past 8 or 9 months or so. She denies any other drug use and states smoking pot is "no big deal."

After discussion with the patient and her parents, Robbin is admitted into a substance abuse hospital to treat her high level of irritability and anxiety and for daily individual and group behavioral counseling.

Upon admission:

PE: Physical examination is remarkable only for a mildly erythematous throat without petechiae. Lungs are slightly congested, and the rest of her exam is normal. Vital signs are also unremarkable. A rapid strep screen is negative.

FIRST DAY—INDIVIDUAL COUNSELING: Discussion with patient about side effects and risks of abusing pot. She states she has tried to quit but can't make it through an entire day without smoking. It is pointed out to her that her pot use is already having a negative impact on her life (absence and lack of interest in school). We discussed options and methodologies for her quitting with reduced effects. Blood is taken to record the levels of THC, and she agrees to regular surveillance.

(continued)

PLAN: Marijuana abuse behavioral counseling; daily individual counseling; daily group counseling. Reevaluation after six (6) full days of residential treatment.

Jennell Goren, MD

556845/mt98328: 03/17/19 09:50:16   T: 03/17/19 12:55:01

Determine the most accurate ICD-10-PCS code(s) for the counseling.

WESTWARD HOSPITAL

591 Chester Road

Masters, FL 33955

PHYSICAL REHABILITATION ASSESSMENT

PATIENT: LEWTER, GENE

DATE OF ADMISSION: 01/15/19

DATE OF DISCHARGE: 01/17/19

DIAGNOSIS: 1. Acute myofascial strain.
              2. Acute exacerbation of chronic low back pain.

SUBJECTIVE: The patient is a 47-year-old male. The patient came in for back pain. He was initially evaluated by Dr. Bruce Allen for back pain for the last 2 days. He said it was in the mid back, going down to the left knee, with some paresthesias in the feet and numbness in the feet. Movement, remaining still, and laying on a side seem to relieve pain. Lying directly on his back increases the pain. No problems with urination. No fever or chills. No nausea, vomiting, or diarrhea. No abdominal pain.

PAST MEDICAL HISTORY: Significant for back injury. He had anterior fusion of L3–L4 in the past. He has had multiple episodes, about one a month, since the surgery of exacerbation of his chronic back pain. This typical pain pattern with numbness and radiation down the leg, he states, is nothing unusual for the last multiple episodes. He has had no bladder or bowel dysfunction.

SOCIAL HISTORY: He is a smoker.

OBJECTIVE: The patient is alert, in no acute distress, obviously uncomfortable however. C-spine is negative. He is tender over the mid back, L2 through L4, with paravertebral muscle spasm that is palpable, also quite tender. Decreased range of motion. The patient is alert and orientated x3. No motor deficits. Strength 5/5. He does have diminished left patellar reflex. Decreased sensory on the left great and little toes, medial aspect of the foot, and lateral aspect on the plantar surface of the foot. Sensory is intact.

INTERVENTION: Motor and nerve function assessment, range of motion, and joint integrity of lower back and lower extremity were performed.

ASSESSMENT:

1. Acute myofascial strain.
2. Acute exacerbation of chronic low back pain.

PLAN: Percocet 5 mg 1–2 q. 4–6 hours as needed for pain, Soma one, three times a day, Indocin SR 75 mg b.i.d. with food. Follow up with the specialist who did his back surgery for reevaluation of his increasing back pain over the last several years. Any acute problems, recheck sooner. Any problems with bladder or bowel, recheck immediately.

Roberta Opell, PT

556839/mt98328: 01/17/19 09:50:16   T: 01/17/19 12:55:01

Determine the most accurate ICD-10-PCS code(s) for the motor function assessment.

WESTWARD HOSPITAL

591 Chester Road

Masters, FL 33955

HISTORY OF PRESENT ILLNESS ADMISSION

PATIENT: JETT, JAMES

DATE OF ADMISSION: 10/07/19

DATE OF DISCHARGE: 10/09/19

ADMITTING DIAGNOSIS: Schizophrenia and polysubstance abuse

HISTORY OF PRESENT ILLNESS: This is a 27-year-old male with a history of schizophrenia and polysubstance abuse referred by his case manager due to increased hallucinations, including auditory, and new onset of olfactory, gustatory, and tactile hallucinations. Since the onset of the hallucinations, the patient has become acutely suicidal with multiple plans. He has a history of polysubstance abuse with alcohol and crack but has been sober for greater than 3 months and has been in rehab. He also complains of headaches recently. The patient presented frightened and tearful and continued to endorse suicidal thoughts.

PAST PSYCHIATRIC HISTORY: Paranoid schizophrenia, substance abuse.

PAST MEDICAL HISTORY: Left shoulder injury with chronic pain and a seizure one time in the past.

FAMILY HISTORY: The patient does have a brother with schizophrenia and a mother who died from complications of diabetes.

SOCIAL HISTORY: The patient currently is in rehab. Divorced. Did finish high school and went to junior college for a little while but did not get a degree. He has been unable to hold a steady job for most of his life.

REVIEW OF SYSTEMS: Included headache and some blurry vision. He denies constitutional symptoms. He denied chest pain, difficulty breathing, GI symptoms, dysuria. He does endorse left shoulder pain. He denied any skin conditions and he does endorse numbness of his distal feet.

MENTAL STATUS EXAMINATION: Neurobehavioral and Cognitive Status Exam: Appearance and Behavior: He had good eye contact, well groomed, fair hygiene. Speech and Language: Normal volume, tone, and rate, nonpressured. Mood and Affect: Mood was depressed and affect was congruent and restricted. Thought processes linear and goal directed. Thought Content: He does have some paranoia, believing that people, including the doctors, are experimenting on him. HI/SI: He denies currently having suicidal ideations. Perceptual Abnormalities: He reports visual, auditory, gustatory, and tactile hallucinations. Orientation: He is alert and oriented x3. Memory and abstractions are fair. Fund of knowledge and IQ are average and insight and judgment are limited and poor. His initial physical exam was significant for pain and decreased range of motion in the left shoulder on passive abduction and extension and a mild paresthesia of the plantar surface of his right second toe; otherwise, neurologic exam was normal.

JOANNE STAFFORD, MD

556845/mt98328: 10/09/19 09:50:16   T: 10/09/19 12:55:01

Determine the most accurate ICD-10-PCS code(s) for the cognitive status test.

Design elements: ©McGraw-Hill

38 Inpatient Coding Capstone

Learning Outcomes

After completing this chapter, the student should be able to:

LO 38.1 Correctly abstract patient records to determine accurate coding using ICD-10-CM and ICD-10-PCS code sets.

Reporting the procedures provided to a patient who has been admitted into an inpatient facility can cover a broad spectrum. The cases in this chapter will support your learning using ICD-10-PCS procedure codes.

Remember, read carefully and completely.

CASE STUDY #1: NESTOR GONZALEZ

H&P

Nestor Gonzalez, a 69-year-old previously healthy male, was seen in my office with a cough productive of thick purulent sputum of 3-days duration. Fever was present and he reported dyspnea on exertion.

Vital signs—BP 96/60 mmHg, P 116 beats/min, RR 24 breaths/min, T 103.5°F rectal. On examination, he appeared acutely ill.

Lung examination revealed scattered ronchi, which were greater on the right than the left.

I determined that the patient needed to be admitted into the hospital right away.

Upon admission: Bronchoscopic aspiration specimen culture, C&S, and gram stain. Blood tests and sputum culture were ordered and a chest x-ray taken.

RESULTS: Chest x-ray showed increased opacity in the lung field indicating pneumonia, as suspected; culture confirmed *E. coli* with Shiga toxin.

Dx: Community-acquired pneumonia due to *Escherichia coli* 0157 with Shiga toxin

Treatment: IV ciprofloxacin 300 mg q 12h, infused over 60 minutes

Dr. Ryan MacDoule

CASE STUDY #2: TINA LEBROCK

H&P

Patient is Tina LeBrock, a 71-year-old female with known unstable angina due to coronary artery disease. During the week prior to admission, she underwent an outpatient procedure of diagnostic heart catheterization. At the time of this heart catheterization procedure, the patient was found to have occlusion of the left anterior descending coronary artery in two separate locations.

Due to the findings from this diagnostic procedure, the patient is now admitted for a scheduled percutaneous transluminal coronary angioplasty (PTCA) with a plan for stent insertions. The patient also has known secondary diagnoses of hypertension,

(continued)

hyperlipidemia, and current tobacco use. The hypertension, hyperlipidemia, and unstable angina are currently being treated with medications.

The patient was taken to the procedure room and underwent a PTCA of the left anterior descending coronary artery with insertion of two Taxus drug-eluting stents, one at each occlusion site.

Dr. Lawrence Marcheon

CASE STUDY #3: GRAYSON CARLYLE

Patient: Grayson Carlyle   15 May 2019

MRN: C18-54662517

Surgeon: Annalissa Brubaker, MD

PREOPERATIVE: gonarthrosis deformans; four ipsilateral periprosthetic fractures

HPI: A 43-year-old otherwise healthy male patient with a diagnosis of osteoarthrosis was admitted in 2016 for elective left-knee arthroplasty. He had a history of three nonsignificant knee traumas, and an arthrotomy with synovectomy had been performed on the left knee due to synovitis in 2017. His physical examination at admission showed severe insufficiency of the medial collateral ligament and rotational instability of the left knee joint. Other joints showed no abnormal findings.

X-ray revealed gonarthrosis deformans stage II with 5° varus angulation. The patient underwent total arthroplasty (Allopro *NPK,* Switzerland) of the left knee on March 4, 2016. Postoperative x-ray revealed good alignment of the prosthesis; both components were centered in the midline of the joint, and overall knee alignment was 8° in valgus.

Two 1-g prophylactic doses of the antibiotic cefuroxime were administered perioperatively. The patient developed a fever on the third postoperative day, and the same antibiotic was administered intravenously (750 mg three times a day, postoperative days 3–10).

The patient was discharged in good general condition on March 18, 2016, and he had no medical problems during the outpatient follow-up period.

A year later, on May 26, 2017, the patient fell at home and was admitted to the hospital with a supracondylar fracture of the left distal femoral metaphysis (displacement in flexion and varus). Skeletal traction with 7 kg was applied primarily, and the patient underwent surgery. The tibial component of the endoprosthesis was loose and was removed; the femoral shaft was fixed with a dynamic condylar screw device, and a revision arthroplasty using a long-stem endoprosthesis was done.

The patient had no postoperative complications. The outpatient follow-up period was uneventful, and after 3 months, he returned to work.

The patient started experiencing pain and swelling in his left knee joint approximately 1 year after the second surgery. An x-ray performed in August 27, 2018, showed radiolucency around the tibial component, which had also migrated anteroinferiorly. Based on these findings and also on clinical and laboratory data, infection of the endoprosthesis was diagnosed, and the patient was admitted for 1-stage revision arthroplasty. Microbiological culture from joint aspirations showed the presence of *Pseudomonas aeruginosa* sensitive to Tazocin (piperacillin sodium and tazobactam sodium), ceftazidime, imipenem, amikacin, gentamicin, and ciprofloxacin.

The patient had surgery on September 1, 2018. Because the previous femoral supracondylar fracture was consolidated, the DCS fixator and endoprosthesis were removed and revision arthroplasty with long-stem rotational endoprosthesis (*Link Endo-Model Total Hinge Knee*) was performed. The tibial defect was additionally filled with 15-mm spacer.

(continued)

Microbiological cultures taken during surgery confirmed the diagnosis of *P. aeruginosa* infection. During the hospital stay, antibiotics were administered intravenously according to microbe sensitivity (antibiogram) and our infection protocol: gentamicin 240 mg once a day and ciprofloxacin 200 mg twice a day for the first 5 postoperative days. Starting on the sixth postoperative day, gentamicin combined with ceftazidime 500 mg twice a day was administered, and was continued for 9 days.

The patient was discharged home with no complaints. He was prescribed oral rifampicin 300 mg twice a day for the next 2 months. Full weight-bearing was allowed after 6 weeks.

Three months later, the patient fell on a slippery street and sustained an axially displaced fracture of proximal metaphysis of tibia and fibula. This time treatment was conservative: closed reduction was achieved and maintained in a long-leg cast. Follow-up x-ray on December 14, 2018, showed that bone fragments were still in satisfactory alignment and there was evidence of callus formation. The patient returned to work and his usual activities in January 2019.

On March 9, 2019, the patient was admitted to the hospital again because of a spiral dislocated fracture in left femoral distal diaphysis. The femur was shortened and displaced axially in varus position. Skeletal traction (5 kg) was applied primarily, and surgery was performed later. Offstripping of femoral periosteum in both fragments was seen during surgery. Internal fixation of the left femoral bone was achieved with an AO plate and screw. The patient recovered and was discharged on March 17, 2019. He was told to limit weight-bearing for the next 2.5 months and to walk with crutches.

Unfortunately the patient didn't follow these instructions, and the plate broke off the bone in its distal part due to walking. An open reosteosynthesis (exchange of screws and repositioning of the plate) was performed this morning (May 15, 2019).

CASE STUDY #4: DAMARIS ALBAQSHI

Patient: Damaris Albaqshi

Date of Admission: 11 June 2019

MRN: D9513597135

Attending Physician: Markesha Cacciola, MD

A 42-year-old female patient was admitted to the hospital with a swelling on the right tibia. Past history revealed that the patient was operated upon 24 years ago for a pathological fracture of the right tibia and the diagnosis at that time had been adamantinoma. The preoperative radiograph of the right leg showed osteolysis of the bone, and the chest radiograph revealed lung metastases. Regional computed tomography (CT) of the right leg showed that the tumor was invading the surrounding soft tissues. The cortex appeared moderately expanded and attenuated. Bone scanning showed intensive positivity in the middle of the right tibia. The CT scan of the thorax demonstrated two lung metastases. One of these was in close contact with the right anterior pulmonary artery and the other was located in the left posterior lobe. Fine needle aspiration (FNA) biopsy confirmed the diagnosis of adamantinoma of right tibia suggesting local recurrence.

The patient underwent surgery wherein the tumor was widely resected and the tibia reconstructed with specific recombined osteosynthesis (salvage surgery). The pathological examination of the excised tumor confirmed the diagnosis of adamantinoma set by FNA biopsy. The histological examination revealed a multiforming adamantinoma with basaloid, spindle cellular, and tubular characteristics. Examination of the adamantinoma that had been excised earlier revealed the same characteristics. The postoperative period was without complications and the patient walked in 15 days.

Patient: Michaela DeMarco   14 July 2019

MRN: K3357151

Attending Physician: Cecilia Rowens, MD

HISTORY: This patient is a 5-year-old female with normal birth history and development with the exception of an episode of maternal hemiplegia during pregnancy. Family history is not significant of any neurologic issues. Her medical history is unremarkable except for celiac disease. Due to this, she is sustained with a gluten-free diet.

Five months ago, she was found to have scarlet fever. Resulting therefrom, she experienced episodes of left hand tremor lasting about 5–7 seconds with no alteration of consciousness. Four weeks later, she had additional events and was taken to the nearby emergency department, where an EEG was performed.

The results of the EEG evidenced a normal background with right centrotemporal spikes. A second EEG, performed the next day, showed similar findings yet recorded sleep and sleep activation of the discharges.

With these results, she was placed on ethosuximide. An MRI of the brain was completed and showed unremarkable results with the exception of "*slight signal alteration involving the posterior periventricular white substance of both sides of a nonspecific nature.*" Opacification of the sinuses and otomastoiditis was also observed.

The patient exhibited some "restlessness of her limbs" during sleep, but has had no additional seizures. However, this past month, she then had two larger events. She was then placed on divalproex sodium at 750 mg divided per day for 14 days.

Family history:

Mother experienced a transitory left hemiplegia during pregnancy. Both the father and 18-month-old sister are reported to be in good health. No family history is known related to epilepsy or mental retardation.

Medical background:

Delivered during normal spontaneous delivery at 39th week + 2.

No pre-, peri- and postnatal anguish reported. Neonate exhibited good suction. Mother breastfed the infant up until 6 months, then weaned.

During physical examination, it was noted that the neonate's psychomotor development was within normal limits. Seated posture at 4.5 months, standing unassisted at 11 months, first words when 8 months. Alvus and diuresis WNL, feeding non-gluten diet due to celiac disease. Her sleep-wake rhythm is also reported within normal limits. NKA. Patient diagnosed previously with celiac disease.

Five months ago, she was placed on a regime of antibiotic therapy due to an episode of scarlet fever. Four weeks later, while under antibiotic therapy, she developed a fever and then started to show brief episodes evidenced by right hand tremors, with a duration of approximately 5–7 seconds each, without any concomitant consciousness alterations.

The parents report that these episodes began approximately 7 months ago, and both described these episodes as occasional. Currently, similar episodes of tremors were observed prompting her parents to take her to urgent care.

The child was transferred and admitted to the hospital's pediatric neurology floor. This is when a diagnosis of "*Focal epilepsy of myoclonic nature in patient with normal psychomotor development*" was determined. During this admission, tests were ordered and completed:

- Blood tests: within normal limits with the exception of Hb (Hemoglobin) 11.03 g/dl (v.n. 12–14), MCV 64.9 fl (v.n. 75–85), Platelets 607 (v.n. 130–400), iron in the blood 39 mcg/dl (v.n. 50–80).

- EEG: Right centrotemporal paroxysmal abnormalities with tendency to omo and contralateral spreading in tracing with normal background rhythm.

- EEG during sleeping: 2 right centrotemporal paroxysmal abnormalities with tendency to spreading and with activation when sleeping.

(continued)

The patient was discharged with prescriptions for:
Ethosuximide 80 mg × 2 a day at 8 a.m. and 8 p.m. for 1 week
Ethosuximide 80 mg + 160 mg at 8 a.m. and 8 p.m. for 1 week
Ethosuximide 160 mg × 2 a day at 8 a.m. and 8 p.m. continuing

Brain MRN was performed under sedation with results within normal limits, except for the "*slight signal alteration involving the posterior peri-ventricular white substance of both sides, of nonspecific nature, and bilateral otomastoiditis, opacification of maxillary sinuses, of ethmoid cells and of sphenoidal sinuses bilaterally. Asymmetry of temporal-basal superficial vessels, due to ectasia of a vessel on the right side, is observed.*"

The child's parents observed some type of restless limbs (both arms and legs) when she was sleeping occasionally, after about 3 hours as well as early in the morning. Additionally, and perhaps more of a concern, these restless limbs in the evenings (about 7 p.m.), as well as when the child goes to bed (approximately 10:00 p.m.). They reported that she often complains about being cold, repeating this multiple times.

This month, she experienced two epileptic seizures. The first one occurred during an afternoon nap — waking up catatonic, staring, with hardly any response to questions. There were times that right-sided rigidity was also noted. These events typically lasted about 10 minutes and she would then fall asleep. Once awaking, the child took about 90 minutes to recover either her mood. At times, she also complained stomach pain.

The second epileptic seizure was noted when the child was being seen in the clinic to check her medication dosage and a follow-up visit. Once awake, she experienced a 25-seconds-long crisis, with remarkable tremors to arms, legs, eyes, and twisted and munching mouth.

Following these events, her attending physician changed her medication regime with:
Valproic acid oral suspension 80 mg at 8 a.m. and 80 mg at 8 p.m. for 7 days
Valproic acid oral suspension 120 mg at 8 a.m. and 120 mg at 8 p.m. for 7 days
Valproic acid oral suspension 160 mg at 8 a.m. and 160 mg at 8 p.m. on-going

No substantial crisis occurred after the first 7 days of treatment with the minimum dosage. During sleep, the child moves constantly, wriggling her limbs at about 3 a.m. (intensely for 30 minutes at a time until she falls back to sleep) or at about 5:00 a.m. In addition, when she wakes up, she moves uncontrollably for approximately 5 minutes.

Evaluation and consultations have determined two possible diagnoses:

1) Focal-Onset Epilepsy.

The patient's seizures began on the right side of her brain (causing the effect to the left side of the body including shaking and rigidity). Should these spread to the entire brain, this could result in the entire body shaking, This was evidenced with her second seizure. The MRI, was unremarkable as to a cause for the seizure (such as a tumor, stroke, or malformation). This is an encouraging indication with an improved opportunity for the child to outgrow seizures. Observations of the sinuses and mastoid showed nothing that would cause the seizures. We recommend that an ENT specialist should evaluate these incidental findings.

2) Benign Rolandic Epilepsy.

This is the most common epilepsy syndrome in childhood (not counting febrile seizures) and onset can occur anywhere from age 1–15 (however, typically by age 7). These seizures are typically similar to the partial seizures described by her parents. It should be noted that these seizures can occur on either side of the brain and commonly occur just after falling asleep or just upon waking. The diagnostic EEG reveals centrotemporal spikes that are more frequent during sleep (similar to this patient's). On an EEG, these spikes can be identified only on one side or they might alternate between the right and left sides, showing from one test to the next. When the spikes are only seen

(continued)

consistently on one side, then subsequent EEGs would reveal discharges on the opposite side. Virtually all children outgrow this type of epilepsy, around puberty if not earlier. The restlessness of the limbs during sleep is not epileptic; however, it is common in epileptic children. They often exhibit restless sleep or jerking motions of the limbs (sleep myoclonus). These are benign.

TREATMENT: A 24-hour EEG is ordered during this current admission.

DISCHARGE: The 24-hour EEG evidenced abnormalities consistently on only the left side, confirming a diagnosis of idiopathic focal-onset epilepsy. Her normal development is very reassuring and can be seen with this type of epilepsy. Some children with this type of seizure can experience problems with attention/focus/memory as they get older, but this is usually mild and gets better as the condition normalizes.

CASE STUDY #6: POPPY BROWNING

Patient: Poppy Browning

DATE: 9 April 2019

MRN: A399523147

Physician: Carla Firmann, MD

Second hospitalization, 1 month later, following appearance of arising colics, difficult to treat with pain medications, high body temperature, and increase in inflammation ratings, symptoms consistent with picture of infective cholangitis. Therefore, the picture was resolved with antibiotic therapy and with carrying out a papillotomy by means of ERCP. Discharged under antibiotic therapy with Ciprofloxacin, Cortisone, and Azathioprine.

Third hospitalization, 3 days after discharge from previous hospitalization, following arising colics with progressive ultrasound scan dilatation of bile ducts and evidence of dropsy of the gallbladder. Moreover, 48 hours following hospitalization, amylase increase (600 UI/l) was detected. The IgG4 dosage (18 mg/dl) was within normal limits, excluding a possible autoimmune hepatitis/pancreatitis syndrome.

ERCP performed with dilatation and cleaning of the common bile duct that involved the spillage of corpuscular material and bile with purulent appearance bringing about a fast improvement of symptomatology and a rapid reduction in the amylase values. Later on, laparoscopic cholecystectomy was carried out. During postsurgery, after a short period of wellness, the patient suffered from an abdominal pain. Reappearance interpreted, at the beginning, as a light pancreatitis (treated with antibiotic therapy). Subsequently, persisting painful crises were observed despite blood tests showing substantial stability.

Therefore, an MR cholangiography was carried out (images enclosed on CD) that has revealed an appearance of intra- and extrahepatic bile duct dilatation, evident also at common bile duct level where the picture seems to reveal a relevant stenosis: "Intrahepatic bile ducts with clear wall irregularity and with minimal stenosis followed by dilatations in a picture to be related to the base pathology. Irregularity at the extrahepatic bile ducts and at the common bile duct level too, the common bile duct distal region appears moderately reduced in diameter, also in papillary region, also as a result of papillotomy."

In light of the aforesaid, a biliary stent was placed during ERCP in order to guarantee bile ducts patency. The clinical picture, after surgery, was stable with occasional presence of pains involving mainly the right hypochondrium without any characteristics of biliary colics. At discharge, blood tests showed evidence of improvement of the hepatic cytolisys index (AST 28, ALT 38) with still elevated values of gammaGt (197) and APC 2.02 mg/dl probably linked to the inflammatory pathology rather than to an infective

(continued)

event. Discharge with indication to follow a therapy with Deltacortene to scale down the Azathioprine and antibiotic therapy with Augmentin.

Fourth hospitalization, 1 month later, in gastroenterology department for clinical test: The patient reported slight painful crisis in epigastric region; at examinations APC negativization (0.59) and a further reduction in GGTs with transaminase substantially stable. Therefore, the therapy with Amoxicillin + Clavulanic Acid was suspended and Metronidazole 250 mg was prescribed three times a day every other week.

Fifth hospitalization during the same month, following an episode of infective cholangitis with blood tests that showed transaminase on the increase (ALT 248, AST 114, GGT 281) with leukocytosis (WBCs 13,000, neutrophils 88%, lymphocytes 7.9%) and elevated APC (4.48). Therapy started with Augmentin (1 g three times a day) for 7 days and then end. At the end of the 7 days, preventive treatment prescribed with Cotrimoxazole (tablet 160 + 800) one tablet twice a day.

Sixth hospitalization, 2 weeks after the previous one, following epigastric pain and nausea, occurred after 1 day from Augmentin interruption and 1 day after the beginning of therapy with Cotrimoxazole.

The most significant lab examinations at admission: CRP = 1.92 mg/dl; GGT 129 U/L; AST = 29 U/L; ALT = 97 U/L.

Abdomen ultrasound scan with evidence of common bile duct dilatation. "Dilatation of the proximal and medial segment of the common bile duct, with diameter up to 10 mm, in whose context binary images are appreciated referable to the well-known stent. A moderate ectasia of intrahepatic bile ducts is connected, in particular in the left parts."

To treat the severe painful symptomatology, a therapy with Ketorolac Tromethamine 90 mg in 250 cc in continuous infusion was started.

Because of the increase in the inflammation ratings and in the dilatation of the common bile duct at the abdominal ultrasound scan, supposing an occlusion of the biliary stent with overlapped cholangitis, an antibiotic therapy has been started with Meropenem 1 g × 3 and a high osmolar ERCP was carried out.

ERCP didn't show any materials obstructing the stent. Biliary washing was within normal limits.

Therapy prescribed at home:
Augmentin (1 g × 3); Ciproxin (500 mg × 2); Folina 5 mg (one tablet every other day); Deltacortene (25 mg daily); Azathioprine (100 mg daily); Lansoprazole (30 mg daily); Ursodesossicolic Acid (300 mg three times a day).

CASE STUDY #7: DAVID CHANG

Patient: David Chang   13 February 2019

MRN: C55359541

Attending Physician: Evangeline DeRupo, MD

HPI: A 13-year-old boy had been well until 4 weeks before admission, when he developed a cough, periorbital edema, ankle swelling, headaches, and upper abdominal discomfort. On admission, he was febrile with facial and ankle edema; there were generalized, superficial lymphadenopathy; numerous adventitial sounds in the lungs; and mild hypertension (BP 140/110). His hemoglobin was 72 g/l with a normal white-cell count and an erythrocyte sedimentation rate (ESR) of 137 mm/h. His blood urea was high (27.5 mmol/l) with a low serum bicarbonate (13.6 mmol/l) and serum albumin (19 g/l). His creatinine clearance was 45 ml/min/m^2 with urinary protein loss of 6.7 g/day. His serum CH_{50} was low (14 U/ml; NR 25–45), as was his C3 level (0.20 g/l; NR 0.8–1.4); his C4 level was normal (0.30 g/l; NR 0.2–0.4). A chest x-ray showed several rounded

(continued)

opacities in both lungs. These were presumed to be infective and treated with amoxycillin and flucloxacillin with resolution of the radiological findings.

The association of a low C3 with acute glomerulonephritis suggested acute poststreptococcal disease as the most likely diagnosis, although no streptococci were isolated and streptococcal antibodies were not raised. Over the following 3 weeks, his blood urea fell but the proteinuria and hypertension persisted.

CURRENT ADMISSION: Although he feels better, he still has heavy proteinuria with a low serum albumin (22 g/l; NR 35–50). Surprisingly, the serum CH_{50} and C3 levels are still low at 18 U/ml and 0.4 g/l, respectively. This pattern was not consistent with the working diagnosis. It suggested continued complement activation via the alternate pathway, either due to some circulating activating factor or because of a regulatory defect caused by absence of the inhibitors I or H. However, his serum levels of I and H are normal. Electrophoresis of fresh serum and plasma showed the presence of C3 breakdown products and his serum was able to break down C3 in normal serum due to the presence of C3 nephritic factor.

C3 nephritic factor shows a strong association with membranoproliferative glomerulonephritis, but not with acute poststreptococcal glomerulonephritis. Because these conditions have different prognoses, a bilateral renal biopsy was performed yesterday. The results show 11 glomeruli, all of which were swollen with proliferation of mesangial, endothelial, and epithelial cells. On electron microscopy, the capillary loops showed basement membrane thickening with electron-dense deposits within the GBM. On immunofluorescence, intense C3 deposition is present in the GBM without immunoglobulin staining. These appearances, together with the finding of circulating C3 nephritic factor, are characteristic of *membranoproliferative glomerulonephritis* with *dense intramembranous deposits* (type II MPGN). Alternate-day prednisolone 10 mg PO per day was started, with prescription for 5 mg PO every other day for 30 days, although this disease nearly always shows a slow progression to chronic renal failure.

CASE STUDY #8: MARYBELLE OSENKOWSKY

Patient: Marybelle Osenkowsky

Physician: Fiona McNally, MD

December 17, 2019

History

This 87-year-old female has been a patient of the McGraw Health Center and Clinic since 2005. Chronic conditions: pernicious anemia, osteoarthritis, and urinary incontinency. She is fully functional and fully independent. She provides care for her homebound husband, who has severe COPD. They live in a home chosen because it was "close to the hospital" to ensure access to house calls for her husband.

In September 2005, the husband died as a result of respiratory arrest. Her only relative is a niece who talks with her about once a month. In October 2017, her home was broken into and our patient was raped and robbed. She was taken to a local hospital specializing in rape. Here, she is distressed, delusional, and reported to be very emotionally distraught.

Examination

I saw the patient about 3 weeks after the rape in a community nursing home, where she was moved after a 4-day stay at the hospital. She was very distressed, delusional, and confused. She slowly improved over 2 months and was discharged to a senior living center.

(continued)

In March of 2019, the patient was seen in the office. She is still very emotionally unstable. She is crying, depressed (not suicidal), and stressed about her new home. She wants to move to a different senior housing unit because it would be on the bus route, making it easier to get around. She has also hired a middle-aged woman as a caregiver.

Today, 9 months after moving to the new facility, she becomes acutely ill with psychotic symptoms and severe paranoia. She hallucinates that men and women are in her bed and calls others all hours of the day. I admitted her into a hospitalized psychiatric unit and she shows improvement over about 14 days without antipsychotic medication. IV Haloperidol 2.5 mg q30 min x3 h.

Diagnosis: Delusional disorder, Acute Post Traumatic Stress Disorder

CASE STUDY #9: ROGER WESTERMAN

Patient: Roger Westerman

Physician: LaTisha Rodriquez, MD

February 3, 2019

H&P

History:
05/13: trouble w balance × 1 year, fatigue, fall × 4 (retropulse × 3)
Walking slowly for few years—getting worse
Trouble going to standing from sitting position
No tremor, handwriting OK, no shuffling gait
Urinary incontinence without urgency—just leaks, not at night
Inattentive per wife
Cooks, but wife must redirect at times
Gave up driving 1 yr ago because he was nervous about his skills
Decline in function—no aerobics × 2–3 yrs
Depressive symptoms—had seen a psychiatrist for years. Had been on Prozac but it "made him feel too great" and he gave it up
Overall, there had been a significant deterioration in function

Past Medical History
2006: Serial TIAs—anterior circulation symptoms—Carotid ultrasound (–), treated with aspirin 81 mg qd
2008: Another TIA—ASA 325 mg. Repeat carotid ultrasound (–)
2013: Right hemisensory symptoms—Left thalamic infarct on MRI
2015: Neurology evaluation—problems with balance, coordination, reduced exercise tolerance
February 1, 2019: MRI—mild prominence 3rd and lateral vents, periventricular white matter changes, old left thalamic lacune. Low normal B12. Normal: TSH, folate, ESR, CBC, HbA1C

Examination
SH: retired kindergarten teacher
Recently moved to an apartment house in the city
Requires help with instrumental activities of daily living

Physical Examination
Cranial nerves normal
Motor: normal × LUE extensor, LE flex 4/5
Normal tone, no cogwheeling, no shuffle, normal facies

(continued)

3+ patellar DTR, 1+ ankles DTR, toes downgoing

- Retropulses with challenge
- Normal cerebellar exam
- Gait—ataxia present

Data and Scans
Review of head MRI/CTs from '06, '08, '13, '15:
Enlarging ventricles over time
Substantial white matter changes
Thalamic infarct
MRI, 02/01/2019 shows differential diagnosis of:
Sequelae of stroke (ataxia) vs. Normal pressure hydrocephalus
Surgery: Open procedure to insert monitoring device into cerebrum. Successful.
Code for monitoring device surgery.

CASE STUDY #10: KARL ATTENDA

DATE OF OPERATION: 05/15/2019

PREOPERATIVE DIAGNOSIS: Bilateral inguinal hernia

POSTOPERATIVE DIAGNOSIS: Bilateral inguinal hernia, direct

OPERATION PERFORMED: Laparoscopic bilateral inguinal hernia repair

SURGEON: Lawrence Podentale, MD

ANESTHESIA: General endotracheal

ESTIMATED BLOOD LOSS: Minimal

DESCRIPTION OF OPERATION: With the patient under general endotracheal anesthesia, the abdomen was prepped with ChloraPrep solution and draped in the usual manner. A transverse skin incision was made below and to the right of the umbilicus to a length of approximately 4 cm. The incision was carried through the subcutaneous tissue. Bleeders were cauterized. The right rectus sheath was identified and incised lateral to the midline. The preperitoneal space was then developed following insertion of a Spacemaker balloon, which was inflated under direct vision.

Following removal of the Spacemaker balloon, a #10 trocar was placed in the preperitoneal space and the preperitoneal space was insufflated with CO_2. Two #5 trocars were placed in the lower midline. Video laparoscope was inserted in the preperitoneal space. Landmarks including symphysis pubis, right Cooper ligament, and right inferior epigastric vessels were identified. Dissection was then continued lateral to the transverse abdominis muscle. The internal ring was then explored for the presence of an indirect hernia sac. No indirect hernia sac was identified. The patient had a cord lipoma, which was reduced under direct vision. Exploration of the medial space showed a medial defect suggesting a direct hernia. A large-size Bard 3D mesh was placed in the preperitoneal space and anchored to the symphysis pubis and anterior abdominal wall along the upper edge of the mesh with a stapler. The lower edge of the mesh was affixed to the abdominal wall with Tisseel fibrin glue.

Following this, the left preperitoneal space was explored in the same fashion. Landmarks including symphysis pubis, Cooper ligament, and inferior epigastric vessels were identified. The dissection was continued laterally to the transverse abdominis muscle. The internal ring was then explored for the presence of an indirect hernia sac. No indirect hernia sac was identified. A cord lipoma was reduced. The patient was found to

(continued)

have a medial defect suggesting a direct hernia. A large-size left 3D Prolene mesh was then placed in the preperitoneal space and placed over the floor of the inguinal canal and stapled to the symphysis pubis and anterior abdominal wall along the upper edge of the mesh with a stapler.

The lower edge was anchored to the abdominal wall with Tisseel fibrin glue. The preperitoneal space was then deflated. All trocars were withdrawn. The defect in the rectus sheath was closed with figure-of-eight 0 Vicryl suture. The skin incisions were closed with subcuticular 5-0 Monocryl suture. Sterile dressings were then applied. The patient tolerated the procedure well and was brought to the recovery room in stable condition. Needle and sponge counts were correct.

PROCEDURE: Laparoscopic repair of bilateral inguinal hernias

Lawrence Podentale, MD

CASE STUDY #11: KEASHA FROENMAN

DATE OF OPERATION: 06/07/2019

PREOPERATIVE DIAGNOSIS: Degenerative joint disease, left shoulder

POSTOPERATIVE DIAGNOSIS: Degenerative joint disease, left shoulder, with degenerative labral tear and chondral flap tear of glenoid

OPERATION PERFORMED: Arthroscopic exam of glenohumeral joint with arthroscopic debridement of labral tears, chondroplasty, and microfracture of glenoid

SURGEON: Cassandra LeRoy, MD

ASSISTANT SURGEON: Rose Carter, MD

ANESTHESIA: General

DESCRIPTION OF OPERATION: The patient was brought to the operating room and placed in a supine position on the operating room table. General anesthetic was administered. The left shoulder was prepped and draped in a sterile orthopedic fashion after she was placed in a beach-chair position. A time-out was performed confirming left shoulder pathology, and she also had 1 gram of Ancef administered intravenously. After the sterile orthopedic prep and drape, a posterior stab wound was created and the arthroscope was introduced into the glenohumeral joint. The joint was inspected. There were degenerative changes of the labrum circumferentially. Through an anterior portal, a full-radius resector was inserted and these areas debrided back to stable tissue, and this was supplemented with use of the ArthroCare wand on a setting of one. There was a flap tear of the anterior portion of the mid glenoid region. This was easily displaceable. Using a 4.2 full-radius resector, this was debrided back to stable tissue and then an awl was used to microfracture the bone. The inflow pump was then stopped and bloody fluid could be seen coming from the microfracture area. The undersurface of the rotator cuff was inspected and found to be without pathology. The arthroscope was then placed into the anterior portal, and through the posterior portal, the ArthroCare wand and a full-radius resector were inserted and the most inferior aspect and posterior aspect of the glenoid and labrum debrided. There were no frank tears of the posterior labrum. The arthroscope was then placed in the subacromial space, which did appear to be pristine. There was no evidence of impingement. All instruments were then removed and the stab wounds were closed with a single Monocryl suture and Steri-Strips. Dry sterile dressings were placed over the wound. The patient was placed in a shoulder sling and then sent to the recovery room in stable condition.

CASE STUDY #12: REISHICA DECLERQUE

DATE OF ADMISSION: 09/09/2019

DATE OF DISCHARGE: 09/11/2019

DISCHARGE DIAGNOSES:

1. Intrauterine gestation at term
2. History of two previous cesarean sections
3. Delivered viable male infant
4. Multiparity, fertility, desired sterilization

PROCEDURES PERFORMED:

1. Repeat low transverse cesarean section
2. Bilateral tubal ligation

COMPLICATIONS: None

PERTINENT FINDINGS/HISTORY AND PHYSICAL: Refer to the detailed admission dictation.

The patient is a 35-year-old gravida 6, now para 3-0-3-3 female, who was admitted at term for repeat cesarean section and sterilization. The patient had previous cesarean sections for labor arrest, for an infant weighing 9 pounds 12 ounces, and elective repeat. The patient strongly desired repeat cesarean section. She also wanted to have a tubal ligation and signed the appropriate consent forms. Patient is well aware of the risks, options, failure rates, and permanency of sterilization procedures. Her antenatal course was significant for development of A1 diabetes with blood sugars in excellent control, on diet only. The patient declined genetic screening because of advanced maternal age.

LABORATORY INVESTIGATIONS: The patient's admission hemoglobin was 11.1 with hematocrit of 33.4 and platelet count 196,000. Her postoperative hematocrit was 32.2.

HOSPITAL COURSE: The patient was admitted on the morning of her scheduled surgery. Detailed informed consent was again obtained. Under spinal anesthesia, uncomplicated repeat low transverse cesarean section and bilateral tubal ligation were performed. A viable male infant with Apgars of 9 and 9 with birth weight of 8 pounds 6 ounces was delivered. The patient's postoperative course was uneventful. She remained afebrile with stable vital signs. She returned quickly to good ambulation and regular diet. She had normal GI function return. Her incision healed nicely. Her lochia was light.

Discharge examination revealed negative HEENT, neck, heart, lung, extremities, and abdominal examinations.

CONDITION ON DISCHARGE: Stable.

DISPOSITION: Discharged to home.

DISCHARGE INSTRUCTIONS:

ACTIVITY: Slow increase as tolerated. No heavy lifting. Strict pelvic rest.

DIET: Regular.

MEDICATIONS: Colace p.r.n., Tylenol p.r.n., and prenatal vitamins. The patient is breast-feeding. Prescriptions for Percocet 325/5 tablets, #30, no refills, 1 to 2 p.o. q.4–6 h. p.r.n. pain and ibuprofen 800 mg, #20, no refills, 1 p.o. q.8 h. p.r.n. pain.

Follow up as an outpatient in the office in 1 week.

The patient has received routine verbal instructions and agrees to comply. She knows to contact us immediately should she develop any signs or symptoms of complications such as fevers, chills, drainage from the incision, abdominal distention, nausea, vomiting, heavy vaginal bleeding, leg redness or swelling, chest pain, chest pressure, or shortness of breath.

DATE OF CONSULTATION: 11/16/2019

REFERRING PHYSICIAN: Charles Craigen, MD

REASON FOR CONSULTATION: Evaluation and management of painful lymphadenitis. Thank you for this infectious disease consultation.

HISTORY OF PRESENT ILLNESS: The patient is a 41-year-old male who about 3 days prior to admission noticed what appeared to be a painful inguinal lymph node on the left that seemed to progressively increase in size. This started while on a business trip, but after he returned to work, he noticed it became a lot more tender and swollen. He finally presented to the emergency department after having a couple of days of onset of fever and was admitted for further evaluation. The patient on arrival did have a low-grade temperature of 100. He was started initially on Flagyl and Cipro, that was changed to doxycycline and Rocephin, and now he is on Zithromax and vancomycin.

The patient does not have any known infection as far as he knows. The patient has not had any exposure to tuberculosis, although he said that he has had weight loss and some night sweats, but this has only started since the onset of his symptoms about a week ago. He has not had any long-term weight loss or long-term night sweats or cough. The patient had traveled for that weekend prior to getting his onset of symptoms, but he did not do any camping. He does have two cats at home but no obvious cat bite or scratches as far as he knows. The patient has also been involved in a new sexual relationship about several months ago and has not had an HIV test recently. He had one 2 years ago that he reports was negative. No other history of sexually transmitted diseases to his knowledge.

REVIEW OF SYSTEMS: Unremarkable other than mentioned above. The patient had diarrhea 1 day prior to admission and currently still has diarrhea.

PAST MEDICAL HISTORY: Hypertension, history of kidney stones, depression, migraines.

PAST SURGICAL HISTORY: Cyst removed from the right leg.

ALLERGIES: No known allergies.

MEDICATIONS: List is currently reviewed and the antibiotics are listed above in the HPI.

SOCIAL HISTORY: The patient does not use tobacco, alcohol, or drugs. He is divorced from his first wife but is living with a new girlfriend. He has four children, all of whom live at home with him.

FAMILY HISTORY: Negative for immune dysfunction.

PHYSICAL EXAMINATION: General: The patient is alert and oriented and in no acute distress. He is afebrile. Temperature 96.5, pulse 70, respirations 19, and blood pressure 115/73. HEENT: Pupils are equal and reactive. Head is normocephalic and atraumatic. Sinuses are nontender. Oropharynx is clear without lesions. Neck: Supple without lymphadenopathy. Heart: Regular rate and rhythm. Lungs: Clear to auscultation bilaterally. Abdomen: Soft, nontender, and nondistended with no rebound or guarding. Good bowel sounds are heard. Genitourinary: The left groin reveals tender adenopathy. There is definite swelling and a mass felt in the left inguinal area. There is no obvious cut or scratches seen. The rest of the inguinal area appears fairly unremarkable without lesions or blisters seen. Lower extremities are without edema, clubbing, or cyanosis, and appeared normal. Skin: Reveals no rashes. Neurologic: Grossly nonfocal.

LABORATORY DATA: Laboratory data have been reviewed and showed an elevated white count of 16. There is a band neutrophilia of 27%. Liver function tests are

(continued)

unremarkable. Creatinine is normal. UA is unremarkable. Chlamydia and gonorrhea DNA probe are negative.

DIAGNOSTIC STUDIES: CT of the abdomen was done that was unremarkable. There is a nonspecific enlargement of a lymph node within the left inguinal region as seen on the CT of the pelvis.

IMPRESSION:

1. Painful lymph node lymphadenitis with a broad differential.
2. Diarrhea, which is new onset, right before admission.

DISCUSSION: The differential is broad. This could be suppurative bacterial process, which is usually due to staph and strep. It is less likely to be tularemia or Yersinia. We also need to consider fungal, TB, and sexually transmitted diseases including HIV. We also need to consider cat scratch disease.

RECOMMENDATIONS:

1. I will do a percutaneous biopsy of the inguinal mass.
2. We will order HIV antibody and quantitative viral load.
3. We will check Bartonella antibodies as well as *Chlamydia trachomatis* titers.
4. We will check PPD.
5. Check *Clostridium difficile* toxin.
6. Daptomycin antibiotic to replace the vancomycin.

We will continue to follow. Thank you for asking us to participate in this patient's care.

Code for the biopsy of the inguinal mass.

CASE STUDY #14: HILLARY ROMINEY

DATE OF STUDY: 02/22/2019

ORDERING PHYSICIAN: Harrison Brady, MD

DATE OF INTERPRETATION OF STUDY:

Echocardiogram was obtained for assessment of left ventricular function. The patient has been admitted with diagnosis of syncope. Overall, the study was suboptimal due to poor sonic window.

FINDINGS:

1. Aortic root appears normal.
2. Left atrium is mildly dilated. No gross intraluminal pathology is recognized, although subtle abnormalities could not be excluded. Right atrium is of normal dimension.
3. There is echo dropout of the interatrial septum. Atrial septal defects could not be excluded.
4. Right and left ventricles are normal in internal dimension. Overall left ventricular systolic function appears to be normal. Eyeball ejection fraction is around 55%. Again, due to poor sonic window, wall motion abnormalities in the distribution of lateral and apical wall could not be excluded.
5. Aortic valve is sclerotic with normal excursion. Color flow imaging and Doppler study demonstrate trace aortic regurgitation.
6. Mitral valve leaflets are also sclerotic with normal excursion. Color flow imaging and Doppler study demonstrate trace to mild degree of mitral regurgitation.

(continued)

7. Tricuspid valve is delicate and opens normally. Pulmonic valve is not clearly seen. No evidence of pericardial effusion.

CONCLUSIONS:

1. Poor quality study.
2. Eyeball ejection fraction is 55%.
3. Trace to mild degree of mitral regurgitation.
4. Trace aortic regurgitation.

CASE STUDY #15: ELENA BEVERLY

DATE OF ADMISSION: 03/01/2019

DATE OF DISCHARGE: 03/09/2019

DISCHARGE DIAGNOSES:

AXIS I:

1. Bipolar disorder, depressed, with psychotic features, symptoms in remission.
2. Attention deficit hyperactivity disorder, symptoms in remission.

AXIS II: Deferred.
AXIS III: None.
AXIS IV: Moderate.
AXIS V: Global assessment of functioning 65 on discharge.

REASON FOR ADMISSION: The patient was admitted with a chief complaint of suicidal ideation. The patient was brought to the hospital after her guidance counselor found a note the patient wrote, which detailed to whom she was giving away her possessions when she dies. The patient told the counselor that she hears voices telling her to hurt herself and others. The patient reports over the last month these symptoms have exacerbated. The patient had a fight in school recently, which the patient blames on the voices. Three weeks ago, she got pushed into a corner at school and threatened to cut herself and others with a knife. The patient was suspended for that remark.

PROCEDURES AND TREATMENT:

1. Individual cognitive and group psychotherapy.
2. Psychopharmacologic management.
3. Family therapy conducted by social work department with the patient and the patient's family for the purpose of education and discharge planning.

HOSPITAL COURSE: The patient responded well to individual and group psychotherapy, milieu therapy, and medication management. As stated, family therapy was conducted.

DISCHARGE ASSESSMENT: At the time of discharge, the patient is alert and fully oriented. Mood euthymic. Affect broad range. She denies any suicidal or homicidal ideation. IQ is at baseline. Memory intact. Insight and judgment good.

PLAN: The patient may be discharged as she no longer poses a risk of harm toward herself or others. The patient will continue on the following medications: Ritalin LA 60 mg q.a.m., Depakote 500 mg q.a.m. and 750 mg q.h.s., Abilify 20 mg q.h.s. Depakote level on date of discharge was 110. Liver enzymes drawn were within normal limits. The patient will follow up with Dr. Petrikas for medication management and Dr. Sanders for psychotherapy. All other discharge orders per the psychiatrist, as arranged by social work.

Design elements: ©McGraw-Hill

PART VI

REIMBURSEMENT, LEGAL, AND ETHICAL ISSUES

INTRODUCTION

A professional coding specialist's responsibilities may not stop when the last code is determined. Remember, the codes you determine are used on requests for payment, known as reimbursement *claims. Whenever money is involved, there are always legal and ethical issues attached, and you must familiarize yourself with all of the aspects for doing a complete and professional job for your facility, whether it is a small physician's office or a huge hospital. Understanding these components ensures that you will have a career draped in honesty, integrity, and success.*

39 Reimbursement

Insurance Premium
The amount of money, often paid monthly, by a policyholder or insured, to an insurance company to obtain coverage.

Learning Outcomes

After completing this chapter, the student should be able to:

LO 39.1 Define the role of health insurance and managed care plans in the delivery of health care services.

LO 39.2 Identify and define the types of health insurance plans.

LO 39.3 Explain the types of compensation used in health care reimbursement.

LO 39.4 Describe the information available for proper coding from NCCI edits and NCD and LCD.

LO 39.5 Utilize Place-of-Service and Type-of-Service codes as required.

LO 39.6 Create a system for organizing claims, understanding denials, and filing appeals.

39.1 The Role of Insurance in Health Care

A health insurance policy is a contractual agreement between an insurance carrier (company) and an individual related to health care issues. And the basis of this contract is risk. Insurance is just like gambling in Las Vegas. Basically, the insurance company is betting that a certain event will *not* happen to you, such as you getting sick. If that happens, it would have to pay your medical bills. On the other side of the table, you are betting (by paying an **insurance premium**) that you *will* have a major illness or health catastrophe. Think about it—if you knew for a fact that you would never get ill or have any injury, and would only have to go to the doctor for your annual checkups, would you pay all that money every month for insurance premiums? Of course not. You are betting that you will, at some point, get all that money back, when you need it to pay for some type of treatment.

When **managed care** was developed, the health insurance industry realized that it could lower its risk (and save money) if it could keep people healthy by encouraging them to go to the doctor for regular checkups, tests, and so forth. This thinking created a major change in the health insurance industry and in the medical care industry, increasing the focus of health care delivery to include preventive care, rather than only therapeutic (medical) care.

Medical care is the identification and treatment of illnesses and injuries—in other words, whatever a health care provider does to help you with a health problem or concern that you have (Figure 39-1).

Preventive care is provision of services designed to prevent the problem from manifesting (developing) or to discover it in early stages when it is more easily corrected. Preventive care includes well-baby visits (Figure 39-2), screenings, diagnostics, and routine checkups.

The term **health care** refers to a combination of these two types of services.

FIGURE 39-1 Treatment of a broken leg is an example of medical care
©ERproductions Ltd/Blend Images LLC

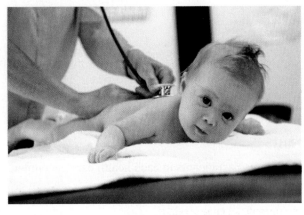

FIGURE 39-2 Well-baby visits are an example of preventive care
©Picture Partners/AGE Fotostock

Managed Care
A type of health insurance coverage that controls the care of each subscriber (or insured person) by using a primary care provider as a central health care supervisor.

Health Care
The total management of an individual's well-being by a health care professional.

CODING BITES

Medical Care + Preventive Care = Health Care

EXAMPLES

Dr. Michaelson examines Paul and gives him a shot of antibiotics to help Paul get rid of an infection. The doctor has identified Paul's illness and is treating that illness. This is medical care.

Dr. Calavari knows Katrina works at a day care center and gives her a flu shot to help her avoid getting the flu. The doctor is preventing Katrina from becoming ill. This is preventive care.

We all know that every organization needs to have money coming in so that it can stay in business. The physician provides a service to his or her patients and expects to be paid for those services. That money is what keeps a practice open and allows it to pay your salary. If enough people don't pay their bills, then an office must lay off people (and that could mean you!). Or you might not be able to get that next raise, even if you deserve it.

By now, you understand how important all of this information is and how you have a personal stake in completing claim forms correctly. As you transfer information from patient registration forms and other documents, be certain to

- Double-check your work to make sure it is accurate.

CODING BITES

The process of getting information and submitting claims to the third-party payer is key to the survival of your health care facility and all the people it employs.

- Confirm that the form is completely filled out, with no necessary information missing.
- Verify the spelling of every name and the accuracy of every number.

It all must be absolutely correct.

Most third-party payers, including Medicare, prefer claim forms to be submitted electronically. An **electronic media claim (EMC)**, also called an electronic claim, is evaluated more quickly than a print claim form. Accepted claims are paid faster. Years ago, it was not unusual for health care facilities to wait 4 to 6 months to receive payment from an insurance company. With electronic claims, this time has been reduced to 2 to 3 weeks.

Increased use of technology in this process also means that there is an excellent chance a computer will be reviewing your claim form. During the initial processing of a claim you have sent, the computer will only compare letter to letter and number to number, looking for an exact match to the letters and numbers in its files. Then, claims with errors, such as invalid policy numbers or missing information, will be rejected and returned to you.

EXAMPLE

The computer cannot scan your claim form and say, "Oh, I can see this is a typo. They really meant to put a *W* instead of a *U*." No, all the computer knows is that the letter is supposed to be a *U* and it is not. And the claim will be rejected.

The Participants

Essentially, there are three participants in each health care encounter, or visit:

1. The physician or health care provider.
2. The patient—the person seeking services.
3. The insurance carrier covering the costs of health care activities for the patient.

Some people get their health insurance policies through a program at their place of employment, some through the government, and others directly with the insurance carriers as individual policyholders. It doesn't matter very much to the health care facility. In any case, a **third-party payer** will pay, in part, the patient's bills for services that your facility will provide. Health insurance carriers are often referred to as third-party payers. This means that someone not directly involved in the health care relationship is paying for the service. The health care provider is party #1, the patient is party #2, and the insurance carrier is party #3—the third party. Therefore, the insurance company is the third-party payer.

39.2 Types of Insurance Plans

There are many types of health plans that people may purchase, or contract for, with companies that specialize in insurance.

Health Maintenance Organization (HMO)

In a **health maintenance organization (HMO)**, members, also called enrollees, prepay for health care services. The members are encouraged to get preventive treatment to promote wellness (and keep medical costs down). In addition, each member has a primary care physician (PCP), also known as a **gatekeeper**. The PCP is responsible for monitoring the individual's well-being and making all decisions regarding care. It is the PCP who determines if a specialist is required for a certain evaluation or procedure. When this occurs, it is the PCP who is responsible for completing the patient referral form and getting approval from the HMO for the patient to visit the specialist. Generally, HMOs do not require a patient to satisfy a deductible before benefits begin. (See the section *Patient/Beneficiary Out-of-Pocket Contributions* later in this chapter.)

Preferred Provider Organization (PPO)

In a **preferred provider organization (PPO)**, physicians, hospitals, and other health care providers join together and agree to offer services to members of a group (often called subscribers) at a lower cost or discount. These plans usually permit the individual subscriber (the patient) to choose the physician or specialist to see, with a discount for staying in the network by using a physician who is a member of the plan. If the individual chooses a physician who does not belong to the network, or is not participating with that PPO, the individual will pay a penalty or receive less of a discount in the cost of those services. This can give the individual more control over his or her health care. It can save time and money, as well.

Some PPO plans require the patient to satisfy a deductible first before benefits begin. (See the section *Patient/Beneficiary Out-of-Pocket Contributions* later in this chapter.) Typically, a higher deductible will translate into a lower monthly premium for this type of insurance coverage.

EXAMPLE

If a person covered under a PPO plan is having problems sneezing and knows the problem is his or her allergies, the individual can choose an allergist—a provider who specializes in the treatment of allergies—from the PPO network without having to go to his or her primary care physician for a referral. If the plan were an HMO, the person would have to make an appointment with the PCP first in order to get the referral to the allergist. Then, the person could make an appointment to see the allergist.

Point-of-Service (POS) Plan

Giving individuals a little more flexibility, a **point-of-service (POS)** plan is almost a combination of an HMO and a PPO. Each insured person has a primary care physician (PCP) and a list of providers that participate in the HMO. When health care providers within the HMO network are used, the insured pays only a regular copayment amount or a small charge. There is no deductible or co-insurance payment involved. However, this plan may also include a self-referral option, in which the individual insured can choose to go to an out-of-network provider. In that case, the individual may be responsible for paying both a deductible and a co-insurance payment.

CODING BITES

POS plans combine features of an HMO and a PPO.

Federal Government Plans

Centers for Medicare & Medicaid Services (CMS)

In 1977, the Health Care Financing Administration (HCFA, pronounced hic-fah) was created to coordinate federal health services programs. On July 1, 2001, HCFA became

Gatekeeper
A physician, typically a family practitioner or an internist, who serves as the primary care physician for an individual. This physician is responsible for evaluating and determining the course of treatment or services, as well as for deciding whether or not a specialist should be involved in care.

Preferred Provider Organization (PPO)
A type of health insurance coverage in which physicians provide health care services to members of the plan at a discount.

Point-of-Service (POS)
A type of insurance plan that will allow an HMO enrollee to choose his or her own nonmember physician at a lower benefit rate, costing the patient more money out-of-pocket.

FIGURE 39-3 Medicare.gov, the official U.S. government site for Medicare
Source: Medicare.gov

CODING BITES

Medica**RE** = **RE**tired people (who are over the age of 65)

Medica**ID** = **I**n**D**igent, or low-income, individuals

the **Centers for Medicare & Medicaid Services (CMS)**. Many health care professionals still refer to this agency as "HicFah" and to the CMS-1500 claim form as the "HicFah 1500." Old habits take a while to change. At least you now understand that these two acronyms refer to the same federal organization.

Medicare is a national health insurance program that pays, or reimburses, for health care services provided to those over the age of 65 (see Figure 39-3). In addition, this plan may cover individuals who are under the age of 65 and are permanently disabled (such as the blind), as well as those with end-stage renal disease (ESRD) who are suffering from permanent kidney failure and require either dialysis or a kidney transplant.

Medicaid is a plan that pays for, or reimburses, medical assistance and health care services for people who are indigent (low-income) (see Figure 39-4). The program is jointly funded by the federal and state governments. Each state government then administers its own plan. This means that each state determines who is eligible and what services are covered. It is important to know that each state has its own requirements, in case you have a patient that has just moved to your state. Each state may even have a unique name or term for its program. For example, in California the program is called Medi-Cal.

TriCare

TriCare offers the most common health care plans you will encounter when caring for individuals in the military and their families (see Figure 39-5). This program was formerly known as CHAMPUS.

TriCare was created to help the following individuals receive better access to improved health care services:

- Active-duty service members (ADSM), also known as sponsors.
- The **dependents** (spouses and children) of ADSMs.
- Surviving spouses and surviving children of deceased ADSMs.
- Retired service members, their spouses, and their children.
- Surviving spouses and children of deceased retired members.

FIGURE 39-4 Medicaid.gov, the official U.S. government website of Medicaid
Source: Medicaid.gov

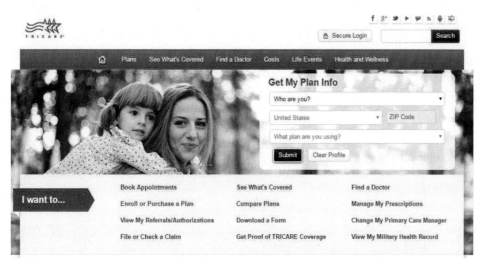

FIGURE 39-5 TriCare.mil, the official U.S. government website of TRICARE
Source: Tricare.gov

TriCare was created to provide health care benefits for the dependents of those serving in the uniformed services and retirees. ADSMs are those from any of the seven uniformed services, including the U.S. military (the Army, Navy, Air Force, Marine Corps, and Coast Guard), as well as those serving in the Public Health Service, National Guard and Reserve, and the National Oceanic and Atmospheric Administration (NOAA). Eligibility for TriCare is determined by the services, and information is maintained in the Defense Enrollment Eligibility Reporting System (DEERS).

Other Insurance Plans

Workers' compensation is an insurance program designed to pay the medical costs for treating those injured, or made ill, at their place of work or by their job. This includes injuries resulting from a fall off a ladder while performing a job-related task, getting hurt in an accident while driving a company car on a business trip, or

Workers' Compensation
An insurance program that covers medical care for those injured or for those who become ill as a consequence of their employment.

developing a lung disorder caused by toxic fumes in the office. Generally, a workers' compensation plan covers only specific medical bills, such as laboratory bills, physicians' fees, and other medical services. Most often, lost income is not covered by this policy. Each state oversees the workers' compensation contracts with particular insurance carriers.

Disability Compensation
A plan that reimburses a covered individual a portion of his or her income that is lost as a result of being unable to work due to illness or injury.

Disability compensation is an insurance plan that reimburses disabled individuals for a percentage of what they used to earn each month. This plan does not pay physicians' bills or for therapy treatments. A disability plan only provides insureds with money to replace a portion of their lost paycheck because they are unable to work. Disability payments might come through a federal government agency such as the Social Security Administration, or patients may have a private insurance plan (such as AFLAC).

YOU INTERPRET IT!

Joe Hines works as an electrician for a small company. One day, he falls off a ladder at work and injures his back severely. He is taken to the emergency room by ambulance, and the attending physician orders x-rays and a CT scan. The tests confirm that Joe's spine is broken in two places and a cast is applied around Joe's entire torso. After a week in the hospital, Joe is discharged. The physician's discharge orders state that Joe is to stay in bed for 7 months, in traction, while the fracture heals. A home health agency is contracted to provide a trained health care professional to go to Joe's house to care for him and attend to his needs around the clock.

1. In this scenario, what type of insurance will be responsible for the payment of each of Joe's expenses due to this accident?

Liability Insurance
A policy that covers loss or injury to a third party caused by the insured or something belonging to the insured.

Liability insurance is commonly part of a person's homeowners or business owners insurance. This type of policy covers losses to a third party caused by the insured or something owned by the insured. In other words, the insurance company will pay for, or reimburse for, any harm or damage done to someone else (not a member of the household or the business).

YOU INTERPRET IT!

Sarah goes over to Margaret's house for dinner. After a delicious meal, Sarah walks toward the door to leave and go home. As she turns to say goodnight to Margaret, Sarah trips and falls. Margaret calls the paramedics, and, at the hospital, the x-rays ordered by the attending physician confirm that Sarah has indeed broken her wrist. A cast is applied, and Sarah is sent home with a prescription for pain medication. The attending physician advises Sarah to see her primary care physician in 1 week for a follow-up.

2. What type of insurance will cover Sarah's medical expenses?

YOU INTERPRET IT!

Kyle, a fifth-grade student, slipped down the stairs at school. Typically, the school's liability policy would cover the damage, or medical expenses. The school is the insured, and the student is the third party.

3. If a faculty member and a student are walking through the cafeteria of the school and both slip and fall, what types of policies will cover any injuries that might be caused by the fall?

Automobile insurance might become an issue for your office if you treat someone for an injury that was caused by the individual's involvement in an automobile accident. Full-coverage automobile policies usually include liability insurance that covers these expenses.

Automobile Insurance
Auto accident liability coverage will pay for medical bills, lost wages, and compensation for pain and suffering for any person injured by the insured in an auto accident.

Details Are Required

As you can see from all this information, different types of insurance policies might be responsible for an individual's medical treatment. Therefore, in your job as medical insurance coder/biller, you must make certain that if an individual comes to the provider for treatment for an *injury* (rather than an *illness*), you must find out the *details* of how and where the injury occurred. This will help determine which carrier will cover the charges.

> **CODING BITES**
>
> And you need these details for determining the external cause codes, too!

39.3 Methods of Compensation

There are several payment plans that insurance carriers (third-party payers) use to pay physicians and other health care providers for their services.

Fee-for-Service (FFS) Plans

In **fee-for-service (FFS) plans**, the insurance company pays the health care provider for each individual service supplied to the patient, as reported by the procedure codes listed on the claim, according to an agreed-upon price list (also known as a fee schedule). When the physician's office agrees to participate in the plan, it is also agreeing to provide services and accept the amount of money indicated on that schedule for each of those services. This is like going to a restaurant with an à la carte menu. The menu lists a price for each item: the salad, the roast beef, the apple pie. The restaurant accepts the amount of money the guest pays for each item received. Different plans may pay different amounts of money for one particular service, just as different restaurants may charge different amounts for a similar dish.

Sometimes, when one insurance carrier pays a provider at a lower rate than other carriers, it is referred to as a **discounted FFS**. In a typical discounted FFS, the payments are reduced from the physician's regular rate. This is similar to the discount you might get at a store when showing your student ID card—you get a discount because you are a member of the school.

Fee-for-Service (FFS) Plans
Payment agreements that outline, in a written fee schedule, exactly how much money the insurance carrier will pay the physician for each treatment and/or service provided.

Discounted FFS
An extra reduction in the rate charged to an insurer for services provided by the physician to the plan's members.

> **EXAMPLE**
>
> Three people, each with a different insurance carrier, go to the same physician for a flu shot (injection). Insurance carrier #1 has agreed to pay the physician $20 for giving the injection. Insurance carrier #2 has agreed to pay the physician $22.50, and insurance carrier #3 has agreed to pay the physician $18 for the same injection. Your office should charge all patients the same amount. This is known as the *charged amount*. However, insurance carriers working with your office on a fee-for-service contract will pay only the amount stated on their fee schedule. That's all they will pay and no more. This is called the *allowed amount*.

Capitation Plans

With **capitation plans**, the insurance company pays the physician a fixed amount of money for every individual covered by that plan (often called members or subscribers) being seen by that physician. Physicians get this amount of money every month, as long as they are listed as the physician of record (primary care physician (PCP)) for that individual. Whether the insured person goes to see that physician once, three

Capitation Plans
Agreements between a physician and a managed care organization that pay the physician a predetermined amount of money each month for each member of the plan who identifies that provider as his or her primary care physician.

Episodic Care

An insurance company pays a provider one flat fee to cover the entire course of treatment for an individual's condition.

Diagnosis-Related Group (DRG)

An episodic care payment system basing reimbursement to hospitals for inpatient services upon standards of care for specific diagnoses grouped by their similar usage of resources for procedures, services, and treatments.

Usual, Customary, and Reasonable (UCR)

The process of determining a fee for a service by evaluating the *usual* fee charged by the provider, the *customary* fee charged by most physicians in the same community or geographical area, and what is considered *reasonable* by most health care professionals under the specific circumstances of the situation.

times, or not at all during a particular month, the physician's office will be paid the same amount. This plan is like the dinner special at your local restaurant. You pay one price, which includes soup, salad, all-you-can-eat entrée, and dessert. If you don't eat your soup, you do not pay any less; if you get seconds on the entrée, you do not pay any more.

Episodic Care

An **episodic care** agreement between insurer and physician means the provider is paid one flat fee for the expected course of treatment for a particular injury or illness. This is like the meal deal of health care. One package price includes all of the services and treatments necessary for the proper care of the patient's condition in accordance with the accepted standards of care.

> **EXAMPLE**
>
> Audrey Callahan fell off her bicycle and broke her arm. The x-ray shows that it is a simple, clean fracture, and the physician applies a cast. The doctor schedules a follow-up appointment for her and expects that she will not need much other attention until the cast comes off in 6 weeks. At that time, an x-ray will confirm that the fracture has healed properly and the cast will be removed. This entire sequence of events, and treatment, is very predictable for a routine simple fracture. Therefore, the insurance company has agreed to pay the physician one flat fee for this event, rather than having the physician's office file a claim for each procedure and service individually: the first encounter; the first x-ray; the application of the cast; the follow-up encounter; the last encounter; the last x-ray; and removal of the cast.
>
> Audrey Callahan's physician is being reimbursed under an episodic care agreement with the insurance carrier.

Diagnosis-related groups (DRGs) are a type of episodic care payment plan used by Medicare to pay for treatments and services provided to beneficiaries who have been admitted into an acute care hospital (inpatients). DRGs are categorized by the principal (first-listed) diagnosis code and take into consideration elements such as the patient's age and gender and the presence of any complications or manifestations (additional diagnoses or conditions). You read more about DRGs in the chapter titled *Inpatient (Hospital) Diagnosis Coding.*

Patient/Beneficiary Out-of-Pocket Contributions

Patients with insurance policies often contribute to reimbursing providers for their health care services, in addition to paying monthly premiums. The following are the most common methods used for the individual's payments:

1. *Copayment (also known as the copay).* The copayment is usually a fixed amount of money that the individual will pay each time he or she goes to a health care provider. It may be $10, $15, $20, or more. Each policy is different. As a matter of fact, the copay on the same policy for the same patient may be different, depending on whether this is a visit to a family physician, a specialist, or the hospital.

2. *Co-insurance.* Co-insurance is different from the copayment because it is based on a percentage of the total charge rather than a fixed amount. The percentage that the patient pays is most often calculated on the **usual, customary, and reasonable (UCR)** charge that has been determined for this type of visit or procedure. Frequently, the individual is required to pay 20% of the total allowed amount by the physician or facility, but that might differ for various types of policies and carriers.

3. *Deductible.* This is the amount of money that patients must pay, out of their own pockets, before the insurance benefits begin. The deductible might be as little as $250 or as much as $1,000 or more. Patients have to pay the total amount until they have paid the whole deductible for that calendar year. After that, they will usually pay just the copayment and/or the co-insurance amount.

> **CODING BITES**
>
> The various amounts for the copay, the co-insurance, and the deductible are good examples of why it is so essential that you contact the insurance carrier for every patient to verify the patient's coverage and eligibility for certain procedures and treatments and to see if the deductible has been met for the year.

MACRA

Medicare Access and CHIP Reauthorization Act (MACRA) has been designed to reward health care providers for quality patient care and to ultimately reduce costs. As a part of this, the Quality Payment Program also was implemented. This program incorporates important advances to ensure that electronic health information will be available when and where clinicians need it so optimal care can be provided.

The Quality Payment Program includes two paths:

- Advanced Alternative Payment Models (APMs)
- Merit-Based Incentive Payment System (MIPS)

Both of these paths require use of certified EHR technology to exchange information across providers and with patients to support improved care delivery, including patient engagement and care coordination. In addition, this program requires EHR manufacturers to publish application programming interfaces (API), which increase interoperability (making it easier for software programs such as smartphone apps to access information from other programs) for certified health IT.

Physicians have options and began participating in this program as early as January 2017.

39.4 NCCI Edits and NCD/LCD

National Correct Coding Initiative (NCCI)

The CMS developed the National Correct Coding Initiative (NCCI) to reinforce accurate and proper coding in addition to preventing reimbursement of inaccurate amounts as the result of noncompliance coding methods in Part B claims (physician and outpatient services). This system was founded with coding policies based on

- The official coding guidelines, as published in the American Medical Association's CPT code book.
- National (NCD) and local (LCD) policies and edits.
- Coding guidelines developed by national societies.
- Analysis of standard medical and surgical practices.
- Review of current coding practices.

There are two types of edits within the NCCI focus: PTP and MUE.

Procedure-to-Procedure (PTP) Edits

Within the long lists of procedures, services, and treatments performed by health care providers, there are those that cannot, or should not, be provided to the same patient on the same date of service. CMS computers evaluate submitted claims to look for pairs of codes being reported that are known to be mutually exclusive procedures, also known as procedure-to-procedure (PTP) edits.

> ### EXAMPLE
>
> 23680   Open treatment of shoulder dislocation, with surgical or anatomical neck fracture, with manipulation
> 20690   Application of a uniplane (pins or wires in 1 plane), unilateral, external fixation system
>
> These codes report two procedures that would not be performed at the same time for the same patient, according to the standards of care. This is an example of a PTP edit.

Medically Unlikely Edits (MUE)

The purpose of the NCCI medically unlikely edits (MUE) is to prevent improper payments when services are reported with incorrect units of service. An MUE for an HCPCS/CPT code is the maximum units of service that a provider would report under most circumstances for a single beneficiary on a single date of service.

> ### EXAMPLE
>
> 72270   Myelography, 2 or more regions, radiological supervision and interpretation
>
> The MUE edit for this code is a maximum of one for a patient per date of service because the code description states "two or more." Therefore, reporting this code more than once for the same patient on the same date would not be accurate.

National Coverage Determinations (NCD) and Local Coverage Determinations (LCD)

In some circumstances, a National Coverage Determination (NCD) is created to clearly establish the criteria for coverage of an item or service applicable to all Medicare beneficiaries nationwide. When there is no NCD, there may be a Local Coverage Determination (LCD) in effect. An LCD is a decision by a fiscal intermediary (FI) or carrier as to when and for what reasons a particular service or item is covered in that area (a state or region). The Medicare Coverage Database (MCD), available at https://www.cms.gov (see Figure 39-6), contains all NCDs and LCDs in a searchable database.

Virtually all third-party payers issue coverage determinations valid nationally or in a particular state or locale. Therefore, you should have the ability to verify coverage for an item or service *prior* to providing it, and certainly before creating and submitting the claim.

Once you find a coverage determination on the service or item the physician wants to provide to the patient, you can obtain the details about the criteria for coverage. In this Medicare NCD on Adult Liver Transplantation (Figure 39-7), the procedure would be categorized (**BENEFIT CATEGORY**) as an Inpatient Hospital Service. Next, the section **ITEM/SERVICE DESCRIPTION** is provided to ensure that everyone understands precisely what procedure, service, or item is being discussed. Read further down the page to the section **INDICATIONS AND LIMITATIONS OF COVERAGE: B. NATIONALLY COVERED INDICATIONS** and you can see the diagnoses considered as medically necessary for this procedure. Earlier in this text, you learned about medical necessity in the chapter *Introduction to the Languages of Coding*. The next section clarifies what types of **FOLLOW-UP CARE** will be covered, as well.

CODING BITES

Submitting a claim for a service or item not covered by the patient's policy is considered fraud . . . even if it gets paid. It is your responsibility to know! Not the patient. Not the doctor. You, the professional coding specialist.

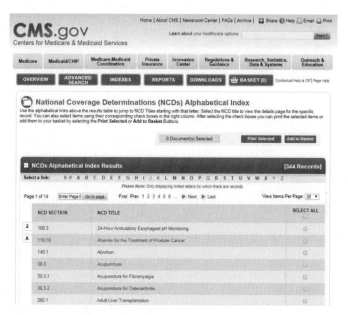

FIGURE 39-6 National Coverage Determinations (NCDs) Alphabetic Index
Source: CMS.gov

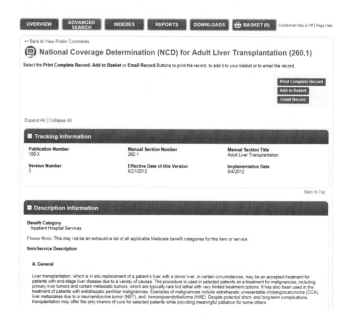

FIGURE 39-7 NCD for Adult Liver Transplantation (in part) Source: CMS.gov

39.5 Place-of-Service and Type-of-Service Codes

Place-of-Service Codes

Place-of-Service (POS) codes are used on professional claims to identify the specific location where procedures, services, and treatments were provided to the patient.

Place of Service Code(s)	Place of Service Name	Place of Service Description
01	Pharmacy	A facility or location where drugs and other medically related items and services are sold, dispensed, or otherwise provided directly to patients.
02	Telehealth	The location where health services and health-related services are provided or received, through a telecommunication system.
03	School	A facility whose primary purpose is education.
04	Homeless Shelter	A facility or location whose primary purpose is to provide temporary housing to homeless individuals (e.g., emergency shelters, individual or family shelters).
05	Indian Health Service Free-Standing Facility	A facility or location, owned and operated by the Indian Health Service, that provides diagnostic, therapeutic (surgical and nonsurgical), and rehabilitation services to American Indians and Alaska Natives who do not require hospitalization.
06	Indian Health Service Provider-Based Facility	A facility or location, owned and operated by the Indian Health Service, that provides diagnostic, therapeutic (surgical and nonsurgical), and rehabilitation services rendered by, or under the supervision of, physicians to American Indians and Alaska Natives admitted as inpatients or outpatients.
07	Tribal 638 Free-Standing Facility	A facility or location, owned and operated by a federally recognized American Indian or Alaska Native tribe or tribal organization under a 638 agreement, that provides diagnostic, therapeutic (surgical and nonsurgical), and rehabilitation services to tribal members who do not require hospitalization.
08	Tribal 638 Provider-Based Facility	A facility or location, owned and operated by a federally recognized American Indian or Alaska Native tribe or tribal organization under a 638 agreement, that provides diagnostic, therapeutic (surgical and nonsurgical), and rehabilitation services to tribal members admitted as inpatients or outpatients.
09	Prison/Correctional Facility	A prison, jail, reformatory, work farm, detention center, or any other similar facility maintained by either federal, state, or local authorities for the purpose of confinement or rehabilitation of adult or juvenile criminal offenders.
10	Unassigned	N/A
11	Office	Location, other than a hospital, skilled nursing facility (SNF), military treatment facility, community health center, state or local public health clinic, or intermediate care facility (ICF), where the health professional routinely provides health examinations, diagnosis, and treatment of illness or injury on an ambulatory basis.
12	Home	Location, other than a hospital or other facility, where the patient receives care in a private residence.
13	Assisted Living Facility	Congregate residential facility with self-contained living units providing assessment of each resident's needs and on-site support 24 hours a day, 7 days a week, with the capacity to deliver or arrange for services including some health care and other services.
14	Group Home	A residence, with shared living areas, where clients receive supervision and other services such as social and/or behavioral services, custodial service, and minimal services (e.g., medication administration).
15	Mobile Unit	A facility/unit that moves from place-to-place equipped to provide preventive, screening, diagnostic, and/or treatment services.
16	Temporary Lodging	A short-term accommodation such as a hotel, camp ground, hostel, cruise ship, or resort where the patient receives care, and that is not identified by any other POS code.

(continued)

Place of Service Code(s)	Place of Service Name	Place of Service Description
17	Walk-in Retail Health Clinic	A walk-in health clinic, other than an office, urgent care facility, pharmacy, or independent clinic and not described by any other Place-of-Service code, that is located within a retail operation and provides, on an ambulatory basis, preventive and primary care services.
18	Place of Employment-Worksite	A location, not described by any other POS code, owned or operated by a public or private entity where the patient is employed, and where a health professional provides ongoing or episodic occupational medical, therapeutic, or rehabilitative services to the individual.
19	Off-Campus Outpatient Hospital	A portion of an off-campus hospital provider-based department that provides diagnostic, therapeutic (both surgical and nonsurgical), and rehabilitation services to sick or injured persons who do not require hospitalization or institutionalization.
20	Urgent Care Facility	Location, distinct from a hospital emergency room, an office, or a clinic, whose purpose is to diagnose and treat illness or injury for unscheduled, ambulatory patients seeking immediate medical attention.
21	Inpatient Hospital	A facility, other than psychiatric, that primarily provides diagnostic, therapeutic (both surgical and nonsurgical), and rehabilitation services by, or under, the supervision of physicians to patients admitted for a variety of medical conditions.
22	On-Campus Outpatient Hospital	A portion of a hospital's main campus that provides diagnostic, therapeutic (both surgical and nonsurgical), and rehabilitation services to sick or injured persons who do not require hospitalization or institutionalization.
23	Emergency Room—Hospital	A portion of a hospital where emergency diagnosis and treatment of illness or injury is provided.
24	Ambulatory Surgical Center	A free-standing facility, other than a physician's office, where surgical and diagnostic services are provided on an ambulatory basis.
25	Birthing Center	A facility, other than a hospital's maternity facilities or a physician's office, that provides a setting for labor, delivery, and immediate post-partum care as well as immediate care of newborn infants.
26	Military Treatment Facility	A medical facility operated by one or more of the Uniformed Services. Military Treatment Facility (MTF) also refers to certain former U.S. Public Health Service (USPHS) facilities now designated as Uniformed Service Treatment Facilities (USTF).
27–30	Unassigned	N/A
31	Skilled Nursing Facility	A facility that primarily provides inpatient skilled nursing care and related services to patients who require medical, nursing, or rehabilitative services but does not provide the level of care or treatment available in a hospital.
32	Nursing Facility	A facility that primarily provides to residents skilled nursing care and related services for the rehabilitation of injured, disabled, or sick persons, or, on a regular basis, health-related care services above the level of custodial care to other than individuals with intellectual disabilities.
33	Custodial Care Facility	A facility that provides room, board, and other personal assistance services, generally on a long-term basis, and that does not include a medical component.
34	Hospice	A facility, other than a patient's home, in which palliative and supportive care for terminally ill patients and their families are provided.
35–40	Unassigned	N/A

(continued)

Place of Service Code(s)	Place of Service Name	Place of Service Description
41	Ambulance—Land	A land vehicle specifically designed, equipped, and staffed for lifesaving and transporting the sick or injured.
42	Ambulance—Air or Water	An air or water vehicle specifically designed, equipped, and staffed for lifesaving and transporting the sick or injured.
43-48	Unassigned	N/A
49	Independent Clinic	A location, not part of a hospital and not described by any other Place-of-Service code, that is organized and operated to provide preventive, diagnostic, therapeutic, rehabilitative, or palliative services to outpatients only.
50	Federally Qualified Health Center	A facility located in a medically underserved area that provides Medicare beneficiaries preventive primary medical care under the general direction of a physician.
51	Inpatient Psychiatric Facility	A facility that provides inpatient psychiatric services for the diagnosis and treatment of mental illness on a 24-hour basis, by or under the supervision of a physician.
52	Psychiatric Facility—Partial Hospitalization	A facility for the diagnosis and treatment of mental illness that provides a planned therapeutic program for patients who do not require full-time hospitalization, but who need broader programs than are possible from outpatient visits to a hospital-based or hospital-affiliated facility.
53	Community Mental Health Center	A facility that provides the following services: outpatient services, including specialized outpatient services for children, the elderly, individuals who are chronically ill, and residents of the CMHC's mental health services area who have been discharged from inpatient treatment at a mental health facility; 24-hour-a-day emergency care services; day treatment, other partial hospitalization services, or psychosocial rehabilitation services; screening for patients being considered for admission to state mental health facilities to determine the appropriateness of such admission; and consultation and education services.
54	Intermediate Care Facility/Individuals with Intellectual Disabilities	A facility that primarily provides health-related care and services above the level of custodial care to individuals but does not provide the level of care or treatment available in a hospital or SNF.
55	Residential Substance Abuse Treatment Facility	A facility that provides treatment for substance (alcohol and drug) abuse to live-in residents who do not require acute medical care. Services include individual and group therapy and counseling, family counseling, laboratory tests, drugs and supplies, psychological testing, and room and board.
56	Psychiatric Residential Treatment Center	A facility or distinct part of a facility for psychiatric care that provides a total 24-hour therapeutically planned and professionally staffed group living and learning environment.
57	Nonresidential Substance Abuse Treatment Facility	A location that provides treatment for substance (alcohol and drug) abuse on an ambulatory basis. Services include individual and group therapy and counseling, family counseling, laboratory tests, drugs and supplies, and psychological testing.
58-59	Unassigned	N/A
60	Mass Immunization Center	A location where providers administer pneumococcal pneumonia and influenza virus vaccinations and submit these services as electronic media claims, paper claims, or using the roster billing method. This generally takes place in a mass immunization setting, such as a public health center, pharmacy, or mall but may include a physician office setting.

(continued)

Place of Service Code(s)	Place of Service Name	Place of Service Description
61	Comprehensive Inpatient Rehabilitation Facility	A facility that provides comprehensive rehabilitation services under the supervision of a physician to inpatients with physical disabilities. Services include physical therapy, occupational therapy, speech pathology, social or psychological services, and orthotics and prosthetics services.
62	Comprehensive Outpatient Rehabilitation Facility	A facility that provides comprehensive rehabilitation services under the supervision of a physician to outpatients with physical disabilities. Services include physical therapy, occupational therapy, and speech pathology services.
63–64	Unassigned	N/A
65	End-Stage Renal Disease Treatment Facility	A facility, other than a hospital, that provides dialysis treatment, maintenance, and/or training to patients or caregivers on an ambulatory or home-care basis.
66–70	Unassigned	N/A
71	Public Health Clinic	A facility maintained by either state or local health departments that provides ambulatory primary medical care under the general direction of a physician.
72	Rural Health Clinic	A certified facility that is located in a rural medically underserved area that provides ambulatory primary medical care under the general direction of a physician.
73–80	Unassigned	N/A
81	Independent Laboratory	A laboratory certified to perform diagnostic and/or clinical tests independent of an institution or a physician's office.
82–98	Unassigned	N/A
99	Other Place of Service	Other place of service not identified above.

Type-of-Service Codes

In addition to providing pre-categorization of procedures, Type-of-Service (TOS) codes are also used to ensure that procedures, services, and treatments, along with the Place-of-Service codes, are used to determine appropriateness of location and service.

Type of Service Indicators

0   Whole Blood
1   Medical Care
2   Surgery
3   Consultation
4   Diagnostic Radiology
5   Diagnostic Laboratory
6   Therapeutic Radiology
7   Anesthesia
8   Assistant at Surgery
9   Other Medical Items or Services
A   Used DME
B   High-Risk Screening Mammography
C   Low-Risk Screening Mammography
D   Ambulance
E   Enteral/Parenteral Nutrients/Supplies

<u>*Type of Service Indicators*</u>

F   Ambulatory Surgical Center (Facility Usage for Surgical Services)

G   Immunosuppressive Drugs

H   Hospice

J   Diabetic Shoes

K   Hearing Items and Services

L   ESRD Supplies

M   Monthly Capitation Payment for Dialysis

N   Kidney Donor

P   Lump Sum Purchase of DME, Prosthetics, Orthotics

Q   Vision Items or Services

R   Rental of DME

S   Surgical Dressings or Other Medical Supplies

T   Outpatient Mental Health Treatment Limitation

U   Occupational Therapy

V   Pneumococcal/Flu Vaccine

W   Physical Therapy

39.6 Organizing Claims: Resubmission, Denials, and Appeals

One thing that is very important for a professional insurance biller to do is to keep track of all the claims sent out on behalf of his or her medical facility, whether it is a physician's office or a hospital. Even with the help of computers and clearinghouses, a claim can get lost. It happens on occasion with letters sent through the post office, and it can happen electronically as well. One little power surge or a computer with a virus can make your claim disappear. The only way you may know about this happening is the absence of a response, such as a payment, a statement of rejection, or a denial. Therefore, you have to keep track of every claim form you submit.

The following are two simple steps for staying organized.

CODING BITES

You are responsible for following up on every claim you send.

1. Keep a log of every claim as you send it. If you are using a clearinghouse, you will receive a report, listing all the claims sent (complete with date and time sent) and to which payer they were forwarded. Place these notices in a file folder on your computer's desktop or print out these reports and place them in a three-ring binder or another type of file. If you are sending claims directly from your office, you should create a separate master index for logging in this information. If you prefer, you can keep a master index in a notebook on your desk and handwrite a notation for each claim you send, indicating the following:

   - Carrier name (the third-party payer to whom you sent the claim)

   - Patient name

   - Date of service

   - Date and time you sent the claim

2. Build into your schedule a specific day and time each week for following up claims. When you set an appointment with yourself, such as every Friday at 9 a.m., or Mondays after the morning staff meeting, you will reduce the number of times that your workday will prevent you from doing this. It is so easy to say, "Once a week I am going to follow up on the claims" and just never have the time for this very important task. Each week, or as often as required by the number of claims you send out, go over the list and separate the claims into three "piles":

- Pile 1: Claims that have been paid by the insurers
- Pile 2: Claims for which you have received rejection or denial notices
- Pile 3: Claims for which you have received no notices or payment

Pile 1: Claims That Have Been Paid by the Insurers

The HIPAA Health Care Payment and Remittance Advice is the electronic transmission of this payment, using HIPAA-approved secure data sets. The transmission has two parts: the transaction and the document.

- The document is a **remittance advice (RA)** or an **electronic remittance advice (ERA)**. Some health care professionals also refer to this document as an **explanation of benefits** or **EOB**. However, an EOB is sent to the patient or beneficiary, not the provider.
- The transaction is an electronic funds transfer (EFT) that sends the payment directly into your facility's bank account, like a direct deposit.

The RA will provide all the details of this payment, including

- The exact amount of monies your office is receiving
- For which patient
- For which procedures performed
- On which service dates

Once you are certain that a claim has been approved and your office has received payment from the third-party payer, the first thing you should do is mark this claim as paid in your master index. Be very careful when doing this.

When you enter the deposits into the computer (and into the bank, if the funds were not electronically transferred), you must be very diligent. You might have two claims for the same patient for different dates or two patients with the same name or similar names. You do not want to mark the wrong claim paid and leave the wrong claim marked unpaid. This will cause a lot of confusion and aggravation in dealing with the insurance carrier.

Pile 2: Claims for Which You Have Received Denial Notices

You have learned how to avoid many denied claims by checking, double-checking, and triple-checking your work. Make certain that

1. Insurance coverage is confirmed (eligibility verification).
2. All the information (such as policyholder and policy number) is entered correctly.
3. The best, most appropriate codes are used.
4. Medical necessity has been established by those codes.
5. All the information has been correctly placed on the correct claim form.

Despite doing everything correctly, some claims are denied and come back unpaid. However, this does not mean that you either have to go after the guarantor for the money or have your office go without the money it deserves. There are many reasons an insurance carrier, or payer, may deny a claim. Let's review some of the most common reasons for a claim to be denied and what you can do about it.

Denied Due to Office Personnel Error

If you discover that the claim has been denied by the insurance carrier due to an error made by you or someone in your office, this can be fixed. Simply find out what the error was and correct it.

Compare the policy number on the claim to the copy of the insurance card that you made when the patient was seen in your office for this encounter. It is important that

Remittance Advice (RA)
Notification identifying details about a payment from the third-party payer.

Electronic Remittance Advice (ERA)
Remittance advice that is sent to the provider electronically.

Explanation of Benefits (EOB)
Another type of paper remittance advice, more typically sent to the policyholder. However, some in the industry use the term *EOB* interchangeably with *RA*.

Eligibility Verification

The process of confirming with the insurance carrier that an individual is qualified for benefits that would pay for services provided by your health care professional on a particular day.

you specifically check it against the copy taken at the encounter for which this claim form is billing the insurance company. The patient may have been in your office more recently with a new policy because his or her insurance changed between the most recent visit and the visit for which this claim was submitted.

You might find that, when you keyed the number into the computer, you inadvertently switched two numbers. It can happen when you are in a busy, hectic, noisy office with many people talking to you at the same time.

If you find that the policy number matches the ID card, you will have to continue looking for the typo, going over the claim form one box at a time to check every piece of information that was entered. Once you find the error, all you have to do is correct it and resubmit a corrected claim form.

You should have caught the error when you double-checked your work, but . . . OK. It happens. You have wasted time (and if you are using a clearinghouse, you have wasted money as well), and you have delayed payment to your office, but follow the third-party payer's procedure for resubmitting corrected claims and the money will arrive.

> ### EXAMPLES
> The policy number or a CPT code is invalid (nonexistent) because it was entered improperly.
> Anyone could look at the number 546998823 and accidentally key in 546999823.

Denied Due to Lack of Coverage

You look at the denial notice and it doesn't make sense. You have documentation in the file that, when you called for **eligibility verification**, the insurance carrier representative confirmed that the patient's coverage was valid and the policy carried no exclusions. The copayment, co-insurance, and deductible were also confirmed. However, the claim was returned as denied, with the reason that the patient was not covered.

What may have happened is that, between your verification of the patient's coverage and the arrival of the claim at the insurance carrier's office, the policy was canceled or changed. When your claim arrived, the computer, or the person, simply looked at the file, saw that the policy was no longer in effect, and therefore denied the claim. If this is the case:

1. You will need to send a letter, not make a phone call, to the insurance carrier. In the letter, carefully state the date and time of the eligibility verification and the name of the insurance representative who told you the patient was covered for services by your office. (Make certain your office's procedure for eligibility verification includes the documentation of all of these details for just this reason.) Emphasize the date of the phone call or print out the electronic verification, as well as the date(s) of treatment or service, and attach a fresh printout of the claim form.

2. Before you mail this letter, call the company and confirm the name, title, and address of the employee responsible for receiving your appeal request. If you send this information to the wrong person, it may get lost within the company or, at the very least, it will delay your satisfaction of this issue.

3. Make certain you keep copies of everything, and follow up in a week or two if you have not heard from the insurer.

In other cases, claims have been denied because the individual's policy was canceled prior to your treatment and the insurance representative did not have (or did not tell you) up-to-date information. Therefore, your office provided treatment based on misinformation. As a matter of policy, typically the insurance carrier will claim that its staff member's confirmation of coverage does not represent a guarantee that your office will be paid. Again, you do not want to take no for an answer.

Both federal and state courts have ordered insurance carriers to pay claims based on their statements of eligibility at the time treatment and services were provided. These courts have established that the insurance representative's, or the electronic, confirmation of benefits serves as encouragement to the physician, or other provider, to offer that treatment or service.

When you think about it, if the insurance carrier had stated that the patient did not have coverage at the time you called for verification, your office may have chosen to not see the patient, to not take an x-ray, or to ask the patient to pay cash at that time. The fact that the insurance carrier told you, or a member of your office, that it would pay the claim encouraged your physician to treat the individual and reasonably expect to be paid for his or her work. Again, you must do the following:

1. Write a letter of appeal to the appropriate person at the insurance company, stating all the details of the verification conversation.

2. If your office does eligibility verification electronically, you should copy the printout of the electronic confirmation and attach it to the letter.

3. Always keep hard copy (paper) documentation or notes indicating to whom you spoke, what was said, and the date and time of the conversation.

If your appeal is denied again, your office may need to enlist the services of an attorney. The bottom line is that your office is entitled to this payment, but there are times you may need to fight for it.

Denied Due to Lack of Medical Necessity

Should your office receive a denial based on lack of medical necessity, there are some things you must do:

1. Go back and confirm the diagnosis (ICD-10-CM) and procedure (CPT or ICD-10-PCS) codes that appear on the claim form are the best, most accurate codes.

   a. There is a possibility that there was a simple error in keying in the code (such as transposing two of the numbers or leaving off a digit). More than once, a health care office and a patient have gone through months of arguing with the insurance carrier for the coverage of a procedure, only to find that the entire problem was a simple typographical error.

   b. Perhaps there was an error in coding. Go back and look at the physician's notes. Start from the beginning and recode the encounter. If there is another coder in your office, you might ask him or her to look at the notes and code the diagnosis and procedure(s). Then compare the other coder's determination of the best, most appropriate codes with yours. If you come up with different and/or additional codes this time, you might go ahead and resubmit the claim with the new codes. Or this review might confirm that the codes were correct on the original claim.

   c. Review the linking of the procedure codes to diagnosis codes (CMS-1500 Box 24E). Confirm the links are correct.

2. Contact the insurance carrier and get a written copy of its definition of medical necessity, or check its website and print it out. Often the list of criteria for medical necessity consists of any treatment or service that

   a. Is commonly performed by health care practitioners (considered accepted standard of care) for the treatment of the condition, illness, or injury as indicated by the diagnosis code(s) provided.

   b. Is provided at the most efficient level of care that ensures the patient's safety.

   c. Is not experimental.

   d. Is not elective.

   Using the criteria for medical necessity from the insurance carrier that denied the claim (different carriers may have different criteria), review the patient's health record to confirm that this individual and this particular encounter meet all of the requirements. Again,

- Double-check the diagnosis and procedure codes to make certain they all accurately represent what occurred during that visit.
- Call and speak with the claims examiner to identify exactly what he or she thought the problem was with the claim. This conversation may give you some insight into what you should be looking for as you review the patient's chart.
- Get support materials from your health care professionals, particularly the attending physician on this case. Copies of articles or pages from credible sources, such as *The Merck Manual,* the *New England Journal of Medicine,* or other qualified sources of research, will help support your claim.
- If this patient encounter was the result of another provider referring the individual to your physician for additional treatment, the referring physician might agree to write a letter supporting your office.

3. Write a letter to the third-party payer's appeals board, or to whomever the claims representative instructs you to send the documentation, outlining all of the information you have gathered to corroborate specifically why the denial should be overturned.

   a. Include copies of supporting documentation, such as pages from the National Library of Medicine's website or a letter from the referring provider.

   b. In addition, request that a qualified health care professional licensed in the area of treatment or service under discussion be the one to review your appeal. This may provide a more agreeable opinion as to the medical necessity of your claim and get it approved.

EXAMPLE

Christopher Novack, a 67-year-old male, is seen by his family physician after stating that he was driving to his office earlier and felt so dizzy he had to pull over. While waiting for the dizziness to pass, he felt his heart beating rapidly, and he began to sweat. He was worried that he was having a heart attack and came right over to see Dr. Bennetti.

Dr. Bennetti, knowing that Chris had been diagnosed with type 2 diabetes mellitus, checked his glucose levels and found them to be grossly abnormal, causing the dizziness and sweating. He administered an injection of insulin. Then, Dr. Bennetti checked Chris's heart with a 12-lead EKG. The results were negative.

When you perform your medical necessity review, you can see that the code for type 2 diabetes mellitus will justify the glucose test and the injection of the insulin.

However, if you do not have a second diagnosis code for his rapid heartbeat, the claim would be rejected. Without the code for rapid heartbeat, there is no medical justification provided on the claim form for performing an EKG.

Denied Due to Preexisting Condition

A denial on the grounds that the patient was treated for a preexisting excluded condition or illness reinforces the need for accurate confirmation of eligibility before the patient is seen and treated by the physician. If, in fact, your physician is about to treat a patient for a specific diagnosis, you must determine if the insurance carrier has excluded that condition, illness, or injury from coverage. This should be done during the eligibility verification. However, if you get to the point at which a submitted claim has been denied due to a preexisting condition that has been excluded, you still have several options to try to get your claim paid:

1. Start by reviewing the diagnosis code. There may be a difference in the diagnosis codes, now and for past treatment, making your claim valid.

2. Request a copy of the insurance carrier's definition of a preexisting condition. Once you clearly understand the requirements, you will be able to better analyze the details of this claim and its validity.

3. A review of the patient's past medical records also may assist you in appealing this denial. Examining specific diagnosis codes and physician's notes' diagnostic statements may find an opportunity to justify the insurance carrier's coverage of this claim.

When you have the information to support your claim, write an appeal letter outlining why the denial should be reversed.

Denied Due to Benefit Limitation on Treatment by an Assistant

Some medical offices have physician's assistants and nurse practitioners treat patients for routine examinations, vaccinations, and other medical services. However, some insurance carriers limit the types of treatments and services for which they will pay when provided by a health care worker who is not a licensed physician. There are a couple of approaches to appeal this type of denial.

1. Begin by authenticating the qualifications of the person who provided the service or treatment. You will also want to reinforce, in your appeal, that having this health care professional perform this procedure, under the supervision of the licensed physician, was the most cost-efficient way to provide the service to the patient.

2. Obtain a copy of the carrier's written policy regarding treatment to patients by assistants and search for language that specifically denies payment for services provided by a professional with the credentials of your staff member. If you do not find any such language, your appeal letter should include that the insurance carrier's policy does not specifically exclude services provided by this level of professional.

Subsequent Denials

There are additional steps that can be taken to appeal a second or third denial. Sometimes an insurance carrier will deny a claim, hoping that you will give up and it will not have to pay. However, most of the time, subsequent denials are just a matter of poor communication between the insurance carrier and the health care facility. Remember, although it is an insurance carrier's responsibility and obligation to pay claims, it is also its responsibility and obligation to protect its assets from fraud. Primarily, it is this intention that creates the circumstance of a falsely denied claim. However, after you have exhausted all efforts within the insurance carrier's organization to get the carrier to see your side and pay the claim, you have additional options:

1. Many states have state boards and/or review panels for this type of situation. Experienced health care providers, with varying areas of specialization, sit on these review boards. Their duty is to go over all the details of the case; examine the patient's health record, the claim form, and all other documentation; and evaluate the insurance carrier's basis for denying the claim. They have the right, empowered by the state government, to override the insurance carrier's decision and force the carrier to pay the claim. Bringing an appeal to this type of review board is an option to both health care professionals and individuals alike.

2. If the patient is covered under an employer's self-insured health plan, the state board is usually not an option for appeal. However, the federal government oversees and regulates self-insured plans and can provide you with an appeals process. At the very least, these insurers are required to have an in-house appeal board that will hear your case.

Surprisingly, you have an excellent chance of winning an appeal when you handle it properly. Researchers have found very high success rates for providers who file appeals. Therefore, if a claim is denied, it is worth the time to look into the reasons for denial and possibly exercise the right to appeal.

Writing Letters of Appeal

When a claim has been denied and you have gathered all the documentation to support your position that the denial is incorrect, you need to write a formal letter of appeal. This letter should contain the following:

Recipient: Call the third-party payer and get the name, title, and address of the person to whom you should address this letter. Make certain you double-check the spelling of the person's name—don't assume. Even a name as straightforward as John can also be spelled Jon or Jahn. Just ask!

RE: In the space between the recipient's name and address, and the salutation, you need to include identification regarding the person to whom this letter refers. This should be indented to your one-inch tab position. The details that should be shown in this area of the letter are

Patient Name:
Policyholder Name:
Policy Number:
Date(s) of Service:
Claim Number:
Total Amount of Claim: $

Salutation: Always begin the letter with a proper business salutation to the recipient by name. For example, Dear Mr. Smith: or Dear Ms. Jones (followed by a colon). Avoid generic salutations such as To Whom It May Concern unless the insurance carrier will not release the name of the person designated to receive appeal letters and has instructed you to address this letter to a department or title.

Paragraph 1: State briefly and directly why you are writing this letter. This is a summary or condensed version of the rest of the letter. Be factual, not emotional. Be specific about when and/or how you were informed that the claim was denied and the reasons stated by the insurance carrier for the denial. This paragraph is to make certain that you and the reader of this letter are on the same page (pardon the pun!). It is difficult to capture and retain someone's attention to what you are saying if he or she doesn't know to what or whom you are referring.

EXAMPLES

1. Our claims service representative, Raul Vega, told us that the above claim was denied due to a lack of medical necessity. This letter is an official notice that we wish to appeal this decision.
2. On November 3, 2019, our office received a notice stating that the above-mentioned claim was denied because of lack of coverage. This letter is to appeal this decision.

Paragraph 2: Itemize all the facts/evidence you have to support your position that you should be paid. Explain what documentation you have to encourage them to change their minds and approve/pay your claim. This list may contain highlights from the physician's notes outlining why the procedure was medically necessary. You might include statistics proving that this procedure is no longer considered experimental but is now widely accepted as the new standard of care. Attach copies (never originals) of documents that contain the information and refer to those attachments in this portion of the letter. In reality, this section of the letter may need to be longer than one paragraph. Write what you need to establish your rationale, but remember that this is not creative writing. Do not use flowery language or get long in your explanation. Be direct and to the point and include just the facts.

Paragraph 3: Use paragraph 3 (the last paragraph) to clearly define where this discussion should go next. Of course, you want them to just reconsider and pay the claim; however, you will need to keep this a bit more open-ended. Offer to provide any additional documentation the insurance carrier may feel necessary. Supply your contact information (office phone number, e-mail address, fax number) even if it is right there on the letterhead. Set an appointment generally (i.e., "I will call you next week") to follow up with this person. The purpose of this statement is to keep this appeal moving in a direction toward acceptance and payment. You do not want this letter to get buried on a busy desk. In addition, mark your calendar and call when you said you would. It is your responsibility to keep this issue on the top of the insurance carrier's priority list. You know that old saying, "The squeaky wheel gets the grease." This means that those that speak up get the attention.

Closing and Signature: All business letters should contain a closing, as well as the signature and title of the person sending the correspondence. *Sincerely* or *Sincerely yours* (followed by a comma) are the most common closings. After leaving four lines blank to make room for your signature, key in your full name. Directly underneath your name, key in your title (e.g., Insurance Specialist). If you are going to attach copies of important documentation to this letter, you need to note this under your signature. Leave one empty line under your title, and key in Enclosure or Enclosures or Enc. This notation points the recipient to the additional pages included in the envelope.

Pile 3: Claims for Which You Have Received No Notices or Payment

If a reasonable time has passed after sending a claim and you have received no notices or payment, you will need to follow up with the insurance carrier. (The term *reasonable time* is specifically defined by each third-party payer.)

1. Go to the third-party payer's website and check the status of the claim, or call and speak with someone in customer service to determine which examiner or representative will be handling your claim. Try to confirm that he or she has received your claim by getting a date and time of receipt and ask which staff member received it. If you cannot get this information, or you get a vague statement, such as "Oh, I'm sure we have it somewhere. We are very busy. We'll get to it soon," you will need to take the next step.
2. Go back over all the paperwork that accompanied claims paid by this carrier in the same time frame, such as an electronic remittance advice (ERA), or a remittance

advice (RA). There may have been a mistake and the wrong claim was marked paid in your file (meaning that this claim has really already been paid) and it is another claim that is still outstanding.

3. Once you are certain the insurance company has not responded to this claim in any way, you may need to send a **tracer**, also known as a duplicate billing or second submission.

Most insurance carriers require you to wait a specific number of days or weeks after the original date of submission before you are permitted to send a tracer claim. Check with the carrier, as each may have a different waiting period. This second version of the same claim must be marked "Tracer." This is to make sure that the insurance carrier knows you are not attempting to bill a second time for the same services. Double billing is against the law; however, sending a bill a second time because you believe that the first claim has been lost is good business.

Make a note in your master index of the date and time that you refiled the claim. That way, you can follow up again if you need to.

Tracer
An official request for a third-party payer to search its system to find a missing health claim form. It is also a term used for a replacement health claim form resubmitted to replace one that was lost.

Chapter Summary

A fundamental part of an insurance coding and medical billing specialist's job is to work with the insurance companies that will reimburse your health care facility for the services and procedures you provide to your patients. You need to understand how your facility will be paid (such as fee-for-service, capitation, or episodic care); be able to distinguish among the types of policies (such as HMOs, PPOs, and managed care policies, as well as Medicare, Medicaid, and TriCare plans); and quickly identify which is responsible for sending payment to you. This will help your billing efforts be more efficient and you get paid more quickly.

The procedures you develop and abide by for tracking the health insurance claim forms you submit is almost as important as the coding process itself. Some health care offices do not have a routine for handling situations, such as lost claims or denied claims. However, you must realize how important this is to the overall financial well-being of your facility.

When you are organized, and keep a tracking log of all the claims you submit, your work is easier and your success rate is higher. Appealing denied claims is a part of your career, and it is an important part of the entire medical billing and insurance claims process.

> ## CODING BITES
>
> The basic reimbursement methods are applicable across all types of health care, and include capitation, fee for service, episodic (global) payment, and cost reimbursement.
>
> It is the provider's responsibility to confirm the method of reimbursement prior to providing services.
>
> For more information on the newest program, MACRA, go to https://www.cms.gov/Medicare/Quality-Initiatives-Patient-Assessment-Instruments/Value-Based-Programs/MACRA-MIPS-and-APMs/MACRA-MIPS-and-APMs.html

You Interpret It! Answers

1. Workers' compensation and disability compensation, **2.** Margaret's liability insurance, **3.** Facility member = workers' compensation; student = school's liability insurance

CHAPTER 39 REVIEW
Reimbursement

Enhance your learning by
completing these exercises and
more at mcgrawhillconnect.com!

CHAPTER 39 REVIEW

Let's Check It! Terminology

Match each term to the appropriate definition.

Part I

1. LO 39.2 A physician, typically a family practitioner or an internist, who serves as the primary care physician for an individual. This physician is responsible for evaluating and determining the course of treatment or services, as well as for deciding whether or not a specialist should be involved in care.

2. LO 39.1 A type of health insurance coverage that controls the care of each subscriber (or insured person) by using a primary care provider as a central health care supervisor.

3. LO 39.2 A type of health insurance that uses a primary care physician, also known as a gatekeeper, to manage all health care services for an individual.

4. LO 39.2 A policy that covers loss or injury to a third party caused by the insured or something belonging to the insured.

5. LO 39.1 The total management of an individual's well-being by a health care professional.

6. LO 39.3 An insurance company pays a provider one flat fee to cover the entire course of treatment for an individual's condition.

7. LO 39.2 The agency under the Department of Health and Human Services (DHHS) in charge of regulation and control over services for those covered by Medicare and Medicaid.

8. LO 39.3 Payment agreements that outline, in a written fee schedule, exactly how much money the insurance carrier will pay the physician for each treatment and/or service provided.

9. LO 39.3 An extra reduction in the rate charged to an insurer for services provided by the physician to the plan's members.

10. LO 39.1 The amount of money, often paid monthly, by a policyholder or insured, to an insurance company to obtain coverage.

11. LO 39.2 Auto accident liability coverage will pay for medical bills, lost wages, and compensation for pain and suffering for any person injured by the insured in an auto accident.

12. LO 39.3 Agreements between a physician and a managed care organization that pay the physician a predetermined amount of money each month for each member of the plan who identifies that provider as his or her primary care physician.

13. LO 39.2 A plan that reimburses a covered individual a portion of his or her income that is lost as a result of being unable to work due to illness or injury.

14. LO 39.2 Individuals who are supported, either financially or with regard to insurance coverage, by others.

A. Automobile Insurance
B. Capitation Plans
C. Centers for Medicare & Medicaid Services (CMS)
D. Dependents
E. Disability Compensation
F. Discounted FFS
G. Episodic Care
H. Fee-for-Service (FFS) Plans
I. Gatekeeper
J. Health Care
K. Health Maintenance Organization (HMO)
L. Insurance Premium
M. Liability Insurance
N. Managed Care

Part II

1. **LO 39.6** An official request for a third-party payer to search its system to find a missing health claim form. It is also a term used for a replacement health claim form resubmitted to replace one that was lost.

2. **LO 39.3** The process of determining a fee for a service by evaluating the _usual_ fee charged by the provider, the _customary_ fee charged by most physicians in the same community or geographical area, and what is considered _reasonable_ by most health care professionals under the specific circumstances of the situation.

3. **LO 39.6** Remittance advice that is sent to the provider electronically.

4. **LO 39.2** A type of insurance plan that will allow an HMO enrollee to choose his or her own nonmember physician at a lower benefit rate, costing the patient more money out-of-pocket.

5. **LO 39.1** An individual or organization that is not directly involved in an encounter but has a connection because of its obligation to pay, in full or part, for that encounter.

6. **LO 39.6** Another type of paper remittance advice, more typically sent to the policyholder. However, some in the industry use the term _EOB_ interchangeably with _RA_.

7. **LO 39.2** A type of health insurance coverage in which physicians provide health care services to members of the plan at a discount.

8. **LO 39.2** A government health plan that covers medical expenses for the dependents of active-duty service members, CHAMPUS-eligible retirees and their families, and the dependents of deceased active-duty members.

9. **LO 39.2** An insurance program that covers medical care for those injured or for those who become ill as a consequence of their employment.

10. **LO 39.1** A health care claim form that is transmitted electronically.

11. **LO 39.6** The process of confirming with the insurance carrier that an individual is qualified for benefits that would pay for services provided by your health care professional on a particular day.

12. **LO 39.6** Notification identifying details about a payment from the third-party payer.

A. Electronic Media Claim (EMC)

B. Electronic Remittance Advice (ERA)

C. Eligibility Verification

D. Explanation of Benefits (EOB)

E. Point-of-Service (POS)

F. Preferred Provider Organization (PPO)

G. Remittance Advice (RA)

H. Third-Party Payer

I. Tracer

J. TriCare

K. Usual, Customary, and Reasonable (UCR)

L. Workers' Compensation

Part III

1. **LO 39.2** May cover medical expenses caused by a car accident.

2. **LO 39.2** Preferred provider organization.

3. **LO 39.3** A fixed amount paid each visit by the individual.

4. **LO 39.3** Payment, per service provided, from the insurance company.

5. **LO 39.2** A government program for indigent and needy people.

6. **LO 39.3** An episodic-care payment system basing reimbursement to hospitals for inpatient services upon standards of care for specific diagnoses grouped by their similar usage of resources for procedures, services, and treatments.

A. Copayment

B. DRG

C. Fee-for-Service

D. PPO

E. Medicaid

F. Auto Insurance Policy

Let's Check It! Concepts

Choose the most appropriate answer for each of the following questions.

1. LO 39.1 Medical care is defined as

   a. identification and treatment of illness and/or injury.

   b. services to prevent illness such as a routine checkup or wellness visit.

   c. laboratory services.

   d. only those services performed by a medical doctor.

2. LO 39.2 An organization that depends on the services of a gatekeeper is

   a. a preferred provider organization.

   b. Medicare.

   c. a health maintenance organization.

   d. a not-for-profit hospital.

3. LO 39.3 A capitation plan pays the provider

   a. per specific service.

   b. per member every month.

   c. for treatments in a hospital only.

   d. one flat fee per illness or condition.

4. LO 39.2 Medicare is a government plan that covers primarily

   a. military personnel.

   c. those over the age of 65.

   b. poor and needy.

   d. government employees.

5. LO 39.4 When CMS computers evaluate submitted claims to look for pairs of codes being reported that are known to be mutually exclusive procedures, this is also known as _____ edits.

   a. LCD

   c. PTP

   b. NCD

   d. MUE

6. LO 39.2 TriCare provides health care benefits for the dependents of

   a. state workers.

   b. those serving in the uniformed services.

   c. athletes.

   d. health care workers.

7. LO 39.5 What specific location does POS code 23 identify?

   a. Urgent Care Facility

   c. Telehealth

   b. Assisted Living Facility

   d. Emergency Room–Hospital

8. LO 39.6 The HIPAA Health Care Payment and Remittance Advice is the electronic transmission of payment, using HIPAA-approved secure data sets. The transmission has two parts: the _____ and the _____.

   a. claim, transaction

   c. document, claim

   b. transaction, document

   d. date, carrier name

9. LO 39.3 When an individual pays a percentage of the total charge, it is called the

   a. deductible.

   c. co-insurance.

   b. copayment.

   d. premium.

10. LO 39.2 CMS stands for

    a. Centers for Medical Services.

    c. Centers for Medicare & Medicaid Services.

    b. Corporation of Medical Systems.

    d. Cycle of Medical Selections.

Let's Check It! Which Type of Insurance?

Match the situation with the type of insurance that would cover the expenses. Answers may be used more than once.

1. LO 39.2 Mrs. Matthews, a teacher at Medical Coder Academy, slipped in her office, fell, and hurt her back.

2. LO 39.2 Ralph broke his leg and must be in traction for 9 months. What plan will help him pay his rent and electric bill?

3. LO 39.2 Mary Lou was at the mall, shopping for a birthday present, when she slipped on a wet floor and broke her hip.

4. LO 39.1 Keith was walking down the stairs in his house, fell over his son's toy, and twisted his ankle.

5. LO 39.2 Marlene was driving to work when another car hit her from behind. The EMTs took her to the hospital with a sprained ankle and sore neck.

6. LO 39.2 Harvey caught a cold when he went fishing last weekend.

7. LO 39.2 Jared enrolled in the insurance coding program at the local college. While leaving after his first class, another student bumped into him, he banged his head on a shelf, and he got a scalp laceration.

8. LO 39.2 At home after his 85th birthday party, Jack tripped on the rug, fell, and broke his hip.

9. LO 39.2 Suzette's husband is in the Marines. She is pregnant with their first child.

10. LO 39.2 James is out of work and has no prospects. He is broke and has a really bad sore throat.

A. Health Insurance
B. Workers' Compensation
C. Medicaid
D. Disability Compensation
E. Liability Insurance
F. TriCare
G. Automobile Insurance
H. Medicare

Let's Check It! Rules and Regulations

Please answer the following questions from the knowledge you have gained after reading this chapter.

1. LO 39.4 What does NCCI stand for, and what is its purpose?

2. LO 39.4 What is a procedure-to-procedure edit, who performs it, and when is it performed?

3. LO 39.4 What is the purpose of medically unlikely edits?

4. LO 39.6 What does it mean when a claim is denied due to an office personnel error, and can it be corrected?

5. LO 39.6 What should you do if your office receives a claim denial due to lack of medical necessity?

Design elements: ©McGraw-Hill

Introduction to Health Care Law and Ethics

40

Learning Outcomes

After completing this chapter, the student should be able to:

LO 40.1 Identify the sources for directives governing behavior.

LO 40.2 Understand the rules for ethical and legal coding.

LO 40.3 Apply the requirements of the False Claims Act.

LO 40.4 Translate the components of the Health Insurance Portability and Accountability Act's Privacy Rule.

LO 40.5 Elaborate the responsibilities of the Health Care Fraud and Abuse Control Program.

LO 40.6 Adhere to the codes of ethics of our industry.

LO 40.7 Analyze the reasons for creating a compliance plan.

Key Terms

Administrative Laws
Civil Law
Coding for Coverage
Common Law
Covered Entities
Criminal Law
Disclosure
Double Billing
Executive Orders
HIPAA's Privacy Rule
Mutually Exclusive Codes
Protected Health Information (PHI)
Release of Information (ROI)
Statutory Laws
Supporting Documentation
Unbundling
Upcoding
Use

40.1 Sources for Legal Guidance

The health care industry is responsible for providing services to maintain and repair the human body. For all of those providing health care services, the federal and state governments have crafted and enacted laws and regulations designed to ensure honest, safe, and appropriate behaviors from all involved. In addition, these laws and regulations provide a remedy—compensation or restitution—when individuals step outside of these approved boundaries. As a health care professional, you must be familiar with the government's directives so you can conduct yourself and your facility accordingly. This text is written to provide you with the necessary foundation of legal and ethical knowledge and understanding to support a successful career in health care. This chapter will introduce you to the basic concepts.

The *Federal Register*

The *Federal Register* is the daily journal of the U.S. federal government. The Office of the Federal Register (OFR), in conjunction with the U.S. Government Printing Office (GPO), created and maintains the website version of this publication.

Created in 1935, the *Federal Register*'s purpose is to inform *"citizens of their rights and obligations, documents the actions of Federal agencies, and provides a forum for public participation, in the democratic process."* Included in its contents are executive orders, presidential proclamations, policy statements, proposed rules, notices of scheduled hearings, and other government actions.

Take a look at a small section of the *Federal Register* in Figure 40-1 and access the full *Federal Register* at https://www.federalregister.gov/.

Sources of Directives

Many different types of laws and regulations exist to direct certain behaviors of those individuals working in health care, on both the clinical side and the administrative side. Federal and state governments and their agencies initiate these directives.

39186   Federal Register / Vol. 78, No. 126 / Monday, July 1, 2013 / Rules and Regulations

List of Subjects

21 CFR Part 21

Privacy.

45 CFR Part 5b

Privacy.

Therefore, the Department of Health and Human Services is amending 21 CFR part 21 and 45 CFR part 5b to read as follows:

Title 21

PART 21—PROTECTION OF PRIVACY

■ 1. The authority citation for 21 CFR part 21 continues to read as follows:

Authority: 21 U.S.C. 371; 5 U.S.C. 552, 552a.

■ 2. Section 21.61 is amended by adding paragraph (d) to read as follows:

§ 21.61 Exempt systems.

*   *   *   *   *

DEPARTMENT OF HEALTH AND HUMAN SERVICES

Office of the Secretary

45 CFR Part 5b

[Docket No. NIH–2011–0001]

Privacy Act; Implementation

ACTION: Final rule.

SUMMARY: The Department of Health and Human Services (HHS or Department), through the National Institutes of Health (NIH), is exempting a system of records from certain requirements of the Privacy Act to protect the integrity of NIH research misconduct proceedings and to protect the identity of confidential sources in such proceedings.

DATES: *Effective Date:* This rule is effective July 31, 2013.

FOR FURTHER INFORMATION CONTACT: Jerry Moore, NIH Regulations Officer, Office of Management Assessment, Division of Management Support, 6011 Executive

support is contrary to the interests of the PHS and the Federal government and to the health and safety of the public, to the integrity of research, and to the conservation of public funds" 42 CFR 93.100(a).

Under the Privacy Act, individuals have a right of access to information pertaining to them that is contained in a system of records. At the same time, the Privacy Act permits certain types of systems to be exempt from some of the Privacy Act requirements. For example, section (k)(2) of the Privacy Act allows Agency heads to exempt from certain Privacy Act provisions a system of records containing investigatory material compiled for law enforcement purposes. This exemption's effect on the record access provision is qualified in that if the maintenance of the material results in the denial of any right, privilege, or benefit that the individual would otherwise be entitled to by federal law, the individual must be granted access to the material except to the extent that the access would reveal

FIGURE 40-1 U.S. Congress's *Federal Register* showing official details relating to the Privacy Act (in part) Source: gpo.gov

There is a hierarchy established that sets the level of authority, which begins at the top with the U.S. Constitution as the first and foremost directive. In 1787, at the Constitutional Convention in Philadelphia, Pennsylvania, the Constitution of the United States was determined to be the highest and foremost of enacted law. Article VI of the Constitution states:

> *"This Constitution, and the Laws of the United States which shall be made in Pursuance thereof; and all Treaties made, or which shall be made, under the Authority of the United States, shall be the supreme Law of the Land; and the Judges in every State shall be bound thereby, any Thing in the Constitution or Laws of any State to the Contrary notwithstanding."*

Following the U.S. Constitution is federal law—those laws established by the U.S. Congress. State constitutions, state statutory laws, and then local laws complete the bottom tiers.

Statutory laws, most often referred to as *statutes,* are created and enacted by the federal and state legislatures (Congress). Members of Congress are responsible for writing the law. Then, once passed by votes in the House and the Senate, it is said to be "enacted." Because federal statutes take precedence over state statutory laws, state and local legislatures are not permitted to enact a law that contradicts any current federal law. This way, no one has to worry about which law takes dominance because this order of priority is already established.

There are circumstances, however, where the federal law provides some flexibility in behavior and the state law is more exact about the required behavior. In these cases, the state law would take precedence. For example, the federal law commonly called HIPAA's Privacy Rule (Health Insurance Portability and Accountability Act) empowers a health care provider to use his or her judgment whether or not to reveal protected health information to authorities when a patient is diagnosed with a contagious disease. However, virtually every state has a law that makes the reporting to authorities of a patient diagnosed with a contagious disease mandatory. The state law does not conflict with the federal law; it is actually more specific in its directive about behavior, so it overrules the federal law. This example is one that illustrates how important it is for all health care professionals to be familiar with both federal and state laws that govern their job responsibilities.

Statutory Laws

Laws that are enacted by federal and state legislature.

EXAMPLES

The Emergency Medical Treatment and Active Labor Act (EMTALA)

The Affordable Care Act (ACA)

Equal Employment Opportunity Act (EEO)

Executive orders are official documents issued by the president of the United States to set policy. They do not require approval from the legislature (Congress); however, they are issued, typically, under statutory authority and, therefore, have the full effect and force of a federal statute. The federal courts have upheld this.

Common law, also referred to as case law, is created by a judicial decision made during a court trial. These decisions, documented in law books for local, state, and federal court cases, create precedents—they establish a position. If you have ever watched a television show or movie with a court scene, you might remember the attorneys stating something like, "In *Brown v. The Board of Education. . . .*" This statement refers to a specific court case (*Brown v. The Board of Education*) and the decision made by that presiding judge. Those decisions are already accepted by the court, and therefore provide the current presiding judge with an established opinion.

You can see an example of the use of case law in the small portion of the Supreme Court opinion shown in Figure 40-2, the last three lines. A previous case—*PLIVA, Inc. v. Mensing,* 564 U.S. ___—is cited and this document goes on to explain the decision determined in that case and how it is related to this current case.

Administrative laws are those created and monitored by administrative agencies that have been given the responsibility to oversee specific areas, such as health care. The creation and implementation of specific rules and regulations have been delegated to those agencies created by Congress, under the Administrative Procedures Act, so each agency can ensure its assigned tasks can be accomplished. For example, Congress created the Centers for Disease Control and Prevention (CDC) as an administrative agency of the federal government to oversee issues related to contagious diseases. The CDC, therefore, has the authority to establish rules and regulations and to enforce those regulations (as long as they are consistent with the statute under which the agency was created). One of these rules is the mandated reporting of infectious diseases. Several surveillance information systems are used to enable the required reporting of these diagnoses; some are direct to the CDC while others are channeled through state departments of health first. However, if a particular diagnosis of an infectious disease is not reported, as required, the CDC has the authority to take action for noncompliance.

In Figure 40-3, you can see a screen shot of the website Regulations.gov. This website provides you with a searchable database of all federal agency regulations.

EXAMPLE

Centers for Medicare & Medicaid Services (CMS) has established its "rules of participation" for health care participating providers.

Criminal law seeks to control the behavior of people and companies when their actions are related to the health, welfare, and safety of an individual or property with the intention of protecting public order. Criminal activity is divided into two types, determined by the severity of the infraction: misdemeanors and felonies.

- A *misdemeanor* is a lesser offense, such as driving under the influence, public nuisances, and certain traffic violations. These infractions are adjudicated in local courts and are punishable with fines, penalties, and possible sentences of incarceration to county jail for up to 364 days.

Executive Orders
Official policies issued by the president of the United States.

Common Law
Also known as case law, this is created by judicial decisions made during court trials.

Administrative Laws
Also known as rules and regulations, these are created and adjudicated by administrative agencies given authority by Congress.

Criminal Law
Laws governing the behavior of the actions of the population related to health and well-being.

SUPREME COURT OF THE UNITED STATES
Syllabus

MUTUAL PHARMACEUTICAL CO., INC. v. BARTLETT

CERTIORARI TO THE UNITED STATES COURT OF
APPEALS FOR THE FIRST CIRCUIT

No. 12-142. Argued March 19, 2013—Decided June 24, 2013

Federal Food, Drug, and Cosmetic Act (FDCA) requires manufacturers to gain Food and
Drug Administration (FDA) approval before marketing any brand-name or generic drug in
interstate commerce. 21 U. S. C. §355(a). Once a drug is approved, a manufacturer is prohibited from making any major changes to the "qualitative or quantitative formulation of the
drug product, including active ingredients, or in the specifications provided in the approved
application." 21 CFR §314.70(b)(2)(i). Generic manufacturers are also prohibited from making any unilateral changes to a drug's label. See §§314.94(a)(8)(iii), 314.150(b)(10).

In 2004, respondent was prescribed Clinoril, the brand-name version of the nonsteroidal
anti-inflammatory drug (NSAID) sulindac, for shoulder pain. Her pharmacist dispensed a
generic form of sulindac manufactured by petitioner Mutual Pharmaceutical. Respondent
soon developed an acute case of toxic epidermal necrolysis. She is now severely disfigured,
has physical disabilities, and is nearly blind. At the time of the prescription, sulindac's label
did not specifically refer to toxic epidermal necrolysis. By 2005, however, the FDA had recommended changing all NSAID labeling to contain a more explicit toxic epidermal necrolysis warning. Respondent sued Mutual in New Hampshire state court, and Mutual removed
the case to federal court. A jury found Mutual liable on respondent's design-defect claim and
awarded her over $21 million. The First Circuit affirmed. As relevant, it found that neither
the FDCA nor the FDA's regulations pre-empted respondent's design-defect claim. It distinguished *PLIVA, Inc. v. Mensing,* 564 U. S. ___—in which the Court held that failure-to-warn
claims against generic manufacturers are pre-empted by the FDCA's prohibition on changes
to generic drug labels—by . . .

FIGURE 40-2 The use of case law is cited in this Supreme Court opinion regarding a drug approval case Source: Supreme Court of the United States Syllabus

---

- A *felony* is much more serious. This is a crime in violation of state or federal law
  and often carries a sentence of anywhere from 1 year to life in prison. Health care
  claims that are fraudulent and abusive of the reimbursement system constitute
  criminal activity and are an example of a felony. The Department of Justice, in conjunction with states' attorneys general, investigates accusations of these improper
  actions.

In Figure 40-4, you can see a release from the FBI reporting a guilty plea from a man
in Ohio who was investigated and found guilty of criminal activity—involving billing
Medicare and Medicaid for home health care services.

Civil law governs the conduct of those involved in a relationship: between private
companies, individuals, and sometimes the government. Most often, a civil complaint

Civil Law
Laws that govern the relationships between people, and
between businesses.

FIGURE 40-3 A snapshot of the website Regulations.gov, which offers a searchable database of federal agency rules and regulations Source: Regulations.gov

---

**Orange Man Pleads Guilty to Health Care
Fraud Charges Related to Overbilling
Medicaid and Medicare by $2.5 Million**

U.S. Attorney's Office   **Northern District of Ohio**
April 15, 2013   (216) 622-3600

A man who lives in Orange, Ohio, admitted to overbilling Medicaid and Medicare by more than $2.5 million, said Steven M. Dettelback, United States Attorney for the Northern District of Ohio.

Divyesh "Davis" C. Patel, age 39, pleaded guilty to one count of conspiracy to commit health care fraud and four counts of health care fraud. Patel is expected to be sentenced later this year.

"This defendant enriched himself and his company by flouting rules designed to protect the public," Dettelbach said.

"Mr. Patel defrauded the taxpayers by scamming Medicaid and Medicare," said Stephen D. Anthony, Special Agent in Charge of the FBI's Cleveland Field Office. "Waste, fraud, and abuse take critical resources out of our health care system and contribute to the rising cost of health care for all Americans."

Patel was the owner and president of Alpine Nursing Care, Inc.

FIGURE 40-4 A brief summary of a case where a man pleads guilty to health care fraud Source: "Orange Man Pleads Guilty to Health Care Fraud Charges Related to Overbilling Medicaid and Medicare by $2.5 Million," FBI, U.S. Attorney's Office, April 15, 2013.

---

or lawsuit will result from one party accusing the other of failure to comply with the terms of a contract. There are many instances of contractual relationships throughout the health care industry. Physicians and health care facilities may contract with a managed care organization; some facilities use contract workers to fill in for staff members on vacation; a family may contract with a home health care agency for services to a homebound patient; and the federal government may contract for health care services from a professional that does not include direct patient care. Figure 40-5 shows specific language that may be included in one of these contracts. The violation of a patient's confidentiality falls into this category because, in the United States, privacy

FIGURE 40-5 A partial example of language used in a contract for health care services that does not always include direct patient contact Source: Acquisition.gov

is considered a civil right. This is why an alleged violation of privacy laws is handled through the Office of Civil Rights (OCR) within the Department of Health and Human Services (DHHS) of the federal government.

40.2 Rules for Ethical and Legal Coding

As a coder, you have a very important responsibility—to yourself, your patients, and your facility. The work you do results in the creation of health claim forms and other reports that are legal documents. What you do can contribute to your facility staying healthy (businesswise) or being fined and possibly shut down by the Office of the Inspector General and your state's attorney general. You might make an error that could cause a patient to be unfairly denied health insurance coverage. It is important that you clearly understand the ethical and legal aspects of your position. Following are some issues, with regard to the ethics and legalities of coding, with which you should become very familiar.

1. It is very important that the codes indicated on the health claim form represent the services actually performed and the reasons why they are provided as supported by the documentation in the patient's health record. Don't use a code on a claim form without ensuring the **supporting documentation** is there in the file.

Supporting Documentation
The paperwork in the patient's file that corroborates the codes presented on the claim form for a particular encounter.

> **EXAMPLE**
>
> Coral Robinson's file indicates that Dr. Longmire ordered a blood test to determine whether or not she is pregnant. There is no report showing the results of the test. You see Dr. Longmire, and he tells you that Coral is pregnant and you should go ahead and code that diagnosis so the claim can be sent in. He promises to place the lab report and update the notes in her file later. Until the physician documents in the patient's chart that the patient is pregnant, you are not permitted to code the pregnancy.

2. Some health care providers may improperly encourage **coding for coverage**. This term refers to the process of determining diagnostic and procedural codes not by the accuracy of the code but with regard to what the insurance company will pay for or "cover." That is dishonest and is considered fraud. If you find yourself in an office or facility that insists you "code for coverage" rather than code to accurately reflect the documentation and the services actually performed, you should immediately discuss your situation with someone you trust. Some providers will rationalize the process by saying they are doing it so the patients can get the treatment they really need paid for by the insurance company. Altruism aside, it is still illegal and, once discovered, financial penalties and possible jail time can be assessed.

Coding for Coverage
Choosing a code on the basis of what the insurance company will cover (pay for) rather than accurately reflecting the truth.

> ### EXAMPLE
> Corbin Bloom wants a nose job (rhinoplasty); however, he cannot afford it. The insurance carrier will not pay for cosmetic surgery, so the coder changes the code to indicate that Corbin has a deviated septum requiring surgical correction so that the insurance carrier will pay for the procedure. That is *coding for coverage* and is fraud.

3. If you find yourself in an office or facility that insists that you include codes for procedures that you know, or believe, were never performed at a level of intensity or complexity as described by the code, this might be fraudulent behavior known as **upcoding**—the process of using a code that claims a higher level of service, or a more severe illness, than is true. Upcoding is considered falsifying records. Even if all you do is fill out the claim form, you are participating in something unethical and illegal.

Upcoding
Using a code on a claim form that indicates a higher level of service than that which was actually performed.

> ### EXAMPLE
> Erica Forney, a 69-year-old female, in the hospital for a broken hip, had her glucose level checked by the nurse, and it was at an abnormal level. Dr. Magnus ordered additional tests to rule out diabetes mellitus. Coding that Erica has diabetes is *upcoding* her condition and will fraudulently increase reimbursement from Medicare by changing the diagnosis-related group (DRG). In addition, placing a chronic disease on her health chart when she doesn't have it will cause her problems later on.

4. It is not permissible to code and bill for individual (also known as *component*) elements when a comprehensive or combination (bundle) code is available. This is referred to as **unbundling** and is illegal.

   For Medicare billing, refer to the Medicare National Correct Coding Initiative (CCI), which lists standardized bundled codes. The CCI is used to find coding conflicts, such as unbundling, the use of **mutually exclusive codes**, and other unacceptable reporting of CPT codes. When these errors are discovered, those claims are pulled for review and may be subject to possible suspension or rejection.

Unbundling
Coding individual parts of a specific procedure rather than one combination, or bundle, that includes all the components.

Mutually Exclusive Codes
Codes that are identified as those that are not permitted to be used on the same claim form with other codes.

Double Billing
Sending a claim for the second time to the same insurance company for the same procedure or service, provided to the same patient on the same date of service.

> ### EXAMPLE
> Dr. Hayden's notes indicate that Rico was experiencing nausea and vomiting. Instead of coding **R11.2 Nausea with vomiting,** the coder unbundles, coding **R11.0 Nausea** alone and **R11.11 Vomiting** alone.

5. If you resubmit a claim that has been lost, identify it as a "tracer" or "second submission." If you don't, you might be found guilty of **double billing**, billing the insurance company twice for a service provided only once. This also constitutes fraud.

6. You must code all conditions or complications that are relevant to the current encounter. Separating the codes relating to one specific encounter and placing them on several different claim forms over the course of several different days is neither legal nor ethical. It not only indicates a lack of organization of the office but also can cause suspicion of duplicating service claims, known as double billing. Even if you are reporting procedures that were actually done for diagnoses that actually exist, remember that the claim form is a legal document. All data on that claim form, including dates of service, must be accurate. Do not submit the claim form until you are certain it is complete, with all diagnoses and procedures listed. If it happens that, after you submit a claim, an additional service provided comes to light (such as a lab report with an extra charge that didn't come across your desk until after you filed the claim), then you must file an amended claim. While not illegal because you are identifying that the claim contains an adjustment, most third-party payers really dislike amended claims. You can expect an amended claim to be scrutinized.

All the activities mentioned here are considered fraud and are against the law. It is not worth breaking the law and being charged with any of these penalties just to hang on to a job.

Office of the Inspector General (OIG) Workplan

The Office of the Inspector General (OIG), in the Department of Health and Human Services, is the agency that investigates and prosecutes failure to comply with the legal requirements for coding. The OIG plans in advance, for the upcoming year, what specific violations will be reviewed and investigated. This is valuable information to support the development of internal policies and procedures as well as foci for internal audits. When you can uncover and correct coding and billing errors *BEFORE* the federal or state auditors show up, this lessens fines and penalties considerably.

The workplan is released each year by October 1 for the upcoming calendar year. It is subsectioned by the type of facility affected, so you don't have to read through everything to find that which applies to your organization. Sometimes the issue is directly related to billing and coding; others may be more administrative.

EXAMPLES

HOSPITALS

Intensity-Modulated Radiation Therapy
We will review Medicare outpatient payments for intensity-modulated radiation therapy (IMRT) to determine whether the payments were made in accordance with federal requirements. IMRT is an advanced mode of high-precision radiotherapy that uses computer-controlled linear accelerators to deliver precise radiation doses to a malignant tumor or specific areas within the tumor. Prior OIG reviews have identified hospitals that have incorrectly billed for IMRT services. In addition, IMRT is provided in two treatment phases: planning and delivery. Certain services should not be billed when they are performed as part of developing an IMRT plan.

Selected Inpatient and Outpatient Billing Requirements
We will review Medicare payments to acute care hospitals to determine hospitals' compliance with selected billing requirements and recommend recovery of overpayments. Prior OIG reviews and investigations have identified areas at risk for noncompliance with Medicare billing requirements. Our review will focus on those hospitals with claims that may be at risk for overpayments.

40.3 False Claims Act

The federal False Claims Act (FCA) was enacted by Congress to make the submission of a claim to a federal agency containing false information an illegal act. After this law was put into place, virtually every individual state passed its own version. This means that an individual may be charged with violation of both the federal law *AND* the state law, magnifying the fines, penalties, and consequences of this fraudulent behavior.

Who Is Liable?

Which staff members are responsible for ensuring that a facility or provider complies with FCA? All individuals and facilities that are involved in the creation and submission of claims—requests for reimbursement—based on coverage provided by governmental programs, such as Medicare or Medicaid, are responsible for complying with this law. Legally, these entities are referred to as federal contractors. Some people read the word *contractor* and immediately think of construction projects. However, in these cases, this phrase refers to one signing a contract to do business with a government program, that is, a participating provider. The Department of Justice takes enforcement of the FCA seriously. (See Figure 40-6 for just one example.)

Department of Justice Office of Public Affairs
FOR IMMEDIATE RELEASE Monday, February 6, 2017

Healthcare Service Provider to Pay $60 Million to Settle Medicare and
Medicaid False Claims Act Allegations

A major U.S. hospital service provider, TeamHealth Holdings, as successor in interest to IPC Healthcare Inc., f/k/a IPC The Hospitalists Inc. (IPC), has agreed to resolve allegations that IPC violated the False Claims Act by billing Medicare, Medicaid, the Defense Health Agency and the Federal Employees Health Benefits Program for higher and more expensive levels of medical service than were actually performed (a practice known as "up-coding"), the Department of Justice announced today. Under the settlement agreement, TeamHealth has agreed to pay $60 million, plus interest.

"This settlement reflects our ongoing commitment to ensure that health care providers appropriately bill government programs vital to patient health care," said Acting Assistant Attorney General Chad A. Readler of the Justice Department's Civil Division. The government contended that IPC knowingly and systematically encouraged false billings by its hospitalists, who are medical professionals whose primary focus is the medical care of hospitalized patients. Specifically, the government alleged that IPC encouraged its hospitalists to bill for a higher level of service than actually provided. IPC's scheme to improperly maximize billings allegedly included corporate pressure on hospitalists with lower billing levels to "catch up" to their peers.

FIGURE 40-6 An extract from a press release from the Department of Justice concerning a case enforcing the False Claims Act Source: "Justice Department Recovers Nearly $6 Billion from False Claims Act Cases in Fiscal Year 2014," Department of Justice, Office of Public Affairs, November 20, 2014.

What Is a Claim?

Needless to say, this law requires the proper behavior of individuals filing claims for reimbursement. So, let's begin with the FCA's specific definition of what a claim is: "*a demand for money or property made directly to the Federal Government or to a contractor, grantee, or other recipient.*"*

Under the requirements of the individual state governments, this would be a demand for reimbursement from the state government or other entity within.

The Knowledge Requirement

In addition, this law includes a "knowledge requirement." This portion of the law states that the simple action of submitting a claim with false information is not a violation. The individual must *know* that the information on the claim is false. What does "*know*" mean?

- *Actual knowledge* . . . knowing for a fact that the information is false.
- *Willful ignorance,* also known as deliberate ignorance . . . those who should know due to their job position, training, or responsibilities within the organization with regard to filing the claim but purposely don't ask about the validity of the information, or ignore the falsity of the information.
- *Disregard* of the truth or falsity . . . behavior that exhibits an indifference to confirming that the information is true.

EXAMPLES

Actual knowledge:

> *"I know that the procedures documented in the patient's record were not actually performed."*

Willful ignorance:

> *"I don't know for a fact, and I don't want to know."*

Disregard of the truth:

> *"It's not my concern. I just do what I am told."*

Essentially, this means that an individual is required to comply with this law if, as part of his or her job, the individual *knows* the accuracy of the information on the claim, or *should know* the accuracy of the information. If your job involves anything to do with the creation and submission of a claim to any third party, it is your responsibility to know for a fact that the information is true. And no court will accept your excuse that you "didn't know."

The Qui Tam Provision

The *qui tam provision* within the FCA, commonly known as the *Whistleblower Statute,* empowers private citizens (typically those who work within organizations that do not comply) to file a lawsuit on behalf of the federal or state government against the facility for noncompliance. Sadly, there are health care professionals who will not listen to a staff member explaining that a particular behavior or sequence of actions is not legal. The intent of this statute is to recruit those honest individuals who witness an organization that is committing, or encouraging, fraudulent activities to step up and help to stop the illegal actions by reporting the fraud or filing a qui tam suit.

The government knows how scary and difficult it can be to come forward. Therefore, they reward the person or persons reporting the fraud with a percentage of the total amount recovered by the federal or state government as a result of the qui tam lawsuit. This reward can be anywhere from 15% to 30%.

*Source: Federal False Claims Act, Department of Justice.

40.4 Health Insurance Portability and Accountability Act (HIPAA)

The Health Insurance Portability and Accountability Act of 1996, known as HIPAA (pronounced *hip-aah*), was enacted by the federal government and directly applies to you as a coding professional. Like most federal laws, HIPAA covers many different issues and concerns. The Privacy Rule is one part of this law that you are obligated to know and understand.

HIPAA's Privacy Rule

HIPAA's Privacy Rule was written to protect an individual's privacy with regard to personal health information, without getting in the way of the flow of data that is necessary to provide appropriate care for that patient. Essentially, the lawmakers tried to make certain that *a patient's information is easily accessible to those who should have access to it* [such as the physician, insurance coder and biller, and therapist] *and, at the same time, keep it secured against unauthorized people* [such as potential employers, coworkers, or neighborhood gossips] so that they do not see things they have no business seeing.

Who Is Responsible for Obeying This Law

HIPAA's Privacy Rule went into effect on April 14, 2003, and concerns every physician's office, clinic, hospital, and health insurance carrier—every type of business that is directly involved in the delivery of and/or payment for health care services, no matter how big or small. The largest of corporations owning hundreds of hospitals around the country and an office with one physician working alone are all included. HIPAA calls these businesses **covered entities**, and they all must comply with the terms of the law.

Covered entities are divided into three categories:

- Health care providers
- Health plans
- Health care clearinghouses

You probably already know the definition of a *health care provider:* any person or organization that gives health care services as the primary business purpose.

HIPAA's Privacy Rule
A portion of HIPAA that ensures the availability of patient information for those who should see it while protecting that information from those who should not.

Covered Entities
Health care providers, health plans, and health care clearinghouses—businesses that have access to the personal health information of patients.

EXAMPLE

Health care providers as defined by HIPAA: physicians, dentists, hospitals, clinics, pharmacies, laboratories, and so on.

Health plans are described as organizations that provide and/or pay for health care services as their main reason for being in business. They include health insurance carriers, HMOs, employee welfare benefit plans, government health plans (such as

Respecting a patient's privacy is also a sign of respect for the person. When you are the patient, you want to be treated with respect. So following HIPAA's Privacy Rule is not just the law of the United States; it is the law of treating people fairly.

TriCare, Medicare, and Medicaid), and group health plans provided through employers and associations. It doesn't matter whether the plan is offered to an individual or a group—all companies offering this coverage are included.

EXAMPLE

Health care plans as defined by HIPAA: Medicare, Medicaid, TriCare, BlueCross BlueShield, Prudential, and so on.

In addition, technology has created another type of organization involved in this process, called a *health care clearinghouse.* These companies help process electronic health insurance claims. Medical billing services, medical review services, and health information management system companies are included in this definition.

EXAMPLE

Health care clearinghouses as defined by HIPAA: National Clearinghouse, NDC Electronic Claims, WebMD Network Services, and others.

The workforces of covered entities are also included under HIPAA. A covered entity's workforce consists of every person who is involved with the company—full time, part time, volunteer, intern, extern, physician, nurse, assistant—and this has nothing to do with whether they are paid. Everyone must comply with the terms of this law.

CODING BITES

HIPAA's Privacy Rule is mostly about protecting your patient's privacy.

EXAMPLE

A covered entity's workforce as defined by HIPAA: full-time staff members, part-time staff members, volunteers, interns, externs, janitorial staff members, and so on.

What This Law Covers

You are certainly familiar with the topic of doctor–patient confidentiality. It means that anything a patient tells his or her doctor must be kept private. The doctor is not allowed, under most circumstances, to reveal to anyone what was said. This includes family members, parents (in many cases), and friends. This is important so that an individual will feel comfortable being open and honest and tell the physician things that are very, very personal, possibly even embarrassing or private facts that this person has never told anyone else. However, in order for the physician to properly treat this individual, the physician must know everything.

In order for you to do your job properly, you have access to all this confidential information. You need to know very personal and private facts about every one of your patients in order to accurately report the data.

You know what is wrong with them (their diagnoses) now and in the past; you know why they came to see this health care provider and why they saw others before they came to your facility; and you know what the health care provider thinks (observations and impressions) about these patients, as well as what has been done, is being done, and will be done to treat them. You know all these things because you have access to patients' health care records, including all the physician's notes. HIPAA calls this personal health care information (past, present, and future conditions) individually identifiable health information. In other words, it is information that anyone could look at and know exactly which individual is being discussed—one specific person. Specific pieces of data, called **protected health information (PHI)**, are pieces of information related to an individual that must be kept confidential, the grouping of facts that might have someone say, "Oh, I know him! Oh, and he has that!"

Protected Health Information (PHI)
Any patient-identifiable health information regardless of the form in which it is stored (paper, computer file, etc.).

Nicholas's private health record is no longer private. His diagnosis of a sexually transmitted disease is health information. After discovering his gender, address, and birth date, someone can connect this diagnosis directly to one particular person. All these details, and any other pieces of information like these, are protected to be private under the law. This means that all this information is confidential, and it is against the law for you to reveal any of it, with only a few exceptions:

1. You can tell other health care professionals who are directly involved in the course of doing your job.
2. You can tell someone when given written permission from the patient to do so.
3. You can tell in situations, as outlined in the law, based on "best professional judgment."

The Use and Disclosure of PHI

HIPAA's Privacy Rule is very specific as to how you can handle the PHI that you work with every day. The guidelines offer two terms to describe how you might deal with these data.

The term **use** (with regard to HIPAA) means that the information is being shared between people who work together in the same office and need to exchange PHI in order to better serve the patient.

The second term is **disclosure**. HIPAA defines the term *disclosure* to mean that PHI is being revealed to someone outside the health care office or facility. For example, you

Use
(1) The sharing of information between people working in the same health care facility for purposes of caring for the patient. (2) Occasional consumption of a substance without clinical manifestations.

Disclosure
The sharing of information between health care professionals working in separate entities, or facilities, in the course of caring for the patient.

prepare a health insurance claim form to send to the patient's insurance company so it will pay your office for the procedures provided. On that claim form, you must put the patient's full name and address, birth date, diagnosis codes, and procedure codes. As you learned earlier in this chapter, each piece of data is not necessarily confidential. When you put all this information together in one place, it becomes PHI because this health information (diagnosis and procedure codes) is now connected to a specific person (identified by the name, address, birth date, etc.) on one piece of paper. However, you must disclose this information to the insurance carrier in order to get paid. You are disclosing the information because the insurance company personnel who will read this claim form do not work for your health care facility—they are an outside company.

> ### EXAMPLE
> Dr. Royan indicates that his patient, Caleb Carter, needs some lab work. Dr. Royan will use Mr. Carter's PHI in his orders for which tests should be performed. Then you need to call the laboratory and disclose Mr. Carter's PHI (his name and diagnosis) along with what specific tests should be performed by the lab.

Remember that everyone in your office and everyone at the insurance carrier and the lab is a member of a covered entity's workforce. You are all bound by the same terms of the HIPAA law and cannot reveal any patient's PHI, except under particular circumstances (such as use and disclosure), unless you have the patient's written permission (Figure 40-7).

Getting Written Approval

In most situations, other than those already mentioned, the health care provider must get a patient's written permission to disclose the PHI. Although there are many preprinted **Release of Information (ROI)** forms that your office or facility may purchase, the Privacy Rule of HIPAA insists that all these documents have the following characteristics:

Release of Information (ROI)
The form (either on paper or electronic) that a patient must sign to give legal permission to a covered entity to disclose that patient's PHI.

1. Are written in plain language (not legalese) so that the average person can understand what he or she is signing.
2. Are very specific as to exactly what information will be disclosed or used.
3. Specifically identify the person or organization that will be disclosing the information.
4. Specifically identify the person(s) who will be receiving the information.
5. Have a definite expiration date.
6. Clearly explain that the person signing this release may retract this authorization in writing at any time.

Figure 40-8 is an example of a form that your facility might use for this purpose.

HHS.gov	Health Information Privacy	U.S. Department of Health & Human Services
$750,000 HIPAA SETTLEMENT UNDERSCORES THE NEED FOR ORGANIZATION WIDE RISK ANALYSIS		
The University of Washington Medicine (UWM) has agreed to settle charges that it potentially violated the Health Insurance Portability and Accountability Act of 1996 (HIPAA) Security Rule by failing to implement policies and procedures to prevent, detect, contain, and correct security violations. The settlement includes a monetary payment of $750,000, a corrective action plan, and annual reports on the organization's compliance efforts.		

FIGURE 40-7 A partial summary of a case where HIPAA violations cost a health care facility big money Source: "$750,000 HIPAA Settlement Underscores the Need for Organization Wide Risk Analysis," HHS Press Office, December 14, 2015.

DEPARTMENT OF HEALTH AND HUMAN SERVICES
Indian Health Service

FORM APPROVED: OMB NO. 0917-0030
Expiration Date: 4/30/2016
See OMB Statement on Reverse.

AUTHORIZATION FOR USE OR DISCLOSURE OF PROTECTED HEALTH INFORMATION

COMPLETE ALL SECTIONS, DATE, AND SIGN

I. I, _____ , hereby voluntarily authorize the disclosure of information from my

health record.   *(Name of Patient)*

II. The information is to be disclosed by: And is to be provided to:

NAME OF FACILITY	NAME OF PERSON/ORGANIZATION/FACILITY
ADDRESS	ADDRESS
CITY/STATE	CITY/STATE

III. The purpose or need for this disclosure is:

☐ Further Medical Care   ☐ Attorney   ☐ School   ☐ Research

☐ Personal Use   ☐ Insurance   ☐ Disability   ☐ Other *(Specify)* _____

IV. The information to be disclosed from my health record: *(check appropriate box(es))*

☐ Only information related to *(specify)* _____

_____

☐ Only the period of events from _____ to _____

☐ Other *(specify) (CHS, Billing, etc.)* _____

☐ Entire Record

If you would like any of the following sensitive information disclosed, check the applicable box(es) below:

☐ Alcohol/Drug Abuse Treatment/Referral   ☐ HIV/AIDS-related Treatment

☐ Sexually Transmitted Diseases   ☐ Mental Health *(Other than Psychotherapy Notes)*

☐ Psychotherapy Notes ONLY (by checking this box, I am waiving any psychotherapist-patient privilege)

V. I understand that I may revoke this authorization in writing submitted at any time to the Health Information Management Department, except to the extent that action has been taken in reliance on this authorization. If this authorization was obtained as a condition of obtaining insurance coverage or a policy of insurance, other law may provide the insurer with the right to contest a claim under the policy. If this authorization has not been revoked, it will terminate one year from the date of my signature unless a different expiration date or *expiration event* is stated.

_____
(Specify new date)

I understand that IHS will not condition treatment or eligibility for care on my providing this authorization except if such care is:
(1) research related or (2) provided solely for the purpose of creating Protected Health Information for disclosure to a third party.

I understand that information disclosed by this authorization, except for Alcohol and Drug Abuse as defined in 42 CFR Part 2, may be subject to redisclosure by the recipient and may no longer be protected by the Health Insurance Portability and Accountability Act Privacy Rule [45 CFR Part 164], and the Privacy Act of 1974 [5 USC 552a].

SIGNATURE OF PATIENT OR PERSONAL REPRESENTATIVE *(State relationship to patient)*	DATE
SIGNATURE OF WITNESS *(If signature of patient is a thumbprint or mark)*	DATE

This information is to be released for the purpose stated above and may not be used by the recipient for any other purpose. Any person who knowingly and willfully requests or obtains any record concerning an individual from a federal agency under false pretenses shall be guilty of a misdemeanor (5 USC 552a(3)).

PATIENT IDENTIFICATION	NAME *(Last, First, MI)*	RECORD NUMBER
	ADDRESS	
	CITY/STATE	DATE OF BIRTH

PSC Graphics (301) 443-1090   EF

FIGURE 40-8 Example of authorization form to release health information   Source: Department of Health and Human Services,
Form IHS-810 (4/09)

Permitted Uses and Disclosures

The Privacy Rule outlines six circumstances in which health care professionals are permitted, with or without written patient permission, to use their best professional judgment as to whether or not they should use and/or disclose a patient's PHI.

1. *To the individual.* Health care professionals can *use their best professional judgment to decide whether or not a patient should be told* certain things contained in his or her health care record. Questions come up especially when mental health issues and terminal conditions (when a patient is almost certain to die in the near future) are concerned and there is doubt if the patient can deal with the medical facts. In almost all cases, providing patients with their own PHI is allowed.

2. *Treatment, payment, and/or operations (TPO).* This means that health care professionals are free to use and/or disclose PHI when it comes to making decisions, coordinating, and managing the *treatment* of a patient's condition.

    In addition, PHI can be disclosed for *payment* activities, such as billing and claims processing, as mentioned earlier in this chapter. In this description, the term *operations* refers to the health care facility's own management of case coordination and quality evaluations.

> **EXAMPLE**
>
> A physician needs to be able to discuss PHI details with a therapist so that, together, they can establish a proper course of treatment for the patient.

3. *Opportunity to agree or object.* This relates to a more informal situation where the patient is present and alert and has the ability to give verbal permission or not with regard to a specific disclosure.

    One important point to remember: Although it is much easier to simply ask someone for his or her oral approval than to go get a form and make the patient sign first, it is in your best interest to get written approval whenever possible. People's memories may fail, or they may change their mind later about what they really did tell you. If there is nothing on paper, you cannot prove what was said. For your own protection, get it in writing whenever possible!

> **EXAMPLE**
>
> Asher Grimm is about to hear Dr. Brant explain his test results. Asher's wife is in the waiting room. Dr. Brant may ask Asher if it is okay to invite his wife in and permit her to hear this information, too. Asher can then say, "Yes, that is fine" or "No, I don't want her to know about this." Dr. Brant then must abide by what the patient requests.

CODING BITES

Incidental is close to the word *accidental*—if someone accidentally overhears what you say.

4. *Incidental use and disclosure.* As long as reasonable safeguards are in place, this portion of the rule addresses the fact that information might accidentally be used or disclosed during the regular course of business.

> **EXAMPLE**
>
> Dr. Holloway comes out of an examining room and approaches Nurse Miller standing at the desk. This is a back area, and patients are not generally in this hallway, so Dr. Holloway speaks to the nurse in a normal tone of voice to instruct her on preparing Mrs. Hunter for a procedure. All of a sudden, another patient comes around the corner, lost on her way back to the waiting room, and overhears the conversation.

This is called incidental use and is understandable in a working environment; therefore, it is not considered a violation of the law.

However, it is important for conversations like this to include only the minimum necessary PHI to accomplish the goal. *Minimum necessary* refers to the caution that should be used to release only the smallest amount of information required to accomplish the task and no more. Not only is it unnecessary to release more, it is unprofessional.

> ### EXAMPLE
>
> In the hallway outside the exam room, the physician would only need to say, "Serita, please prepare Mrs. Hunter for her examination." She would not need to include other details about Mrs. Hunter, such as, "Serita, please prepare Mrs. Hunter for her examination. You know she has a terrible rash on her thighs. I suspect that it's poison ivy. However, it could be a sexually transmitted disease. We'll have to find out how many sexual partners she has had in the last 6 months." All that extra information is unnecessary to the proper care of Mrs. Hunter at this moment.

5. *Public interest.* There are times when the public's best interest may prompt disclosing what you know about a patient. Very often, this is mandated by state laws, which would then take priority over the federal HIPAA law. In other words, if the federal law says you are allowed to tell, and your state's law says you must tell–then, you must! These situations include the reporting of suspected abuse (child abuse, elder abuse, neglect, domestic violence) and the reporting of sexually transmitted and other contagious diseases. You are included in the health care team and must think about the community, which must be warned if someone is walking around with a contagious (communicable) disease. Most states require notification to the police in cases where the patient has been shot or stabbed. It is your responsibility to find out what the laws are in your state and how to correctly file a report.

   If the physician does not report suspected child abuse of one of your patients, it is your obligation to pick up the phone and call.

6. *Limited data set.* For research, public health statistics, or other health care operations, PHI can be revealed, but only after it has been depersonalized. In other words, if the data that connect this information to a specific individual are removed or blacked out, the information is no longer individually identifiable health information, so it does not need to be protected any longer.

> ### CODING BITES
>
> Remember that, when there is a state or federal mandate to report (that means you have no choice; you must report to the proper authorities), this does not apply *only* to the physician of your practice but also applies to you.

> ### EXAMPLE
>
> You can release a health record that has no name, address, telephone number, e-mail address, Social Security number, or photographs attached to it. Even certain physician's notes can be released after they have been stripped of personal data. Following is a sample portion of a record that can be shown without fear of violating anyone's privacy:
>
> "_____ is 33 years old. Back in April, _____ was in a motor vehicle accident while he was on the job. _____ is complaining about some neck pain. _____ has tingling into the left hand."
>
> The example above is a direct quote from the medical record of an actual patient after the specified direct identifiers have been removed. You cannot connect this health information to any one particular person. Therefore, the information is no longer protected and can be used for research and in other ways that may help the community.

> ### CODING BITES
>
> This law simply assures every person coming to your health care facility that his or her personal and private information will be protected and treated with respect.

Privacy Notices

HIPAA instructs all its covered entities to create policies and procedures with regard to the use and disclosure of PHI. In addition, the law actually states that, once policies and procedures are developed, the facilities must follow these policies. Copies of the written policy must be given to every patient and posted in a general area where it can be seen by all patients.

Notices of Privacy written in compliance with HIPAA's Privacy Rule must contain the following points:

1. A full description of how the covered entity may use and/or disclose a patient's PHI.

2. A statement about the covered entity's responsibility to protect a patient's privacy.

3. Complete information about the patient's rights, including contact information for the Department of Health and Human Services (DHHS), should the patient wish to lodge a complaint that his or her privacy was violated.

4. The name of a specific employee of the covered entity, who must be named as *privacy officer.* This person's name, as well as contact information, must be included in the written notice to handle patients' questions and complaints.

The covered entity must receive written acknowledgment from each patient stating that he or she received the written privacy practices notice. This is usually one of the papers that a patient has to sign when going to a health care facility for the first time.

One of the most important aspects of this portion of the Privacy Rule is that the law specifically says that the covered entity not only has to create these policies and procedures but also has to abide by them. If it doesn't, it is considered to be in violation of federal law and punishable by fines and/or imprisonment.

Although some health care staff members feel that HIPAA and its Privacy Rule are a pain in the neck, think about what this law actually means: respecting your patients' privacy and dignity. Isn't that what you expect from your health care professionals when you go for help? It is not enough that only the doctor be bound to protect the patient's information as confidential because the doctor is no longer the only person who has access. Your health care facility is no place for gossip. You might find this person's hemorrhoids funny or that person's rash gross. As a professional, you should not be concerned with entertaining your friends with your patients' private circumstances. How would you feel if it were *your* personal problem that your health care team members were giggling about with their friends? Or you might consider telling your brother that his girlfriend came in with a sexually transmitted disease. You cannot! Everyone is entitled to privacy. As difficult as it may be, you must remain a professional.

CODING BITES

Just because you *can* take a look at any patient's chart doesn't mean you should. In your facility, you will probably be granted permission to access patients' charts so you can do your work. Under certain circumstances you may be tempted to look, not for your job but because the patient is your friend or neighbor or a celebrity. You may think no harm is being done, just caring or curiosity. But there is harm, and you are prohibited, by law, to do this.

Back in October 2007, 27 employees of a New Jersey hospital were fired or put on suspension for looking at George Clooney's file after he was brought into the emergency department (ED) following a motorcycle accident.

You could be the president of the hospital and have your best friend come into the ED of your hospital. Without specific permission from that patient, you would be forbidden from looking at the record. Every individual has the right to make his or her own decision about who should know what about his or her own health information.

Violating HIPAA's Privacy Rule

Any individual who discovers that his or her privacy has been misused or disclosed without permission can file a complaint with the Department of Health and Human Services (DHHS) that the health care provider, health plan, or clearinghouse has not followed HIPAA's regulations. When writing this law, Congress included specifications for both civil and criminal penalties to be applied against any covered entity that fails to protect its patients' PHI. These penalties include fines—up to $250,000—and up to 10 years in prison (Figure 40-9).

A covered entity is responsible for any violation of HIPAA requirements by any of its employees, business associates, or other members of its workforce, such as interns and volunteers. Generally, the senior officials of the covered entity may be punished for the lack of compliance; however, middle managers and staff members are not exempt.

HHS requires California medical center to protect patients' right to privacy

FOR IMMEDIATE RELEASE   HHS Press Office
Thursday, June 13, 2013   (202) 690-6343

News Release

Shasta Regional Medical Center (SRMC) has agreed to a comprehensive corrective action plan to settle a U.S. Department of Health and Human Services (HHS) investigation concerning potential violations of the Health Insurance Portability and Accountability Act (HIPAA) Privacy Rule.

The HHS Office for Civil Rights (OCR) opened a compliance review of SRMC following a Los Angeles Times article which indicated two SRMC senior leaders had met with media to discuss medical services provided to a patient. OCR's investigation indicated that SRMC failed to safeguard the patient's protected health information (PHI) from impermissible disclosure by intentionally disclosing PHI to multiple media outlets on at least three separate occasions, without a valid written authorization. OCR's review indicated that senior management at SRMC impermissibly shared details about the patient's medical condition, diagnosis and treatment in an email to the entire workforce. In addition, SRMC failed to sanction its workforce members for impermissibly disclosing the patient's records pursuant to its internal sanctions policy.

"When senior level executives intentionally and repeatedly violate HIPAA by disclosing identifiable patient information, OCR will respond quickly and decisively to stop such behavior," said OCR Director Leon Rodriguez. "Senior leadership helps define the culture of an organization and is responsible for knowing and complying with the HIPAA privacy and security requirements to ensure patients' rights are fully protected."

In addition to a $275,000 monetary settlement, a corrective action plan (CAP) requires SRMC to update its policies and procedures on safeguarding PHI from impermissible uses and disclosures and to train its workforce members. The CAP also requires fifteen other hospitals or medical centers under the same ownership or operational control as SRMC to attest to their understanding of permissible uses and disclosures of PHI, including disclosures to the media.

The Resolution Agreement can be found on the OCR website at:
http://www.hhs.gov/ocr/privacy/hipaa/enforcement/examples/shasta-agreement.pdf

FIGURE 40-9 A press release from the Department of Health and Human Services with details about violators of HIPAA facing consequences Source: "HHS Requires California Medical Center to Protect Patients' Right to Privacy," U.S. Department of Health and Human Services, June 13, 2013

Civil Penalties

1. $100 with no prison for each single violation of a HIPAA regulation with a maximum of $25,000 for multiple violations of the same portion of the regulation during the same calendar year.

> ### EXAMPLE
>
> You tell your best friend that Oliver Tesca, whom you both went to school with, came into your physician's office and tested positive for a sexually transmitted disease. You, of course, swear her to secrecy. Later that day, she bumps into Oliver's fiancée and feels obligated to tell her about Oliver's condition. Oliver puts two and two together, after his fiancée breaks up with him, and he files a complaint that you disclosed his PHI without permission. You and/or your physician is fined $100.

Criminal Penalties

2. Up to $50,000 *and* up to 1 year in jail for the unauthorized or inappropriate disclosure of individually identifiable health information.

> ### EXAMPLE
>
> After you are fined the $100 civil penalty for the inappropriate disclosure of Oliver Tesca's PHI, you and/or your physician is charged with criminal penalties for the same disclosure, including a fine of $50,000 and a year in jail.

3. Up to $100,000 *and* up to 5 years in prison for the unauthorized or inappropriate disclosure of individually identifiable health information through deception.

> ### EXAMPLE
>
> Your best friend since high school, Sally-Anne Hoskins, just got a great job as a pharmaceutical representative. To help her, you give her a list of 250 patients from your facility who have been diagnosed with diabetes so she can advertise her company's new drug to them. You and she both know this is illegal, so you tell Sally-Anne that you got permission from each of the patients to release the information (and that is a lie). After a patient complains to DHHS, the investigation discovers your relationship with Sally-Anne. You and your physician are fined $100,000 per occurrence (that's for each person on the list), as well as sentenced to 5 years in prison. FYI: 250 × $100,000 = $25 million!

4. Up to $250,000 *and* up to 10 years in prison for the unauthorized or inappropriate disclosure of individually identifiable health information through deception with intent to sell or use for business-related benefit, personal gain, or hateful detriment.

> ### EXAMPLE
>
> A famous television star is a patient of the physician's office down the hall from yours. You get a call from a tabloid newspaper offering you $50,000 for any information on the celebrity's health. So you call the manager of the pathology lab and tell him you are filling in at the other physician's office and need test results for Mr. TV. Then you call the tabloid reporter and tell him what you found out. You used deception (you lied about working in the other physician's office) to gain PHI, which you then sold for personal financial gain. You (and possibly your physician) are fined a quarter of a million dollars and sentenced to 10 years in prison—definitely not worth it!

Refusing to Release Patient Information

Sometimes, it seems that everyone agrees with the importance of protecting a patient's privacy until he or she asks for someone's details and is refused. It happens with parents and spouses all too often, and you must be prepared for how to say "no" and deal with the impact that may ensue.

When asked *why* you will not release details about a man's wife or mother's teenage daughter, educate the individual with the facts. Frequently, simply replying, "That is our policy" accomplishes little more than infuriating them, so instead, explain why you cannot share the information. Explain that health care staff are all required, by federal law, to protect our patients' privacy with no exceptions. Say that, as soon as possible, he or she should speak with the patient and enable the patient to tell the story about his or her health care encounter. Ask nicely for the individual's understanding.

40.5 Health Care Fraud and Abuse Control Program

The Health Insurance Portability and Accountability Act (HIPAA) created the Health Care Fraud and Abuse Control Program (HCFACP). This program, under the direction of the attorney general and the secretary of the DHHS, acts in accordance with the Office of the Inspector General (OIG) and coordinates with federal, state, and local law enforcement agencies to discover those who attempt to defraud or abuse the health care system, including Medicare and Medicaid patients and programs.

By catching those who submitted fraudulent claims, approximately $2.3 billion was won or negotiated by the federal government during fiscal year 2014. The federal government deposited approximately $1.9 billion to the Medicare Trust Fund in fiscal year 2014, plus more than $523 million of federal Medicaid funds were brought into the U.S. Treasury. Since it was created in 1997, the HCFACP has collected more than $27.8 billion for the Medicare Trust Fund—money improperly received by health care professionals filing fraudulent claims. The statistics show that for every $1 spent to pay for these investigations and prosecutions, the government actually brings in about $4 in money returned.

Also, in 2014, 496 criminal indictments were filed in health care fraud cases, and 805 defendants were convicted for health care fraud–related crimes, resulting in 734 defendants convicted of health care fraud–related crimes. In addition, 782 new civil cases were filed and 957 more civil matters were pending during this same year. These investigations also prohibited 4,017 individuals and organizations from working with any federally sponsored programs (such as Medicare and Medicaid). Most of these were as a result of convictions for Medicare- or Medicaid-related crimes, including patient abuse and patient neglect, or as a result of providers' licenses having been revoked.

When you look at these 2014 numbers, you can see that people are being caught trying to get money for health care services to which they are not entitled. This is an important reminder that if individuals try to get you to participate in illegal or unethical behaviors, the question is not "Will you be caught?" but "*When* will you be caught?"

CODING BITES

From *Fact Sheet: The Health Care Fraud and Abuse Control Program Protects Consumers and Taxpayers by Combating Health Care Fraud*, dated February 26, 2016.

"*In Fiscal Year (FY) 2015, the government recovered $2.4 billion as a result of health care fraud judgements, settlements and additional administrative impositions in health care fraud cases and proceedings. Since its inception in 1997, the Health Care Fraud and Abuse Control (HCFAC) Program has returned more than $29.4 billion to the Medicare Trust Funds. In this past fiscal year, the HCFAC program has returned $6.10 for each dollar invested.*"

Source: justice.gov

40.6 Codes of Ethics

There are two premier trade organizations for professional coding specialists. Each has published a code of ethics to guide members of our industry on the best professional way to conduct themselves.

American Health Information Management Association Code of Ethics

The American Health Information Management Association (AHIMA) is the preeminent professional organization for health information workers, including insurance coding specialists. The AHIMA House of Delegates designated the elements as being critical to the highest level of honorable behavior for its members.

In this era of reimbursements based on diagnostic and procedural coding, the professional ethics of health information coding professionals continue to be challenged. Standards of ethical coding practices for coding professionals were developed by AHIMA's Coding Policy and Strategy Committee and approved by AHIMA's board of directors.

AHIMA Standards of Ethical Coding

Coding is one of the foundational functions of the health information management department. As complex as is the process of coding accurately, there are multipart, intricate regulations that impact that process. In addition, professional coding specialists must make ethical decisions that would benefit from an appropriate and knowledgeable source. The AHIMA Standards of Ethical Coding are presented to all members of the industry to support their ethical and legal decisions and behaviors, as well as to reinforce and evidence the commitment of coding professionals to integrity. These Standards are offered for use to all AHIMA members or nonmembers, in all types of health care facilities and organizations.

AAPC Code of Ethical Standards

American Academy of Professional Coders (AAPC) is an influential organization in the health information management industry. Its members, and their certifications, are well respected throughout the United States and the world. Its Code of Ethical Standards also illuminates the importance of an insurance coding and billing specialist's exhibiting the most ethical and moral conduct.

GUIDANCE CONNECTION

AHIMA Code of Ethics

You can find the AHIMA Code of Ethics at:

http://bok.ahima.org/doc?oid=105098#.XFM6hlxKg3U

GUIDANCE CONNECTION

AHIMA Standards of Ethical Coding

The Standards of Ethical Coding can be found at:

http://bok.ahima.org/CodingStandards#.XFTCCs9Kg8Y

 GUIDANCE CONNECTION

AAPC Code of Ethical Standards

Members of the American Academy of Professional Coders shall be dedicated to providing the highest standard of professional coding and billing services to employers, clients and patients. Professional and personal behavior of AAPC members must be exemplary.

AAPC members shall maintain the highest standard of personal and professional conduct. Members shall respect the rights of patients, clients, employers and all other colleagues.

Members shall use only legal and ethical means in all professional dealings and shall refuse to cooperate with, or condone by silence, the actions of those who engage in fraudulent, deceptive or illegal acts.

Members shall respect and adhere to the laws and regulations of the land and uphold the mission statement of the AAPC.

Members shall pursue excellence through continuing education in all areas applicable to their profession.

(continued)

Members shall strive to maintain and enhance the dignity, status, competence and standards of coding for professional services.

Members shall not exploit professional relationships with patients, employees, clients or employers for personal gain.

Above all else we will commit to recognizing the intrinsic worth of each member.

This code of ethical standards for members of the AAPC strives to promote and maintain the highest standard of professional service and conduct among its members. Adherence to these standards assures public confidence in the integrity and service of professional coders who are members of the AAPC.

Failure to adhere to these standards, as determined by AAPC, will result in the loss of credentials and membership with the American Academy of Professional Coders.

Source: American Academy of Professional Coders.

40.7 Compliance Programs

A formal compliance program has been strongly recommended by the OIG (Office of Inspector General) of the DHHS (Department of Health and Human Services) to help all health care facilities establish their organizations' respect for the laws and their agreement to follow the direction from those laws. However, there are certain health care providers for whom this is not only suggested but mandated by law.

The Deficit Reduction Act of 2005, which went into effect January 1, 2007, mandates a compliance program for all health care organizations that receive $5 million or more a year from Medicaid. This law is very specific that the facility's compliance program include written guidance and policies about employees' responsibilities under the False Claims Act.

On March 23, 2010, President Obama signed the Patient Protection and Affordable Care Act into law. Among the many other elements of health care covered by this law, there is a provision in Section 6401 that providers participating in Medicare and Medicaid create compliance programs. This includes physicians' offices and suppliers.

A compliance program will officially create policies and procedures, establish the structure to adhere to those policies, set up a monitoring system to ensure that it works, and correct conduct that does not comply. The foundation of the compliance program is the creation of an organizational culture of honesty and compliance with the laws; the discouragement of fraud, waste, and abuse; the discovery of any fraudulent activities as soon as possible using internal policies and audits; and immediate corrective action when fraud and abuse do occur.

The federal sentencing guidelines manual provides a seven-step list of the components of an effective compliance program.

GUIDANCE CONNECTION

Federal Sentencing Guidelines Manual: The Seven Steps to Due Diligence

1. Establish compliance standards and procedures
2. Assign overall responsibility to specific high-level individual(s)
3. Use due care to avoid delegation of authority to individuals with an inclination to get involved in illegal actions
4. Effectively communicate standards and procedures to all staff
5. Utilize monitoring and auditing system to detect non-compliant conduct
6. Enforce adequate disciplinary sanctions when appropriate
7. Respond to episodes of non-compliance by modifying program, if necessary

Source: United States Sentencing Commission, *2014 USSC Guidelines Manual* (November 1, 2014), ussc.gov.

Chapter Summary

Knowing your legal and ethical responsibilities as a health care professional will give you a strong foundation for a healthy career. HIPAA's Privacy Rule, along with the codes of ethics from both AHIMA and AAPC, should help guide you through any challenges.

For all of those providing health care services, the federal and state governments have crafted and enacted laws and regulations designed to ensure honest, safe, and appropriate behaviors from all involved. The *Federal Register* is the daily journal of the U.S. federal government, used to inform citizens of the actions of the federal government. The hierarchy established for the levels of authority begin with the U.S. Constitution, followed by federal statutory law, state constitutions, state statutory laws, and local laws. Executive orders, issued by the president of the United States, have the same authority as federal statutes. Common law, also known as case law, is created by judicial decisions made during court trials, establishing precedents. Administrative laws are the rules and regulations established by administrative agencies in their efforts to encourage compliance so they can complete their assigned tasks. The violation of criminal law may be a misdemeanor (lessor offense) or a felony (more serious offense). Civil laws govern the conduct of two individuals or entities in a contractual agreement or a civil wrongdoing, known as a tort.

Confidentiality, honesty, and accuracy are the watchwords that all health information management professionals should live by.

CODING BITES

Medical records, also known as patient charts, whether in paper or electronic form, are legal documents. As business records, they can be used as evidence in a court of law, and can be required by issuance of a *subpoena duces tecum*.

As per the HIPAA Privacy Rule, a "designated record set" must be specified by each health care organization. Essentially, this is a collection of files (paper or electronic) that include:

- the medical records and billing records about individuals maintained by, or for, a covered health care provider;
- the enrollment, payment, claims adjudication, case study, or medical management record systems maintained by or for a health plan; or
- documentation used for the provider or plan to make decisions about individuals.

CHAPTER 40 REVIEW
Introduction to Health Care Law and Ethics

Enhance your learning by completing these exercises and more at mcgrawhillconnect.com!

Let's Check It! Terminology

Match each term to the appropriate definition.

1. **LO 40.2** Choosing a code on the basis of what the insurance company will cover (pay for) rather than accurately reflecting the truth.

2. **LO 40.1** Laws governing the behavior of the actions of the population related to health and well-being.

3. **LO 40.2** Coding the individual parts of a specific diagnosis or procedure rather than one combination or bundle that includes all of those components.

A. Administrative Law

B. Coding for Coverage

C. Common Law

D. Covered Entities

E. Criminal Law

4. LO 40.1 Official policies issued by the president of the United States.

5. LO 40.1 Also known as rules and regulations, these are created and adjudicated by administrative agencies, given authority by Congress.

6. LO 40.4 Health care providers, health plans, and health care clearinghouses—businesses that have access to the personal health information of patients.

7. LO 40.4 Any patient-identifiable health information regardless of the form in which it is stored (paper, computer file, etc.).

8. LO 40.1 Laws that are enacted by federal and state legislature.

9. LO 40.2 Using a code on a claim form that indicates a higher level of service or a more severe aspect of disease or injury than that which was actual and true.

10. LO 40.4 A portion of HIPAA that ensures the availability of patient information for those who should see it while protecting that information from those who should not.

11. LO 40.4 The sharing of information between people working in the same health care facility for purposes of caring for the patient.

12. LO 40.4 The sharing of information between health care professionals working in separate entities, or facilities, in the course of caring for the patient.

13. LO 40.1 Also known as case law, this is created by judicial decisions made during court trials.

14. LO 40.2 The paperwork in the patient's file that corroborates the codes presented on the claim form for a particular encounter.

15. LO 40.2 Sending a claim for the second time to the same insurance company for the same procedure or service, provided to the same patient on the same date of service.

F. Disclosure

G. Double Billing

H. Executive Orders

I. HIPAA's Privacy Rule

J. Protected Health Information (PHI)

K. Statutory Laws

L. Supporting Documentation

M. Unbundling

N. Upcoding

O. Use

Let's Check It! Concepts

Choose the most appropriate answer for each of the following questions.

1. LO 40.4 The intent of HIPAA's Privacy Rule is to

    a. protect an individual's privacy.

    b. not interfere with the flow of information necessary for care.

    c. restrict health care professionals from doing their jobs.

    d. protect an individual's privacy and not interfere with the flow of information necessary for care.

2. LO 40.4 Protected health information (PHI) is

    a. any health information that can be connected to a specific individual.

    b. a listing of diagnosis codes.

    c. current procedural terminology.

    d. covered entity employee files.

3. LO 40.4 According to HIPAA, covered entities include all *except*

    a. health care providers.

    b. health plans.

    c. health care computer software manufacturers.

    d. health care clearinghouses.

4. LO 40.4 The term *use* per HIPAA's Privacy Rule refers to the exchange of information between health care personnel

   a. and health care personnel in other health care facilities.

   b. and family members.

   c. in the same office.

   d. and the pharmacist.

5. LO 40.4 The term *disclosure* per HIPAA's Privacy Rule refers to the exchange of information between health care personnel

   a. and health care personnel in other covered entities.

   b. and family members.

   c. in the same office.

   d. and the patient.

6. LO 40.4 Which of the following is *not* a covered entity under HIPAA?

   a. County hospital

   b. BlueCross BlueShield Association

   c. Physician Associates medical practice

   d. Computer technical support

7. LO 40.6 There are two premier trade organizations for professional coding specialists. Each organization has a code of ethics to guide members on the best professional way to conduct themselves. These two organizations are

   a. AHIMA and OFR.

   b. GPO and AAPC.

   c. AHIMA and AAPC.

   d. HIPAA and EEO.

8. LO 40.4 According to HIPAA's rules and regulations, a covered entity's workforce includes

   a. only paid, full-time employees.

   b. only licensed personnel working in the office.

   c. volunteers, trainees, and employees, part time and full time.

   d. business associates' employees.

9. LO 40.4 HIPAA's Privacy Rule has been carefully crafted to

   a. protect a patient's health care history.

   b. protect a patient's current medical issues.

   c. protect a patient's future health considerations.

   d. all of these.

10. LO 40.4 A written form to release PHI should include all *except*

    a. specific identification of the person who will be receiving the information.

    b. the specific information to be released.

    c. legal terminology so it will stand up in court.

    d. an expiration date.

11. LO 40.4 Those who are permitted to file an official complaint with DHHS are

    a. health care providers.

    b. any individual.

    c. health plans.

    d. clearinghouses.

12. **LO 40.4** Penalties for violating any portion of HIPAA apply to

   a. patients.

   b. patients' families.

   c. all covered entities.

   d. health care office managers.

13. **LO 40.3** An individual who files a false claim can be charged for violations by

   a. federal law.

   b. state law.

   c. both federal and state law.

   d. Filing a false claim is not a violation of law.

14. **LO 40.1** DHHS stands for

   a. Department of Home and Health Services.

   b. Division of Health and Health Care Sciences.

   c. Department of Health and Human Services.

   d. District of Health and HIPAA Systems.

15. **LO 40.2** Changing a code from one that is most accurate to one you know the insurance company will pay for is called

   a. coding for coverage.

   b. coding for packaging.

   c. unbundling.

   d. double billing.

16. **LO 40.2** Unbundling is an illegal practice in which coders

   a. bill for services never provided.

   b. bill for services with no documentation.

   c. bill using several individual codes instead of one combination code.

   d. bill using a code for a higher level of service than what was actually provided.

17. **LO 40.2** Upcoding is an illegal practice in which coders

   a. bill for services never provided.

   b. bill for services with no documentation.

   c. bill using several individual codes instead of one combination code.

   d. bill using a code for a higher level of service than what was actually provided.

18. **LO 40.2** Medicare's CCI investigates claims that include

   a. unbundling.

   b. the improper use of mutually exclusive codes.

   c. unacceptable reporting of CPT codes.

   d. all of these.

19. **LO 40.5** During fiscal year 2014, the federal government won or negotiated approximately _____ billion from those who submitted fraudulent claims.

   a. $1.3

   b. $1.75

   c. $2.3

   d. $2.5

20. **LO 40.7** According to the federal sentencing guidelines manual, all of the following are components of the seven steps to due diligence for an effective compliance program *except*

    a. establish compliance standards and procedures.

    b. assign overall responsibility to specific high-level individual(s).

    c. utilize monitoring and auditing systems to detect noncompliant conduct.

    d. cease disciplinary sanctions.

Let's Check It! Rules and Regulations

Please answer the following questions from the knowledge you have gained after reading this chapter.

1. **LO 40.4** Why was HIPAA's Privacy Rule written?
2. **LO 40.2** Explain double billing. Is it permissible practice for a professional coding specialist?
3. **LO 40.1** Explain civil law in relation to the health care industry.
4. **LO 40.3** What is the False Claims Act's definition of a claim and what is the knowledge requirement?
5. **LO 40.7** What are the federal sentencing guidelines manual's seven steps to due diligence for an effective compliance program?

YOU CODE IT! Application

Following are some health care scenarios. Determine the best course of action that you, as the health information management professional for the facility, should take. Identify any legal and/or ethical issues that may need to be considered and explain how you would deal with the situation.

PRADER, BRACKER, & ASSOCIATES

A Complete Health Care Facility

159 Healthcare Way • SOMEWHERE, FL 32811 • 407-555-6789

PATIENT: HOLLAND, FELECIA

ACCOUNT/EHR #: HOLLFE001

DATE: 04/26/19

Attending Physician: Oscar R. Prader, MD

This 31-year-old female is 32-weeks pregnant. She presents today in tears. She is suffering from hemorrhoids and cannot stand it anymore. The pain and itching are making life difficult for her, as it hurts to sit for any length of time, and she cannot sleep. As it is difficult for her to lie on her stomach, due to the pregnancy, she can only find some comfort by either walking around or lying on her side. She is asking (more like begging) for a hemorrhoidectomy—a simple surgical procedure that can be done in the office and will almost immediately provide her with complete relief.

(continued)

The correct CPT code for the treatment of Felecia's condition is

46260   Hemorrhoidectomy, internal and external, 2 or more columns/groups

However, Felecia's insurance carrier will not pay for a hemorrhoidectomy with a diagnosis that indicates there are no complications. According to the insurance customer service representative, it will only pay in full for the procedure

46250   Hemorrhoidectomy, external, 2 or more columns/groups

Felecia's husband, Ben, is a civilian who works for a defense contractor and is currently in Iraq supporting the troops. Money is tight for the family because Ben's paycheck has been delayed due to a mix-up in paperwork when he was transferred to the Middle East. There is no way they can afford to pay cash for the hemorrhoidectomy.

All you need to do is change the one number of the code and Felecia can have the relief she so desperately needs. As the professional coding specialist in this office, what should you do?

PRADER, BRACKER, & ASSOCIATES

A Complete Health Care Facility

159 Healthcare Way • SOMEWHERE, FL 32811 • 407-555-6789

PATIENT: OKONEK, MARC

ACCOUNT/EHR #: OKONMA001

DATE: 08/12/19

Attending Physician: Andrew Bracker, MD

As the coding specialist for this facility, you are given the chart for this patient after his recent encounter with Dr. Bracker. On the face sheet you notice that Dr. Bracker has indicated the procedure provided to this patient to be Excision dermoid cyst, nose; simple, skin, subcutaneous. However, there is nothing at all in the rest of the documentation, including the encounter notes and lab reports, to support medical necessity for this procedure.

As a professional coding specialist in this office, what should you do?

PRADER, BRACKER, & ASSOCIATES

A Complete Health Care Facility

159 Healthcare Way • SOMEWHERE, FL 32811 • 407-555-6789

PATIENT: RIALS, ELIZABETH

ACCOUNT/EHR #: RIALEL001

DATE: 12/08/19

Attending Physician: Oscar R. Prader, MD

(continued)

Today, Tonya Baliga comes into your office. She states that she is Elizabeth Rials's sister and that she has been asked by her sister to collect a copy of her complete medical record. Ms. Baliga tells you that her sister has moved to another town and needs the records for an upcoming medical appointment with her new doctor. She hands you a printout of an e-mail, supposedly from Ms. Rials, to serve as documentation that she should have the records.

As a professional coding specialist in this office, what should you do?

PRADER, BRACKER, & ASSOCIATES

A Complete Health Care Facility

159 Healthcare Way • SOMEWHERE, FL 32811 • 407-555-6789

PATIENT: SINGELTON, SANDRA

ACCOUNT/EHR #: SINGSA001

DATE: 03/13/19

Attending Physician: Andrew Bracker, MD

The patient is a 17-year-old female who came in for counseling on birth control.

Today, Angela Thurman came into the office. She stated that she is Sandra's mother and found an appointment card for this facility in her daughter's jeans. She demands to know why her daughter came to see the physician. She is angry and frustrated and states that she will not leave until she is told why her daughter saw the doctor.

As a professional coding specialist in this office, what should you do?

PRADER, BRACKER, & ASSOCIATES

A Complete Health Care Facility

159 Healthcare Way • SOMEWHERE, FL 32811 • 407-555-6789

PATIENT: EVERFIELD, CARL

ACCOUNT/EHR #: EVERCA001

DATE: 06/28/19

Attending Physician: Oscar R. Prader, MD

The patient came to see the physician because he hates his nose. His self-esteem is very low, and, as a teenage boy, he has developed severe social anxiety. His family does not have the money to pay for

(continued)

a rhinoplasty (nose job), and the only way that the insurance company will pay for this cosmetic surgery is for medical necessity, such as a deviated septum.

You have been told to code the diagnosis of deviated septum to support medical necessity for the rhinoplasty. The doctor and office manager both tell you that this is the "right" thing to do.

As a professional coding specialist in this office, what should you do?

E/M Coding Rubric Worksheet

Begin by narrowing down the entire E/M chapter to the appropriate subsection:

Step 1. Location	New Patient/Initial	Established/Subsequent
Office/Outpatient	99347–99350	99211–99215
Hospital—Observation	99218–99220	99224–99226
Hospital—Inpatient	99221–99223	99231–99233
Emergency Department	99281–99285	
Nursing Facility	99304–99306	99307–99310
Domiciliary (Assisted Living)	99324–99328	99334–99337
Home Services	99341–99345	99347–99350

Step 2. Key Components	New Patient/ Initial	Established/ Subsequent
History		
<u>Problem-Focused:</u> Chief complaint; brief history of present illness or problem.		
<u>Expanded Problem-Focused:</u> Chief complaint; brief history of present illness; problem-pertinent system review		
<u>Detailed:</u> Chief complaint; extended history of present illness; problem-pertinent system review extended to include a review of a limited number of additional systems; pertinent past, family, and/or social history directly related to patient's problem(s).		
<u>Comprehensive:</u> Chief complaint; extended history of present illness; review of systems that are directly related to the problem(s) identified in the history of the present illness plus a review of all additional body systems; complete past, family, and social history.		

CodePath: For more information on determining level of history, see *Let's Code It!* Chapter 23, Section 23.4 *Types of E/M Services – Level of Patient History.*

Step 3. Key Components	New Patient/ Initial	Established/ Subsequent
Physical Examination		
Problem-Focused: A limited exam of the affected body area or organ system		
Expanded Problem-Focused: A limited exam of the affected body area or organ system and other symptomatic or related organ system(s)		
Detailed: An extended exam of the affected body area(s) and other symptomatic or related organ system(s)		
Comprehensive: A general multisystem exam -or- a complete exam of a single organ system		

CodePath: For more information on determining level of Physical Examination, see *Let's Code It!* Chapter 23, Section 23.4 *Types of E/M Services – Level of Physical Examination.*

Step 4. Key Components	New Patient/ Initial	Established/ Subsequent
Medical Decision Making		
Straightforward: Minimal number of possible diagnoses and/or treatment options; minimal quantity of information to be obtained, reviewed, and analyzed; and minimal risk of significant complications, morbidity, and/or mortality		
Low Complexity: Limited number of possible diagnoses and/or treatment options; limited quantity of information to be obtained, reviewed, and analyzed; and limited risk of significant complications, morbidity, and/or mortality		
Moderate Complexity: Multiple number of possible diagnoses and/or treatment options; moderate quantity of information to be obtained, reviewed, and analyzed; and moderate risk of significant complications, morbidity, and/or mortality		
High Complexity: Extensive number of possible diagnoses and/or treatment options; extensive quantity of information to be obtained, reviewed, and analyzed; and high risk of significant complications, morbidity, and/or mortality		

CodePath: For more information on determining level of Medical Decision Making, see *Let's Code It!* Chapter 23, Section 23.4 *Types of E/M Services – Level of Medical Decision Making.*

Combining Multiple Levels in One Code

Once you have determined what level of history was taken, what level of physician exam was performed, and what level of MDM was provided by the physician as documented in the case notes, this all needs to be put together into one code. When all three key components point to the same code, this is a piece of cake. But what about when the three levels point toward different E/M codes? How do you mesh them all into one code? The CPT guidelines state, ". . . *must meet or exceed the stated requirements to qualify for a particular level of E/M service.*"

You must find the one level that is satisfied by ALL THREE levels of care when you are reporting for a NEW patient, or TWO out of THREE for established patients. Find the only code that has ALL THREE levels equal to or greater than the code's key component descriptors, as identified on your above worksheets, to determine which one E/M code should be reported.

CodePath: For new Patients . . . You can only code as high as your lowest key component.

GLOSSARY

A

Ablation The destruction or eradication of tissue.

Abnormal Findings Test results that indicate a disease or condition may be present.

Abortifacient A drug used to induce an abortion.

Abortion The end of a pregnancy prior to or subsequent to the death of a fetus.

Abstracting The process of identifying the relevant words or phrases in health care documentation in order to determine the best, most appropriate code(s).

Abuse This term is used in different manners: (a) extreme use of a drug or chemical; (b) violent and/or inappropriate treatment of another person (child, adult, elder); (c) Regular consumption of a substance with manifestations.

Accessory Organs Organs that assist the digestive process and are adjacent to the alimentary canal: the gallbladder, liver, and pancreas.

Accommodation Adaptation of the eye's lens to adjust for varying focal distances.

Acute Severe; serious.

Administration To introduce a therapeutic, prophylactic, protective, diagnostic, nutritional, or physiological substance.

Administrative Laws Also known as rules and regulations, these are created and adjudicated by administrative agencies given authority by Congress.

Advanced Life Support (ALS) Life-sustaining, emergency care provided, such as airway management, defibrillation, and/or the administration of drugs.

Adverse Effect An unexpected bad reaction to a drug or other treatment.

Agglutination The process of red blood cells combining together in a mass or lump.

Allogeneic The donor and recipient are of the same species, e.g., human → human, dog → dog (also known as an *allograft*).

Allotransplantation The relocation of tissue from one individual to another (both of the same species) without an identical genetic match.

Alphabetic Index The section of a code book showing all codes, from A to Z, by the short code descriptions.

Alphanumeric Containing both letters and numbers.

Alphanumeric Section The section of the HCPCS Level II code book listing all of the codes in alphanumeric order.

Ambulatory Surgery Center (ASC) A facility specially designed to provide surgical treatments without an overnight stay; also known as a *same-day surgery center.*

AMCC Automated Multi-Channel Chemistry—Automated organ disease panel tests performed on the same patient, by the same provider, on the same day.

Anatomical Site A specific location within the anatomy (body).

Anemic Any of various conditions marked by deficiency in red blood cells or hemoglobin.

Anesthesia The loss of sensation, with or without consciousness, generally induced by the administration of a particular drug.

Anesthesiologists Physicians specializing in the administration of anesthesia.

Angina Pectoris Chest pain.

Angiography The imaging of blood vessels after the injection of contrast material.

Anomaly An abnormal, or unexpected, condition.

Antibodies Immune responses to antigens.

Anticipatory Guidance Recommendations for behavior modification and/or other preventive measures.

Antigen A substance that promotes the production of antibodies.

Anus The portion of the large intestine that leads outside the body.

Anxiety The feelings of apprehension and fear, sometimes manifested with physical manifestations such as sweating and palpitations.

Anxiolytic A drug used to reduce anxiety.

Approach This term is used in different manners: (a) the specific technique used for the procedure; (b) the path the physician took to access the body part upon which the treatment or procedure was targeted.

Arthrodesis The immobilization of a joint using a surgical technique.

Arthrography The recording of a picture of an anatomical joint after the administration of contrast material into the joint capsule.

Arthropathy Disease or dysfunction of a joint [plural: arthropathies].

Articulation A joint.

Ascending Colon The portion of the large intestine that connects the cecum to the hepatic flexure.

Assume Suppose to be the case, without proof; guess the intended details.

Asymptomatic No symptoms or manifestations.

Atherosclerosis A condition resulting from plaque buildup on the interior walls of the arteries, causing reduced blood flow; also known as *arteriosclerosis.*

Atrium A chamber that is located in the top half of the heart and receives blood.

Audiology The study of hearing, balance, and related disorders.

Autologous The donor tissue is taken from a different site on the same individual's body (also known as an *autograft*).

Automobile Insurance Auto accident liability coverage will pay for medical bills, lost wages, and compensation for pain and suffering for any person injured by the insured in an auto accident.

Avulsion Injury in which layers of skin are traumatically torn away from the body.

Axis of Classification A single meaning within the code set; providing a detail.

B

Bacteria Single-celled microorganisms that cause disease.

Basic Life Support (BLS) The provision of emergency CPR, stabilization of the patient, first aid, control of bleeding, and/or treatment of shock.

Basic Personal Services Services that include washing/bathing, dressing and undressing, assistance in taking medications, and assistance getting in and out of bed.

Behavioral Disturbance A type of common behavior that includes mood disorders (such as depression, apathy, and euphoria), sleep disorders (such as insomnia and hypersomnia), psychotic symptoms (such as delusions and hallucinations), and agitation (such as pacing, wandering, and aggression).

Benign Nonmalignant characteristic of a neoplasm; not infectious or spreading.

Benign Prostatic Hyperplasia (BPH) Enlarged prostate that results in depressing the urethra.

Biofeedback Training to gain voluntary control of automatic bodily functions.

Bladder Cancer Malignancy of the urinary bladder.

Blepharitis Inflammation of the eyelid.

Blister A bubble or sac formed on the surface of the skin, typically filled with a watery fluid or serum.

Blood Fluid pumped throughout the body, carrying oxygen and nutrients to the cells and wastes away from the cells.

Blood Type A system of classifying blood based on the antigens present on the surface of the individual's red blood cells; also known as *blood group.*

Body Part The anatomical site upon which the procedure was performed.

Body System The physiological system, or anatomical region, upon which the procedure was performed.

Bulbar Conjunctiva A mucous membrane on the surface of the eyeball.

Bulla A large vesicle that is filled with fluid.

Burn Injury by heat or fire.

C

Capitation Plans Agreements between a physician and a managed care organization that pay the physician a predetermined amount of money each month for each member of the plan who identifies that provider as his or her primary care physician.

Carbuncle A painful, pus-filled boil due to infection of the epidermis and underlying tissues, often caused by staphylococcus.

Carcinoma A malignant neoplasm or cancerous tumor.

Care Plan Oversight Services E/M of a patient, reported in 30-day periods, including infrequent supervision along with preencounter and postencounter work, such as reading test results and assessment of notes.

Carrier An individual infected with a disease who is not ill but can still pass it to another person; an individual with an abnormal gene that can be passed to a child, making the child susceptible to disease.

Cataract Clouding of the lens or lens capsule of the eye.

Category I Codes The codes listed in the main text of the CPT book, also known as CPT codes.

Category II Codes Codes for performance measurement and tracking.

Category II Modifiers Modifiers provided for use with Category II CPT codes to indicate a valid reason for a portion of a performance measure to be deleted from qualification.

Category III Codes Codes for emerging technology.

Catheter A thin, flexible tube, inserted into a body part, used to inject fluid, to extract fluid, or to keep a passage open.

Cecum A pouchlike organ that connects the ileum with the large intestine; the point of connection for the vermiform appendix.

Centers for Medicare & Medicaid Services (CMS) The agency under the Department of Health and Human Services (DHHS) in charge of regulation and control over services for those covered by Medicare and Medicaid.

Cerebral Infarction An area of dead tissue (necrosis) in the brain caused by a blocked or ruptured blood vessel.

Cerebrovascular Accident (CVA) Rupture of a blood vessel causing hemorrhaging in the brain or an embolus in a blood vessel in the brain causing a loss of blood flow; also known as *stroke.*

Certified Registered Nurse Anesthetist (CRNA) A registered nurse (RN) who has taken additional, specialized training in the administration of anesthesia.

Character A letter or number component of an ICD-10-PCS code.

Chelation Therapy The use of a chemical compound that binds with metal in the body so that the metal will lose its toxic effect. It might be done when a metal disc or prosthetic is implanted in a patient, eliminating adverse reactions to the metal itself as a foreign body.

Chief Complaint (CC) The primary reasons why the patient has come for this encounter, in the patient's own words.

Cholelithiasis Gallstones.

Chondropathy Disease affecting the cartilage [plural: chondropathies].

Choroid The vascular layer of the eye that lies between the retina and the sclera.

Chronic Long duration; continuing over an extended period of time.

Chronic Kidney Disease (CKD) Ongoing malfunction of one or both kidneys.

Chronic Obstructive Pulmonary Disease (COPD) An ongoing obstruction of the airway.

Ciliary Body The vascular layer of the eye that lies between the sclera and the crystalline lens.

Civil Law Laws that govern the relationships between people, and between businesses.

Class A Finding Nontraumatic amputation of a foot or an integral skeletal portion.

Class B Finding Absence of a posterior tibial pulse; absence or decrease of hair growth; thickening of the nail, discoloration of the skin, and/or thinning of the skin texture; and/or absence of a posterior pedal pulse.

Class C Finding Edema, burning sensation, temperature change (cold feet), abnormal spontaneous sensations in the feet, and/or limping.

Classification Systems The term used in health care to identify ICD-10-CM, CPT, ICD-10-PCS, and HCPCS Level II code sets.

Clinical Laboratory Improvement Amendment (CLIA) Federal legislation created for the monitoring and regulation of clinical laboratory procedures.

Clinically Significant Signs, symptoms, and/or conditions present at birth that may impact the child's future health status.

Closed Treatment The treatment of a fracture without surgically opening the affected area.

Co-morbidity A separate diagnosis existing in the same patient at the same time as an unrelated diagnosis.

Coagulation Clotting; the change from a liquid into a thickened substance.

Coding for Coverage Choosing a code on the basis of what the insurance company will cover (pay for) rather than accurately reflecting the truth.

Coding Process The sequence of actions required to interpret physician documentation into the codes that accurately report what occurred during a specific encounter between health care professional and patient.

Common Bile Duct The juncture of the cystic duct of the gallbladder and the hepatic duct from the liver.

Common Law Also known as case law, this is created by judicial decisions made during court trials.

Complex Closure A method of sealing an opening in the skin involving a multilayered closure and a reconstructive procedure such as scar revision, debridement, or retention sutures.

Complication An unexpected illness or other condition that develops as a result of a procedure, service, or treatment provided during the patient's hospital stay.

Computed Tomography (CT) A specialized computer scanner with very fine detail that records imaging of internal anatomical sites; also known as computerized axial tomography (CAT).

Computed Tomography Angiography (CTA) A CT scan using contrast materials to visualize arteries and veins all over the body.

Concurrent Coding System in which coding processes are performed while a patient is still in the hospital receiving care.

Condition The state of abnormality or dysfunction.

Cone A receptor in the retina that is responsible for light and color.

Confirmed Found to be true or definite.

Congenital A condition existing at the time of birth.

Conjunctivitis Inflammation of the conjunctiva.

Conscious Sedation The use of a drug to reduce stress and/or anxiety.

Consultation An encounter for purposes of a second physician's opinion or advice, requested by another physician, regarding the management of a patient's specific health concern. A consultation is planned to be a short-term relationship between a health care professional and a patient.

Cornea Transparent tissue covering the eyeball; responsible for focusing light into the eye and transmitting light.

Corneal Dystrophy Growth of abnormal tissue on the cornea, often related to a nutritional deficiency.

Corrosion A burn caused by a chemical; chemical destruction of the skin.

Covered Entities Health care providers, health plans, and health care clearinghouses—businesses that have access to the personal health information of patients.

CPT Code Modifier A two-character code that may be appended to a code from the main portion of the CPT book to provide additional information.

Criminal Law Laws governing the behavior of the actions of the population related to health and well-being.

Critical Care Services Care services for an acutely ill or injured patient with a high risk for life-threatening developments.

Cushing's Syndrome A condition resulting from the hyperproduction of corticosteroids, most often caused by an adrenal cortex tumor or a tumor of the pituitary gland.

Cyst A fluid-filled or gas-filled bubble in the skin.

Cytology The investigation and identification of cells.

D

Dacryocystitis Lacrimal gland inflammation.

Decubitus Ulcer A bedsore or wound created by lying in the same position, on the same irritant without relief.

Deformity A size or shape (structural design) that deviates from that which is considered normal.

Demographic Demographic details include the patient's name, address, date of birth, and other personal details, not specifically related to health.

Densitometry The process used to measure bone density, most often done to assess the patient's risk for osteopenia or osteoporosis.

Dependence Ongoing, regular consumption of a substance with resulting significant clinical manifestations, and a dramatic decrease in the effect of the substance with continued use, therefore requiring an increased quantity of the substance to achieve intoxication.

Dependents Individuals who are supported, either financially or with regard to insurance coverage, by others.

Depressive An emotional state that includes sadness, hopelessness, and gloom.

Dermis The internal layer of the skin; the location of blood vessels, lymph vessels, hair follicles, sweat glands, and sebum.

Descending Colon The segment of the large intestine that connects the splenic flexure to the sigmoid colon.

Detoxification The process of removing toxic substances or qualities.

Device The identification of any materials or appliances that may remain in or on the body after the procedure is completed.

Diabetes Mellitus (DM) A chronic systemic disease that results from insulin deficiency or resistance and causes the body to improperly metabolize carbohydrates, proteins, and fats.

Diagnosis A physician's determination of a patient's condition, illness, or injury.

Diagnosis-Related Group (DRG) An episodic care payment system basing reimbursement to hospitals for inpatient services upon standards of care for specific diagnoses grouped by their similar usage of resources for procedures, services, and treatments.

Differential Diagnosis When the physician indicates that the patient's signs and symptoms may closely lead to two different diagnoses; usually written as "diagnosis A vs. diagnosis B."

Disability Compensation A plan that reimburses a covered individual a portion of his or her income that is lost as a result of being unable to work due to illness or injury.

Disclosure The sharing of information between health care professionals working in separate entities, or facilities, in the course of caring for the patient.

Discounted FFS An extra reduction in the rate charged to an insurer for services provided by the physician to the plan's members.

Dislocation The movement of a muscle away from its normal position.

DMEPOS Durable medical equipment, prosthetic, and orthotic supplies.

Donor Area (Site) The area or part of the body from which skin or tissue is removed with the intention of placing that skin or tissue in another area or body.

Dorsopathy Disease affecting the back of the torso [plural: dorsopathies].

Double Billing Sending a claim for the second time to the same insurance company for the same procedure or service, provided to the same patient on the same date of service.

Duodenum The first segment of the small intestine, connecting the stomach to the jejunum.

Duplex Scan An ultrasonic scanning procedure to determine blood flow and pattern.

Durable Medical Equipment (DME) Apparatus and tools that help individuals accommodate physical frailties, deliver pharmaceuticals, and provide other assistance that will last for a long time and/or be used to assist multiple patients over time.

Durable Medical Equipment Regional Carrier (DMERC) A company designated by the state or region to act as the fiscal intermediary for all DME claims.

Dyslipidemia Abnormal lipoprotein metabolism.

E

Early and Periodic Screening, Diagnostic, and Treatment (EPSDT) A Medicaid preventive health program for children under 21.

Ectopic Out of place, such as an organ or body part.

Edema An overaccumulation of fluid in the cells of the tissues.

Edentulism Absence of teeth.

Electronic Media Claim (EMC) A health care claim form that is transmitted electronically.

Electronic Remittance Advice (ERA) Remittance advice that is sent to the provider electronically.

Elevated Blood Pressure An occurrence of high blood pressure; an isolated or infrequent reading of a systolic blood pressure above 120 mmHg and/or a diastolic blood pressure above 80 mmHg.

Eligibility Verification The process of confirming with the insurance carrier that an individual is qualified for benefits that would pay for services provided by your health care professional on a particular day.

Embolus A thrombus that has broken free from the vessel wall and is traveling freely within the vascular system.

End-Stage Renal Disease (ESRD) Chronic, irreversible kidney disease requiring regular treatments.

Enteral Within, or by way of, the gastrointestinal tract.

Epidermis The external layer of the skin, the majority of which is squamous cells.

Episodic Care An insurance company pays a provider one flat fee to cover the entire course of treatment for an individual's condition.

Eponym A disease or condition named for a person.

Esophagus The tubular organ that connects the pharynx to the stomach for the passage of nourishment.

Established Patient A person who has received professional services within the last 3 years from either this provider or another provider of the same specialty belonging to the same group practice.

Etiology The original source or cause for the development of a disease; also, the study of the causes of disease.

Evaluation and Management (E/M) Specific components of a meeting between a health care professional and a patient.

Exacerbation An increase in the severity of a disease or its symptoms.

Excision The full-thickness removal of a lesion, including margins; includes (for coding purposes) a simple closure.

Executive Orders Official policies issued by the president of the United States.

Experimental A procedure or treatment that has not yet been accepted by the health care industry as the standard of care.

Explanation of Benefits (EOB) Another type of paper remittance advice, more typically sent to the policyholder. However, some in the industry use the term *EOB* interchangeably with *RA*.

Extent The percentage of the body that has been affected by the burn or corrosion.

External Cause An event, outside the body, that causes injury, poisoning, or an adverse reaction.

Extra-articular Located outside a joint.

Extracorporeal Outside of the body.

Extraocular Muscles The muscles that control the eye.

F

Fee-for-Service (FFS) Plans Payment agreements that outline, in a written fee schedule, exactly how much money the insurance carrier will pay the physician for each treatment and/or service provided.

First-Degree Burn Redness of the epidermis (skin).

First-Listed "First-listed diagnosis" is used, when reporting outpatient encounters, instead of the term "principal diagnosis."

Fluoroscope A piece of equipment that emits x-rays through a part of the patient's body onto a fluorescent screen, causing the image to identify various aspects of the anatomy by density.

Fornix The conjunctival fornix is the area between the eyelid and the eyeball. The superior fornix is between the upper lid and eyeball; the inferior fornix is between the lower lid and the eyeball [plural: fornices].

Fracture Broken cartilage or bone.

Full-Thickness A measure that extends from the epidermis to the connective tissue layer of the skin.

Functional Activity Glandular secretion in abnormal quantity.

Fundus The domed section of an organ farthest from its opening.

Fungi Group of organisms, including mold, yeast, and mildew, that cause infection [singular: fungus].

Furuncle A staphylococcal infection in the subcutaneous tissue; commonly known as a *boil*.

G

Gallbladder A pear-shaped organ that stores bile until it is required to aid the digestive process.

Gangrene Necrotic tissue resulting from a loss of blood supply.

Gatekeeper A physician, typically a family practitioner or an internist, who serves as the primary care physician for an individual. This physician is responsible for evaluating and determining the course of treatment or services, as well as for deciding whether or not a specialist should be involved in care.

General Anesthesia The administration of a drug in order to induce a loss of consciousness in the patient, who is unable to be aroused even by painful stimulation.

Genetic Abnormality An error in a gene (chromosome) that affects development during gestation; also known as a *chromosomal abnormality.*

Gestation The length of time for the complete development of a baby from conception to birth; on average, 40 weeks.

Gestational Diabetes Mellitus (GDM) Usually a temporary diabetes mellitus occurring during pregnancy; however, such patients have an increased risk of later developing type 2 diabetes.

Gestational Hypertension Hypertension that develops during pregnancy and typically goes away once the pregnancy has ended.

Glands of Zeis Altered sebaceous glands that are connected to the eyelash follicles.

Glaucoma The condition that results when poor draining of fluid causes an abnormal increase in pressure within the eye, damaging the optic nerve.

Global Period The length of time allotted for postoperative care included in the surgical package, which is generally accepted to be 90 days for major surgical procedures and up to 10 days for minor procedures.

Global Surgical Package A group of services already included in the code for the operation and not reported separately.

Glomerular Filtration Rate (GFR) The measurement of kidney function; used to determine the stage of kidney disease. GFR is calculated by the physician using the results of a creatinine test in a formula with the patient's gender, age, race, and other factors; normal GFR is 90 and above.

Gross Examination The visual study of a specimen (with the naked eye).

Gynecologist (GYN) A physician specializing in the care of the female genital tract.

H

Hair A pigmented, cylindrical filament that grows out from the hair follicle within the epidermis.

Hair Follicle A saclike bulb containing the hair root.

Harvesting The process of taking skin or tissue (on the same body or another).

HCPCS Level II Modifier A two-character alphabetic or alphanumeric code that may be appended to a code from the main portion of the CPT book or a code from the HCPCS Level II book.

Health Care The total management of an individual's well-being by a health care professional.

Health Maintenance Organization (HMO) A type of health insurance that uses a primary care physician, also known as a gatekeeper, to manage all health care services for an individual.

Hematopoiesis The formation of blood cells.

Hemoglobin (hgb or Hgb) The part of the red blood cell that carries oxygen.

Hemolysis The destruction of red blood cells, resulting in the release of hemoglobin into the bloodstream.

Hemorrhage Excessive or severe bleeding.

Hemostasis The interruption of bleeding.

Hernia A condition in which one anatomical structure pushes through a perforation in the wall of the anatomical site that normally contains that structure.

High Osmolar An ionic water-soluable iodinated contrast medium.

HIPAA's Privacy Rule A portion of HIPAA that ensures the availability of patient information for those who should see it while protecting that information from those who should not.

History of Present Illness (HPI) The collection of details about the patient's chief complaint, the current issue that prompted this encounter: duration, specific signs and symptoms, etc.

Hospice A facility that provides care to terminally ill patients and their families.

Hospital-Acquired Condition (HAC) A condition, illness, or injury contracted by the patient during his or her stay in an acute care facility; also known as *nosocomial condition.*

Human Immunodeficiency Virus (HIV) A condition affecting the immune system.

Hyperglycemia Abnormally high levels of glucose.

Hypertension High blood pressure, usually a chronic condition; often identified by a systolic blood pressure above 140 mmHg and/or a diastolic blood pressure above 90 mmHg.

Hypnotic A drug that induces sleep.

Hypoglycemia Abnormally low glucose levels.

Hypoglycemics Prescription, non-insulin medications designed to lower a patient's glycemic level.

Hypotension Low blood pressure; systolic blood pressure below 90 mmHg and/or diastolic measurements of lower than 60 mmHg.

Hypothyroidism A condition in which the thyroid converts energy more slowly than normal, resulting in an otherwise unexplained weight gain and fatigue.

I

Ileum The last segment of the small intestine.

Immunization To make someone resistant to a particular disease by vaccination.

Index to External Causes The alphabetic listing of the external causes that might cause a patient's injury, poisoning, or adverse reaction.

Infarction Tissue or muscle that has deteriorated or died (necrotic).

Infection The invasion of pathogens into tissue cells.

Infectious A condition that can be transmitted from one person to another.

Inflammation The reaction of tissues to infection or injury; characterized by pain, swelling, and erythema.

Influenza An acute infection of the respiratory tract caused by the influenza virus.

Infusion The introduction of a fluid into a blood vessel.

Injection Compelling a fluid into tissue or cavity.

Inpatient An individual admitted for an overnight or longer stay in a hospital.

Inpatient Facility An establishment that provides health care services to individuals who stay overnight on the premises.

Insurance Premium The amount of money, often paid monthly, by a policyholder or insured, to an insurance company to obtain coverage.

Intermediate Closure A multilevel method of sealing an opening in the skin involving one or more of the deeper layers of the skin. Single-layer closure of heavily contaminated wounds that required extensive cleaning or removal of particulate matter also constitutes intermediate closure.

Interpret Explain the meaning of; convert a meaning from one language to another.

Interval The time measured between one point and another, such as between physician visits.

Intervertebral Disc A fibrocartilage segment that lies between vertebrae of the spinal column and provides cushioning and support.

Intravascular Optical Coherence A high-resolution, catheter-based imaging modality used for the optimized visualization of coronary artery lesions.

Iris The round, pigmented muscular curtain in the eye.

Isogeneic The donor and recipient individuals are genetically identical (i.e., monozygotic twins).

J

Jejunum The segment of the small intestine that connects the duodenum to the ileum.

K

Keratitis An inflammation of the cornea, typically accompanied by an ulceration.

L

Laboratory A location with scientific equipment designed to perform experiments and tests.

Laceration Damage to the epidermal and dermal layers of the skin made by a sharp object.

Lacrimal Apparatus A system in the eye that consists of the lacrimal glands, the upper canaliculi, the lower canaliculi, the lacrimal sac, and the nasolacrimal duct.

Laminaria Thin sticks of kelp-related seaweed, used to dilate the cervix, that can induce abortive circumstance during the first 3 months of pregnancy.

Laminectomy The surgical removal of a vertebral posterior arch.

Laterality The right or left side of anatomical sites that have locations on both sides of the body; e.g., right arm or left arm; *unilateral* means one side and *bilateral* means both sides.

Lens A transparent, crystalline segment of the eye, situated directly behind the pupil, that is responsible for focusing light rays as they enter the eye and travel back to the retina.

Level of Patient History The amount of detail involved in the documentation of patient history.

Level of Physical Examination The extent of a physician's clinical assessment and inspection of a patient.

Liability Insurance A policy that covers loss or injury to a third party caused by the insured or something belonging to the insured.

Linking Confirming medical necessity by pairing at least one diagnosis code to at least one procedure code.

Liters per Minute (LPM) The measurement of how many liters of a drug or chemical are provided to the patient in 60 seconds.

Liver The organ, located in the upper right area of the abdominal cavity, that is responsible for regulating blood sugar levels; secreting bile for the gallbladder; metabolizing fats, proteins, and carbohydrates; manufacturing some blood proteins; and removing toxins from the blood.

Local Anesthesia The injection of a drug to prevent sensation in a specific portion of the body; includes local infiltration anesthesia, digital blocks, and pudendal blocks.

Locum Tenens Physician A physician who fills in, temporarily, for another physician.

Low Birth Weight (LBW) A baby born weighing less than 5 pounds 8 ounces, or 2,500 grams.

Low Osmolar A non-ionic water-soluble iodinated contrast medium.

M

Macule A flat lesion with a different pigmentation (color) when compared with the surrounding skin.

Magnetic Resonance Arthrography (MRA) MR imaging of an anatomical joint after the administration of contrast material into the joint capsule.

Magnetic Resonance Imaging (MRI) A three-dimensional radiologic technique that uses nuclear technology to record pictures of internal anatomical sites.

Main Section The section of the CPT code book listing all of the codes in numeric order.

Major Complication and Co-morbidity (MCC) A complication or co-morbidity that has an impact on the treatment of the patient and makes care for that patient more complex.

Malformation An irregular structural development.

Malignant Invasive and destructive characteristic of a neoplasm; possibly causing damage or death.

Malunion A fractured bone that did not heal correctly; healing of bone that was not in proper position or alignment.

Managed Care A type of health insurance coverage that controls the care of each subscriber (or insured person) by using a primary care provider as a central health care supervisor.

Manic An emotional state that includes elation, excitement, and exuberance.

Manifestation A condition that develops as the result of another, underlying condition.

Manipulation The attempted return of a fracture or dislocation to its normal alignment manually by the physician.

Mass Abnormal collection of tissue.

Measurement To determine a level of a physiological or physical function.

Medical Decision Making (MDM) The level of knowledge and experience needed by the provider to determine the diagnosis and/ or what to do next.

Medical Necessity The assessment that the provider was acting according to standard practices in providing a procedure or service for an individual with a specific diagnosis.

Meibomian Glands Sebaceous glands that secrete a tear film component that prevents tears from evaporating so that the area stays moist.

Mesentery A fold of a membrane that carries blood to the small intestine and connects it to the posterior wall of the abdominal cavity.

Metastasize To proliferate, reproduce, or spread.

Microscopic Examination The study of a specimen using a microscope (under magnification).

Modifier A two-character code that affects the meaning of another code; a code addendum that provides more meaning to the original code.

Moll's Glands Ordinary sweat glands.

Monitored Anesthesia Care (MAC) The administration of sedatives, anesthetic agents, or other medications to relax but not render the patient unconscious while under the constant observation of a trained anesthesiologist; also known as "twilight" sedation.

Morbidity Unhealthy.

Morphology The study of the configuration or structure of living organisms.

Mortality Death.

Mutually Exclusive Codes Codes that are identified as those that are not permitted to be used on the same claim form with other codes.

Myalgia Pain in a muscle.

Myocardial Infarction (MI) Malfunction of the heart due to necrosis or deterioration of a portion of the heart muscle; also known as a *heart attack*.

Myopathy Disease of a muscle [plural: myopathies].

N

Neoplasm Abnormal tissue growth; tumor.

Neoplasm Table The Neoplasm Table lists all possible codes for benign and malignant neoplasms, in alphabetic order by anatomical location of the tumor.

Nevus An abnormally pigmented area of skin. A birthmark is an example.

New Patient A person who has not received any professional services within the past 3 years from either the provider or another provider of the same specialty who belongs to the same group practice.

Nodule A tissue mass or papule larger than 5 mm.

Nonessential Modifiers Descriptors whose inclusion in the physician's notes are not absolutely necessary and that are provided simply to further clarify a code description; optional terms.

Nonphysician A nonphysician can be a nurse practitioner, certified registered nurse anesthetist, certified registered nurse, clinical nurse specialist, or physician assistant.

Nonunion A fractured bone that did not heal back together; no mending or joining together of the broken segments.

Nosocomial A hospital-acquired condition; a condition that develops as a result of being in a health care facility.

Not Elsewhere Classifiable (NEC) Specifics that are not described in any other code in the ICD-10-CM book; also known as *not elsewhere classified*.

Not Otherwise Specified (NOS) The absence of additional details documented in the notes.

Notations Alerts and warnings that support more accurate use of codes in a specific code set.

NSTEMI A nontransmural elevation myocardial infarction—a heart event during which the coronary artery is partially occluded (blocked).

Nuclear Medicine Treatment that includes the injection or digestion of isotopes.

Nursing Facility A facility that provides skilled nursing treatment and attention along with limited medical care for its (usually long-term) residents, who do not require acute care services (hospitalization).

O

Obstetrics (OB) A health care specialty focusing on the care of women during pregnancy and the puerperium.

Obstruction A blockage or closing.

Official Guidelines A listing of rules and regulations instructing how to use a specific code set accurately.

Open Treatment Surgically opening the fracture site, or another site in the body nearby, in order to treat the fractured bone.

Ophthalmologist A physician qualified to diagnose and treat eye disease and conditions with drugs, surgery, and corrective measures.

Optometrist A professional qualified to carry out eye examinations and to prescribe and supply eyeglasses and contact lenses.

Oral Cavity The opening in the face that begins the alimentary canal and is used for the input of nutrition; also known as the *mouth*.

Orbit The bony cavity in the skull that houses the eye and its ancillary parts (muscles, nerves, blood vessels).

Orthotic A device used to correct or improve an orthopedic concern.

Other Specified Additional information the physician specified that isn't included in any other code description.

Otorhinolaryngology The study of the human ears, nose, and throat (ENT) systems.

Outpatient A patient who receives services for a short amount of time (less than 24 hours) in a physician's office or clinic, without being kept overnight.

Outpatient Facility Includes a hospital emergency room, ambulatory care center, same-day surgery center, or walk-in clinic.

Outpatient Services Health care services provided to individuals without an overnight stay in the facility.

Overlapping Boundaries Multiple sites of carcinoma without identifiable borders.

P

Palpebrae The eyelids [singular: palpebra].

Palpebral Conjunctiva A mucous membrane that lines the palpebrae.

Pancreas A gland that secretes insulin and other hormones from the islet cells into the bloodstream and manufactures digestive enzymes that are secreted into the duodenum.

Pancreatic Islets Cells within the pancreas that secrete insulin and other hormones into the bloodstream.

Papule A raised lesion with a diameter of less than 5 mm.

Parasites Tiny living things that can invade and feed off other living things.

Parathyroid Glands Four small glands situated on the back of the thyroid gland that secrete parathyroid hormone.

Parenteral By way of anything other than the gastrointestinal tract, such as intravenous, intramuscular, intramedullary, or subcutaneous.

Parenteral Enteral Nutrition (PEN) Nourishment delivered using a combination of means other than the gastrointestinal tract (such as IV) in addition to via the gastrointestinal tract.

Past, Family, and Social History (PFSH) Collection of details, related to the chief complaint, regarding possible signs, symptoms, behaviors, genetic connection, etc.

Patch A flat, small area of differently colored or textured skin; a large macule.

Pathogen Any agent that causes disease; a microorganism such as a bacterium or virus.

Pathology The study of the nature, etiology, development, and outcomes of disease.

Percutaneous Skeletal Fixation The insertion of fixation instruments (such as pins) placed across the fracture site. It may be done under x-ray imaging for guidance purposes.

Perforation An atypical hole in the wall of an organ or anatomical site.

Perinatal The time period from before birth to the 28th day after birth.

Personnel Modifier A modifier adding information about the professional(s) attending to the provision of this procedure or treatment to the patient during this encounter.

Phalanges Fingers and toes [singular: phalange or phalanx].

Phobia Irrational and excessive fear of an object, activity, or situation.

Physical Status Modifier A two-character alphanumeric code used to describe the condition of the patient at the time anesthesia services are administered.

***Physicians' Desk Reference* (PDR)** A series of reference books identifying all aspects of prescription and over-the-counter medications, as well as herbal remedies.

Placement To put a device in or on an anatomical site.

Plasma The fluid part of the blood.

Platelets (PLTs) Large cell fragments in the bone marrow that function in clotting; also known as *thrombocytes*.

Pneumonia An inflammation of the lungs.

Pneumothorax A condition in which air or gas is present within the chest cavity but outside the lungs.

Point-of-Service (POS) A type of insurance plan that will allow an HMO enrollee to choose his or her own nonmember physician at a lower benefit rate, costing the patient more money out-of-pocket.

Polydipsia Excessive thirst.

Polyuria Excessive urination.

Preferred Provider Organization (PPO) A type of health insurance coverage in which physicians provide health care services to members of the plan at a discount.

Prematurity Birth occurring prior to the completion of 37-weeks gestation.

Prenatal Prior to birth; also referred to as *antenatal*.

Present-On-Admission (POA) A one-character indicator reporting the status of the diagnosis at the time the patient was admitted to the acute care facility.

Pressure Ulcer An open wound or sore caused by pressure, infection, or inflammation.

Preventive A type of action or service that stops something from happening or from getting worse.

Preventive Care Health-related services designed to stop the development of a disease or injury.

Principal Diagnosis The condition, after study, that is the primary, or main, reason for the admission of a patient to the hospital for care; the condition that requires the largest amount of hospital resources for care.

Problem-Pertinent System Review The physician's collection of details of signs and symptoms, as per the patient, affecting only those body systems connected to the chief complaint.

Procedure Action taken, in accordance with the standards of care, by the physician to accomplish a predetermined objective (result); a surgical operation.

Products of Conception The zygote, embryo, or fetus, as well as the amnion, umbilical cord, and placenta.

Proptosis Bulging out of the eye; also known as *exophthalmos*.

Prostatitis Inflammation of the prostate.

Prosthetic Fabricated artificial replacement for a damaged or missing part of the body.

Protected Health Information (PHI) Any patient-identifiable health information regardless of the form in which it is stored (paper, computer file, etc.).

Psychotherapy The treatment of mental and emotional disorder through communication or psychologically rather than medical means.

Puerperium The time period from the end of labor until the uterus returns to normal size, typically 3 to 6 weeks.

Pupil The opening in the center of the iris that permits light to enter and continue on to the lens and retina.

Push The delivery of an additional drug via an intravenous line over a short period of time.

Pustule A swollen area of skin; a vesicle filled with pus.

Q

Qualifier Any additional feature of the procedure, if applicable.

Qualitative The determination of character or essential element(s).

Quantitative The counting or measurement of something.

Query To ask.

R

Radiation The high-speed discharge and projection of energy waves or particles.

Recipient Area The area, or site, of the body receiving a graft of skin or tissue.

Rectum The last segment of the large intestine, connecting the sigmoid colon to the anus.

Red Blood Cells (RBCs) Cells within the blood that contain hemoglobin responsible for carrying oxygen to tissues; also known as *erythrocytes*.

Regional Anesthesia The administration of a drug in order to interrupt the nerve impulses without loss of consciousness.

Rehabilitation Health care that is committed to improving, maintaining, or returning physical strength, cognition, and mobility.

Reimbursement The process of paying for health care services after they have been provided.

Relationship The level of familiarity between provider and patient.

Release of Information (ROI) The form (either on paper or electronic) that a patient must sign to give legal permission to a covered entity to disclose that patient's PHI.

Remittance Advice (RA) Notification identifying details about a payment from the third-party payer.

Respiratory Disorder A malfunction of the organ system relating to respiration.

Retina A membrane in the back of the eye that is sensitive to light and functions as the sensory end of the optic nerve.

Retinal Detachment A break in the connection between the retinal pigment epithelium layer and the neural retina.

Retinopathy Degenerative condition of the retina.

Rh (Rhesus) Factor An antigen located on the red blood cell that produces immunogenic responses in those individuals without it.

Risk Factor Reduction Intervention Action taken by the attending physician to stop or reduce a behavior or lifestyle that is predicted to have a negative effect on the individual's health.

Rod An elongated, cylindrical cell within the retina that is photosensitive in low light.

Root Operation Term The category or classification of a particular procedure, service, or treatment.

Rule of Nines A general division of the whole body into sections that each represents 9%; used for estimating the extent of a burn.

S

Salivary Glands Three sets of bilateral exocrine glands that secrete saliva: parotid glands, submaxillary glands, and sublingual glands.

Saphenous Vein Either of the two major veins in the leg that run from the foot to the thigh near the surface of the skin.

Scale Flaky exfoliated epidermis; a flake of skin.

Schizophrenia A psychotic disorder with no known cause.

Sclera The membranous tissue that covers all of the eyeball (except the cornea); also known as *the white of the eye.*

Screening An examination or test of a patient who has no signs or symptoms that is conducted with the intention of finding any evidence of disease as soon as possible, thus enabling better patient outcomes.

Second-Degree Burn Blisters on the skin; involvement of the epidermis and the dermis layers.

Secondary Diabetes Mellitus Diabetes caused by medication or another condition or disease.

Secondary Hypertension The condition of hypertension caused by another condition or illness.

Sedative A tranquilizer; a drug used to calm or soothe.

Self-Administer To give medication to oneself, such as a diabetic giving herself an insulin injection.

Sepsis Condition typified by two or more systemic responses to infection; a specified pathogen.

Septic Shock Severe sepsis with hypotension; unresponsive to fluid resuscitation.

Septicemia Generalized infection spread through the body via the bloodstream; blood infection.

Sequela A cause-and-effect relationship between an original condition that has been resolved with a current condition; also known as a late effect.

Sequela (Late Effects) A condition directly caused by another condition which may not appear until after the initial condition has cleared; (2) cause-and-effect relationship between an original condition, illness, or injury and an additional problem caused by the existence of that original condition. Time is not a requirement for a diagnosis as a late effect because the additional concern may be present at any time.

Service Spending time with a patient and/or family about health care situations.

Service-Related Modifier A modifier relating to a change or adjustment of a procedure or service provided.

Severe Sepsis Sepsis with signs of acute organ dysfunction.

Severity The level of seriousness.

Sigmoid Colon The dual-curved segment of the colon that connects the descending colon to the rectum; also referred to as the *sigmoid flexure.*

Signs Measurable indicators of a patient's health status.

Simple Closure A method of sealing an opening in the skin (epidermis or dermis), involving only one layer. It includes the administration of local anesthesia and/or chemical or electrocauterization of a wound not closed.

Site The specific anatomical location of the disease or injury.

Skin The external membranous covering of the body.

Somatic Related to the body, especially separate from the brain or mind.

Somatoform Disorder The sincere belief that one is suffering an illness that is not present.

Sonogram The use of sound waves to record images of internal organs and tissues; also called an *ultrasound.*

Specialty Care Transport (SCT) Continuous care provided by one or more health professionals in an appropriate specialty area, such as respiratory care or cardiovascular care, or by a paramedic with additional training.

Specimen A small part or sample of any substance obtained for analysis and diagnosis.

Sphincter A circular muscle that contracts to prevent passage of liquids or solids.

Spondylopathy Disease affecting the vertebrae [plural: spondylopathies].

Standard of Care The accepted principles of conduct, services, or treatments that are established as the expected behavior.

Status Asthmaticus The condition of asthma that is life-threatening and does not respond to therapeutic treatments.

Statutory Laws Laws that are enacted by federal and state legislature.

STEMI An ST elevation myocardial infarction—a heart event during which the coronary artery is completely blocked by a thrombus or embolus.

Stomach A saclike organ within the alimentary canal designed to contain nourishment during the initial phase of the digestive process.

Subcutaneous The layer beneath the dermis; also known as the *hypodermis.*

Substance Abuse Regular consumption of a substance with manifestations.

Supplemental Report A letter or report written by the attending physician or other health care professional to provide additional clarification or explanation.

Supporting Documentation The paperwork in the patient's file that corroborates the codes presented on the claim form for a particular encounter.

Surgical Approach The methodology or technique used by the physician to perform the procedure, service, or treatment.

Surgical Pathology The study of tissues removed from a living patient during a surgical procedure.

Symbols Marks, similar to emojis, that provide additional direction to use codes correctly and accurately.

Symptom A subjective sensation or departure from the norm as related by the patient.

Systemic Spread throughout the entire body.

Systemic Condition A condition that affects the entire body and virtually all body systems, therefore requiring the physician to consider this in his or her medical decision making for any other condition.

Systemic Inflammatory Response Syndrome (SIRS) A definite physical reaction, such as fever, chills, etc., to an unspecified pathogen.

T

Table of Drugs and Chemicals The section of the ICD-10-CM code book listing drugs, chemicals, and other biologicals that may poison a patient or result in an adverse reaction.

Tables The section of the ICD-10-PCS code book listing all of the codes in alphanumeric order, based on the first three characters of the code.

Tabular List The section of the ICD-10-CM code book listing all of the codes in alphanumeric order.

Teeth Small, calcified protrusions with roots in the jaw [singular: tooth].

Third-Degree Burn Destruction of all layers of the skin, with possible involvement of the subcutaneous fat, muscle, and bone.

Third-Party Payer An individual or organization that is not directly involved in an encounter but has a connection because of its obligation to pay, in full or part, for that encounter.

Thrombus A blood clot in a blood vessel [plural: thrombi].

Thyroid Gland A two-lobed gland located in the neck that reaches around the trachea laterally and connects anteriorly by an isthmus. The thyroid gland produces hormones used for metabolic function.

Topical Anesthesia The application of a drug to the skin to reduce or prevent sensation in a specific area temporarily.

Topography The classification of neoplasms primarily by anatomical site.

Tracer An official request for a third-party payer to search its system to find a missing health claim form. It is also a term used for a replacement health claim form resubmitted to replace one that was lost.

Transfer of Care When a physician gives up responsibility for caring for a patient, in whole or with regard to one specific condition, and another physician accepts responsibility for the care of that patient.

Transfusion The provision of one person's blood or plasma to another individual.

Transplantation The transfer of tissue from one site to another.

Transverse Colon The portion of the large intestine that connects the hepatic flexure to the splenic flexure.

Treatment The provision of medical care for a disorder or disease.

TriCare A government health plan that covers medical expenses for the dependents of active-duty service members, CHAMPUS-eligible retirees and their families, and the dependents of deceased active-duty members.

Tuberculosis An infectious condition that causes small rounded swellings on mucous membranes throughout the body.

Type 1 Diabetes Mellitus A sudden onset of insulin deficiency that may occur at any age but most often arises in childhood and adolescence; also known as *insulin-dependent diabetes mellitus (IDDM), juvenile diabetes,* or *type I.*

Type 2 Diabetes Mellitus A form of diabetes mellitus with a gradual onset that may develop at any age but most often occurs in adults over the age of 40; also known as *non-insulin-dependent diabetes mellitus (NIDDM)* or *type II.*

U

Ulcer An erosion or loss of the full thickness of the epidermis.

Unbundling Coding individual parts of a specific procedure rather than one combination, or bundle, that includes all the components.

Underlying Condition One disease that affects or encourages another condition.

Uniform Hospital Discharge Data Set (UHDDS) A compilation of data collected by acute care facilities and other designated health care facilities.

Unlisted Codes Codes shown at the end of each subsection of the CPT used as a catch-all for any procedure not represented by an existing code.

Unspecified The absence of additional specifics in the physician's documentation.

Upcoding Using a code on a claim form that indicates a higher level of service than that which was actually performed.

Urea A compound that is excreted in urine.

Urea Reduction Ratio (URR) A formula to determine the effectiveness of hemodialysis treatment.

Urinary System The organ system responsible for removing waste products that are left behind in the blood and the body.

Urinary Tract Infection (UTI) Inflammation of any part of the urinary tract: kidney, ureter, bladder, or urethra.

Use (1) The sharing of information between people working in the same health care facility for purposes of caring for the patient. (2) Occasional consumption of a substance without clinical manifestations.

Usual, Customary, and Reasonable (UCR) The process of determining a fee for a service by evaluating the *usual* fee charged by the provider, the *customary* fee charged by most physicians in the same community or geographical area, and what is considered *reasonable* by most health care professionals under the specific circumstances of the situation.

Uveal Tract The middle layer of the eye, consisting of the iris, ciliary body, and choroid.

V

Vascular Referring to the vessels (arteries and veins).

Venography The imaging of a vein after the injection of contrast material.

Ventricle A chamber that is located in the bottom half of the heart and receives blood from the atrium.

Vermiform Appendix A long, narrow mass of tissue attached to the cecum; also called *appendix*.

Vertebra A bone that is a part of the construction of the spinal column [plural: vertebrae].

Viruses Microscopic particles that initiate disease, mimicking the characteristics of a particular cell; viruses can reproduce only within the body of the cell that they have invaded.

Vitreous Chamber The interior segment of the eye that contains the vitreous body.

W

White Blood Cells (WBCs) Cells within the blood that help to protect the body from pathogens; also known as *leukocytes*.

Withdrawal Abruptly stopping the use of a drug that has been used continuously prior to the cessation, which can result in both physical and psychological conditions.

Workers' Compensation An insurance program that covers medical care for those injured or for those who become ill as a consequence of their employment.

X

Xenogeneic The donor and recipient are of different species, e.g., bovine cartilage → human (also known as a *xenograft* or *heterograft*).